Modern System of Ophthalmology (MSO) Series

Principles and Practice of Glaucoma

Second Edition

Modern System of Ophthalmology (MSO) Series

Principles and Practice of Glaucoma

Second Edition

Editor-in-Chief

AK Khurana MS, FAICO, CTO (London)
Fellow, Moorfields Eye Hospital, London
Director, Institute of Ophthalmology and Health Sciences, KEC, Rohtak
Former Professor and Head, Department of Ophthalmology
SGT Medical College, Hospital and Research Institute Gurugram, Haryana, India
Former Senior Professor and Head
Regional Institute of Ophthalmology
Postgraduate Institute of Medical Sciences, Rohtak, Haryana

Honorary Editors

Tanuj Dada MD
Professor, Glaucoma Services
Dr RP Centre for Ophthalmic Sciences
All India Institute of Medical Sciences
New Delhi

Sushmita Kaushik MS
Professor, Glaucoma Services
Advanced Eye Centre
Postgraduate Institute of Medical Education and Research, Chandigarh

Associate Editors

Parul Ichhpujani MS
Professor
Glaucoma Services
Government Medical College and Hospital
Chandigarh

Aruj K Khurana DNB, FICO
Assistant Professor
Department of Ophthalmology
Vitreo-Retinal Services
SGT Medical College, Hospital and Research Institute
Gurugram, Haryana, India

Bhawna P Khurana MS, DNB, FICO
Associate Professor
Squint, Paediatric Ophthalmology
Orbit and Oculoplasty Services
Department of Ophthalmology
SGT Medical College, Hospital and Research Institute
Gurugram Haryana, India

Foreword by

Prof Tin Aung

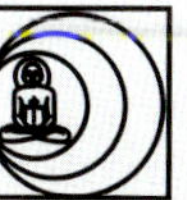

CBS Publishers & Distributors Pvt Ltd

New Delhi • Bengaluru • Chennai • Kochi • Kolkata • Lucknow • Mumbai
Hyderabad • Jharkhand • Nagpur • Patna • Pune • Uttarakhand

Disclaimer

Science and technology are constantly changing fields. New research and experience broaden the scope of information and knowledge. The editors have tried their best in giving information available to them while preparing the material for this book. Although, all efforts have been made to ensure optimum accuracy of the material, yet it is quite possible some errors might have been left uncorrected. The publisher, the printer and the editors will not be held responsible for any inadvertent errors, omissions or inaccuracies.

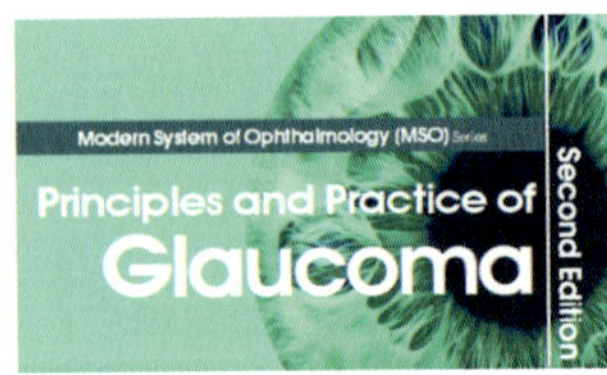

ISBN: 978-93-5466-568-4

Second Edition 2024
Reprint **2025**
First Edition 2015
Reprint 2021

Published by Satish Kumar Jain and produced by Varun Jain for
CBS Publishers & Distributors Pvt Ltd
4819/XI Prahlad Street, 24 Ansari Road, Daryaganj, New Delhi 110 002, India.
Ph: 011-23289259, 23266838 Website: www.cbspd.com
e-mail: delhi@cbspd.com

Corporate Office: 204 FIE, Industrial Area, Patparganj, Delhi 110 092
Ph: 011-4934 4934 Fax: 011-4934 4935 e-mail: publishing@cbspd.com; publicity@cbspd.com

Branches

- **Bengaluru:** Seema House 2975, 17th Cross, KR Road, Banasankari 2nd Stage, Bengaluru 560 070, Karnataka, India
  Ph: +91-80-26771678/79 Fax: +91-80-26771680 e-mail: bangalore@cbspd.com
- **Chennai:** 7, Subbaraya Street, Shenoy Nagar, Chennai 600 030, Tamil Nadu, India
  Ph: +91-44-26680620, 26681266 Fax: +91-44-42032115 e-mail: chennai@cbspd.com
- **Kochi:** 42/1325, 1326, Power House Road, Opp KSEB, Power House, Ernakulum Kochi 682 018, Kerala, India
  Ph: +91-484-4059061-65,67 Fax: +91-484-4059065 e-mail: kochi@cbspd.com
- **Kolkata:** 147, Hind Ceramics Compound, 1st Floor, Nilgunj Road, Belghoria, Kolkata-700056, West Bengal, India
  Ph: +033-25633055, 033-25633056 e-mail: kolkata@cbspd.com
- **Lucknow:** Basement, Khushnuma Complex, 7 Meerabai Marg (Behind Jawahar Bhawan), Lucknow-226001, UP, India
  Ph: +0522-4000032 e-mail: tiwari.lucknow@cbspd.com
- **Mumbai:** PWD Shed, Gala no 25/26, Ramchandra Bhatt Marg, Next to JJ Hospital Gate no. 2, Opp. Union Bank of India, Noorbaug, Mumbai-400009, Maharashtra, India
  Ph: 022-66661880/89 e-mail: mumbai@cbspd.com

Representatives

- Hyderabad 0-9885175004
- Jharkhand 0-9811541605
- Nagpur 0-8692091830
- Patna 0-9334159340
- Pune 0-9664372571
- Uttarakhand 0-9716462459iv

Printed at HT Media Ltd, Greater Noida

to

---

the teachers and residents in ophthalmology for
their endeavor to dissipate and acquire knowledge
our parents and teachers for their blessings
our families for their understanding and encouragement
our patients for letting us learn

Foreword

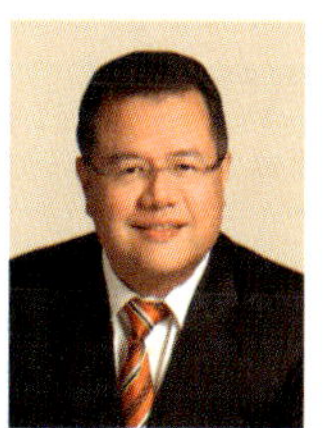

I am pleased to write the foreword to second edition of *Principles and Practice of Glaucoma*, one of the thirteen books in the series *Modern System of Ophthalmology* by Sr Prof AK Khurana (Editor-in-Chief). With ophthalmology becoming an increasingly complex subspecialty, focussed textbooks are a necessity. Therefore, a textbook that encompasses comprehensive knowledge and recent advances on glaucoma will be an excellent resource for trainees/residents and general ophthalmologists; and will also serve as a handbook for glaucoma fellows. The book has been aptly organized into well-planned and comprehensive sections; Section I. Glaucoma: Introduction, Basics and Epidemiology; Section II. Glaucoma Diagnostic: Clinical Evaluation and Investigations; Section III. Glaucoma: The Clinical Entities and Section IV. Glaucoma: Management. Leading glaucoma experts including Professor Tanuj Dada from Dr RP Centre of Ophthalmic Sciences, AIIMS, New Delhi, and Dr Sushmita Kaushik, Professor from Advanced Eye Centre PGIMER, Chandigarh, have contributed as Honorary Editors; with Dr Parul Ichhpujani, Professor from GMCH, Chandigarh, Dr Aruj K Khurana and Dr Bhawna P Khurana from Department of Ophthalmology, SGT Medical College, Hospital and Research Institute, Budhera, Gurugram, as Associate Editors. They all are dedicated teachers, outstanding academicians and faculty of international repute on glaucoma. The contributors present a lucid and easy to comprehend text, supplemented by superb clinical photographs, line diagrams, tables and flow charts. I know Prof Khurana is a highly sought-after author whose books are being received with great enthusiasm by specialists and students of ophthalmology. I am confident that readers will benefit greatly from second edition textbook and I wish Prof Khurana and his team best of luck for the success of their academic venture.

Professor Tin Aung

MBBS (Singapore), M Med (Ophth), FRCS (Ed), FRC Ophth, FAMS, PhD (London)

Executive Director, Singapore Eye Research Institute
Deputy Medical Director (Research), Singapore National Eye Centre
Senior Consultant and Head, Glaucoma Department, Singapore National Eye Centre
Professor, Department of Ophthalmology, Yong Loo Lin School of Medicine
National University of Singapore

Preface to the Second Edition

Modern System of Ophthalmology (MSO) series comprises separate volumes on different subspecialties of ophthalmology. Each volume is planned with a very specific aim to cater to the needs of postgraduate students and fellows in respective subspeciality of ophthalmology. Salient Features of MSO Series are:.

Salient Features of MSO Series

- Each volume is edited by different editors, yet the layout and organization has been kept identical.
- Editors of different volumes are masters in their subspecialty with an uncanny knack of picking up the right perspectives.

Principles and Practice of Glaucoma. A volume of MSO series in its second edition presents an updated and thoroughly revised text. To remain abreast with recent advances in Glaucoma diagnostics and medical Lasers and surgical management techniques is essential and must for each and every ophthalmologist in making and in practice. Such an endeavor will go a long way in timely and effective management of glaucoma and thus prevention of blindness that might ensue.

Salient Features of this book:

Section I. Glaucoma: Introduction, Basics and Epidemiology, introduces the subject with a workable classification of glaucoma. Basic and applied aspects of the related anatomy and physiology have been highlighted. Pathophysiology of glaucomatous damage and epidemiological aspects have also been covered briefly in this section.

Section II. Glaucoma Diagnostics: Clinical Evaluation and Investigations, covers from history taking to the most recent diagnostic tests developed over the years for an early diagnosis of glaucoma.

Section III. Glaucoma: The Clinical Entities, is devoted to common clinical types of glaucoma with recent concepts about their understanding, diagnosis and management.

Section IV. Glaucoma: Management, describes medical, laser and surgical therapy of different types of glaucoma in depth and, comprehensively yet concisely.

Organization and exposition of text matter

- Text matter is designed to meet the needs of residents in ophthalmology with a comprehensive coverage in a concise manner. Text is complete and up-to-date with recent advances incorporated.
- Text is organized in such a way that the students can easily understand, retain and reproduce it.
- Various levels of headings, subheadings, bold face and italics given in the text will be helpful for a quick revision of the subject.
- A brief list of chapter contents given in the beginning of each chapter provides a clear layout of the text.
- Text has been profusely illustrated with high quality coloured photographs and computer drawn colour diagrams which provide vivid details.
- Exposition of the text is such that an average postgraduate student will find it easy to glean through and assimilate the facts for longer retention.

Acknowledgements. Second edition of the book has been possible as a result of active criticism, suggestions and generous help of many teachers and students. Surely, I owe sincere thanks to them all. Those who need special mention are Prof RC Nagpal, Former Head, RIO, PGIMS, Rohtak; Prof Jagat Ram, Ex-Dean, PGIMER, Chandigarh; Prof and Head Swapan Samanta, Governement Medical College, Raigarh; Prof Atul Kumar, Prof JS Titiyal, Prof Namrata Sharma and Prof Tanuj Dada from Dr RP Centre for Ophthalmic Sciences, AIIMS, New Delhi; Prof SP Singh, Faridkot; Prof CS Dhull, WCMSR, Jhajjar; Prof Sanjiv Mittal, AIIMS, Rishikesh, Uttarakhand; Prof Subhash Dadeya, MAMC, New Delhi; Prof Harsh Bahadur and Prof Renu Dhasmana from HIMS, Jolly Grant, Dehradun; Prof Manisha Gupta, SGRRIHMS, Dehradun; Prof SP Singh and Prof Kamaljeet Singh from Allahabad; Prof Rupali Chopra and Prof Nitin Batra, CMC, Ludhiana; Prof Gursatinder Singh, Head, Department of Ophthalmology, Adesh Medical College and Hospital, Shahbad, Kurukshetra; Prof Anand Aggarwl, Head, Department of Ophthalmology, Government Medical College, Patiala; Prof Prempal Kaur, Head, Department of Ophthalmology, Government Medical College, Amritsar; Prof Manjeet Kaur from SHKM Government Medical College, Mewat; Dr Sumeet Khanduja from Karnal; and Dr Mahipal S Sachdev, Medical Director, Centre for Sight, New Delhi. I acknowledge the special help rendered by Dr Rashmi S, Associate Professor, Yenepoya Medical College, Mangaluru; Dr Supriya, Dr Harmanjot Singh, Dr Divya Rana, Dr Amandeep Arora, Dr Sareeta, Dr Srishti, Dr Niharika, Residents from SGT Medical College, for their sincere help in updating this edition. I acknowledge with thanks, the respect, affection and cooperation of faculty members of Department of Ophthalmology, SGT Medical College, Hospital and Research Institute, Gurugram namely Prof JP Chugh, Prof Neeraj Sharma, Dr Tulika Gupta, and Faculty of Regional Institute of Ophthalmology (RIO), PGIMS, Rohtak namely, Dr RS Chauhan, Senior Professor and Head, Dr Manisha Rathi, Dr Neebha Anand, Dr Manisha Nada, Dr Urmil Chawla, Dr Ashok Rathi, Dr Sumit Sachdeva, Dr Reena Gupta, Dr Jitender Phogat, Dr Jyoti Deswal, and Dr Ruchi Dabas. The contribution made by Dr Aruj K Khurana and Dr Bhawna P Khurana in completion of this edition is duly acknowledged. The love and moral support, in addition to the editorial help, rendered by my daughter Dr Arushi and son-in-law Dr Gurukripa, Assistant Professors of Medicine, Mayo Clinic College of Medicine and Science, Rochester, Minnesota, USA, and my wife Dr Indu Khurana, Emeritus Professor, SGT University, and Former Professor of Physiology and Dean-cum Principal, World College of Medical Sciences and Research, Gurawar, Jhajjar, and Former Professor and Head, Department of Physiology, PGIMS, Rohtak, made my task untiring.

I also thank Shri Manmohan Singh Chawla, Managing Trustee; Ms Madhupreet Chawla, Chairperson; Shri Ram Bahadur Rai, Chancellor; Prof Sham Lal Singla, Advisor; Prof OP Kalra, Vice-Chancellor; Prof Gen. SPS Kochar, Dean, FHMS; GL Khanna, Head, HR Department, SGT University, for providing atmosphere conducive to such academic activities. Sincere efforts have been made to verify the correctness of the text.

The enthusiastic co-operation received from Mr SK Jain, Managing Director; Mr YN Arjuna, Senior Vice President–Publishing, Editorial and Publicity, and Mrs Ritu Chawla, AGM, Production. CBS Publishers & Distributors, New Delhi, needs special acknowledgement. Mr Sanju, Graphic artist, Mr Sunil Dutt, who initially made hand drawings and Mrs Jyoti Kaur, DTP Operator, need special mention because of their efforts to provide considerable beauty to this volume.

However, in spite of best efforts, ventures of this kind are not likely to be free from human errors, some inaccuracies, ambiguities and typographic mistakes. Users are therefore requested to send their feedback and suggestions. The importance of such views in improving the future editions of the book cannot be overemphasized. Feedbacks received will be highly appreciated and duly acknowledged.

AK Khurana

Editorial Board and Contributors

Editor-in-Chief

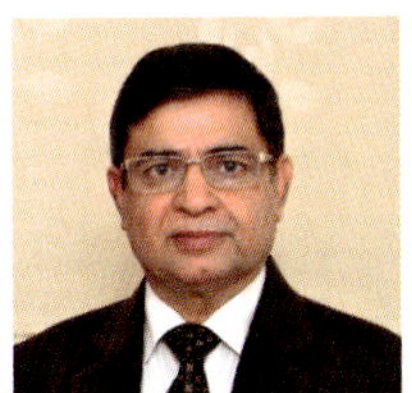

AK Khurana MS, FAICO, CTO (London)
Fellow, Moorfields Eye Hospital, London
Senior Professor and Head
Regional Institute of Ophthalmology
Postgraduate Institute of Medical Sciences (PGIMS)
Rohtak, Haryana

Honorary Editors

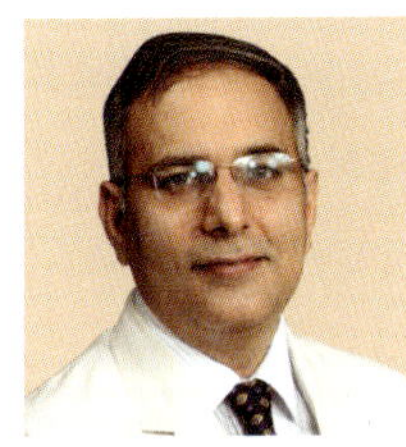

Tanuj Dada MD
Professor
Glaucoma Services
Dr RP Centre for Ophthalmic Sciences, AIIMS
New Delhi

Sushmita Kaushik MS
Professor
Glaucoma Services
Advanced Eye Centre
PGIMER, Chandigarh

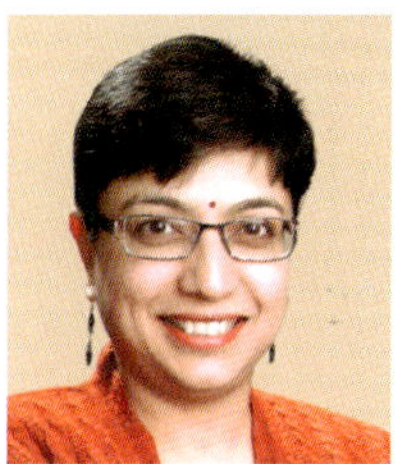

Associate Editors

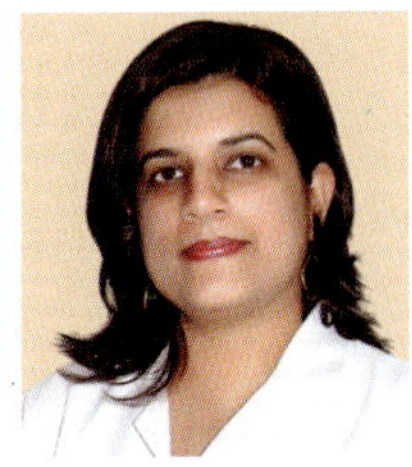

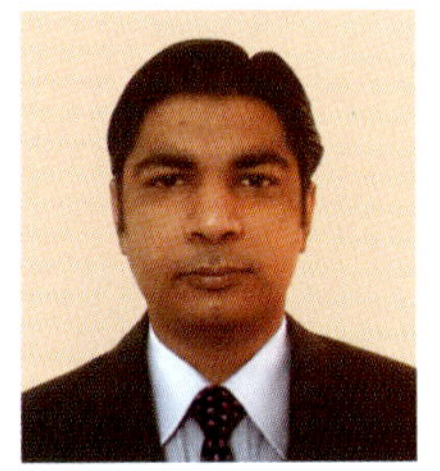

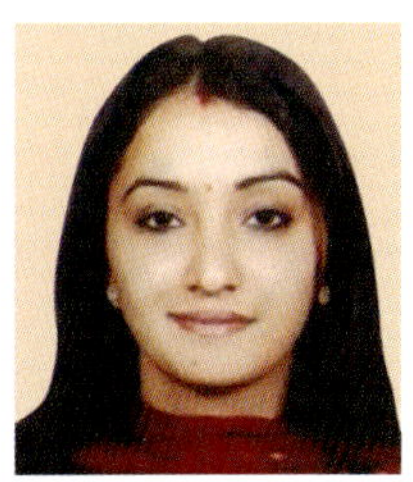

Parul Ichhpujani MS
Professor
Government Medical College and Hospital
Chandigarh

Aruj K Khurana DNB, FICO
Assistant Professor
Department of Ophthalmology
Vitreo-Retinal Services
SGT Medical College, Hospital and Research Institute
Gurugram, Haryana, India

Bhawna P Khurana MS, DNB, FICO
Associate Professor
Squint, Paediatric Ophthalmology
Orbit and Oculoplasty Services
Department of Ophthalmology
SGT Medical College, Hospital and Research Institute
Gurugram, Haryana, India

List of Contributors

AK Khurana MS, FAICO, CTO
Director, Institute of Ophthalmology and Health Sciences, KEC, Rohtak
Former Professor and Head, Department of Ophthalmology
SGT Medical College, Hospital and Research Institute Gurugram, Haryana, India

CS Dhull MS DCEH
Former Professor and Head
Department of Ophthalmology
WCMSR, Jhajjar

Indu Khurana MD
Emeritus Professor
SGT University
Gurugram

Pardeep K Khanna MD
Former Senior Professor and Head
Department of Community Medicine
PGIMS, Rohtak

Manisha Nada MS
Senior Professor
Regional Institute of Ophthalmology
PGIMS, Rohtak

Reema Raval MS
Professor
Department of Ophthalmology
Smt. NHL Municipal Medical College
Ahmedabad

Bhawna P Khurana MS, DNB, FICO
Associate Professor
Department of Ophthalmology
SGT Medical College, Hospital and Research Institute
Gurugram

Shilpa Aggarwal MS
Former Senior Resident
RIO, PGIMS, Rohtak

Arushi Khurana MD
Assistant Professor
Medical Oncology, Lymphoma Services
Department of Medicine, Mayo Clinic College of Medicine and Science
Rochester, Minnesota, USA

Shweta Goel
Medical Director
Vinod Eye Centre
Noida

Tanuj Dada MD
Professor
Glaucoma Services
Dr RP Centre for Ophthalmic Sciences
AIIMS, New Delhi

SS Pandav MS
Chief
Professor and Head
Glaucoma Services
Advanced Eye Centre
PGIMER, Chandigarh

Sushmita Kaushik MS
Professor
Glaucoma Services
Advanced Eye Centre
PGIMER, Chandigarh

Prateep Vyas MS
Medical Director and Head
Glaucoma Services
Centre for Sight, Indore

Sushma Tejwani DOMS, DNB
Head, Glaucoma Services
Narayana Nethralay-2,
Bengaluru

Parul Ichhpujani MS
Professor
Government Medical College and Hospital, Chandigarh

Aruj K Khurana DNB, FICO
Assistant Professor
Department of Ophthalmology
SGT Medical College, Hospital and Research Institute
Budhera, Gurugram

Ankita Phougat MS
Glaucoma Consultant
Department of Ophthalmology
York and Scarborough,
NHS Hospital Group, UK

Ankur Singh MS
Senior Resident
Advanced Eye Centre
PGIMER, Chandigarh

Sujay Chauhan DO, DNB, FICO
Associate Consultant
Centre for Sight
Faridabad

Contents

Section III. Glaucoma: The Clinical Entities

Section IV. Glaucoma: Management

GLAUCOMA: INTRODUCTION, BASICS AND EPIDEMIOLOGY

SECTION I

GLAUCOMA: INTRODUCTION AND CLASSIFICATION

CHAPTER 1

INTRODUCTION

Although the modern concepts of glaucoma can be traced back to the middle of 19th century, this group of ill-understood disorders was recognized as early as 400 BC by the Greeks when Hippocrates coined the term 'glaucosis' for the bluish-green hue of the affected eye. It was in 10th century that an association with raised intraocular pressure was found.

Glaucoma is a leading cause of irreversible blindness throughout the world. Although it more commonly affects older adults, it occurs in all segments of society, with significant health and economic consequences, making it a major public health problem. Being characterized by widely diverse clinical and histopathologic manifestations, it is not commonly appreciated by the general public, or even by a portion of the medical community, which frequently leads to confusion. Once the blindness of glaucoma has occurred, there is no known treatment that will restore the lost vision. In nearly all cases, however, blindness due to glaucoma is preventable making it prudent for the ophthalmologists to recognize the early clinical manifestations of the various glaucomas. Appropriate treatment requires an understanding of the pathogenic mechanisms involved, as well as a detailed knowledge of the drugs and surgeries that are used to control the IOP.

GLAUCOMA TERMINOLOGIES

DEFINITION

- *Glaucoma is not a single disease process* but a group of disorders characterized by a progressive optic neuropathy resulting in a characteristic appearance of the optic disc and a specific pattern of irreversible visual field defects that are associated frequently but not invariably with raised intraocular pressure (IOP).
- *Common denominator of the glaucoma* is a characteristic optic neuropathy, which derives from various risk factors that include but are not limited to increased IOP.
- *IOP is thus the most common risk factor* but not the only risk factor for development of glaucoma.
- Consequently, the term *'Ocular Hypertension'* is used for cases having constantly raised IOP (>21 mm Hg) without any associated glaucomatous optic disc or visual field damage.
- Conversely, the term *normal* or *low tension glaucoma (NTG/LTG)* is suggested for the

typical cupping of the disc and/or visual field defects associated with a normal or low IOP.

GLAUCOMA AND IOP

- *Level of IOP* is unimportant for the diagnosis of glaucoma, although in equivocal cases an abnormal IOP makes the diagnosis more certain.
- *IOP contributes significantly* to the development and progression of glaucoma.
- *Non-IOP factors* also contribute to the aetiology of glaucoma and must be considered.
- *IOP is the only modality,* we currently have available to reduce the risk of glaucoma even in the presence of non-IOP contributing factors.

GLAUCOMA AND OPTIC NEUROPATHY

Glaucoma has a characteristic pattern of damage to the optic nerve head; prominently recognised at the superior and inferior poles of the optic disc. The vertical cup:disc ratio (VCDR) has been used as an index of glaucomatous loss of the neuroretinal rim. But it should be kept in mind that just like intraocular pressure, VCDR is a continuous variable within the population.

VCDR is not a very robust defining feature for glaucoma as there exists variation in the size of the optic disc between individuals, variation in the number of axons in the optic nerve, from a minimum of 8,16,000 to a maximum of 15,02,000 (mean 11,59,000 plus or minus 1,96,000) and the observation that larger optic nerves have a larger neuroretinal rim area and contain more axons. Hence, correction for variation in disc size when assessing the VCDR has been suggested.

GLAUCOMA AND VISUAL FIELD DEFECTS

For all practical purposes, for a visual field defect to be labelled as glaucomatous, the glaucoma hemifield test must be graded "outside normal limits" along with a cluster of three contiguous points at the 5% level on the pattern deviation plot, using the threshold test strategy with the 24-2 test pattern of the Zeiss-Humphrey field analyser 2. We do not imply that this device is the only acceptable tool for field analysis but we consider it the standard as most centres in India and across the globe use this device.

GLAUCOMA: PREDISPOSING AND RISK FACTORS

Everyone should be concerned about glaucoma and its effects. It is important for each of us, from infants to senior citizens, to have our eyes checked regularly, because early detection and treatment of glaucoma are the only way to prevent vision impairment and blindness.

Primary open-angle glaucoma (POAG)

1. *Heredity*. POAG has a polygenic inheritance. The approximate risk of getting disease is 10% in the siblings, and 4% in the offspring of patients with POAG.
2. *Age*. The risk increases with increasing age. The POAG is more commonly seen in elderly between 5th and 7th decades.
3. *Race*. POAG is significantly more common, develops earlier and is more severe in black people than in white.
4. *Myopes* are more predisposed than the normals.
5. *Diabetics* have a higher prevalence of POAG than non-diabetics.
6. *Cigarette smoking* is also thought to increase its risk.
7. *High blood pressure* is not the cause of rise in IOP, however, the prevalence of POAG is more in hypertensives than the normotensives.
8. *Thyrotoxicosis* is also not the cause of rise in IOP, but the prevalence of POAG is more in patients suffering from Graves' ophthalmic disease than the normals.

Primary angle-closure glaucoma (PACG)

Predisposing factors for **PACG** can be divided into anatomical and general factors:

I. *Anatomical factors.* Eyes anatomically predisposed to develop primary angle-closure glaucoma (PACG) include:

- Hypermetropic eyes with shallow anterior chamber.
- Eyes in which iris–lens diaphragm is placed anteriorly.
- Eyes with narrow angle of anterior chamber, which may be due to: small eyeball, relatively large size of the lens and smaller diameter of the cornea or bigger size of the ciliary body.
- Plateau iris configuration.

II. ***General factors*** include:

- *Age*. PACG is comparatively more common in 5th decade of life.
- *Sex*. Females are more prone to get PACG than males (male to female ratio is 1 : 4)
- *Type of personality*. It is more common in nervous individuals with unstable vasomotor system.
- *Season*. Peak incidence is reported in rainy season.
- *Family history*. The potential for PACG is generally believed to be inherited.
- *Race*. In Caucasians, PACG accounts for about 6% of all glaucomas and presents in sixth to seventh decades. It is more common in South-East Asians, Chinese and Eskimos but uncommon in Blacks. In Asians, it presents in the 5th to 6th decades and accounts for 50% of primary adult glaucomas in this ethnic group.

CLASSIFICATION OF GLAUCOMA

Glaucoma can be classified variously, but all classification schemes are considered arbitrary and limited. However, till the complete understanding, it will be worthwhile to stick to the traditional clinico-etiological classification, which is as below.

A. DEVELOPMENTAL GLAUCOMAS

I. ***Primary developmental glaucomas*** (without associated anomalies)

- Newborn glaucoma (true congenital glaucoma)
- Infantile glaucoma
- Juvenile glaucoma

II. ***Developmental glaucoma associated with ocular abnormalities***

III. ***Developmental glaucoma associated with systemic abnormalities***

B. PRIMARY ACQUIRED GLAUCOMAS

I. ***Primary open-angle glaucoma (POAG)***

- Classical POAG with IOP, higher than normal range, and
- Normal tension glaucoma (NTG) with IOPs within normal range

II. ***Primary angle-closure disease***

Stages based on natural history

- Primary angle-closure suspect (PACS)
- Primary angle-closure (PAC), and
- Primary angle-closure glaucoma (PACG)

Types based on mechanism of angle-closure

- Pupillary block,
- Plateau iris syndrome, and
- Phacomorphic mechanism.

C. SECONDARY GLAUCOMAS

I. Depending upon the mechanism of rise in IOP

1. ***Secondary open-angle glaucomas*** in which aqueous outflow may be blocked by:

- Pretrabecular membrane
- Trabecular clogging
- Oedema and scarring, or
- Elevated episcleral venous pressure.

2. ***Secondary angle-closure glaucoma*** which may or may not be associated with pupil block.

- Anterior 'pulling mechanism': The iris is pulled forward by some process in the angle, often by the contraction of a membrane or peripheral anterior synechiae.
- Posterior 'pushing mechanism': The iris is pushed forward by some condition in the posterior segment. Often the ciliary body is rotated anteriorly, allowing the lens to come forward also.

II. Depending upon the causative primary disease, secondary glaucomas are named as follows:

1. Lens-induced (phacogenic) glaucomas.
2. Inflammatory glaucoma (glaucoma due to intraocular inflammation).
3. Pigmentary glaucoma.
4. Neovascular glaucoma.
5. Glaucomas associated with iridocorneal endothelial syndromes.
6. Pseudoexfoliative glaucoma.
7. Glaucomas associated with intraocular haemorrhage.
8. Steroid-induced glaucoma.
9. Traumatic glaucoma.
10. Glaucoma-in-aphakia.
11. Glaucoma associated with intraocular tumours.

SUGGESTED READING

1. Casson RJ, Chidlow G, Wood JP, et al. Definition of glaucoma: Clinical and experimental concepts. Clin Experiment Ophthalmol 2012; 40(4):341–9.
2. Classification of glaucomas. The glaucomas, 2nd edition. St. Louis, Mosby, 1996.
3. Comprehensive Adult Medical Eye Evaluation (Preferred Practice Pattern). San Francisco: American Academy of Ophthalmology (2010). Available online: *http://aao.org/ppp*.
4. Glaucoma: Classification, causes, and surgical control—results of microgonioscopic research. American J Ophthalmol 1938;21: 1099–117.
5. Introduction and Classification of Glaucomas. Becker-Shaffer's diagnosis and therapy of the glaucomas, 8th edition. Pennysylvania St. Louis, Mosby, 2009.
6. Molecular genetics of glaucoma: Effects on the future of disease classification. 100 years of progress in glaucoma. Philadelphia: Lippincott-Raven; 1997:143.
7. Primary Angle Closure (Preferred Practice Pattern). San Francisco: American Academy of Ophthalmology (2010). Also available online: *http://aao.org/ppp*.

ANATOMY AND PHYSIOLOGY OF AQUEOUS HUMOUR DYNAMICS AND INTRAOCULAR PRESSURE

CHAPTER 2

ANATOMICAL CONSIDERATIONS

Maintenance of intraocular pressure (IOP) and pathophysiology of glaucoma revolves around the aqueous humour dynamics. The aqueous humour is involved with virtually all portions of the eye, although the principal ocular structures concerned with it are:

- Ciliary body
- Posterior chamber
- Anterior chamber
- Angle of the anterior chamber, and
- Aqueous outflow system.

CILIARY BODY

Ciliary body is the site of aqueous production. It is the forward continuation of the choroid at ora serrata. In cut section, it is triangular in shape. The anterior side of triangle forms the part of the angle of anterior and posterior chamber. In its middle, it is attached to the iris. The outer side of the triangle lies against the sclera with a suprachoroidal space in between. The inner side of the triangle is divided into two parts. The anterior part (about 2–2.5 mm) having finger-like ciliary processes is called *pars plicata* (corona ciliaris) and the posterior smooth part (about 5 mm wide temporally and 3 mm wide nasally) is called *pars plana* (orbicularis ciliaris) (Fig. 2.1).

Microscopic structure

From without inwards, ciliary body consists of following five layers (Fig. 2.2):

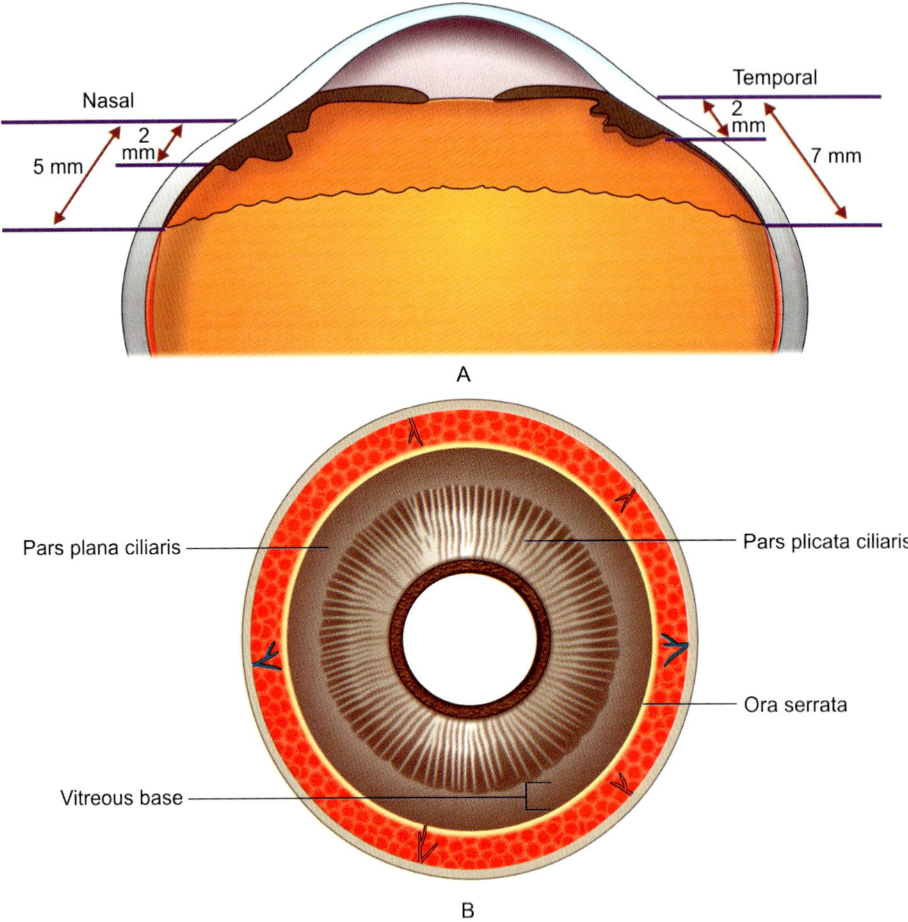

Fig. 2.1 *Showing region of the pars plana and pars plicata: (A) As seen in the axial section of the eyeball; (B) As seen from inside the eyeball posteriorly*

1. ***Supraciliary lamina.*** It is the outermost condensed part of stroma and consists of pigmented collagen fibres. Posteriorly, it is a continuation of the suprachoroidal lamina and anteriorly it becomes continuous with the anterior limiting membrane of the iris.

2. ***Stroma of the ciliary body.*** It consists of connective tissue of collagen and fibroblasts. Embedded in the stroma are ciliary muscle, vascular stroma, nerves, pigment cells and other cells.

Ciliary muscle. It is non-striated muscle which occupies most of the outer part of the ciliary body. In cut section, it is triangular in shape. It consists of three parts:

- *The longitudinal or meridional fibres* take origin largely by tendinous fibres from the scleral spur and adjacent trabeculae and run posteriorly to insert into the suprachoroidal lamina as far back as equator or even beyond.
- *The circular fibres* occupy the anterior and inner portion of the ciliary body and run parallel to the limbus. These fibres lie nearest to the lens.
- *Radial fibres* are described as the obliquely placed fibres which become continuous with the circular fibres.

Actions: Main action of all the parts of the ciliary muscle is to slacken the suspensory ligaments of the lens and thus help in accommodation. Circular fibres act directly as a sphincter.

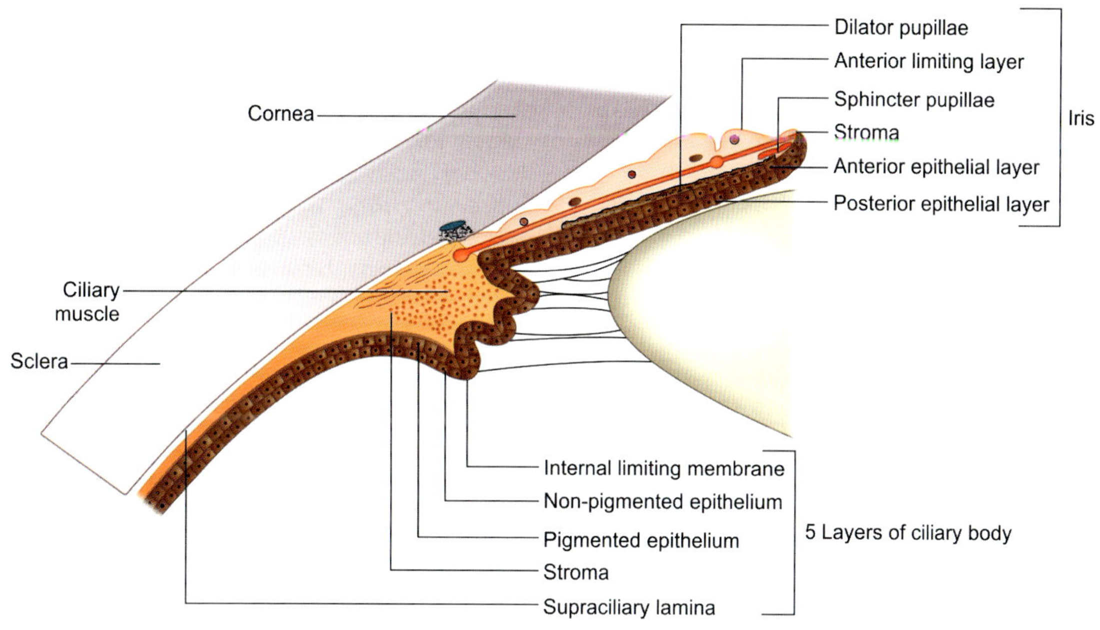

Fig. 2.2 *Microscopic structure of iris and ciliary body*

Radial fibres also act in the same way. Longitudinal fibres' mode of action is disputed. Some say these act by drawing the choroid forward. Due to their attachment to the scleral spur, these fibres also help in aqueous outflow.

Nerve supply. The ciliary muscle is innervated by the parasympathetic fibres from ciliary ganglion which reach the eyeball along the short ciliary nerves.

Vascular stroma of the ciliary body. *The major arterial circle* lies in the connective tissue stroma of ciliary body just in front of the circular fibres of the muscle. It is formed by anastomosis between the long posterior ciliary artery and anterior ciliary arteries and sends branches to the iris and ciliary body.

Vascular stroma forming ciliary processes is described separately.

3. *Layer of pigmented epithelium.* It is a forward continuation of the retinal pigment epithelium. Anteriorly, it is continuous with the anterior pigmented epithelium of the iris.

4. *Layer of non-pigmented epithelium.* It consists mainly of low columnar or cuboidal cells, and is a forward continuation of the sensory retina which stops at the ora serrata. It continues anteriorly with the posterior (internal) pigmented epithelium of the iris.

5. *Internal limiting membrane.* It lines the non-pigmented epithelium and is the forward continuations of the internal limiting membrane of the retina.

Ciliary processes

Ciliary processes are whitish finger-like projections from the pars plicata part of the ciliary body. They are about 70–80 in number and form the site of aqueous production. Each process is about 2 mm long and 0.5 mm in diameter.

Ultrastructure of the ciliary process

Each ciliary process is composed of three basic components: the network of capillaries, stroma and two layers of the epithelium (Fig. 2.3).

1. *The network of capillaries* occupies the centre of each process. Each capillary consists of a very thin endothelium with fenestrae or false pores (the site of increased permeability) which is lined by a basement membrane. Mural cells or pericytes are present within the basement membrane.

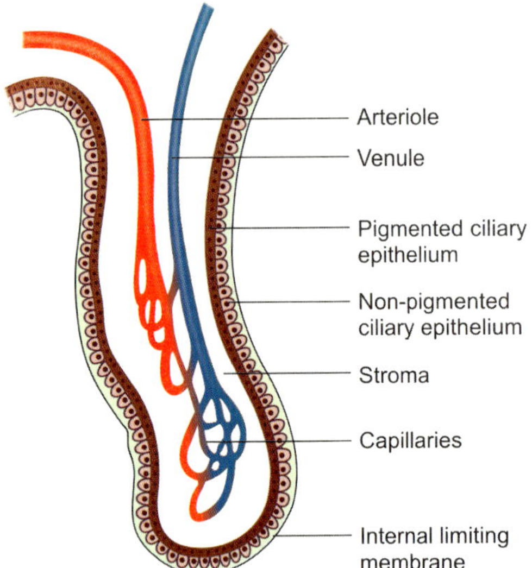

Fig. 2.3 *Microscopic structure of a ciliary process*

2. ***Stroma of ciliary processes*** is very thin and separates the capillary network from the epithelial layers. It consists of ground substance (containing mucopolysaccharides, proteins and solute of plasma), a few collagen connective tissue fibres and wandering cells.

3. ***Two layers of epithelium*** are arranged with their apical surfaces in apposition to each other. The outer pigmented epithelium contains numerous melanin granules. The inner non-pigmented epithelium is characterized by mitochondria (M), zonula occludens (ZO) and lateral and surface interdigitations (I). The tight junctions between the cells of this layer create part of the blood-aqueous barrier. Basement membrane lines the double cell layer and constitutes the internal limiting membrane (ILM) on the inner surface (Fig. 2.4).

BLOOD SUPPLY OF THE UVEAL TRACT

Arterial supply

The uveal tract is supplied by three sets of arteries (Fig. 2.5).

1. ***Short posterior ciliary arteries.*** These arise as two trunks from the ophthalmic artery. Each trunk divides into 10–20 branches which pierce the sclera around the optic nerve and supply the choroid in a segmental manner.

2. ***Long posterior ciliary arteries.*** These are two in number (nasal and temporal). These pierce the sclera obliquely on medial and lateral side of the optic nerve and run forward in the suprachoroidal space to reach the ciliary muscle, without giving any branch. At the anterior end of ciliary muscle, these anastomose with each other and with the anterior ciliary arteries to form the major arterial circle and also give branches which supply the ciliary body.

3. ***Anterior ciliary arteries.*** These are derived from the muscular branches of ophthalmic artery. These are 7 in number: 2 each from the arteries of superior rectus, inferior rectus and medial rectus muscles and one from that of lateral rectus muscle. These arteries pass anteriorly in the episclera, give branches to sclera, limbus and conjunctiva, and ultimately pierce the sclera near the limbus to enter the ciliary muscle where they anastomose with the two long posterior ciliary arteries to form the *circulus arteriosus major,* near the root of the iris. Several branches arise from the circulus arteriosus major and supply the ciliary processes (one branch for each process). Similarly, many branches from this major arterial circle run radially through the iris towards pupillary margin where they anastomose with each other to form *circulus arteriosus minor.*

Venous drainage

Veins draining uveal blood are (Fig. 2.5):

1. ***Anterior ciliary veins.*** These are tributaries of the muscular veins. Since they carry blood only from the ciliary muscle, they are smaller than the corresponding arteries.

2. ***Smaller veins from the sclera.*** These correspond to the scleral branches of the short ciliary arteries. They only carry blood from the sclera and not from the choroid, and are, therefore, smaller than the corresponding arteries.

3. ***Venae verticosae (vortex veins or posterior ciliary veins).*** These are usually 4 in number (superior temporal, inferior temporal, superior nasal and inferior nasal). They pierce the sclera obliquely on each side of the superior rectus and inferior rectus muscles, about 6 mm behind the equator of the globe. Of these, superior temporal

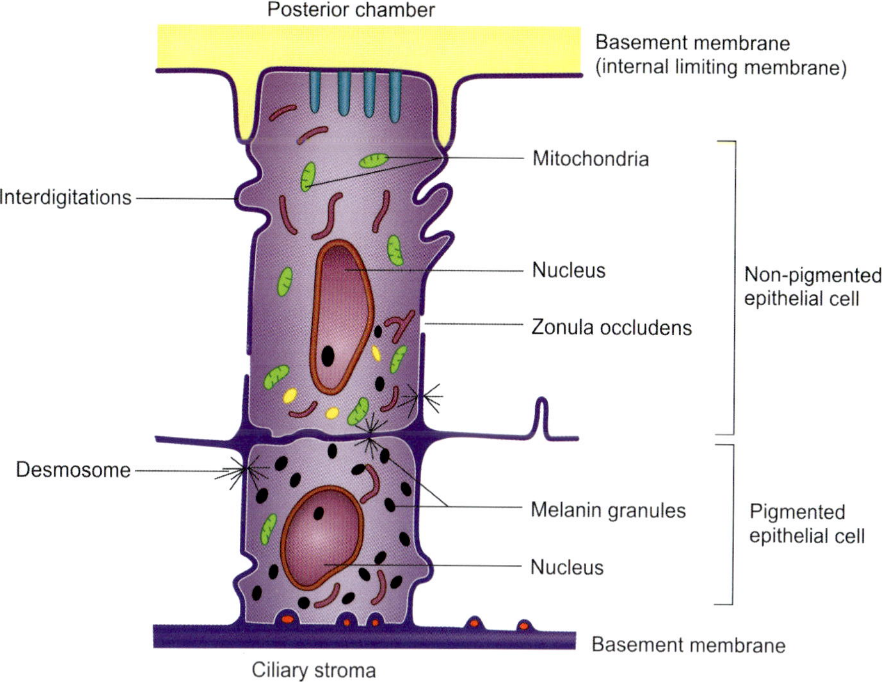

Fig. 2.4 *Microscopic details of the cells of two layers of ciliary epithelium*

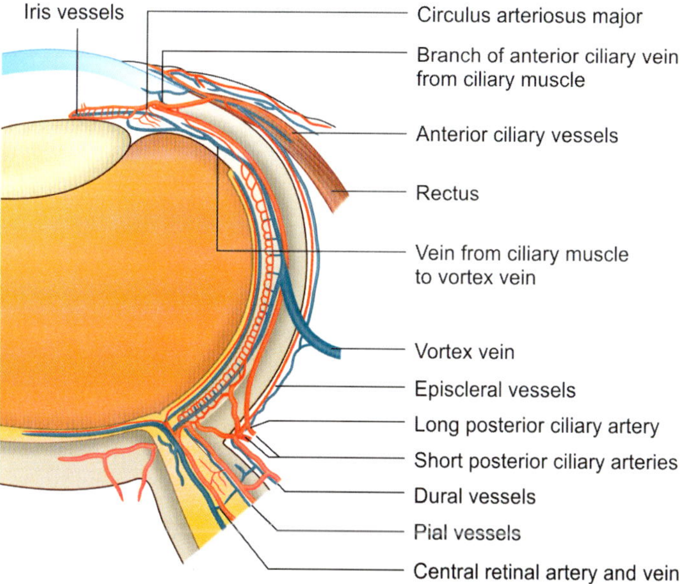

Fig. 2.5 *Blood supply of uveal tract*

vein is most posterior (8 mm behind the equator) and inferior temporal is most anterior (5.5 mm behind the equator).

At their choroidal end, the vortex veins have an ampulliform dilatation. Venae vorticosae drain blood from:

- Whole of the choroid
- Receive small veins from optic nerve head
- Sometimes small veins from retina also join it
- Anterior tributaries come from the iris, ciliary processes, ciliary muscle and anterior part of the choroid. There is no major venous circle corresponding to major arterial circle.

The oblique scleral canals through which the vortex veins pass are about 4 mm long and directed posteriorly in such a way that the four veins appear to converge towards the apex of the orbit.

The two superior vortex veins open into the superior ophthalmic vein directly or through its muscular or lacrimal tributaries. The two inferior vortex veins open into the inferior ophthalmic veins.

POSTERIOR AND ANTERIOR CHAMBERS

Posterior chamber

Posterior chamber is a triangular space containing about 0.06 ml of aqueous humour. The freshly formed aqueous humour from the ciliary processes is poured into this space. Posterior chamber is bounded *anteriorly* by the posterior surface of the iris and part of ciliary body, *posteriorly* by the crystalline lens and its zonules, and *laterally* by the ciliary body (Fig. 2.2). It can be divided into the following three compartments.

1. ***Prezonular space.*** It lies between the posterior surface of the iris and anterior surface of the zonular fibres.

2. ***Zonular space.*** It is also known as circumlental or ciliolental space. It is bounded centrally by equator of the lens, peripherally by the ciliary processes, anteriorly by the posterior surface of anterior zonular fibres and posteriorly by the anterior surface of posterior zonular fibres.

3. ***Retrozonular space.*** It lies between the posterior surface of zonules and the peripheral part of anterior vitreous face.

Anterior chamber

Anterior chamber is bounded *anteriorly* by the back of cornea and *posteriorly* by the anterior surface of iris and part of ciliary body (Fig. 2.2). Anterior chamber is about 3 mm deep in the centre in normal adults. It is comparatively shallow in very young children and old people. Its depth is determined genetically with a dominant inheritance. It contains about 0.25 ml of the aqueous humour. Through pupil, it communicates with the posterior chamber. Its peripheral recess is called angle of the anterior chamber, which is mainly formed by the trabecular meshwork.

ANGLE OF THE ANTERIOR CHAMBER

Structures forming angle recess

Angle of the anterior chamber plays an important role in the process of aqueous drainage. Clinically, the angle structures can be visualized by gonioscopic examination. Starting from posterior to anterior, the angle recess is formed by following structures (Fig. 2.6).

1. ***Ciliary body band.*** It is the most posterior landmark in the angle recess. It is formed by the anterior most part of the ciliary body between its attachment to the scleral spur and insertion of iris. Therefore, its width depends upon the level of iris insertion, and tends to be wider in myopes and narrow in hypermetropes. Usually, it appears as a grey or dark brown band.

2. ***Scleral spur.*** It is the posterior portion of the scleral sulcus which usually appears as a prominent white line on gonioscopy. On it are attached ciliary body posteriorly and corneo-scleral meshwork anteriorly.

3. ***Trabecular meshwork.*** It is seen as a band just anterior to the scleral spur. Its appearance varies considerably, since it has no pigment at birth and develops pigment with increasing age; therefore, with age its colour varies from faint tan to dark brown.

4. ***Schwalbe's line.*** It is a fine ridge seen just in front of the trabecular meshwork. It is formed by the prominent end of the Descemet's membrane of the cornea. It marks the anterior limit of the structures forming the angle of the

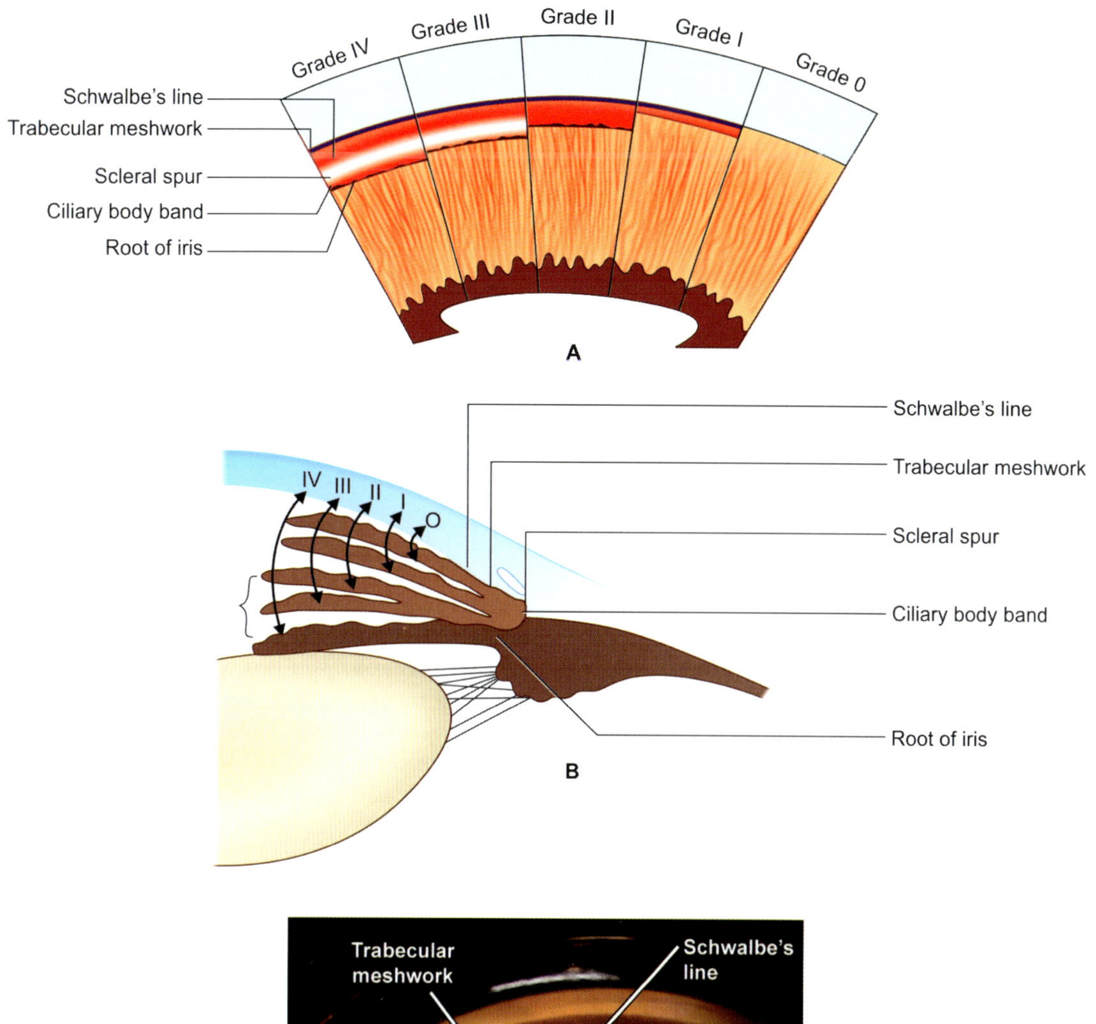

Fig. 2.6 *Depiction of various angle structures as seen in different grades of angle width (Shaffer's grading system): (A) Structures forming angle recess; (B) configuration of the angle in cross-section of anterior chamber; (C) Gonioscopic view.*

anterior chamber. It usually lies in the plane of the posterior corneal surface, but in 15–20% of normal subjects, it may be variably hypertrophied and project as a delicate, glistening ridge into the anterior chamber (posterior embryotoxon).

Gonioscopic grading of the angle width

Various systems have been suggested to grade the angle width. The most commonly used is modified Shaffer's system of grading. The grading of angle width is given in Table 2.1 and is shown diagrammatically in Fig. 2.6.

Table 2.1 *Gonioscopic grading of angle*

	Grade 0	*Grade I*	*Grade II*	*Grade III*	*Grade IV*
Shaffer	Closed	10°	20°	30°	40°
Modified Shaffer	Schwalbe's line not visible	Schwalbe's line visible	Anterior TM visible	Scleral spur visible	Ciliary body band visible

The Shaffer's system is based on the width of the angle recess, but marked intra- and interobserver variability has been noted with this system and hence a modified system where the angle structure visible on gonioscopy is used to grade the angle.

AQUEOUS OUTFLOW SYSTEM

It includes the trabecular meshwork, Schlemm's canal, collector channels, aqueous veins and the episcleral veins (Fig. 2.7).

Trabecular meshwork

It is a sieve-like structure through which aqueous humour leaves the eye. It bridges the scleral sulcus and converts it into a tube, which accommodate Schlemm's canal. The trabecular meshwork is complex connective tissue, the components of which directly or indirectly affect aqueous outflow. Hyaluronic acid is an endogenous glycosaminoglycan (GAG) of the trabecular meshwork. Degradation of hyaluronic acid by hyaluronidase in experiment models enables increased aqueous outflow. Other GAGs including chondroitin, heparin, dermatan and keratan sulphates, are constituents of trabecular meshwork and they too may influence aqueous outflow. Fibronectin, elastin, laminin, collagen (types I, III, IV, V, and VI), and smooth muscle myosin containing cells are other integral components of the trabecular meshwork. Fibronectin secretion by cultured trabecular meshwork cells doubles after treatment with dexamethasone. The significance of this finding with respect to steroid responsiveness has yet to be determined. Composition of the trabecular meshwork is not constant throughout life. Changes in the composition with advancing age

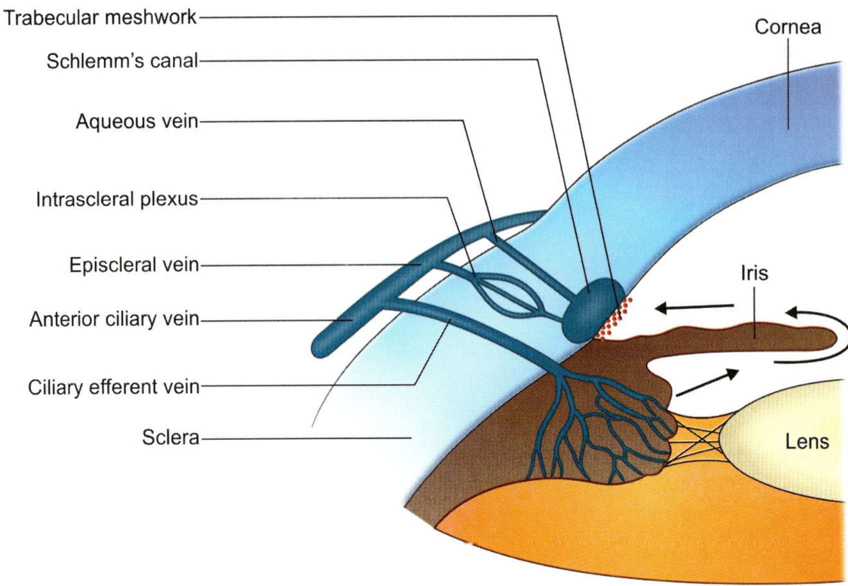

Fig. 2.7 *The aqueous outflow system*

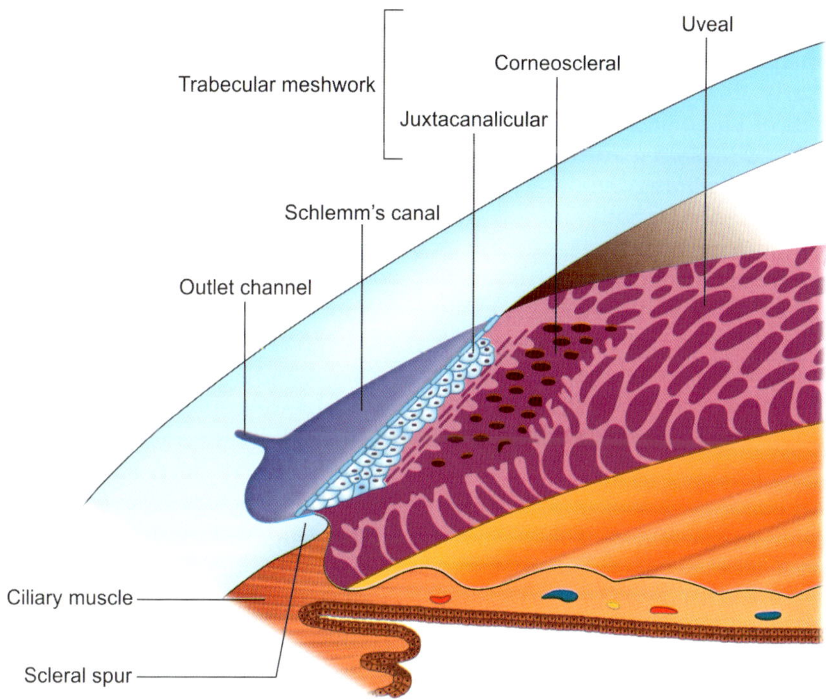

Fig. 2.8 *Schematic drawing showing microscopic structure of trabecular meshwork*

have been implicated in the pathogenesis of primary open-angle glaucoma. The trabecular meshwork consists of three portions (Fig. 2.8).

i. *Uveal meshwork*

It is the innermost part of trabecular meshwork and extends from the iris root and ciliary body to the Schwalbe's line. The trabeculae of uveal meshwork are cord-like and two to three layers thick. The arrangement of uveal trabecular bands creates irregular openings which vary in size from 25 to 75 µ.

On electron microscopy, each trabeculae is seen to have three concentric layers: a central collagenous core, a middle layer of a basement membrane-like material with a periodicity of 1000 Å, and enclosing trabecular cells.

ii. *Corneoscleral meshwork*

It forms the larger middle portion and extends from the scleral spur to the lateral wall of the scleral sulcus. It consists of flat sheets of trabeculae which are perforated by elliptical openings which are smaller than those in the uveal meshwork (5–50 µm). These holes become progressively smaller as the trabecular sheets approach Schlemm's canal and holes of deepest layer may be even 1–2 µ min size. Electron microscopic structure of each trabecula is similar to that of trabeculae of uveal meshwork.

iii. *Juxtacanalicular (endothelial) meshwork*

It forms the outermost portion of the trabecular meshwork. It is that part of the trabecular meshwork which mainly offers the normal resistance to aqueous outflow. It consists of a layer of connective tissue (containing 2–5 layers of loosely arranged cells, embedded in an extracellular matrix) lined on either side by endothelium. This narrow part of trabeculum (thickness 2–20 µm) connects the corneoscleral meshwork with Schlemm's canal. In fact, the outer endothelial layer of the juxtacanalicular meshwork comprises the inner wall of Schlemm's canal and the inner endothelial layer of the juxtacanalicular meshwork becomes continuous with the endothelium of corneoscleral meshwork.

Schlemm's canal

It is an endothelial lined oval channel present circumferentially in the scleral sulcus. The endothelial cells of its inner wall are irregular, spindle-shaped and contain giant vacuoles.

The endothelial cells lining the outer wall of the Schlemm's canal are smooth and flat. The outer wall of the canal contains numerous openings of the collector channels. Torus or lip-like thickenings have been observed around the openings of the outlet (collector) channel and septa have been noted to extend from these openings to the inner wall of Schlemm's canal, which presumably help to keep the canal open.

Collector channels

Collector channels, also called intrascleral aqueous vessels, are about 25–35 in number and leave the Schlemm's canal at oblique angles to terminate ultimately into episcleral veins. They are lined by vascular endothelium similar to that of the outer wall of Schlemm's canal. They are relatively wide at their origin (20–90 μm), but taper towards their anastomoses with the venous channels. No valves are present in the collector channels. These intrascleral aqueous vessels can be divided into two systems:

1. ***Direct system.*** It is formed by about eight larger vessels which run a short intrascleral course and terminate directly into the episcleral veins. On slit-lamp examination, they appear as clear vessels with aqueous and have been called *aqueous veins* by Ascher. Since these aqueous vessels terminate into episcleral and conjunctival veins in a laminated junction, these are also referred to as the *laminated veins of Goldmann*.

2. ***Indirect system.*** It is constituted by numerous finer collector channels which drain into three interconnecting venous plexuses—the deep intrascleral plexus, mid-intrascleral plexus and the episcleral venous plexus—before eventually going into the episcleral veins.

Episcleral veins

Most of the aqueous vessels drain into the episcleral veins. The episcleral veins ultimately drain into the cavernous sinus via the anterior ciliary and superior ophthalmic veins.

Innervation of aqueous outflow system

Many workers now believe that both parasympathetic and adrenergic autonomic fibres and sensory fibres innervate the aqueous outflow system. Both myelinated and non-myelinated nerve fibres have been demonstrated in the trabecular meshwork and Schlemm's canal. Although, it is tempting to designate a role for such innervation in the homeostasis of intraocular pressure, however, no such function has been established till date.

Nerve endings with structural characteristics of mechanoreceptors have also been reported to exist in the human scleral spur. Following functions have been hypothesized for these presumed mechanoreceptors:

- They might be acting as proprioceptive tendon organs for the ciliary muscle fibres inserted on the scleral spur.
- They might be influencing the contraction of the myofibroblastic scleral spur cells. They might perform a baroreceptor function in response to changes in intraocular pressure.

PHYSIOLOGICAL CONSIDERATIONS

FUNCTIONS, PROPERTIES AND COMPOSITION OF AQUEOUS HUMOUR

FUNCTIONS OF AQUEOUS HUMOUR

Aqueous humour is a clear, colourless, watery solution, continuously circulated from the posterior chamber of the eye throughout the anterior chamber. This continuous circulation results from a dynamic equilibrium. The aqueous humour serves following functions:

1. **Maintenance of intraocular pressure.** It is the primary function of the aqueous. By virtue of this, the aqueous humour helps in maintaining the shape and internal structural arrangement of the eye.

2. **Metabolic role.** In addition to its role in maintaining a proper intraocular pressure, it also plays an important metabolic role by providing substrates and removing metabolites from the avascular ocular structures as follows:

i. *Cornea* takes glucose and oxygen from the aqueous and releases lactic acid and carbon dioxide into the aqueous.

ii. *Lens* uses oxygen, glucose, amino acids and potassium from the aqueous and releases lactate, pyruvate and sodium into the aqueous.

iii. *Vitreous and retinal metabolism* also appears to be associated with the aqueous humour in that substances, such as amino acids and glucose, pass into the vitreous from the aqueous.

3. Optical function. Under normal conditions, aqueous is optically clear. The cornea–aqueous interface acts as a diverging lens of low power.

4. Clearing function. The aqueous humour serves as a mechanism to clear blood, macrophages, remnants of lens matter and products of inflammation from the anterior chamber of the eye.

PHYSICOCHEMICAL PROPERTIES

1. *Volume* of the aqueous is about 0.31 ml (0.25 ml in anterior chamber and about 0.06 ml in the posterior chamber).
2. *Refractive index* of the aqueous is 1.336, slightly lower than that of the cornea, so there is a slight divergence of the light rays as they pass the cornea–aqueous interface.
3. *Density* of the normal aqueous is slightly greater than that of water. Relative to water, its viscosity is 1.025 to 1.040.
4. *Osmotic pressure.* Aqueous is slightly hyperosmotic to plasma by 3 to 5 mOsm/L.
5. *pH:* Aqueous is acidic with a pH of 7.2 in the anterior chamber.
6. *Rate of formation.* The normal aqueous production rate is 2.3 μl/min (about 1% of the anterior chamber volume/min).

BIOCHEMICAL COMPOSITION

Chemical analysis of the aqueous humour has revealed many important facts. For many years, Leber's theory, that the aqueous was formed by simple filtration from the blood, was generally accepted. However, study of biochemical composition of the aqueous has revealed that such a simple hypothesis cannot explain the facts. In addition to it, many other facts have surfaced which will be discussed after knowing the constituents of the aqueous humour which are as follows:

Water. It constitutes about 99.9% of the normal aqueous humour.

Proteins (colloid content). The most obvious chemical difference between aqueous humour and blood plasma is in the level of protein content of the two fluids. In the plasma, it is of the order of 6–7 g/100 ml, whereas in the aqueous humour, it is only 5–16 mg/100 ml in human (i.e. about 1/500 that of plasma, protein level) and some 50 mg/100 ml in the rabbit (Table 2.2). This is because of the blood–aqueous barrier; and any disruption of this barrier will increase protein influx. The albumin/globulin ratio is the same as in plasma, although there are less gammaglobulins.

Human aqueous has been found to contain IgG and IgM but no IgD and IgA. Plasminogen and its proactivator are present, but none of their inhibitors or other clotting factors are detectable in the aqueous. Numerous growth factors including FGF, TGF-B and insulin-like growth factor I have also been demonstrated in the aqueous.

Amino acids. The relative concentration of free amino acids in human aqueous varies with aqueous/plasma concentrations ranging from 0.08 to 3.14 supporting the concept of active transport of amino acids.

Non-colloidal constituents. Non-colloids are the dissolved solids that give an absolutely clear solution—one in which a beam of light would not be seen. The non-colloid content of the rabbit aqueous humour, compared to plasma, is given in Table 2.3. Although cursory inspection shows that the non-colloidal composition of the

Table 2.2 *Comparison of protein content of plasma and aqueous humour for human and rabbit*

	Protein levels	
Species	*Plasma*	*Aqueous humour*
Human	7 g/100 ml	5–16 mg/100 ml
Rabbit	6–7 g/100 ml	50 mg/100 ml

(*Source*: After Darson H (ed). The Eye, vol. 1, New York, Academic Press) (1969).

Table 2.3 *Composition of plasma and aqueous humour of the anterior and posterior chambers of rabbits*

Substance	*mmol/kg water*		
	Anterior aqueous	*Posterior aqueous*	*Plasma*
Inorganic constituents			
Sodium	146.5	144.5	146
Potassium	4.7	—	4.8
Chloride	105.1	100.0	111.8
Bicarbonate	27.7	34.1	24
Phosphate	0.89	0.52	1.49
Hydrogen ion (pH)	7.6	7.57	7.4
Organic constituents			
Ascorbate	0.96	1.30	0.02
Lactate	12.1	11.2	8.2
Glucose	6.7	7.1	8.3
Non-protein nitrogen	13.4	13.5	17.6
Urea	6.3	5.8	7.3

(*Source:* Kinsey VE, Reddy DVN. In: Prince JH (ed). The Rabbit in Eye Research, Springfield, III, Charles Thomas 1966).

aqueous humour is similar in its broad outlines to that of plasma, careful review reveals some striking differences that are inconsistent with aqueous being simply a filtrate. For example, the concentrations of ascorbate (vitamin C), pyruvate and lactate are much higher than in plasma, while those of urea and glucose are much less.

Inulin and steroid. These hormones are also present and enter the aqueous humour by simple diffusion.

Prostaglandins. They appear to be actively released into the aqueous by the iris.

Cyclic AMP. It has been detected in the aqueous at a level about the same as found in serum.

Composition of aqueous humour of the anterior and posterior chambers

The composition of aqueous humour in anterior chamber differs from that of the aqueous humour in posterior chamber because it depends not only on the nature of production, but also on the constant metabolic interchange that occurs throughout its intraocular course. Diffusional exchange across the iris is a significant factor in changing the composition, since iris vessels are permeable to anions and non-electrolytes. Composition of aqueous humour of anterior vis-à-vis posterior chamber and plasma as studied by Kinsey and Reddy are shown in Table 2.3. The striking differences are as follows:

- The bicarbonate concentration in posterior chamber aqueous is higher than in the anterior. This is because the freshly secreted fluid has a much higher concentration than in the plasma, but due to diffusion into the vitreous and into the blood from iris and decomposition by the acids formed by the lens and cornea metabolism, its level decreases in the anterior aqueous.
- The chloride concentration in the newly formed aqueous of posterior chamber is lower than the plasma. Diffusion of chloride from the blood raises the chloride levels of anterior chamber aqueous.
- Ascorbate concentration in posterior aqueous is much higher than the plasma. The gradient of diffusion for ascorbic acid from the anterior chamber to the blood reduces the concentration of ascorbic acid in the anterior aqueous.

Factors affecting composition of the aqueous humour

1. *Blood–ocular barrier*

By virtue of blood–ocular barrier, the protein and other large molecular size substances are largely prevented from entering the cavities (anterior chamber, posterior chamber and in tear cavity) of the eyes. This mechanism is essential to maintain the clarity of the media of the eye.

Blood–ocular barrier consists of two parts—the posterior blood–retinal barrier and the anterior blood–aqueous barrier.

Blood–retinal barrier in turn consists of two parts—the inner and the outer. The inner blood–retinal barrier is composed of the tight junction of retinal capillaries, endothelial cells and the outer blood–retinal barrier consists of tight junctional complexes (zonula occludens and zonula adherens) which are located between adjacent RPE cells (Fig. 2.9).

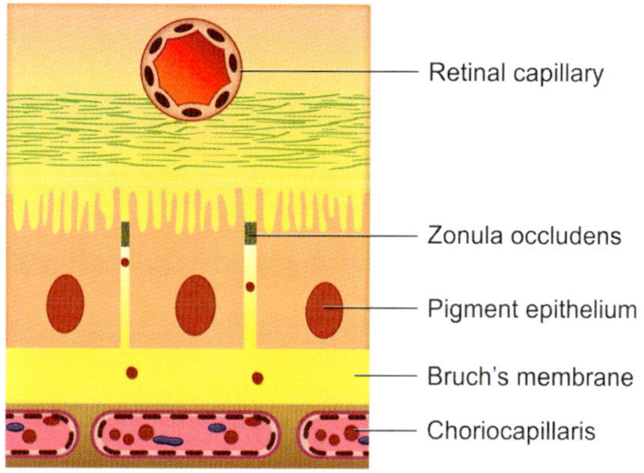

Fig. 2.9 *Blood–retinal barrier*

Blood–aqueous barrier is formed by the tight junctions (zonula occludens and zonula adherens) between the cells of the inner non-pigmented epithelium of the ciliary body (Fig. 2.4) and the non-fenestrated endothelium of the iris capillaries. However, the endothelial cells of iris capillaries are not joined by tight junctions and in inflammatory conditions they become leaky, causing an aqueous flare.

The blood–ocular barrier is not absolute. Medium-sized, water-soluble substances may penetrate it but at much slower rate than their transit across capillary walls. Examples of such substances include urea creatinine and some sugars. Further, lipid solubility greatly facilitates the ability of a substance to penetrate the blood–ocular barrier.

Clinical applications of blood–ocular barrier

i. *Hyperosmotic agents,* like mannitol, penetrate the eye poorly because of the blood–ocular barrier, but are distributed fairly widely in the extracellular spaces of the body. Thus, water is drawn from the cells and the ocular fluids (vitreous more than the aqueous), resulting in a fall in the intraocular pressure.

ii. *Ocular penetration of systemically administered antibiotics.* Only low molecular weight drugs, such as chloramphenicol, cephalothin and ampicillin can cross the blood–aqueous barrier. Very poor passage is allowed to large-sized molecules, such as penicillin, methicillin and erythromycin. Out of the borderline molecular weight drugs, those with high lipid solubility can pass easily, e.g. sulfonamides have the same molecular weight as sucrose but are 16 times more permeable due to their lipid solubility.

Breakdown of the blood–aqueous barrier

Factors interrupting blood–aqueous barrier. The blood–aqueous barrier is rather fragile. Certain conditions which can disturb the blood–aqueous barrier are listed below:

I. *Ocular trauma*

1. Mechanical
   i. Paracentesis
   ii. Corneal abrasion
   iii. Intraocular surgery
   iv. Stroking iris
2. Physical
   i. X-rays
   ii. Atomic radiation
3. Chemical
   i. Alkali
   ii. Irritants, e.g. nitrogen mustard

II. *Pathophysiologic*

1. Vascular dilatation
   i. Histamine
   ii. Sympathectomy
2. Corneal and intraocular infections
3. Intraocular inflammations
4. Prostaglandins
5. Anterior segment ischaemia

III. *Pharmacologic*

1. Melanocyte-stimulating hormone (MSH)
2. Nitrogen mustard
3. Cholinesterase inhibitors
4. Cholinergic drugs
5. Plasma hyperosmolality

Effect of breakdown of blood–aqueous barrier on aqueous humour composition

- With the breakdown of blood–aqueous barrier, substances, such as proteins that are normally almost completely excluded from penetration, appear in the aqueous humour in measurable amounts. Thus, proteins and antibodies in the aqueous equilibrate with those in plasma to form plasmoid aqueous *(secondary aqueous).* Increased protein in the slit-lamp microscope as a pronounced Tyndall beam.

- The ionic composition of the aqueous approaches that of simple dialysate of plasma.
- The rates of penetration of the smaller molecules, such as sucrose or p-amino-hippurate (which were previously partly blocked from aqueous), are increased greatly. In fact, the rapid rate of entry into aqueous of such substances as fluorescein and Evans blue dye can be used as diagnostic indicators of barrier breakdown.
- Fibrinogen appears in the aqueous, which may allow the aqueous actually to clot.

2. *Haemodynamic factors influencing stromal pool*

Formation of plasma filtrate in the stroma of ciliary processes (stromal pool) is the first step in the production of aqueous humour. Thus, the haemodynamic factors will affect the ultrafiltration at the level of ciliary epithelium.

3. *Diffusional exchange across the iris*

Diffusional exchange across the iris is a significant factor in changing the composition of aqueous humour, since iris vessels are permeable to anions and non-electrolytes.

4. *Metabolites*

The metabolic processes ongoing in the cornea, lens, vitreous and retina can also modify the composition of aqueous humour.

5. *Rate of aqueous drainage*

Since the steady state levels of the different constituents of aqueous humour are maintained at a dynamic equilibrium between aqueous formation and aqueous drainage, therefore, decrease or increase in the rate of aqueous drainage will influence the aqueous composition.

6. *Quality of aqueous*

The formation process and factors (neurohormonal and others) regulating this process also influences the aqueous humour composition.

AQUEOUS HUMOUR FORMATION

The ciliary processes are the site of aqueous production. The aqueous humour is primarily derived from the plasma within the capillary network of the ciliary processes. The Leber's theory (which was generally accepted for many years) that aqueous is a simple filtrate from the blood does not hold true any more. Presently, by and large, it is agreed that three mechanisms namely, diffusion, ultrafiltration and secretion play a part in aqueous production at different levels. Salient features of these processes and the steps involved in the production of aqueous humour are discussed below.

FORMATION PROCESSES

The various constituents of the aqueous humour have to traverse the three tissue layers of the ciliary processes, viz. the capillary wall, the stroma and two layers of the epithelium. The various substances appear to pass through these layers by following processes.

1. Diffusion

Diffusion is a biophysical process by which molecules of a gas or solution distribute themselves uniformly throughout the space in which they are contained, by motion of its particles (Fig. 2.10). In this process, there occurs a net flux of the particles from areas of high concentration to areas of low concentration.

Diffusion also occurs across a semipermeable membrane. Quantitatively, the net movement of a substance across a semipermeable membrane where only diffusion is occurring is expressed by Fick's law of diffusion as follows:

$$\text{Rate of movement} = K (C_1 - C_2)$$

C_1 = Concentration of substance on side with higher concentration.

C_2 = Concentration of substance on side with lower concentration.

K = Constant which depends on nature and permeability of membrane, nature of solute and solvent, and the temperature.

In the process of aqueous production, the lipid-soluble substances are transported by diffusion through the lipid portions of the cell membrane of the ciliary processes, propor-

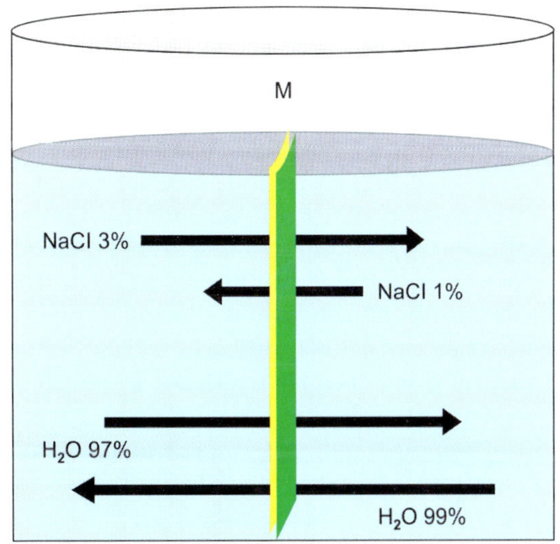

Fig. 2.10 *Diffusion phenomenon through a membrane (M), permeable to NaCl and H_2O. Note a net flux of particles from areas of high concentration to areas of low concentration*

tional to a concentration gradient across the membrane.

2. Ultrafiltration

Dialysis: When a solution of protein and salt is separated from plain water or a less concentrated salt solution by a membrane permeable to salt and water and not to proteins, there will be a net movement of water on the protein side by diffusion and a movement of the salt away from the protein side. This process is called dialysis (Fig. 2.11A).

Ultrafiltration refers to occurrence of dialysis under hydrostatic pressure (Fig. 2.11B).

In the process of aqueous formation, water and water-soluble substances (limited by size and charge) flow through the theoretical micropores in the protein part of the cell membrane in response to osmotic gradient or hydrostatic pressure.

3. Secretion (active transfer)

Secretion implies an active process that selectively transports some substances across the cell membrane. Since energy is consumed, substances can be moved across a concentration gradient in a direction opposite to what would be expected by passive mechanism alone. In the process of aqueous formation, water-soluble substances of larger size or greater charge are actively transported across the cell membrane. This mechanism is believed to be mediated by globular proteins in the membrane and requires the expenditure of energy.

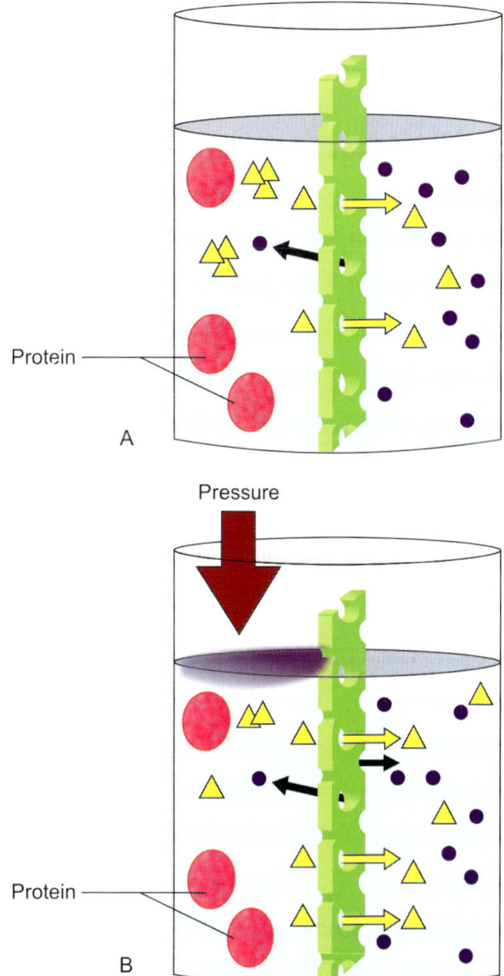

Fig. 2.11 *(A) Phenomenon of dialysis: Note a net movement of water molecules (small solid circles) on the proteins (large circles) side and that of soft molecules (triangles) away from the protein; (B) Phenomenon of ultrafiltration: Note that the hydrostatic pressure increases the rate of net movement of water and salt molecules across the semipermeable membrane (c.f. dialysis—Fig. 2.11A). The final equilibrium concentrations on either side of the membrane are the same as in dialysis*

STEPS OF AQUEOUS FORMATION

The major factor in aqueous production (approximately 70%) is active secretion.

Ultrafiltration accounts for 20% and osmosis 10%. The various constituents of the aqueous humour reach the posterior chamber from the plasma within the capillary network of ciliary processes as follows:

1. Formation of stromal pool

It is the first step in the formation of aqueous. By ultrafiltration, most substances pass easily from the capillaries of the ciliary processes, across the stroma and between the pigmented epithelium cells before accumulating behind the tight junctions of the non-pigmented epithelium. Protein is to be expected in the filtrate because of the fenestrated nature of the ciliary capillaries.

2. Active transport of stromal filtrates

The tight junctions between the non-pigmented epithelial cells create part of blood–aqueous barrier. Evidence of active transport occurring across these non-pigmented epithelial cells, especially in the cell membrane of the lateral interdigitations, comes from observations of the following in these areas:

- Abundant Na^+–K^+-active ATPase,
- Presence of more mitochondria,
- Higher adenyl cyclase activity,
- Higher specific activity for glycolytic enzymes, and
- Preferential incorporation of labelled sulphate into macromolecules (primarily glycolipids and glycoproteins).

Until recently, active aqueous secretion was thought to be carried out solely by the mitochondria rich non-pigmented epithelium as described above. However, recent studies have shown that the pigmented epithelium also plays an active role in the aqueous production. The basolateral membranes of the pigmented epithelial cells contain numerous Na^+ ion dependent cotransporters and exchangers (Fig. 2.12) and carbonic anhydrase activity is also present in these cells. The net effect of these ion transport systems is a low level of Na^+ in both epithelial layers (facilitated by numerous gap junctions between the pigmented and non-pigmented cells), a high level of ascorbate and K^+, and control of intracellular pH.

Following substances from the stromal filtrate are actively transported across epithelial cells:

- *Sodium:* Approximately 70% of the sodium found in the posterior chamber is actively transported by a specific secretory pump. Remaining 30% enters the posterior chamber by diffusion or ultrafiltration. The active transport of sodium is ATPase-dependent but does not appear to be related to the concentration of sodium in plasma.
  Whether carbonic anhydrase works on the sodium pump as a facilitator, as a catalyst or as part of a parallel but related process remains to be demonstrated. It is possible that carbonic anhydrase acts to maintain the proper pH for the Na^+–K^+-ATPase system.
- *Chloride:* A smaller percentage of the chloride ion is actively transported and this appears to be dependent upon the presence of sodium as well as pH. The remaining amount of Cl^- enters into lateral intercellular space by diffusion.
- *Potassium* is transported by secretion and diffusion.
- *Ascorbic acid* is secreted against a large concentration gradient.
- *Amino acids* are secreted by at least three carriers, one each for acidic, basic and neutral molecules.
- *Bicarbonate:* Its formation is catalysed by carbonic anhydrase. The rapid interconversion between bicarbonate and CO_2 makes it difficult to determine the relative proportions of these two substances. It influences fluid transport through its effect on sodium, possibly by regulating the pH for optimum active transport of sodium.

3. Passive transport across non-pigmented ciliary epithelium

Active transport of the substances as described above, across the non-pigmented ciliary epithelium results in an osmotic and electrical gradient. To maintain the balance of osmotic and electrical forces, water, chloride and other small plasma constituents move into the posterior chamber by ultrafiltration and diffusion; sodium is primarily responsible for movement of water into the posterior chamber and its secretion is a

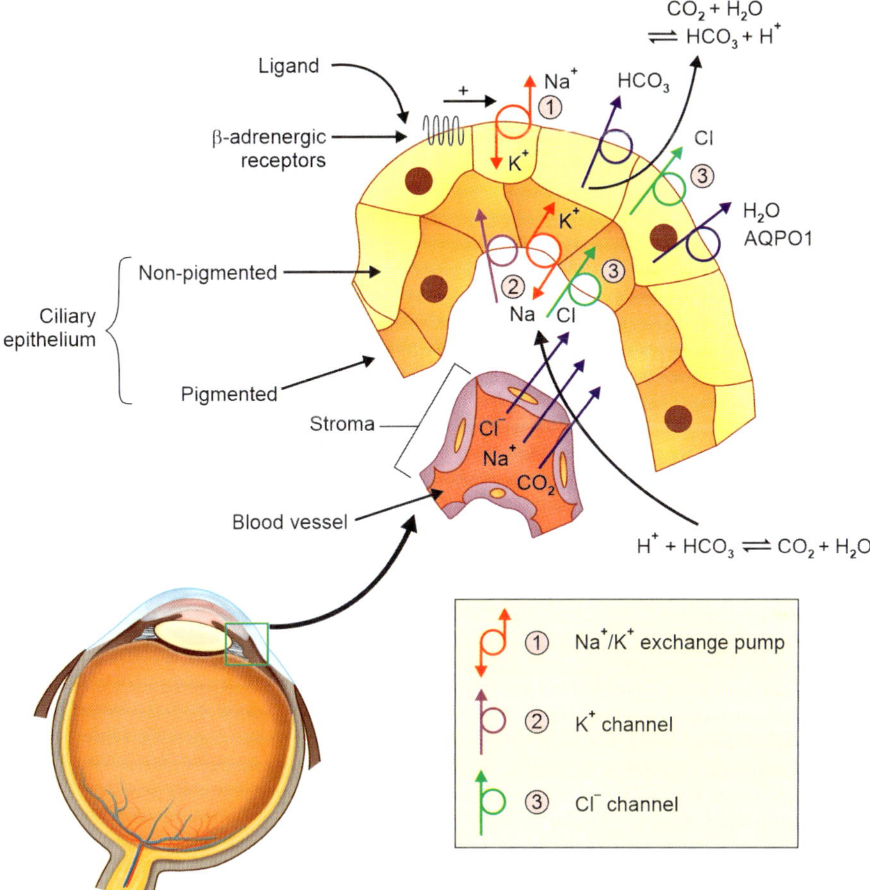

Fig. 2.12 *Mechanism of aqueous humour formation*

major factor in the formation of aqueous. Some authors have suggested that the primary event in the aqueous formation is the production of hydroxyl ions, which depends upon the catalytic action of carbonic anhydrase. However, much of the evidences accumulated till now indicate that the secretion of sodium into the posterior chamber is the key event in aqueous formation. The following evidences support this view:

- Presence of large concentration of $Na–K^+$-activated ATPase especially at the lateral interdigitations of the non-pigmented epithelium.
- Ouabain which is an inhibitor of $Na^+–K^+$-activated ATPase effectively reduces aqueous formation.
- Shrinkage of ciliary processes is inhibited by ouabain.
- Sodium accumulates in the posterior chamber after parenteral administration of radioactive sodium.

RATE OF AQUEOUS HUMOUR PRODUCTION

Normal values

The rate of aqueous humour formation in the human varies somewhat according to the measurement technique used. However, a figure of 2 µl/min is generally used. The corresponding figures in rabbits are about 3–4 µl/min. Fluorophotometric studies which may provide the most reliable estimates, give a value of approximately 2.5 µl/min in the undisturbed human eye.

Methods of measurement

The methods of measuring rate of aqueous humour production are all indirect and can be divided into two:

Class 1 methods

These are based on measuring a chemical substance's rate of appearance in or disappearance from the aqueous and include the following:

1. ***Fluorescein techniques***. These involve instillation of fluorescein into the anterior chamber by iontophoresis through cornea with subsequent measurement of either the flow of unstained aqueous from the posterior to anterior chamber using photographic methods or the change in concentration of fluorescein in the anterior chamber by photofluorometry.
2. ***Radioactive labelled isotopes*** can be used to measure inflow in animals by observing either the accumulation of the isotope in the anterior chamber or the decay rate of the intracamerally injected isotopes.
3. ***Techniques employing intravenous ion of para-aminohippurate (PAH) or fluorescein.*** Either of the above agents is injected intravenously and the rate of fresh aqueous formation can be calculated by measuring the declining concentration either by sampling the aqueous first in one eye then later in the second eye, as in the case of PAH as by optical means or in the case of fluorescein.

Class 2 methods

These methods involve physical measurements and depend upon the following equation:

$$\text{Flow} = C\,(P_0 - P_v)$$

P_0 = Intraocular pressure
P_v = Episcleral venous pressure
C = Facility of outflow

A few class 2 methods are as follows:

1. *Perfusion of eyes* at a constant pressure can be used to determine the inflow in experimental animals.
2. *Tonography* can also be used to determine the rate of aqueous flow.
3. *Perilimbal suction cup method:* The perilimbal suction cup theoretically occludes the outflow channels of the eye, and intraocular pressure then rises. The rate of aqueous formation can be estimated from the rate of increase in intraocular pressure.

CONTROL OF AQUEOUS FORMATION

The role of various endogenous factors which control the aqueous formation is yet to be clearly understood. The diurnal variation in IOP certainly indicates that some endogenous factors do influence the aqueous formation. These factors may be neural or neurohumoral in nature and include the following:

1. ***Adrenergic innervations.*** The ciliary epithelium does not show presence of nerve supply but the vessels of ciliary processes have a dense adrenergic innervation which may influence the aqueous formation by influencing the permeability of these vessels.
2. ***Role of vasopressin:*** The pituitary vasopressin at physiological level supports the active transport of Na^+ ions across ciliary epithelium and thereby an increase in aqueous formation. The levels of vasopressin in plasma depend upon the total body hydration. Increased body hydration would reduce plasma osmolarity which would result in increased water influx through ciliary epithelium. But at the same time the reduced plasma osmolarity would cause a reduction in pituitary vasopressin production and now vasopressin level will reduce the Na^+ transport across the ciliary epithelium.
3. ***Role of adenylcyclase:*** Adenylcyclase activity has been demonstrated on the tips of ciliary processes. Catecholamines cause increased formation of cAMP by stimulating adenylcyclase. Adrenergic receptors have also been demonstrated in ciliary processes. cAMP activates a specific protein kinase and thereby results in specific protein phosphorylation which affects aqueous formation. Another view is that this protein kinase activity induced by cAMP may cause a change permeability of non-pigmentary ciliary epithelium (NPCE). It has also been suggested that the activated Na/K-ATPase and adenylcyclase may not be coupled in series. The Na/K-ATPase may regulate the extraction of Na from stroma and PCE while the adenylcyclase regulates the secretory activity in NPCE.

Adrenergic receptors regulate IOP via adenylate cyclase. The majority of receptors in the ciliary body are α_2, while more than 90% of β-receptors are β_2. Stimulation of α_2-receptors lowers the intraocular pressure via a reduction in aqueous humour production through inhibition of adenylate cyclase. Epinephrine, a preferential α-adrenergic agonist, stimulates prostaglandin synthesis, particularly that of PGE2 and PGF2α, the latter having potent ocular hypotensive activity.

Stimulation of β-receptors, particularly β_2-receptors, leads to an increase in aqueous secretion via activation of adenylate cyclase.

The dual control of aqueous secretion through activation (β) or inhibition of adenylate cyclase (α) is mediated by their respective stimulatory and inhibitor G proteins. Thus, IOP can be lowered by β_2-agonists (e.g. clonidine) or β_2-antagonists (β-blockers, e.g. timolol). α_2-receptors are also linked to vasoactive intestinal peptide receptors, which are costimulated and lead to a reduction in cAMP levels, which in itself may also lower IOP. β-antagonists have no effect on aqueous flow when aqueous production is at its lowest I level, whereas α_2-agonists and carbonic anhydrase inhibitors do.

The mechanisms whereby changes in intracellular cAMP levels alter aqueous secretion are not known but appear to involve transport of the HCO_3^- ion across the cells. In addition, a number of other components appear to be involved in aqueous secretion, such as protein kinase C, which is linked to adenylate cyclase activation and thus may act as a bridge between the two main second messenger systems.

4. ***Ultrafiltration and diffusion.*** The passive mechanisms of aqueous formation are dependent upon the level of blood pressure in the ciliary capillaries, the plasma osmotic pressure and the level of intraocular pressure.

AQUEOUS HUMOUR DYNAMICS

Aqueous humor dynamics includes aqueous inflow (i.e. formation) and outflow (i.e. drainage). Aqueous production remains constant till IOP is raised to 50 mm Hg and over. Aqueous humour flows from the posterior chamber into the anterior chamber through the pupil against slight physiologic resistance. In the anterior chamber, there exists convection (thermal) current which results from a temperature gradient between the anterior and posterior parts of the anterior chamber. The anterior part of the anterior chamber is cooler (since evaporation of tears from the corneal surface causes cooling of the cornea, which being avascular is already cooler) than the posterior part (which is closer to the warm vascular iris). Due to the effect of convection current, the aqueous in posterior part of the anterior chamber moves up along the warmer iris and in the anterior part moves down along the cooler cornea.

From the anterior chamber, the aqueous is drained out by two routes: uveoscleral (unconventional) outflow and the trabecular (conventional) outflow.

1. TRABECULAR (CONVENTIONAL) OUTFLOW

Trabecular outflow is the main outlet for aqueous from the anterior chamber. Approximately, 75 to 90% of the total aqueous is drained via this route. Free flow of aqueous occurs from the trabecular meshwork in the angle of anterior chamber up to juxtacanalicular tissue, which along with the inner wall of the Schlemm's canal, appears to provide some resistance to the outflow.

The process of aqueous transport across the trabecular meshwork cells and the inner wall of Schlemm's canal is partially understood. Before reviewing the suggested mechanisms of aqueous transport, it will be worthwhile to review the salient features of trabecular meshwork cells and Schlemm's canal endothelial cells.

Trabecular meshwork cells and Schlemm's canal cells

Trabecular meshwork cells line the aqueous channels and their activities promote aqueous outflow. Trabecular meshwork endothelial cells have special characteristics, namely active phagocytic properties, high levels of cytoskeletal actin (which in cultured cells are particularly sensitive to cytochalasin B) and lower levels of microtubules (which appear to be relatively nonresponsive to colchicine). These cells also contain vimentin and desmin, thus showing some similarity to smooth muscle cells. Taken together, these findings suggest that trabecular meshwork endothelial cells are specialized both for endocytic transport of water and solutes and contractility. Actin mobilization appears to be mediated via adrenergic receptors, probably of the β_2 type which are highly responsive to epinephrine. Energy metabolism in the trabecular meshwork endothelium is predominantly glycolytic rather than oxidative, although both enzyme systems are present and functional. Transport of water may be achieved not merely by passive transportation of H_2O packets but by activation of a water channel protein, aquaporin 1 (AQPO 1), found in corneal endothelial cells.

Metabolic labelling studies have shown that most of the matrix components in the trabecular meshwork are synthesized and degraded by the endothelial cells. In addition, these cells have high levels of surface tissue plasminogen activator (tPA), higher even than in vascular endothelial cells, and this is likely to play a role in maintaining patency and reducing the resistance of the outflow passages. Phagocytic activity of trabecular meshwork cells is associated with several other enzymatic activities, such as GAG-degrading enzymes and acid phosphatase.

Trabecular meshwork cells have receptors for a variety of agents including epinephrine (β_2-adrenergic receptors, decrease phagocytosis) and glucocorticoids. Both steroids and oxidative damage induce the expression of the trabecular meshwork inducible glucocorticoid response (TIGR) protein. Mutations in the *TIGR* gene have been found in patients with glaucoma. In addition, TGF-β appears to be involved in the glucocorticoid cell response and in the production of trabecular meshwork extracellular material. Steroids inhibit prostaglandin production by trabecular meshwork cells at concentrations as low as 10^{-8} M. Prostaglandin synthesis by trabecular meshwork accounts for a significant proportion of its arachidonic acid metabolism (70% compared with less than 5% in other cells) suggesting that prostaglandins play a major role in trabecular meshwork cell physiology. In addition to substantial amounts of PGE and PGF2α, leukotriene B_4 appears to be produced in high amounts.

Trabecular meshwork cells contain the free radical and hydrogen peroxide detoxifying enzyme systems present in other tissues, such as the ciliary body. Both a catalase and a glutathione-dependent system are active in handling hydrogen peroxide, which can reach levels as high as 25 mmol/L in the aqueous humour.

Various mechanisms of aqueous transport across inner wall of Schlemm's canal

Based on the above description of trabecular meshwork and canal of Schlemm's endothelial cells. Various theories have been put forward from time to time, to explain the flow of aqueous humour across the inner wall of Schlemm's canal. These theories can be grasped as below:

I. *Passive filter mechanisms*

Earlier it was believed that from the juxtacanalicular space, the aqueous enters the Schlemm's canal against slight resistance. Following mechanisms were postulated which are now discarded and have become part of historical interest only:

- *Leaky endothelial cells:* Some workers have suggested that the leaky endothelial cells might allowing aqueous drainage. However, it has not been substantiated by evidence.
- *Sonderman's channels:* These have been described as small tubules. It was suggested that channels help aqueous to flow from inner trabecular spaces of the corneoscleral trabecular mesh into the lumen of Schlemm's canal. But importance and exact role in the aqueous outflow have not been substantiated.
- *Contractile microfilaments:* These have been described by some workers to be present in the inner wall endothelium of Schlemm's canal and also in the endothelial lining of trabeculae. Their disruption by EDTA has been reported to result in decrease in the resistance to outflow. However, the exact role of microfilaments in the aqueous drainage is not yet clear.

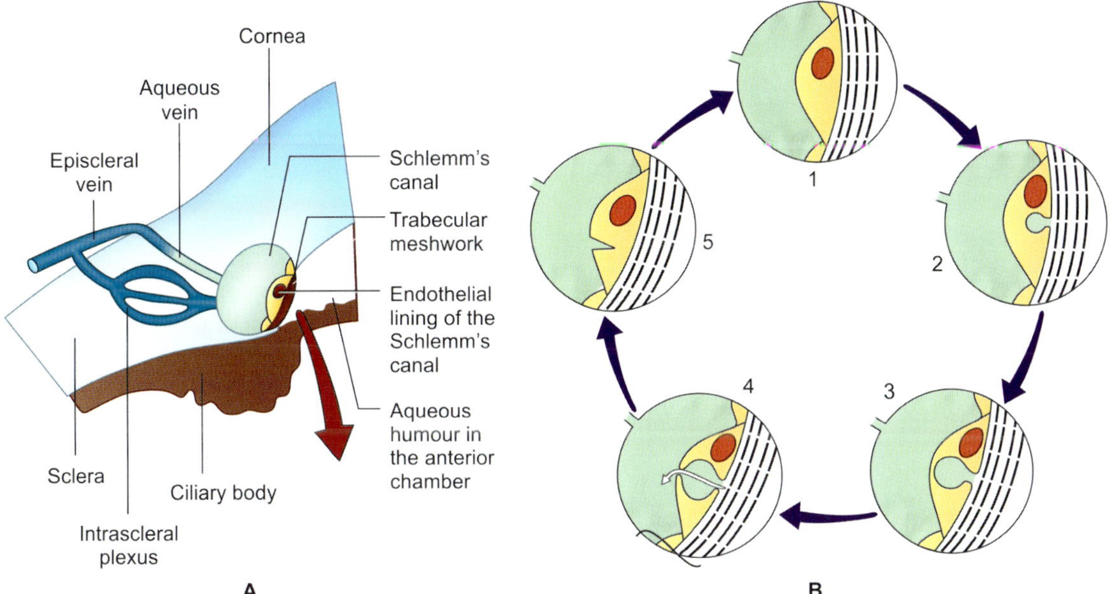

Fig. 2.13 *Vacuolation theory of aqueous transport across the inner wall of Schlemm's canal: 1. Non-vacuolated state; 2. Stage of early infolding of basal surface of the endothelial cell; 3. Stage of macrovacuolar structure formation; 4. Stage of vacuolar transcellular channel formation; 5. Stage of occlusion of the basal infolding*

- *Pores in endothelial cells:* Bill and Svedbergh have shown that the endothelial cells have a total of 20,000 pores with diameter up to 3 µ and that calculations based on this reveal that the pores could be responsible for all the bulk aqueous flow. Perhaps these pores might be part of pores and vacuoles of transcellular system of aqueous outflow as described by Tripathi.
- *Vacuolation theory* (pores and giant vacuole system): Vesicles and larger vacuoles are frequently seen in the endothelium. Tripathi has suggested that these vacuoles open and close intermittenty to transport aqueous from the juxtacanalicular tissue to Schlemm's canal (Fig. 2.13). Whether process is active or passive is still controversy. But at present majority of the workers believe it be a pressure-dependent passive transport.

II. *Aqueous outflow active pump mechanism*

Aqueous outflow through the aqueous outflow system has long been considered a passive filter mechanism against the pressure gradient as described above. However, recently it has been reported that aqueous outflow system acts as *biomechanical pump* as described below:

- *Oscillatory pressure transients*, caused by the ocular pulse, blinking and eye movement, forms the operating force for the biochemical pump.
- *Trabecular meshwork* actively moves outward and recoils back in response to the oscillatory pressure transients. Thus, trabecular meshwork flexibility is essential for aqueous outflow pump mechanism.
- *Aqueous valve mechanism* has been reported to operate at the level of inner wall of Schlemm's canal (SC). These valves are oriented circumferentially in SC and their lumen is continuous with the juxtacanalicular space. These valves allow one way passage of aqueous humour from the juxtacanalicular space to inside the SC and not vice versa.

Working of aqueous outflow pump

The aqueous outflow system is a part of *vascular circulatory loop* as explained below:

i. *Flow of aqueous humour from juxtacanalicular space to inside the Schlemm's canal* as shown in Fig. 2.14A, during cardiac diastole, the IOP is slightly decreased due to less blood flow to choroidal vasculature. As a consequence, the trabecular meshwork is retracted inward leading to a negative pressure inside the Schlemm's canal and opening of the aqueous valves. This is followed by flow of aqueous inside the SC (Fig. 2.14A).

ii. *Aqueous humour flow from SC to collector's channels and episcleral veins* as shown in Fig. 2.14B, during cardiac systole, the choroidal vasculature expansion leads to transient rise in IOP. The aqueous pulse wave distends the trabecular meshwork (TM) forcing it outward against the SC. As a consequence of this pressure push, the aqueous valves close and the aqueous from SC is pushed through the collector channels in its outer wall into the aqueous veins (Fig. 2.14B).

iii. *From aqueous veins, the aqueous is pushed into the episcleral veins by the same mechanism.* The pressure gradient between IOP (12–16 mm Hg + 2.5 mm Hg) and episcleral venous pressure (about 10 mm Hg) also facilitates this unidirectional pulsatile flow of aqueous humour.

Pulsatile aqueous outflow. From the above, it is clear that during diastole aqueous enters into the SC and during systole flows out of it. Thus, Schlemm's canal is the origin of pulsatile aqueous flow. Aqueous pulse wave then enters the aqueous veins through the collector channels. During diastole, the episcleral venous pressure (EVP) is slightly higher than collector channels. During AVP, this causes episcleral venous blood to move toward or even into the aqueous mixing veins (Fig. 2.14A). During next systole, the AVP is transiently raised and the aqueous flows into the episcleral veins (Fig. 2.14B).

2. UVEOSCLERAL (UNCONVENTIONAL) OUTFLOW

The uveoscleral outflow is responsible for some 10–25% of the total aqueous outflow. Aqueous passes across the ciliary body into the suprachoroidal space and is drained by the venous circulation in the ciliary body, choroid, sclera and into the orbital tissues. Uveoscleral outflow is approximately 0.3 µl/min and is surprisingly independent of intraocular pressure changes.

The localization of matrix metalloproteinases-1 (MMP-1) suggests a role for this enzyme in uveoscleral outflow. Uveoscleral drainage is possible owing to the fact that the pressure in the suprachoroid is 2–4 mm Hg lower than in the anterior chamber; this can be reversed after trabeculectomy and can lead to choroidal

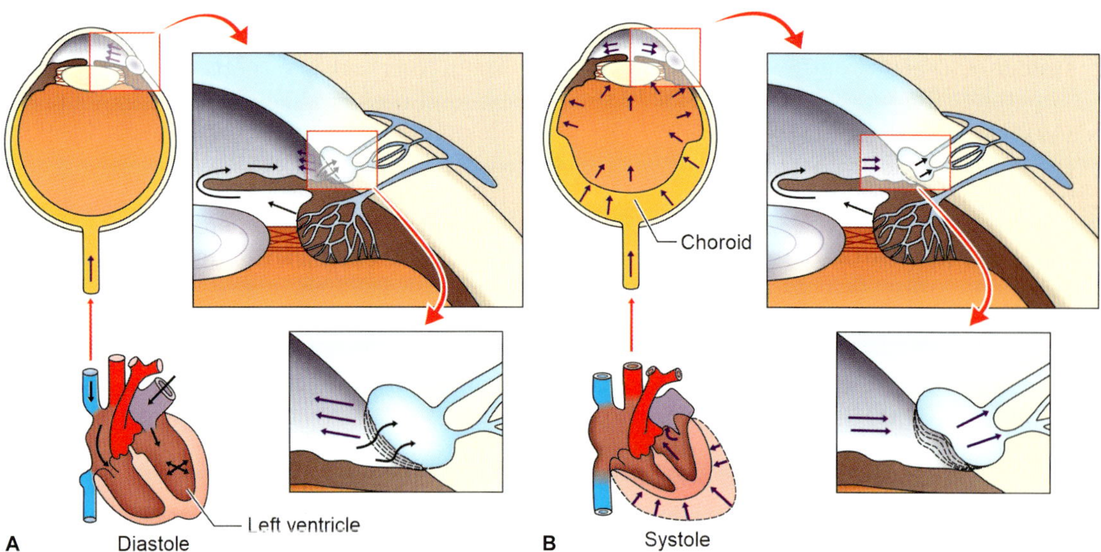

Fig. 2.14 *Aqueous outflow pump mechanism, a part of mascular circulatory loop: (A) during diastole; (B) during systole (for explanation, see text)*

effusion. This pressure differential is also less with age, leading to greater risk of choroidal effusion in such patients. Prostaglandins may decrease the intraocular pressure by increasing the uveoscleral outflow.

Summary of aqueous humour outflow

The drainage of aqueous humour is summarised in Fig. 2.15.

Does aqueous contain components that contribute to flow resistance?

Although aqueous has the same viscosity as isotonic saline, its passage through microporous filters *in vitro* is slower than that of saline. This effect can be abolished by proteolytic agents and detergents, but not by hyaluronidase. It has, therefore, been suggested that some forms of glaucoma may be caused by a build up of a surfactant-like material with age.

AQUEOUS OUTFLOW FACILITY

The facility of aqueous outflow (C-value) is expressed as aqueous outflow in micro-litres per minute per millimetre of mercury

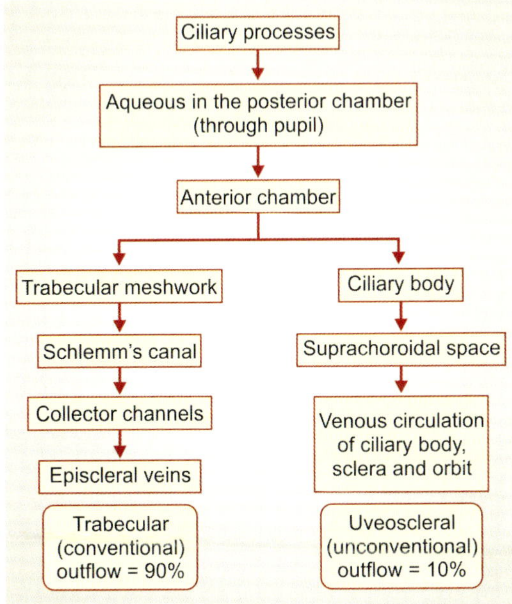

Fig. 2.15 *Flowchart depicting summary of aqueous humour drainage*

(µl/min/mm Hg). It (C-value) represents a quantitative approximation of the state of the aqueous drainage system.

MEASUREMENT OF C-VALUE

The C-value can be measured by three methods: perfusion method, tonography and suction cup method.

1. Perfusion method

This method is not suited for clinical practice but is useful in the laboratory studies with enucleated human eye, or in the animal experiments. In this technique, the eye is cannulated and known volume of fluid is injected at a known pressure (p_1). The outflow facility is then calculated from the following equation:

$$C = \text{Flow rate}/P_1 - P_0$$

In an enucleated eye, P_0 (initial baseline IOP) is 0 mm Hg.

The average C-value obtained by perfusion method in human enucleated eye is 0.28 µl/min/mm Hg, which matches the C-value obtained by perfusion studies *in vivo*, tonography technique and suction cup method. The perfusion studies are independent of the ocular rigidity and corneal curvature.

Sources of error in perfusion method

- A significant artefact is produced by introduction of cannula into the anterior chamber of the eye.
- Deepening of the anterior chamber by the extra fluid injected also produces significant artefact.
- Postmortem tissue changes (in the enucleated eyes), such as lack of blood flow and alteration of aqueous secretion, affect the values.

2. Tonography

Tonography is a non-invasive technique for determining the facility of aqueous outflow, and is thus, the most commonly used method in clinical practice.

Technique

C-value is estimated by placing Schiotz tonometer on the eye for 4 minutes. For a graphic record, the electronic Schiotz tonometer is used. P_0 is determined from the initial scale reading and a standard calibration table. P_0 and the change in scale reading over a few minutes (ΔR) are then used to obtain the C-value from the special tonographic tables.

Sources of error in addition to those discussed under the errors of indentation tonometry (which will also apply here, page 64) are as follows:

- *Variations in line voltage* may produce an apparent drift in the IOP measurements which can be minimized with line voltage stabilizers and by avoiding magnetic fields.
- *Consensual pressure drop.* The IOP may drop by 1 mm Hg in the fellow eye. It has been reported to result from evaporation which occurs when the eye is kept open for fixation during the 4 minutes test.
- *Patient relaxation effect.* The IOP is reported to fall as the patient relaxes during first 15 to 20 seconds, after the tonometer is placed on the cornea. Therefore, 4 minutes tracing should be taken after 30 seconds.
- *Other patient-related factors,* such as blinking, squeezing or lack of fixation during the test, can also lead to poor tonographic record.
- Operator errors including improper cleaning, calibration or positioning of the instrument, as well as improper calculation of the tracing can also lead to inaccurate results.

Normal versus abnormal C-value

- The average C-value is 0.28 ± 0.05 µl/min/mm Hg.
- About 97.5% of the population have values higher than 0.18 and 99.9 to greater than 0.13.
- Most glaucoma patients have C-values less than 0.17.
- A low C-value with a normal P_0 may be due to a sticky tonometer, low ocular rigidity and hyposecretion.
- A high C-value with elevated P_0 may be due to an artificially elevated P_0, high ocular rigidity, elevated episcleral venous pressure and angle closure glaucoma (the force of the tonometer may open the angle).

Clinical value of tonography

There was a time when C-value was considered extremely important for the diagnosis of glaucoma. Presently, C-value is being considered to play not much role in the diagnosis and management of glaucoma.

However, under following conditions, tonography is felt by some physicians to have a clinical value:

- *As an adjunct* in the diagnosis of borderline glaucoma, C-value has very limited role. Though the abnormal tonometric and tonographic results do not make the diagnosis of glaucoma, but do alert the ophthalmologist to follow the patient more closely.
- *In angle-closure glaucoma,* once an acute attack is broken, a C-value of 0.10 or less suggests that a peripheral iridectomy alone may not be sufficient.
- As an adjunct in the diagnosis of myasthenia gravis.
- As an adjunct in the diagnosis of carotid insufficiency.
- May help to assess therapy of glaucoma.
- Evaluation of drug mechanism and study of abnormalities of the various influences on aqueous humour dynamics.

3. Suction cup method

This method is no better than tonography and so not used clinically. In this technique, a suction cup is applied to the perilimbal area, which occludes the episcleral vein and thus, trabecular outflow from the eye, and results in rise of IOP. After the suction cup is removed, the rate of return to normal IOP is noted. The faster the return to baseline IOP, the greater the outflow facility; and conversely, the slower the return to baseline, the lower the outflow facility.

INTRAOCULAR PRESSURE

GENERAL CONSIDERATIONS

Features of normal intraocular pressure

Intraocular pressure refers to the pressure exerted by intraocular contents on the coats of the eyeball. The normal level of IOP is essentially maintained by a dynamic equilibrium between the aqueous humour formation, aqueous humour outflow, and episcleral venous pressure. IOP is distributed evenly throughout the eye, so that the pressure is always the same in the posterior vitreous as it is in the aqueous humour. The intraocular pressure is important in maintaining the shape of the eyeball and thus also the optical integrity.

- Normal IOP varies between 10.5 and 20.5 mm Hg with a mean pressure of 15.5 ± 2.57 mm Hg.
- IOP is created by aqueous formation which has two components: First, a hydrostatic component from the arterial blood pressure and ciliary body tissue pressure, and second, an osmotic pressure induced by the active secretion of sodium and other ions by the ciliary epithelium.
- IOP serves as the tissue pressure of the vascularized internal structures of the eye, and is thus, much higher than the tissue pressure elsewhere in the body (5 mm Hg).
- Normal IOP is pulsatile, reflecting in part its vascular origin and the effects of blood flow on the internal ocular structures.

The IOP is a dynamic function. Any single measurement of IOP is just a momentary sample and may or may not reflect the average pressure for the patient in that hour, day or week.

Frequency distribution of IOP in the population

Several population-based studies have been done to comment upon the frequency distribution of the normal IOP. Despite the use of different instruments and differing ethnic groups, the studies show remarkably close correlation. The most frequently cited population study is that of Leydhecker and associates, in which 10,000 persons with no known eye disease were tested with Schiotz tonometer. The conclusions drawn from the study regarding frequency distribution of IOP in the population are as follows:

- The distribution of pressures observed resembled a Gaussian curve, but was skewed towards the right (Fig. 2.16).

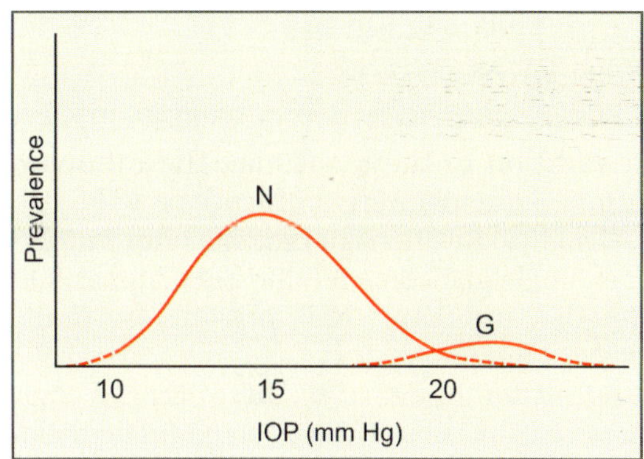

Fig. 2.16 *Distribution of intraocular pressure in non-glaucomatous (N) and glaucoma (G) populations, showing overlap between the two groups (dotted lines represent uncertainty of extreme value in both populations*

- It has been assumed that perhaps two different population groups account for the skewed distribution: a large 'normal' group (having a true Gaussian-shaped curve) and a smaller group that was felt to be glaucomatous without optic nerve head damage (causing a long tail on the right hand side of the distribution curve).
- The mean IOP of normal group was 15.5 ± 2.57 mm Hg.
- 95% of the population had an IOP between 10.5 and 20.5 mm Hg.
- If one chooses a point 2 SD above the mean as the upper limit of normal (about 20.5 mm Hg), then 2.5% of the normal will be included as "abnormal". However, if one chooses 2.5 SD above the mean as the upper limit of normal (about 24 mm Hg), then less than 1% of normal population will be included as "abnormal".

Some of the important conclusions drawn from the other population-based studies are as follows:

- A slight increase of mean IOP in each decade over 40 years.
- A slightly higher pressure exists in women than men in population above 40 years of age.
- IOP difference between right and left eye rarely exceeds 4 mm Hg.
- Level of IOP is inherited as a polygenic multifactorial trait.

FACTORS INFLUENCING THE INTRAOCULAR PRESSURE

A. Factors causing long-term changes in IOP

In addition to the glaucoma, the following factors cause long-term influence on IOP:

1. ***Heredity.*** Relations of patients with primary open-angle glaucoma tend to have higher IOP. Heredity influences IOP, possibly by multi-factorial modes.

2. ***Age.*** After the age of 40, there occurs a slight increase in the mean IOP and standard deviation after each decade. This probably occurs due to age-related reduction in aqueous outflow facility, despite a concomitant reduction in the aqueous production.

3. ***Sex.*** IOP is equal between the sexes in ages of 20–40 years. In older age group, increase in mean IOP with age is greater in females than males.

4. ***Race.*** Though population-based studies in different ethnic groups do not show significant difference in mean IOP, the race may occasionally influence IOP distribution. For example, full blood Indians in a New Mexican tribe were found to have significantly lower mean IOP than a control population.

5. ***Refractive error.*** Myopes tend to have slightly higher IOP as compared to emmetropes.

B. Factors causing short-term changes in intraocular pressure

1. ***Arterial blood pressure.*** The IOP is generally not affected by physiological changes in the arterial blood pressure; however, sudden large swings may affect the IOP accordingly. For example, ligating one carotid can cause a fall in IOP on the ipsilateral side (due to decreased blood flow) and an increase in IOP on the contralateral side (due to increased blood flow).

2. ***Systemic venous pressure (SVP).*** Changes in SVP can cause a profound effect on IOP by affecting ipsilateral venous pressure, for about 1 mm Hg rise in episcleral venous pressure (EVP) raises the IOP by 0.8 mm Hg. Common clinical conditions in which EVP is raised include external pressure of jugular veins, compression of superior vena cava by tumour (thoracic outlet syndrome), cavernous sinus thrombosis and neoplasms, inflammatory or dysthyroid changes at the apex of the orbit. The Valsalva manoeuvre also increases the IOP by raising the EVP. Postural variations in IOP when going from sitting or upright position to the supine position and also the changes in IOP during coughing, straining are related to changes in EVP.

3. ***Mechanical pressure on the globe*** from outside initially raises the IOP by indentation but after some time due to acceleration of aqueous outflow the IOP returns to normal and by prolonged pressure decreases below the initial levels. This forms the basis of ocular massage to lower the IOP. Transient rise due to external pressure on the globe is associated with conditions, like forced eyelid closure, mechanical pull on the restricted extraocular muscle and simultaneous contraction of extraocular muscles in conditions, like Duane's syndrome.

4. ***Plasma osmolarity.*** Plasma osmolarity affects the IOP profoundly. When the total concentration of solute molecules in the blood exceeds, the water from the eye (vitreous and perhaps aqueous also) is withdrawn, lowering the IOP. This effect is used clinically to lower the IOP by use of hyperosmotic agents, like mannitol.

Conversely, when the concentration of solutes in plasma is lower than the ocular fluids, the water will enter the eye from plasma and raise the IOP. This forms the basis of water drinking test used as provocative test for glaucoma. A fall in IOP noted after prolonged exercise, such as running or bicycling, has been attributed to increased serum osmolarity and metabolic acidosis.

5. ***Blood pH.*** Systemic acidosis lowers the IOP. Bietti has postulated that it is the metabolic acidosis induced by carbonic anhydrase inhibition that is responsible for their pressure lowering effect.

6. ***Diurnal variation in IOP.*** Like many other biological parameters, the IOP also fluctuates cyclically throughout the day. The most common pattern is for the pressure to be highest in the early morning and lowest in the late evening (Fig. 2.17). The mean amplitude of daily fluctuation is usually less than 5 mm Hg in normal individual. A diurnal variation in IOP of more than 8 mm Hg is considered pathogno-

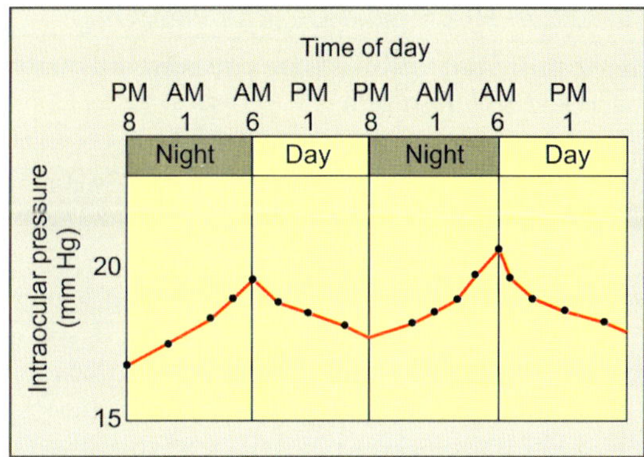

Fig. 2.17 *Diurnal variation of intraocular pressure*

monic of glaucoma. The exact mechanism of diurnal IOP variation is uncertain, however, it has been related to a diurnal variation in the level of plasma cortisol.

7. *Seasonal variation* in IOP has also been described with the highest pressure recorded in winter and lowest in summer.

8. *Systemic hyperthermia* has been shown to cause an increased IOP in rabbits. Similarly, a drop in body temperature will cause a decrease in the IOP, probably by inhibition of aqueous secretion.

9. *Effect of general anaesthesia on IOP* has been widely studied. Intraocular pressure (IOP) may be affected under general anaesthesia by premedication, induction agents, muscle relaxants, inhalation anaesthetics and other drugs administered during preoperative period. Apart from drugs, venous congestion or increased venous pressure, hypertension and changes in blood gas tension also affect the IOP. These changes in IOP basically occur due to alteration of physiological determinants of intraocular pressure which include the following:

- Aqueous humour dynamics
- Vitreous volume
- Extraocular muscle tone, and
- Choroidal blood volume.

Some of the facts about effect of general anaesthesia on IOP are as below:

i. *Acute changes in the volume of blood* present in the eye due to increase in venous pressure as a result of coughing, retching, vomiting and bucking on endotracheal tube cause a serious increase in IOP and is a factor of cardinal importance to anaesthetist. *Hypertension* occurring during laryngoscopy and intubation under general anaesthesia for the same reason may cause a temporary increase in IOP.

ii. *Hypercapnia and hypoxia* during general anaesthesia produce an increase in IOP, while hypocapnia and hyperoxia produce a decrease in IOP due to changes in volume of blood in the eye.

iii. *Drugs* used in general anaesthesia produce a decrease in IOP provided haemodynamic parameters and blood gases are kept in their normal limits. Premedicants, such as diazepam, morphine, pethidine, pentazocine, fentanyl, buprenorphine, produce a decrease in IOP. Thiopentone sodium, an induction agent, reduces IOP and so do most of the gaseous and volatile anaesthetic agents with the possible exception of nitrous oxide. Ketamine, a dissociative agent, has little effect on IOP when given intramuscularly and may transiently raise the IOP when given intravenously. Parenteral use of atropine does not cause a significant rise in IOP, even in the predisposed eye. Suxamethonium is a notorious drug and cause rise in IOP, which can be clinically important. The eyeball is compressed by the extraocular muscles. The other possible mechanisms include a rise in arterial pressure, sharp increase in venous pressure and rotation of eyes in divergent position.

iv. *In general, once the patient is under the effect of general anaesthesia,* the IOP is decreased. This effect occurs regardless of the type of anaesthetic. Possible mechanisms for the decreased IOP include muscle relaxation, decreased pressure, increased carbon dioxide levels in the blood, and/or direct effect of anaesthetic agent.

10. *Effects of drugs on IOP.* In addition to the well-established antiglaucoma drugs and effect of general anaesthetic agents as discussed, many other drugs also affect the IOP. Alcohol, heroin, and systemic vasodilators have been reported to lower the IOP. While tobacco smoking, caffeine, LSD, and corticosteroids may raise the IOP.

11. ***Blockage of the circulation of aqueous*** has a profound effect in raising the intraocular pressure. Such a block may occur at two places:

i. At the pupil where the flow of fluid from the posterior to the anterior chamber may be impeded, and
ii. At the angle of the anterior chamber.

CONTROL OF INTRAOCULAR PRESSURE

Although there are minor physiological variations of IOP, there exists more or less a constant steady level of IOP, in spite of the fact that there is continuous drainage of the aqueous humour or in other words there is continuous leakage from the eye. As already discussed, this steady level of IOP is the result of a dynamic equilibrium between the aqueous humour formation, the normal resistance offered by the drainage channels for the outflow of fluid from the eye and the episcleral venous pressure. The homeostatic mechanisms locally help in maintaining the steady state level of IOP. For example, when IOP rises, there occurs a decrease in the aqueous inflow (pseudo-facility) maintaining the equilibrium.

It is now being assumed that there exists some central controlling mechanisms that tend to maintain pressure homeostasis within the eye. The nature of location(s) of such a centre have still not been delineated. However, the evidences have accumulated which suggest that the controlling centre operates through the sympathetic, parasympathetic and diencephalic influences. The above conclusions are based on the following observations of various workers:

- *Pressure sensitive afferent fibres* have been found in the long posterior and short ciliary nerves.
- *Diencephalon's* stimulation has been reported to cause a fall or rise in IOP, depending upon the area stimulated.
- *Cervical sympathetic ganglion's* stimulation produces a drop in IOP due to diminished aqueous secretion.
- *Beta-adrenergic stimulation* causes inhibition of aqueous secretion and alpha-adrenergic stimulation causes an improvement in aqueous outflow facility.
- *Parasympathetic system* stimulation decreases IOP by an increase in aqueous outflow facility.

MEASUREMENT OF INTRAOCULAR PRESSURE

Measurement of intraocular pressure has been described in Chapter 6.

SUGGESTED READING

1. Armaly MF. The genetic determination of ocular pressure in the normal eye. Arch Ophthal 1967; 78:187.
2. Armaly MF. Studies on intraocular effects of the orbital parasympathetic pathway-effect on intraocular pressure. Arch Ophthalmol 1959; 62:117–24.
3. Becker B. The decline in aqueous secretion and outflow facility with age. Am J Ophthal 1958; 46:731.
4. Bill A, Lutjen-Drecoll E, Svedbergh B. Effects of intracameral Na2 EDTA and EGTa on aqueous outflow routes in the monkey eye. Invest Ophthal Vis Sci 1980;19:492.
5. Bill A, Svedbergh B. Scanning electron microscopic studies of the trabecular meshwork and the canal of Schlemm—an attempt to localize the main resistance to outflow of aqeuous humor in man. Acta Ophthal 1972;50:295.
6. Bill A. The albumin exchange in the rabbit eye. Acta Physiol Scand 1964;60:18.
7. Bills A: Effects of cervical sympathetic tone on blood pressure and uveal blood flow after carotid occlusion. Exp Eye Res 1963;2:203–09.
8. Bito L, Davson H. Steady-State concentrations of potassium in the ocular fluids. Exp Eye Res 1964;3:283.
9. Bonting SL, Becker B. Studies on sodium-potassium-activated adenosine triphosphatase. XIV. Inhibition of enzyme activity and aqueous humor flow in the rabbit eye after intravitreal injection of ouabain. Invest Ophthal 1964;3:523.
10. Chandler PA, Grant WM. Glaucoma, 2nd edition, Lea and Febiger, Philadelphia, 1979;16–22, 30–56.
11. Cole DF. Effects of some metabolic inhibitors upon the formation of the aqueous humour in rabbits. Br J Ophthalmol. 44: 739, 1960.
12. Davson H: The Eye-Vegetative Physiology and Biochemistry, Vol 12nd ed. New York, Academic Press, 1969.
13. Duke-Elder S, Jay B. Glaucoma and hypotony. In: Duke-Elder, S (ed). System of Ophthalmology. Vol XI Diseases of the Lens and Vitreous; Glaucoma and Hypotony, Henry Kimpton, London, 456, 1969.

14. Duke-Elder S. The Physiology of the Eye and of Vision, Vol IV System of Ophthalmology. St Louis, CV Mosby, 1968.
15. Fine BS. Structure of the trabecular meshwork and the canal of Schlemm. Trans Am Acad Ophthal Otol 1966;70:777.
16. Friedenwald JS. Contribution to the theory and practice oftonometry. Am J Ophthal 1937;20:985.
17. Friedenwald JS. Some problems in the calibration of tonometers. Am J Ophthal 1948;31:935.
18. Friedenwald JS. Tonometer calibration: An attempt to remove discrepancies found in the 1954 calibration scale for Schiotz tonometers. Trans Am Acad Ophthal Otol 1957;61:108.
19. Goldmann MH, Schmidt T. Uber applanations-tonometrie. Ophthalmologies 1957;134:221.
20. Kass MA, Zimmerman TJ, Alton E, Lemon L, Becker B. Intraocular pressure and glaucoma in the Zuni Indians. Arch Ophthal 1978;96:2212.
21. Kinsey VE, Reddy DVN. Chemistry and dynamics of aqueous humor. In: Prince JH: (ed.) The Rabbit in Eye Research, Springfield, III., Charles C Thomas, Publisher 215–316, 1964.
22. Kornblueth WAladjimoff IC, Magora F, et al. Influence of general anesthesia on intraocular pressure in man. Arch Ophthalmol 1959;61:84–87.
23. Langham ME, Palewicz K. The pupillary, the intraocular pressure and the vasomotor responses to noradrenaline in rabbits. J Physiol 1977;267:339–55.
24. Leydhecker W, Akiyama K, Neumann HG. Der intraokulare Druck gesunder menschlicher Augen. Klin\Monatsbl Augenheilkd 1958;133: 662.
25. Macri FJ. Interdependence of venous and eye pressure. Arch Ophthalmol 1961;65:442–49.
26. Maren TH. The rates of movement of Na^+, CI^-, and HCO_3^- from plasma to posterior chamber: effect of acetazolamide and relation to the treatment of glaucoma. Invest Ophthal 1976; 15:356.
27. Moses R. Tonometry-effect of tonometer footplate hole on scale reading. Further studies. Arch Ophthal 1959;61:373.
28. Perkins ES. Sensory mechanisms and intraocular pressure. Exp Eye Res 1961,1.160–67.
29. Reddy VN. Dynamics of transport systems in the eye. Invest Ophthal Vis Sci 1979;18:1000.
30. Sears M, Neufeld A. Adrenergic modulation of the outflow of aqueous humor. Invest Ophthalmol 1975;14:83–86.
31. Sears ML. The aqueous. In Moses RA (ed). Adler's Physiology of the Eye, 6th edition. CV Mosby Co, St Louis, 1975;232.
32. Shiose Y. Electron microscopic studies on blood-retinal and blood–aqueous barriers. Jpn J Ophthalmol 1970;14:73.
33. Smelser GK. Electron microscopy of a typical epithelial cell and of the normal human ciliary process. Trans Am Acad Ophthal Otol 1966; 70:738.
34. Smith RS, Rudt LA. Ultrastructural studies of the blood–aqueous barrier. 2 The barrier to horseradish peroxidase in primates. Am J Ophthal 1973;76:937.
35. Sonderman R. Beitrag zur entwicklung and moorphologie des Schlemmschen kanals. Albrecht v J Graefes. Arch Klin Exp Ophthal 1930;124:521.
36. Tamm ER, Flugel C, Stefani FH et al. Nerve endings with structural characteristics of mechoreceptors in human scleral spur. Invest Ophthalmol Vis Sci, 1994;35:1157.
37. Tripathi RC. Mechanism of the aqueous outflow across the trabecular wall of Schlemm's canal. Exp Eye Res 1971;11:116.
38. Von Sallman L, Lowenstein O. Responses of intraocular pressure, blood pressure and cutaneous vessels to electric stimulation of the diencephalon. Am J Ophthalmol 39 (Part II) 1955;11:29.
39. Waitzman MB, Woods WD. Some characteristics of an adenyl cyclase preparation. Exp Eye Res 1971;12:99.

CHAPTER 3

ANATOMY OF OPTIC NERVE HEAD AND PATHOPHYSIOLOGY OF GLAUCOMATOUS DAMAGE

ANATOMICAL CONSIDERATIONS

NERVE FIBRE LAYER OF RETINA

Features of nerve fibre layer

Nerve fibre layer consists of the unmyelinated axons of the ganglion cells which converge at the optic nerve head, pass through lamina cribrosa and become ensheathed by myelin posterior to lamina. In addition to axons of the ganglion cells (*centripetal nerve fibres*), this layer also contains the following:

- *Centrifugal nerve fibres*, which are thicker than the centripetal nerve fibres. Their exact origin and termination is not known.
- Processes of *Müller's cells*, which interweave with the axons of the ganglion cells.
- The *neuroglial cells* that are present in the nerve fibre layer are categorized as macroglia and microglia. Macroglia are constituted by two types of astrocytes (fibrous and protoplasmic) derived from the neural crest. Microglia are small cells that are derived from the mesodermal invasion of the retina at the time of vascularization. Macroglia have a structural role in the retina while microglial cells take the role of wandering tissue histiocytes in response to tissue injury and phagocytose debris which is carried to the vasculature for removal from the retina.
- *Retinal vessels* lie in the nerve fibre layer but as a rule do not project on the surface of retina. A rich bed of superficial capillary network is present in this layer (Fig. 3.1).

Characteristics of nerve fibre layer. The nerve fibres vary in their thickness from 0.5 to 2 μm and are non-myelinated. The cytoplasm of the axons contains microtubules, fine fibrils, mitochondria and occasional vesicles.

Arrangement of nerve fibres

Retina. In contrast to the remaining fibres of the sensory retina, which course perpendicular to the surface of the retina, the fibres within the nerve fibre layer course parallel to the surface in the following manner (Fig. 3.2):

- *Fibres from the nasal half of the retina* come directly to the optic disc as superior radiating fibres and inferior radiating fibres (Srf and Irf).

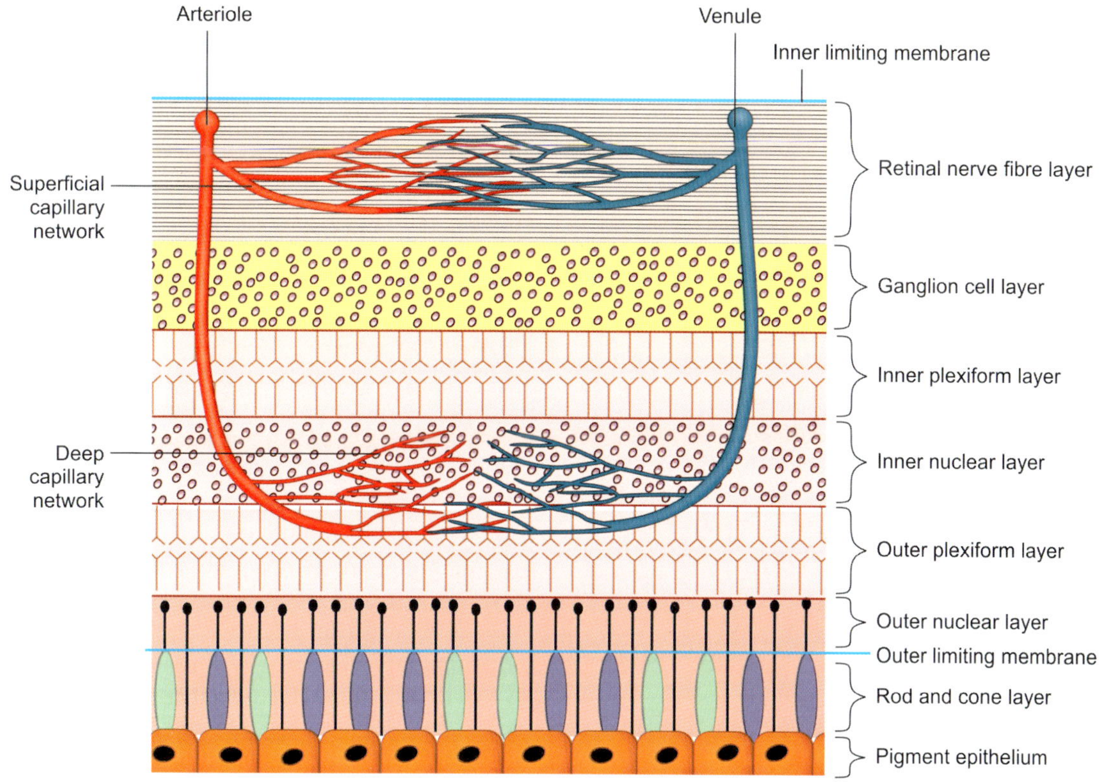

Fig. 3.1 *Arrangement of retinal capillaries*

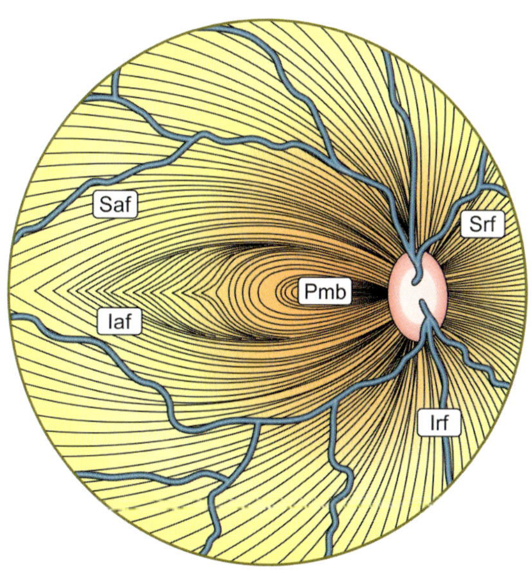

Fig. 3.2 *Arrangement of nerve fibres in the retina*

- *Fibres from the macular region* pass straight in the temporal part of the disc as papillomacular bundle (pmb).
- *Fibres from the temporal retina* arch above and below the macular and papillomacular bundle as superior arcuate fibres and inferior arcuate fibres (saf and iaf) with a horizontal median raphe in between.

Optic nerve head. Fibres from the peripheral part of the retina lie deep in the retina but occupy the most peripheral (superficial) part of the optic disc. While the fibres originating closer to the optic nerve head lie superficially in the retina and occupy a more central (deep) portion of the disc (Fig. 3.3).

Thickness of nerve fibre layer at the optic disc

Thickness of the nerve fibre layer around the different quadrants of the optic disc margin progressively increases in the following order:

- Most lateral quadrant (thinnest)

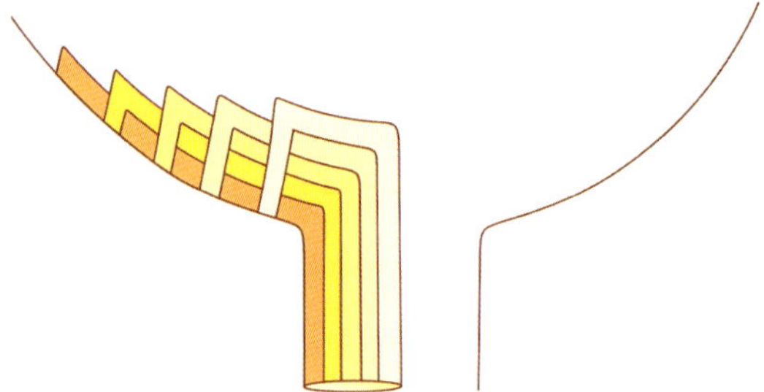

Fig. 3.3 *Arrangement of nerve fibres at the optic nerve head*

- Upper temporal and lower temporal quadrant
- Most medial quadrant
- Upper nasal and lower nasal quadrant (thickest)

Clinical significance of distribution and thickness of nerve fibres at the optic disc margin

- Papilloedema appears first of all in the thickest quadrant (upper nasal and lower nasal) and last of all in the thinnest quadrant (most lateral).
- Arcuate nerve fibres which occupy the superior temporal and inferior temporal quadrants of optic nerve head are most sensitive to glaucomatous damage, accounting for an early loss in corresponding regions of visual field.
- Macular fibres occupying the lateral quadrant are most resistant to glaucomatous damage and explain the retention of the central vision till end.

OPTIC NERVE HEAD

Gross anatomy

Optic nerve head was also known as "papilla"; the term "papilla" was coined based on an impression that the normal optic nerve head was elevated like a papilla. But it is a misnomer. Similarly, the term "optic disc" is also a misnomer as disc refers to a two-dimensional structure but on the contrary optic nerve head is a three-dimensional structure. The optic nerve head may be defined as the intraocular portion of the optic nerve. It extends anteriorly from the retinal surface to the myelinated portion of the optic nerve that begins just behind the sclera, posterior to the lamina cribrosa. It is also the site of entry and exit of the retinal vessels.

The borders of the optic nerve head include:

- *Anteriorly:* Vitreous humour
- *Peripherally:* Retina and sclera
- *Posteriorly:* Pia, arachnoid and dura maters with cerebrospinal fluid present between the arachnoid and dura meninges.
- *Diameter* of optic nerve head varies from 1.66 to 1.92 mm horizontally and 1.57 to 1.76 mm vertically.
- *Area* of the nerve head may range from 0.68 to 4.42 mm^2.

In the context of a discussion on glaucoma, the optic nerve head is defined as the distal portion of the optic nerve that is directly susceptible to intraocular pressure elevation.

In comparison to the rest of retina, the optic disc appears white due to lamina cribrosa and medullated nerve fibres behind it and absence of vascular choroid. In the centre, where the nerve fibres are thinnest, the white lamina shines more brightly. The grey spots in the lamina, when they are seen, are due to the non-medullated nerve fibres reflecting less light than the white connective tissue fibres.

The physiological cup of the optic disc is a depression seen in it. The central retinal vessels emerge through the centre of this cup. The cup varies in size, shape, position and depth in different eyes. Sometimes there is scarcely any physiological cup, in which case the disc is more uniformly pink and the central vessels may have already divided before they come to the surface. Increase in the size of the cup and/or difference in the size of cup of two eyes should be watched with suspicion and investigated to exclude glaucoma.

Microscopic anatomy

The optic nerve head may be arbitrarily divided into four portions from anterior to posterior as defined by light microscopy, scanning electron microscopy and immunohistochemistry (Fig. 3.4).

1. ***Surface nerve fibre layer.*** This part is essentially composed of axonal bundles, i.e. nerve fibres originating from ganglion cell layer of the retina (94%) which converge on the optic disc and astrocytes (5%). The optic disc is covered by a thin layer of astrocytes, the *internal limiting membrane of Elschnig*, which separates it

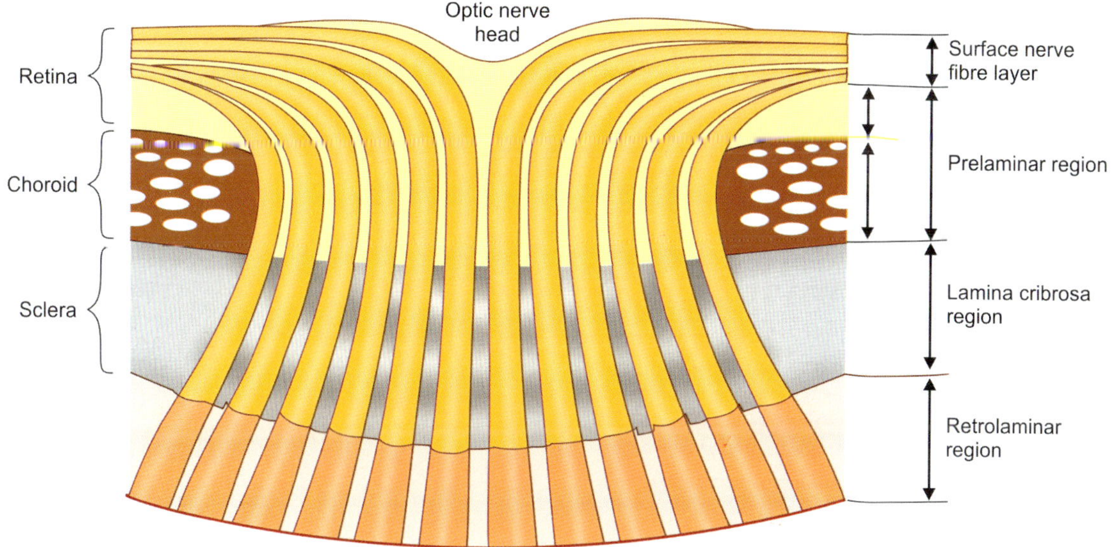

Fig. 3.4 *Schematic drawing of optic nerve head*

from the vitreous and is continuous with the internal limiting membrane of the retina. When the central portion of this membrane is thickened, it is referred to as the *central meniscus of Kuhnt*.

All the layers of retina, apart from nerve fibre layer, near the optic nerve, are separated from it by a partial rim of glial tissue called *intermediate tissue of Kuhnt*.

2. *Prelaminar region.* The predominant structures at this level are neurons and a significantly increased quantity of astroglial tissue. The type 1B astrocytes segregate RGC axons into fascicles (also called bundles). Each fascicle consists of approximately 1000 axons. The *border tissue of Jcoby* (a cuff of astrocytes) separates the nerve from the choroid.

3. *Lamina cribrosa.* It is a fibrillar sieve-like structure made up of fenestrated sheets of scleral connective tissue lined by glial tissue. It bridges the posterior scleral foramina or the scleral canal. The bundles of optic nerve fibres leave the eye through these fenestrations. A rim of collagenous connective tissue with some admixture of glial cells which intervenes between the choroid and sclera and optic nerve fibers is called *border tissue of Elschnig*. The lamina cribrosa gets its rich blood supply from the circle of Zinn.

4. *Retrolaminar region.* This area is characterized by a decrease in astrocytes and the acquisition of myelin that is supplied by oligodendrocytes. The addition of myelin sheath nearly doubles the diameter of the optic nerve (from 1.5 to 3.0 mm) as it passes through the sclera. The axonal bundles are surrounded by connective tissue septa. The posterior extent of the retrolaminar region is not clearly defined.

Blood supply of optic nerve head

Arterial supply

Posterior ciliary artery circulation is the main source of blood supply to the optic nerve head, except for the nerve fibre layer which is supplied by the retinal circulation. The blood supply in the optic nerve head has a sectoral distribution (Fig. 3.5).

- *The surface nerve fibre layer* is mainly supplied by the arterioles derived from central retinal artery, which anastomose with vessels of the prelaminar region and are continuous with the peripapillary retinal and long radial peripapillary capillaries. Occasionally, a ciliary-derived vessel from the prelaminar region may enlarge to form the cilioretinal artery.
- *The prelaminar region* is supplied by vessels of ciliary region. There is lack of agreement as to

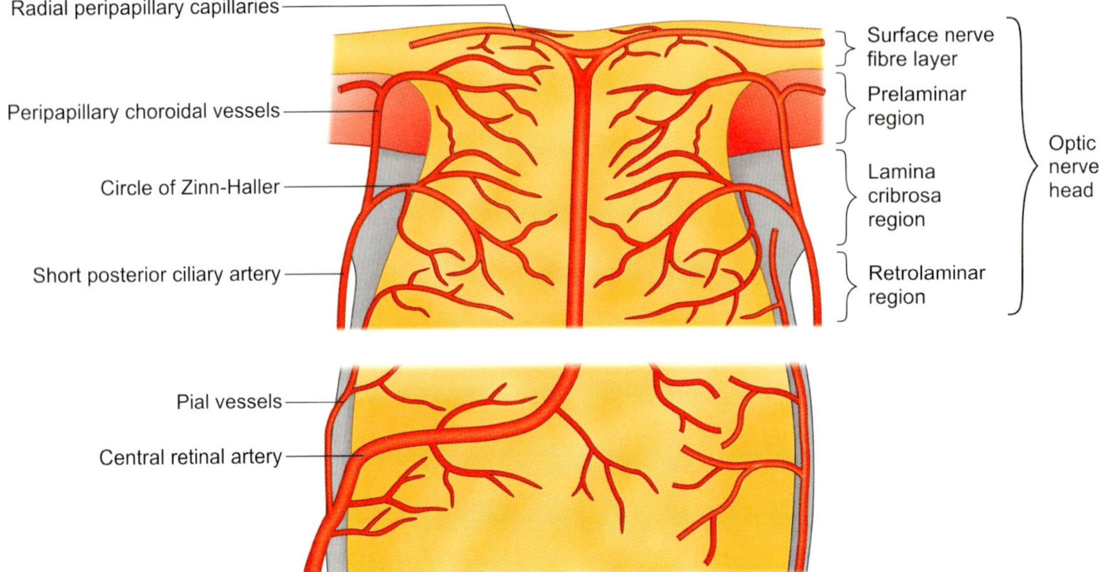

Fig. 3.5 *Blood supply of the optic nerve head*

whether these vessels are derived primarily from the peripapillary choroidal system or from separate branches of the short posterior ciliary arteries.

- *The lamina cribrosa region* is also supplied by the ciliary vessels which are derived from the short posterior ciliary arteries and arterial circle of Zinn-Haller.
- *The retrolaminar region* is supplied by both the ciliary and retinal circulations with the former coming from recurrent pial vessels. The central retinal artery provides centripetal branches from the pial plexus and also centrifugal branches.

Capillaries

Although derived from both the retinal and ciliary circulations, the capillaries of the optic nerve head resemble more closely the features of retinal capillaries than of the choriocapillaries. These characteristics include:

- Tight junctions,
- Abundant pericytes, and
- Non-fenestrated endothelium

They represent a *blood–nerve barrier*. The capillaries decrease in number posterior to the lamina, especially along the margins of the larger vessels.

The rich capillary beds of each of the 4 anatomic regions within the anterior optic nerve are anatomically confluent.

Venous drainage

The venous drainage from the optic nerve head is almost entirely through the central retinal vein, although a small portion may occur through the choroidal system. Occasionally, these communications are enlarged as *retinociliary veins*, which drain from the retina to the choroidal circulation, or *cilio-optic veins*, which drain from the choroid to the central retinal vein.

PATHOPHYSIOLOGY OF GLAUCOMATOUS OPTIC NEUROPATHY

The pathogenesis of glaucomatous optic atrophy has remained a matter of controversy since the mid-19th century. In 1858, Müller proposed that the elevated IOP led to direct compression and death of the neurons. The same year, von Jaeger suggested that a vascular abnormality was the underlying cause of the optic atrophy. In 1892, Schnabel proposed another concept in the pathogenesis, suggesting that atrophy of neural elements created empty spaces, which pulled the nerve head posteriorly (Schnabel cavernous atrophy).

It has now been recognized that progressive optic neuropathy results from the death of retinal ganglion cells (RGCs) in a typical pattern which results in characteristic optic disc appearance and specific visual field defects.

PATHOGENESIS OF RETINAL GANGLION CELL DEATH

Retinal ganglion cell (RGC) death is initiated when some pathologic event blocks the transport of growth factors (neurotrophins) from the brain to the RGCs.

The blockage of these neurotrophins initiates a damaging cascade, and the cell is unable to maintain its normal function. The RGCs losing their ability to maintain normal function undergo apoptosis and also trigger apoptosis of adjacent cells. Apoptosis is a genetically controlled cell suicide programme whereby irreversibly damaged cells die, and are subsequently engulfed by neighbouring cells, without eliciting any inflammatory response.

Retinal ganglion cell death is, of course, associated with loss of retinal nerve fibres. As the loss of nerve fibres extends beyond the normal physiological overlap of functional zones, the characteristic optic disc changes and specific visual field defects become apparent over the time.

Etiological factors

Factors involved in the etiology of retinal ganglion cell death and thus causing glaucomatous optic neuropathy can be grouped as below.

A. *Primary insults*

1. *Raised intraocular pressure (mechanical theory).* Raised intraocular pressure causes mechanical stretch on the lamina cribrosa leading to axonal deformation and ischaemia by altering capillary blood flow. As a result of this, neurotrophins (growth factors) are not able to reach the retinal ganglion cell bodies in sufficient amount needed for their survival.

Concept of translaminar pressure. The mechanical theory stresses on the effect of raised IOP on lamina cribrosa, which is considered the initiating site of glaucomatous optic nerve damage. Now the stress is being laid on the concept of *translaminar pressure.* The lamina separates the higher IOP space anteriorly from the lower subarachnoid pressure space posteriorly. The pressure difference between the two spaces is called *translaminar pressure,* it has been suggested that this pressure accounts for the damage to the ganglion cells' axons at the level of lamina. In this context, a reduced CSF pressure in the subarachnoid space would exert the same effect as raised IOP. A low CSF pressure has been reported in patients with POAG as well as NTG as compared to control. This data, although preliminary, suggest that the dynamic interplay between these fluid spaces may explain why some individuals with normal IOP may develop glaucoma and others with elevated IOP may not.

Mechanism involved in RGC apoptosis secondary to elevated IOP is summarized in Fig. 3.6.

2. *Pressure-independent factors (vascular insufficiency theory).* Factors affecting vascular perfusion of optic nerve head in the absence of raised IOP have been implicated in the glaucomatous optic neuropathy in patients with normal tension glaucoma (NTG). However, these may be the additional factors in cases of raised IOP as well. These factors include:

i. *Failure of autoregulatory mechanism of blood flow.* The retina and optic nerve share a peculiar mechanism of autoregulation of blood flow with rest of the central nervous system. Once the autoregulatory mechanisms are compromised, blood flow may not be adequate beyond some critical range of IOP (which may be raised or in normal range).

ii. *Vasospasm* is another mechanism affecting vascular perfusion of optic nerve head. This hypothesis gets credence from the convincing association between NTG and vasospastic disorders (migranous headache and Raynaud's phenomenon).

iii. *Systemic hypotension* particularly nocturnal dips in patients with night time administration of antihypertensive drugs has been implicated for low vascular perfusion of optic nerve head

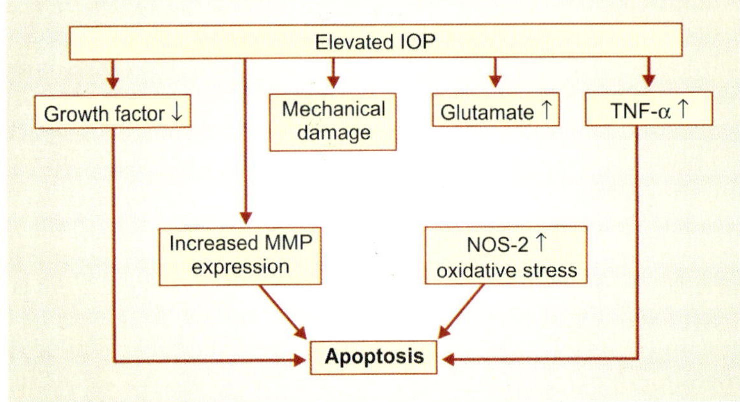

Fig. 3.6 *Mechanism involved in RGC apoptosis secondary to elevated IOP*

resulting in NTG and progression of damage in patients with POAG.

iv. *Other factors,* such as acute blood loss and abnormal coagulability profile, have also been associated with NTG.

Mechanism involved in RGC apoptosis secondary to vascular dysregulation is summarized in Fig. 3.7.

The observed differences in glaucomatous visual field defects between patients with low-tension and high-tension glaucomas have led to the suggestion that ischaemia may be the predominant factor in those glaucomas at the lower end of the IOP scale, whereas a more direct mechanical effect of the pressure may prevail in cases with higher IOP.

B. *Secondary insults (excitotoxicity theory)*

Neuronal degeneration is believed to be driven by toxic factors, such as glutamate (excitatory toxin), oxygen free radicals, or nitric oxide which are released when RGCs undergo death due to primary insults as described above. In this way, the secondary insult leads to continued apoptosis, even after the primary insult has been controlled.

Role of glutamate. Upon exposure to hypoxic conditions, retinal cells are known to release glutamate. Concentrations of glutamate higher than the physiological concentration are toxic to neurons depending upon the duration and extent of increase in concentration. Glutamate-

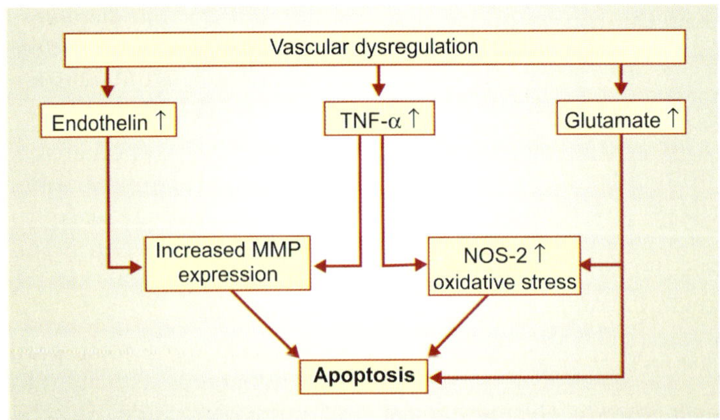

Fig. 3.7 *Mechanism involved in RGC apoptosis secondary to vascular dysregulation*

induced excitotoxicity is primarily mediated by ionotropic NMDA subtype receptors. NMDA receptor activation leads to opening of associated ion channels and the entry of extracellular Ca^{++} and Na^{+} into the neurons. Glutamate-mediated neuronal toxicity is dependent on the influx of extracellular Ca^{+}, which in turn acts as second messenger to activate downstream signaling pathways finally leading to cell death.

In the past, calcium channel blockers were suggested to provide neuroprotection by improving the optic nerve head blood flow. But there were concerns that these agents reduce the systemic blood pressure and might worsen the optic nerve head ischaemia by reducing the perfusion pressure.

Role of nitric oxide. Nitric oxide synthase (NOS) produces NO by oxidation of L-arginine and has been detected in three isoforms. NOS-2 is the inducible form of the enzyme (iNOS), which produces excessive quantities of NO under diverse conditions, such as exposure to cytokines and pressure. The excess of NO thus produced enters freely into the cells after diffusion through the local microenvironment. It is a free radical of moderate reactivity and after entering the cell leads to the production of highly reactive free radicals, such as peroxynitrite after combining with superoxide (a product of mitochondrial metabolism). These highly reactive free radicals cause massive destruction of cell components and macromolecules.

The primary factors responsible for apoptotic cell death in glaucoma include elevated IOP and vascular dysregulation. The molecular mechanisms involved include glutamate excitotoxicity, increased MMP expression, TNF-α upregulation, increased NOS-2 expression and oxidative stress.

Interplay of primary and secondary factors leading to RGC apoptosis is summarized in Fig. 3.8.

Summary

It seems that the glaucomatous optic neuropathy is multifactorial, and at different times and in different eyes, may involve:

- Genetic susceptibility factors
- Mechanical factors including concept of translaminar pressure
- Loss of neuropathic factors, and neurotoxicity, and

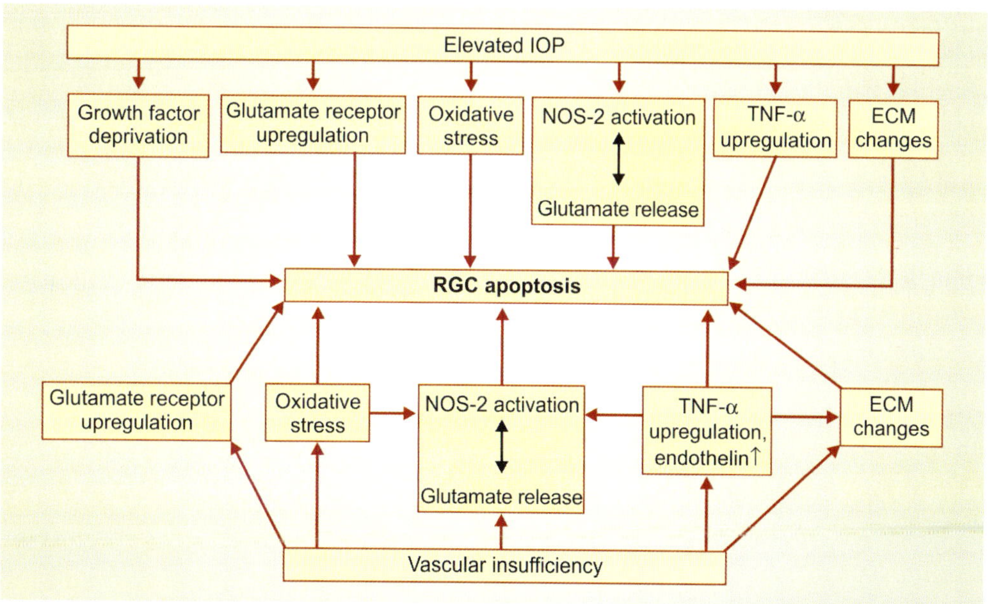

Fig. 3.8 *Interplay of primary and secondary factors leading to RGC apoptosis*

- Inability of the astroglial cells to prevent or repair injury to the ganglion cells or its extracellular matrix regardless of the source of initial insult.

SUGGESTED READING

1. Anderson DR. Ultrastructure of the optic nerve head. Arch Ophthalmol 1970;83(1):63–73.
2. Burgoyne CF, Downs JC, Bellezza AJ, Suh JK, Hart RT. The optic nerve head as a biomechanical structure: a new paradigm for understanding the role of IOP-related stress and strain in the pathophysiology of glaucomatous optic nerve head damage. Prog Retin Eye Res 2005;24:39–73.
3. Cioffi GA. Three common assumptions about ocular blood flow and glaucoma. Survey of ophthalmology 2001;45(Suppl 3):S325-31; discussion S332–34.
4. Chauhan BC, Pan J, Archibald ML et al. Effect of intraocular pressure on optic disc topography, electroretinography, and axonal loss in a chronic pressure-induced rat model of optic nerve damage. Invest Ophthalmol Vis Sci. 2002;43:2969–76.
5. Chen JZ, Kadlubar FF. A new clue to glaucoma pathogenesis. Am J Med 2003;114:697–98.
6. Halpern DL. Grosskreutz CL. Glaucomatous optic neuropathy: mechanisms of disease. Ophthalmology Clinics of North America 2002;15:61–68.
7. Hayreh SS. Blood supply of the optic nerve head and its role in optic atrophy, glaucoma and oedema of the optic disc. Br J Ophthalmol 1969;53:721–48.
8. Hayreh SS, Vrabec F. The structure of the head of the optic nerve in rhesus monkey. Am J Ophthalmol 1966;61(1):136–50.
9. Fechtner RD, Weinreb RN. Mechanisms of optic nerve damage in primary open angle glaucoma. Survey of ophthalmology 1994;39:23–42.

EPIDEMIOLOGY OF GLAUCOMA

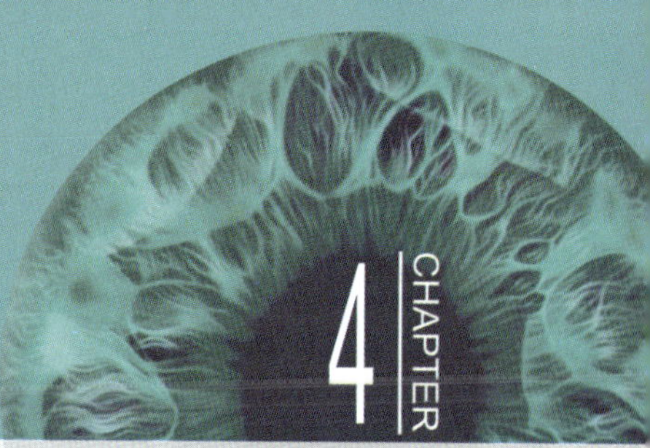

INTRODUCTION

EPIDEMIOLOGICAL TERMS

Before studying the epidemiology of glaucoma, it will be worthwhile to be familiar with some important epidemiological terms.

Epidemiology

Epidemiology has been defined as 'the study of the distribution and determinants of health-related states or events in specified populations, and the application of this study to the control of health problems'.

Tools of measurement

The epidemiologist usually expresses disease magnitude as a rate, ratio or proportion. A clear understanding of the term is required for proper interpretation of epidemiological data. The basic tools of measurement in epidemiology are:

- *Rate* measures the occurrence of some particular event (development of disease or the occurrence of death) in a population during a given time period. It is expressed per thousand or some other round figure (10,000; 1,00,000) selected according to convenience or convention to avoid fractions.
- *Ratio* expresses a relation in size between two random quantities. The numerator is not a component of the denominator.
- *Proportion* is a ratio which indicates the relation in magnitude of a part of the whole. The numerator is always included in the denominator. It is usually expressed as a percentage.

Incidence

Incidence rate is defined as 'the number of new cases occurring in a defined population during a specified period of time'. It is given by the formula:

$$\text{Incidence} = \frac{\text{Number of new cases of specific disease during a given time period}}{\text{Population at risk during that period}} \times 1000$$

It is expressed per 1000 per year.

Prevalence

The term disease prevalence refers specifically to 'all current cases (old and new) existing at a given point in time, or over a period of time in a given population'. It is given by the formula:

$$\text{Prevalence} = \frac{\text{Number of all current cases (old and new) of a specified disease existing at a given point in time}}{\text{Estimated population at the same point in time}} \times 100$$

Relationship between incidence and prevalence

Given the assumption that the population is stable, and incidence and duration are unchanging, the relationship between incidence and prevalence can be expressed as:

$$P = I \times D$$

EPIDEMIOLOGICAL STUDIES

Epidemiological studies can be classified as observational studies and experimental studies with further subdivisions:

1. *Observational studies*
   - Descriptive studies
   - Analytical studies
2. *Experimental studies*
   - Randomised control trials
   - Field trials
   - Community trials

Descriptive epidemiology

These studies are concerned with observing the distribution of disease or health-related characteristics in human populations and identifying the characteristics with which the disease in question seems to be associated. These describe the occurrence and distribution of disease by time, place and person.

- *Time distribution.* The pattern of disease may be described by the time of its occurrence and fluctuations which can be short-term, periodic or long-term (Figs 4.1 and 4.2).
- *Place distribution.* It studies the distribution and occurrence of a specific disease in various geographical areas (Fig. 4.3).

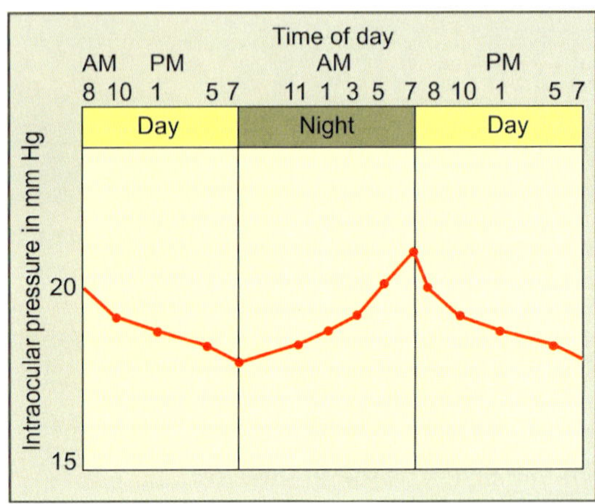

Fig. 4.1 *Diurnal variation in IOP (an example of time distribution)*

- *Person distribution.* It defines the persons who develop the disease by age, sex, occupation, marital status, habits, social class and other host factors (Fig. 4.4).

Analytical epidemiology

Case control study

Often called 'retrospective study', this method has three distinct features:

- Both exposure and outcome have occurred before the start of the study,
- The study proceeds backwards from effect to cause, and
- It uses a control group to support or refute an inference.

Cohort study

It is usually undertaken to obtain additional evidence to refute or support the existence of an association between suspected cause and disease. It is known by a variety of names: prospective study, longitudinal study, incidence study and forward looking study. The distinguishing features of cohort studies are:

- The cohorts are identified prior to the appearance of the disease under investigation.
- The study groups are observed over a period of time to determine the frequency of disease among them.

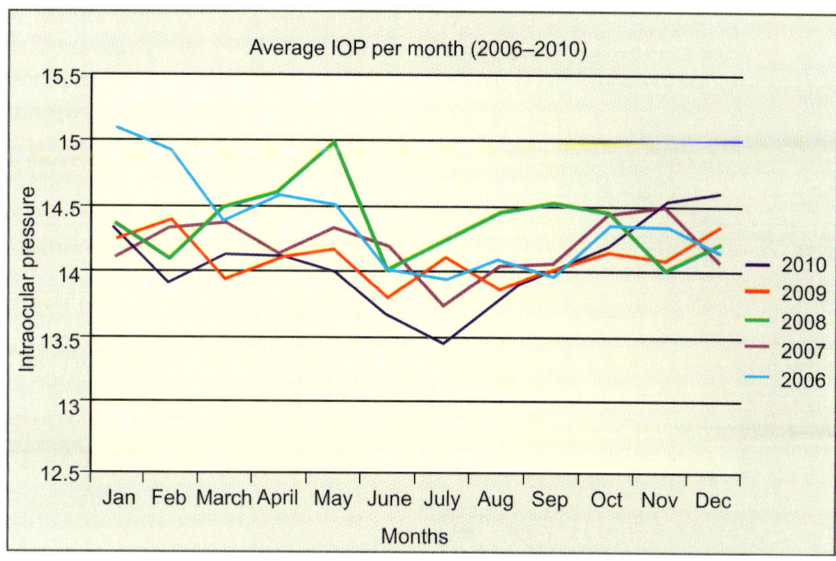

Fig. 4.2 *Average intraocular pressure (IOP) over a 5-year period from 2006 to 2010*

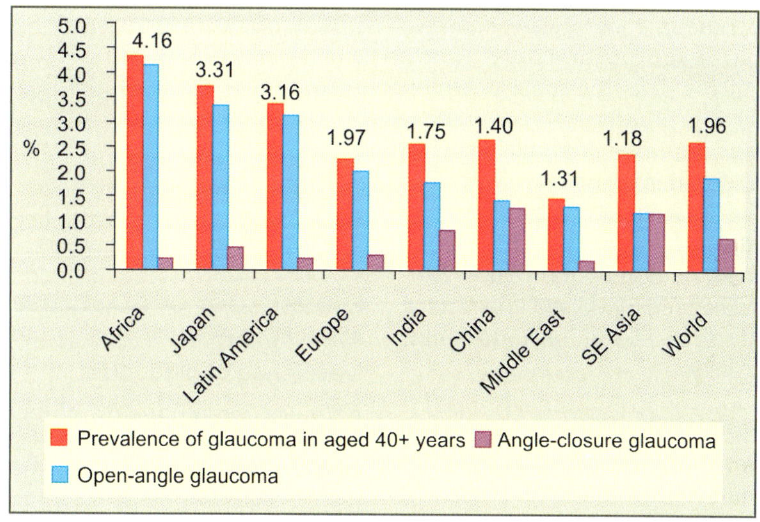

Fig. 4.3 *Prevalence of glaucoma in different countries (an example of place distribution)*

- The study proceeds forwards from cause to effect.

Risk factor, relative risk and attributable risk

Risk factor

Risk factor is an attribute or determinant that is significantly associated with the development of a disease.

Relative risk

It is the ratio of the incidence of the disease among exposed and the incidence among non-exposed.

Attributable risk

It is the difference in incidence rates of disease between an exposed group and non-exposed group.

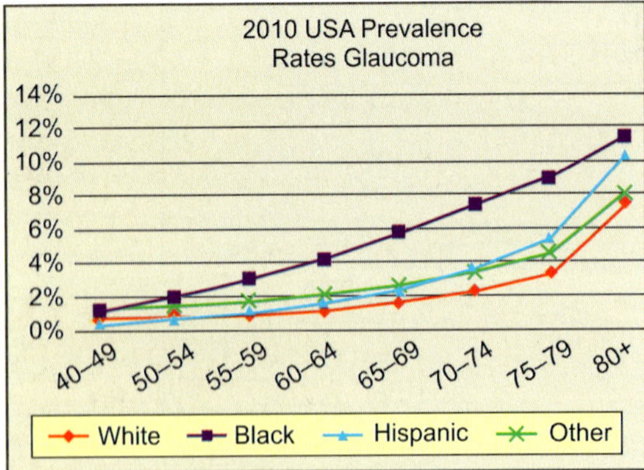

Fig. 4.4 *Prevalence rates of glaucoma in USA (2010) in different races (an example of person distribution)*

EPIDEMIOLOGY OF GLAUCOMA: AN OVERVIEW

EPIDEMIOLOGY OF GLAUCOMA: GLOBAL SCENARIO

- Globally, glaucoma is a significant cause of vision loss that disproportionately affects women and Asians. It is the most common cause of irreversible blindness in the world.
- *Second most frequent cause of blindness,* after cataract, in the world is glaucoma.
- Number of glaucoma blinds in 2002 were 37 million worldwide which is estimated to become almost 80 million by the year 2020.
- Bilateral blindness from glaucoma is projected to affect greater than 11 million individuals worldwide by 2020.

Primary open-angle glaucoma

- Worldwide around 4.5 million people are bilaterally blind because of POAG.
- *Prevalence ratio of POAG versus PACG* reported for different ethnic groups is as below:

Ethnic group	*POAG : PACG*
Europian, African and Hispanics	5 : 1
Indian	1 : 1
Urban Chinese	1 : 2
Mongolian	1 : 3

- *Most common single form* of glaucoma worldwide is POAG. More than two million people develop the disease each year.
- *Prevalence in general population* older than 40 years worldwide is between 1 and 2% in the most studies. However, reports vary considerably according to the population studied, the diagnostic criteria and screening techniques used.
- *Prevalence increases with increasing age,* i.e. from 1–2% in above 40 years to 11% in those above 80 years.
- *Prevalence of POAG in blacks* is three times the prevalence in whites.
- *Prevalence of congenital glaucoma.* In contrast to a prevalence of 1:10,000 in the West, prevalence is as high as 1:1250 among the Romany population of Slovakia, and 1:2500 in the Middle East, suggesting a genetic etiology. In the Indian state of Andhra Pradesh, the prevalence is 1:3300, and the disease accounts for 4.2% of all childhood blindness.

Primary angle-closure glaucoma

- *Prevalence of PACG* is 0.5% worldwide.
- Current estimates of the number of persons who are blind worldwide because of PACG is 3.9 million.
- Highest rates have been reported among Eskimos (Inuits).
- High prevalence has also been reported from China, Mongolia, South-East Asia and India.

EPIDEMIOLOGY OF GLAUCOMA: ASIAN SCENARIO

Prevalence of glaucoma

Primary angle-closure glaucoma (PACG) is more prevalent than *primary open-angle glaucoma (POAG)* in East Asian population. A reverse trend is reported in European and African derived peoples. Asians are expected to represent 47% of those with glaucoma and 87% of those with ACG.

Incidence of acute angle-closure (cases/1,00,000 persons/year for the population aged 30 years and over) reported are as below:

- Europe (Finland): 4.7
- Chinese Singaporeans: 15.5
- Malaya and Indian Singaporeans: 6.0

Glaucomatous optic neuropathy (GON) is reported to be most prevalent among people of

African origin, least in Australian aborigines and intermediate in Asians.

Chinese origin people have higher rate of GON, probably due to higher incidence of PACG.

Risk factors for glaucoma

Risk factors for glaucoma reported from Asian surveys are:
- *Advancing age:* For all types of glaucoma.
- *Positive family* history for all types of glaucoma.
- *Female gender* preponderance is reported for PACG. No gender preponderance reported for POAG.
- *Race:* Chinese ethnic origin at a higher risk for PACG as compared to Malaya descent and South Indian population.
- *Raised IOP* is an important reported risk factor for glaucomatous optic neuropathy in Chinese population.
- *Shallow anterior chamber (AC):* Risk factor for PACG with AC becomes more shallower in females than males.
- *Myopia* is reported to be associated with POAG.
- *Pseudoexfoliation* is reported in 26.7% of POAG from India.

Glaucoma blindness

Glaucoma blindness reported figures from Asia are:
- *Mongolia:* 35% of adult blinds
- *Chinese Singaporeans:* 60% of adult blinds
- *China:* Total 1.7 million blinds due to glaucoma out of which 91% are due to PACG
- *Hong Kong:* 23% of registered permanent blinds are due to glaucoma
- *Japan:* 15% are blind due to glaucoma
- *India:* As per Hyderabad survey (12%); and as per Aravind survey (10.2%), blinds are due to glaucoma. As per National Blindness and Visual Impairment Survey (2015–19), glaucoma a counts for 5.5% cases of blinds in India in a population aged ≥50 years.

EPIDEMIOLOGY OF GLAUCOMA IN INDIA

Population-based studies for glaucoma in India

Population-based studies on which epidemiological data of glaucoma from India is based are the following:
- Vellore Eye Survey (VES)
- Andhra Pradesh Eye Disease Survey (APEDS)
- Chennai Glaucoma Study (CGS)
- West Bengal Glaucoma Study (WBGS), and
- Aravind Comprehensive Eye Survey (ACES).

Note. Though the methodology employed in each of these population-based studies differs widely. All the studies-based diagnosis of glaucoma on the appearance of optic discs and matching visual field defects on automated perimetry. No study relied on measurement of IOP for diagnosis of glaucoma except in situations where optic disc or visual field criteria were unavailable owing to lack of media clarity. Since the above mentioned studies had methodological differences in disease definition which needs to be kept in mind while interpreting the results.

Ocular hypertension (OHT)

Prevalence of OHT (IOP >21 mm Hg, normal disc and visual field) reported in APEDS is 0.42%.

Primary open-angle glaucoma

Prevalence of POAG reported in various studies is as follows:
- CGS (Urban): 3.51
- CGS (Rural): 1.62
- WBGS: 2.99
- ACES: 1.7
- APEDS (Urban): 4
- APEDS (Rural): 1.6

Higher prevalence is reported in urban population as compared to rural (CGS and APEDS).

Risk factors for POAG reported in various studies are:
- *Increasing IOP and increasing age* are reported in all studies
- *Myopia* is reported only in ACES study
- *No association* with central corneal thickness (CCT), gender, myopia and hypertension in CGS and APEDS

Primary angle-closure disease

Prevalence of primary angle-closure disease (PACD) reported in various studies is shown in Table 4.1:

Table 4.1 *Prevalence of primary angle-closure disease in various studies*

Study	*Stage of PACD*			*Total*
	PACS	*PAC*	*PACG*	
CGS (Urban)	7.24	2.75	0.88	–
CGS (Rural)	6.27	0.71	0.87	–
APEDS (Urban)	3.50	0.80	1.80	–
APEDS (Rural)	1.50	0.20	0.70	–
VES	–	–	–	4.32
ACES	–	–	–	0.50
WBGS	–	–	–	0.24

- *Disparities in prevalence rates* are mainly due to the varied classification systems used.
- *Lower prevalence* in rural population may be due to higher cataract surgical rate, i.e. aphakia.

Risk factors reported are as below:

- *Increasing age and increasing IOP* were significant association
- *Female gender* showed preponderance (male : female = 1 : 3)
- *Diabetes and hyperopia* were associated with urban cohort only
- *Hypertension* was not an association both in urban and rural cohort.

Secondary glaucomas

The prevalence of secondary glaucoma in the population has also been reported to be highly variable in the studies as depicted below:

- WBGS: 0.8%
- ACES: 0.3%
- APED: Only in one eye (angle recession)
- CGS: 1.38% in aphakic/pseudophakic population.

Pseudoexfoliation glaucoma

Exfoliation has been recognised to be the most common identifiable risk factor for ocular hypertension and glaucoma. The prevalence of exfoliation glaucoma from hospital-based data in India has been reported to be between 1.87 and 13.5%.

Prevalence of pseudoexfoliation glaucoma is as below:

- CGS: 3.8%
- ACES: 6%
- APEDS: 3.02%

Glaucoma blindness in India

Glaucoma has been declared to be the second common cause of blindness in adult population in India. As per Rapid assessment of Avoidable Blindness (RAB) in 2006, glaucoma is responsible for 5.8% of blindness in India. Scenario of glaucoma blindness as per the population based studies is as below:

- *ACES.* About one-fifth (20.9%) of all POAG patients were blind.
- *APEDS.* Bilateral blindness in 20% and unilateral blindness in 28.7% of PACG patients.
- *CGS.* Bilateral blindness in 5.9% and unilateral blindness in 8.8% of PACG patients.

SUGGESTED READING

1. Glaucoma in a rural population of Southern India: the Aravind Comprehensive Eye Survey. Ophthalmology 2003;110:1484–90.
2. Open angle glaucoma in an urban population in Southern India. The Andhra Pradesh Eye Disease Survey. Ophthalmology 2000;107:1702–09.
3. Prevalence of primary glaucoma in an urban South Indian population. Indian J Ophthalmol 1998;46:81–86.
4. Prevalence of primary open-angle glaucoma in an urban South Indian population and comparison with a rural population. The Chennai Glaucoma Study. Ophthalmology 2008;115(4):648–54.
5. Neena J, Rachel J, Praveen V, Murthy GVS, for the RAAB India Study Group Rapid Assessment of Avoidable Blindness in India. PLoS ONE 3(8): e2867. doi:10.1371/journal.pone.0002867 (2008).
6. Quigley HA, Broman AT. The number of people with glaucoma worldwide in 2010 and 2020. Br J Ophthalmol 2006;90:262–67.
7. The number of people with glaucoma worldwide in 2010 and 2020. Br J Ophthalmol 2006; 90(3):262–67.

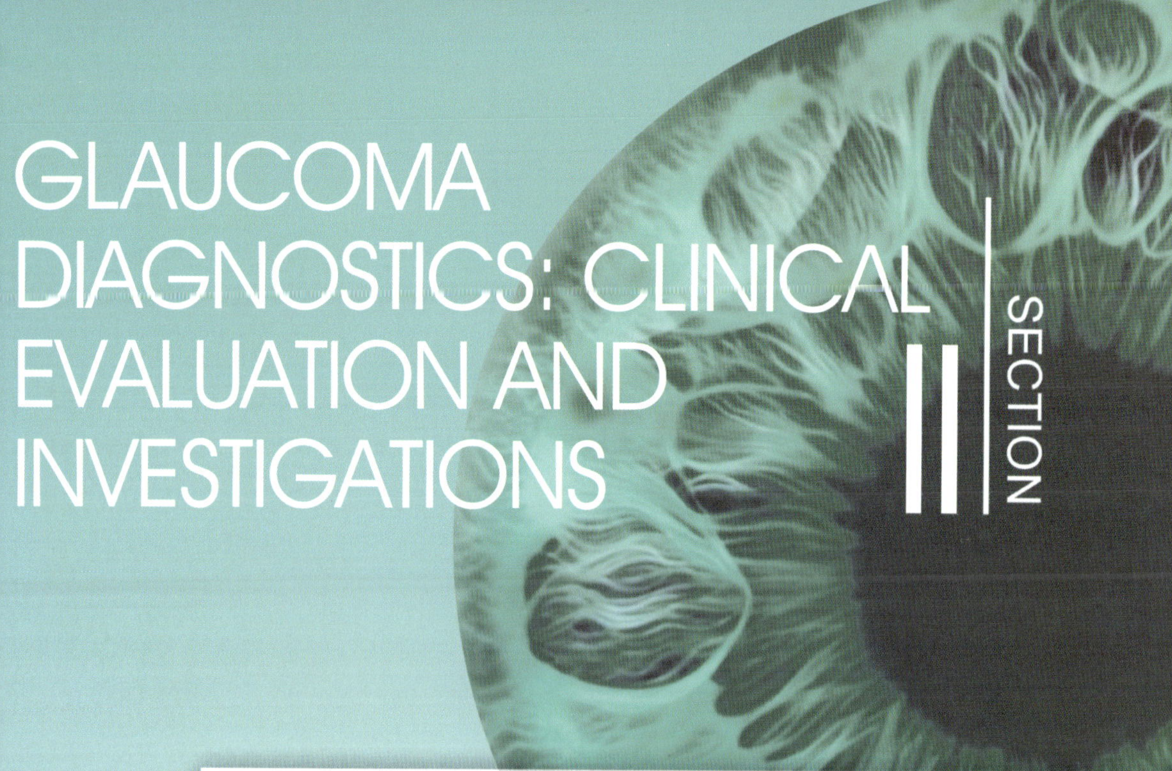

GLAUCOMA DIAGNOSTICS: CLINICAL EVALUATION AND INVESTIGATIONS

SECTION II

CLINICAL EVALUATION OF GLAUCOMA: AN OVERVIEW

CHAPTER 5

INTRODUCTION

GOALS OF CLINICAL EVALUATION

Goals of clinical evaluation during the initial assessment are to know:

- *Glaucoma is present or not*, or is likely to develop (assessment of risk factors)
- *Type of glaucoma,* when present
- *Severity of glaucoma* mild, moderate or severe
- *Underlying mechanism of damage*—intraocular pressure (IOP) or non-IOP factors
- *Planning a strategy for management* and to identify suitable form of treatment.

OUTLINES OF CLINICAL EVALUATION

Clinical evaluation of glaucoma patients, like any other disease, involves:

A. *History taking* in a meticulous and thorough manner

B. *General physical and systemic examinations* relevant to glaucoma

C. *Ocular examination* in a comprehensive way, and

D. *Specific investigations* meant for a case of glaucoma.

HISTORY TAKING

The importance of painstaking meticulous history cannot be overemphasized. The complete history taking should be structured as:

- Demographic data
- Chief presenting complaints and history of present illness
- History of past medical illness
- History of drug intake
- History of past ocular complaints
- Family history
- Social history

I. DEMOGRAPHIC DATA

Demographic data should include patient's name, age, sex, occupation and religion.

Name and address are primarily required for patient's identification and also prove useful for demographic research.

Age and sex. Primary open-angle glaucoma (POAG) usually affects about 1 in 100 of the general population (of either sex) above the age of 40 years. Primary angle-closure glaucoma (PACG) usually presents between 50 and 60 years. It occurs more commonly in females than males in a ratio of 4 : 1.

Ethnicity. The ratio of POAG versus PACG reported for different ethnic groups is as below:

Ethnic group	*POAG : PACG*
Europian, African and Hispanics	5 : 1
Indian	1 : 1
Urban Chinese	1 : 2
Mongolian	1 : 3

Religion. Recording the religion helps in knowing the aptitude and practices prevalent in different communities.

II. CHIEF PRESENTING COMPLAINTS AND HISTORY OF PRESENT ILLNESS

Primary open-angle glaucoma (POAG)

Presenting symptoms. The disease is insidious and usually asymptomatic. Mild symptoms experienced by the patients include:

- Mild headache and eyeache.
- Difficulty in reading (patients usually give history of frequent change in near vision glasses).
- Occasionally, an observant patient may notice a defect in the visual field (scotoma).
- In late stages, patient may complain of delayed dark adaptation.

Primary angle-closure disease

Chronic PACD (asymptomatic) is more common than acute PACD (symptomatic) (3 :1); meaning thereby that most patients do not know they have disease justifying need for glaucoma screening. Presenting symptoms of PACD, depending upon the clinical stage are summarized below.

Primary angle-closure glaucoma suspect (PACGS)/latent glaucoma. Patient does not present in this stage as there are no symptoms. PACGS is diagnosed:

- On routine slit-lamp examination in patients presenting with some other eye disease, and
- In fellow eye of the patients presenting with subacute or acute angle closure.

Primary angle closure. Primary angle-closure (PAC) may manifest as subacute or acute PAC.

Subacute PAC/intermittent glaucoma. Patient presents with transient blurring of vision, coloured haloes around the light due to corneal oedema and mild headache. These symptoms are due to transient rise in intraocular pressure (IOP) and occur in intermittent attacks at irregular intervals. The attacks are usually precipitated by overwork in the evening, anxiety and fatigue.

Acute PAC (old name: acute angle-closure glaucoma). Patient presents with an attack of sudden onset of very severe pain in the eye which radiates along the branches of fifth nerve. Frequently, there is history of associated nausea, vomiting and prostrations. There is history of rapidly progressive loss of vision, redness, photophobia and watering. About 5% patients give history of typical previous intermittent attacks.

Primary angle-closure glaucoma (PACG). PACG may present as chronic congestive PACG or chronic non-congestive PACG.

Chronic congestive PACG. Patients have dull and constant pain in the eye along with marked diminution of vision. Patients usually give history of preceding attack of acute congestive glaucoma or repeated attacks of intermittent glaucoma.

Chronic non-congestive PACG. Typically presents as POAG except that the chamber is shallow and gonioscopy shows narrow angles with synechiae.

Absolute glaucoma. Such patients present with:

- Pain in the eye which is severe and irritating
- Constant headache

- Watering and redness of the eye
- Complete loss of vision (no perception of light)

This stage results, if the chronic phase is left untreated

Secondary glaucoma

Secondary glaucoma may present as acute or chronic disease. History should be taken to rule out the common causes, such as:

- *Uveitis,* acute or chronic
- *Steroids administration*—topical or systemic for a prolonged time
- *Ocular ischaemic diseases,* such as CRVO, proliferative diabetic retinopathy, Eales' disease, which can cause neovascular glaucoma
- *Ocular trauma* including trivial trauma in the past
- *Cataract,* may be complicated by either phacomorphic or phacolytic glaucoma

History from a diagnosed patient of glaucoma under treatment

History taken from a diagnosed patient of glaucoma under treatment should include:

- Type of glaucoma diagnosed
- Date of diagnosis of glaucoma
- Highest IOP recording
- Glaucoma therapy taken in the past and currently being used should be recorded with specific dates
- History of adverse reactions to glaucoma agents used should be recorded in detail.
- Any history of laser therapy and intraocular surgery

Note. It will be prudent to obtain past medical records including previous visual field charts and optic disc photographs.

III. PAST MEDICAL ILLNESS

Medical history relevant for glaucoma cases, which need to be ascertained is summarized below:

Respiratory diseases, such as asthma, chronic obstructive lung diseases associated with hyperresponsive airway and/or reduced lung capacity are contraindications for β-blockers.

Cardiovascular diseases, which need to be probed in a patient with glaucoma are:

- *History of past haemodynamic crisis* (e.g. post-partum haemorrhage, ruptured abdominal aneurysms, severe bleeding loss with trauma) may be responsible for optic disc pallor and cupping that mimics glaucoma but is not progressive.
- *Cardiac arrhythmias,* e.g. heart blocks, are contraindications for use of topical β-blockers and β-agonists.
- *Systemic hypertension,* when overtreated may worsen glaucoma risk and progression. Further systemic β-blocker may mask elevated IOP.
- *Vasospastic disorders,* e.g. migraine, Raynaud's syndrome may be associated with an increased incidence and severity of glaucoma, specially normal tension glaucoma (NTG).

Endocrinal disorders having relevance in glaucoma patients are:

- *Diabetes* may be associated with POAG and may be responsible for neovascular glaucoma in patients with diabetic eye diseases.
- *Thyrotoxicosis* is not the cause of rise in IOP but the prevalence of POAG is more in patients suffering from Graves' ophthalmic disease than the normal. Secondary glaucoma can also occur in thyroid ophthalmopathy.
- *Pituitary tumours* may be responsible for the optic disc pallor mimicking glaucoma.

Central nerve system (CNS) disorders

- Previous head injury, cerebrovascular accidents (CVA) and pituitary lesions may be responsible for the optic disc pallor and/or visual field defects.
- *Carotid-cavernous fistula* and intracranial arteriovenous malformations may cause elevated episcleral venous pressure and secondary glaucoma.
- *Early dementia* may affect compliance, understanding and insight into the disease.

Musculoskeletal diseases, such as osteoarthritis or rheumatoid arthritis may affect the ability to administer the eyedrops.

Urogenital problems, such as urinary stones, may limit use of systemic carbonic anhydrase inhibitors (CAIs).

Pregnancy and lactation may render all interventions hazardous.

IV. HISTORY OF DRUG INTAKE

Certain drugs being used by the patients presently or used in the past may have influence on glaucoma:

- *Steroids* used by any route, as also mentioned earlier, may be associated with steroid-induced glaucoma.
  Note. Steroid may be found in some traditional medicine especially being used by quacks.
- *Antiglaucoma drugs,* after prolonged use, may increase chances of trabeculectomy failure.
- *Anticholinergics/tricyclic* antidepressant drugs can cause angle-closure glaucoma.
- *Anticonvulsants (vigabatrin)* are reported to cause nasal peripheral field loss without disc changes.
- *Systemic beta blocker* and calcium channel blockers may interact with topical beta-blockers.

V. HISTORY OF PAST OCULAR COMPLAINTS

A probe into history of past illness should be made to know:

- *Frequent change of glasses may be seen.* Myopes are at higher risk for POAG and hypermetropes are at higher risk for PACD.
- *History of similar complaints in the past* may be present in recurrent conditions, such as intermittent attacks of primary angle-closure glaucoma, recurrent attacks of glaucomatocyclitic crisis, inflammatory glaucoma especially associated with viral keratouveitis.
- *History of similar complaints in other eye* may be present in patients with primary angle-closure disease.
- *History of trauma to eye in the past* may be present in patients with angle recession glaucoma, cyclodialysis cleft.
- *History of ocular diseases in the past* which may or treatment of which may cause secondary glaucoma, such as uveitis; use of steroids for VKC, intraocular surgery; ocular ischaemic diseases, e.g. CRVO, Eale's disease, proliferative diabetic retinopathy.
- *History of systemic diseases in the past* which may cause secondary glaucoma includes epidemic dropsy, tuberculosis, syphilis, etc.

VI. FAMILY HISTORY

- *Several genes* [e.g. TIGR/MYOC (myocillin), OPTN (optineurin)] and modes of inheritance have been implicated in the development of POAG, juvenile and developmental forms of glaucoma.
- *Family history of glaucoma when positive* should be aimed at knowing the age of diagnosis, presentation, systemic association, progression, and visual status of the affected relative. It is unequivocal that positive family history is *an important risk factor* for the POAG, with greater risk being first degree relatives of glaucoma.
- *Examination of the patient's relative can* also provide important information regarding the appearance of the optic nerve, in particular the cup-to-disc ratio, which has been shown to be inherited.

VII. SOCIAL HISTORY

Social history helps to reveal a patient's ability to understand and successfully manage the challenge of a chronic disease, e.g.,

- How regularly the patient can attend for follow-up?
- Can the patient afford and comply with treatment?
- How the glaucoma will affect the patient's work/family?

GENERAL PHYSICAL AND SYSTEMIC EXAMINATIONS

General physical and systemic examinations should be carried out in each case of glaucoma. The conditions relevant to management of glaucoma are summarized in medical history (see page 55).

COMPREHENSIVE OCULAR EXAMINATION AND SPECIFIC TESTS FOR GLAUCOMA

COMPREHENSIVE OCULAR EXAMINATION

A thorough ocular examination in a suspected case of glaucoma should include:

- Testing of visual acuity and refraction
- Slit-lamp biomicroscopy.

TESTING OF VISUAL ACUITY AND REFRACTION

Visual acuity should be tested both for far and near. Refraction should be carried out to record the best corrected visual acuity as baseline evaluation.

SLIT-LAMP BIOMICROSCOPY

A thorough and meticulous ocular examination should be carried with slit-lamp biomicroscopy. Special attention should be given to the signs of primary as well as secondary glaucoma.

1. Conjunctival signs

- *Episcleral congestion* may occur due to elevated episcleral venous pressure.
- *Ciliary flush* may occur due to congestion of deep conjunctival vessels in acute congestive glaucoma.
- *Conjunctival filtration blebs* may be noted in old operated cases of glaucoma.

2. Corneal signs

- *Oedema*with epithelial vesicles may be noted in acute rise of IOP.
- *Krukenberg'sspindle*and pigment on corneal endothelium is seen in pigment dispersion syndrome.
- *Keratic precipitates* (KPs) may be seen in inflammatory glaucoma.
- *Fuch's corneal dystrophy* may be associated with POAG.
- *Corneal diameter*is increased in buphthalmos.
- *Breaks in Descemet's membrane* (Haab's striae) is a sign of buphthalmos.
- *Central corneal thickness (CCT)* lower than normal is being considered an important risk factor for conversion from ocular hypertension to glaucoma. CCT should be measured in every glaucoma and glaucoma suspect patient. Average CCT lies between 520 and 580 mm. Thinner cornea gives false low reading of IOP on Goldmann applanation tonometry (GAT) and conversely thicker cornea gives false high reading of IOP.

3. Anterior chamber signs

- *Peripheral anterior chamber depth* (van Herring's technique) is shallow in primary angle-closure disease.
- *Aqueous flare and cells* may be seen in acute primary angle closure and in inflammatory glaucoma.
- *Lens proteins* in the anterior chamber (post-cataract surgery or following ocular trauma) may cause lens particle glaucoma.
- *Hyphaema* is a cause of haemorrhagic glaucoma.

4. Iris signs

- *Iris atrophy patch* may be seen of exfoliative glaucoma, old attack of acute PAC.
- *Dilated and congested iris vessels* may be seen in acute PAC.
- *Rubeosis iridis* is a sign of neovascular glaucoma.
- *Posterior synechiae may be seen in post-inflammatory glaucoma.*
- *Transillumination defect* may be seen is iridocorneal endothelial syndrome.

5. Pupillary signs

- *Mid-dilated, vertically oval and poorly reactive pupil* is seen post an angle-closure attack.
- *Relative afferent pupillary defect (RAPD)* may be seen in glaucomatous optic neuropathy.
- *Mildly dilated round pupil* with sluggish reaction may be seen in advanced POAG.

6. Lens signs

- Pseudoexfoliative material (exfoliative glaucoma)
- Glaukomflecken (post-angle-closure attack)
- Swollen intumescent lens may cause phacomorphic glaucoma
- Phacodonesis may be seen in glaucoma due to subluxation and phacolytic glaucoma.

SPECIFIC TESTS FOR GLAUCOMA

Specific tests for glaucoma patients should include:

- Tonometry
- Gonioscopy
- Optic nerve head evaluation
- Visual field testing and other psychophysical tests

- Optic nerve blood flow
- Electrophysiological tests for glaucoma, and
- Genetic testing.

Specific tests for glaucoma patients are deliberated in detail in the coming text and just mentioned briefly here.

1. TONOMETRY

- Tonometry needs to be performed on each follow-up visit, since IOP is the only modifiable risk factor for glaucoma.
- Till date the preferred method is Goldmann-style Applanation Tonometry (GAT). Tonopen may be used, if GAT is increased by taking multiple measurement and averaging the results.
- Central corneal thickness (CCT) need to be considered with GAT in patients with ocular hypertension and glaucoma. Although available formulae to correct IOP based on CCT do not improve prediction of glaucoma development, it is important to account for a thin cornea.
- For details of tonometry, see page 62–75.

2. GONIOSCOPY

- Gonioscopy, visualization of the angle of anterior chamber with the help of a gonioscope is essential to classify glaucoma into open-angle glaucoma and angle-closure glaucoma based on the configuration of the angle.
- Small indentation gonioscopy (e.g. Zeiss 4 mirror).
- Initially the gonioscopy need to be performed in each case of glaucoma and then regularly on each follow-up in angle-closure patients.
- The ideal testing conditions include dim room illumination, minimal intensity of the slit-lamp illumination, a low slit-beam height such that light does not impinge on the pupil and no pressure on the eye with the gonioscope. Then, wait for 30–45 seconds for the pupil to dilate before deciding, if the angle is open.
- Gonioscopy is useful in dividing angle-closure patient into:
  - Primary angle-closure suspects (PACS)
  - Primary angle-closure (PAC), and
  - Primary angle-closure glaucoma (PACG)
- For details of gonioscopy, see Chapter 7.
- Additional diagnostic tools, such as anterior segment optical coherence tomography (OCT) and ultrasound biomicroscopy (UBM) can be supplementary, but are not necessary in routine evaluation of glaucoma suspects.

3. OPTIC NERVE HEAD EVALUATION

Optic disc changes, usually observed on routine fundus examination, provide an important clue for suspecting POAG.

- Optic nerve head changes are typically progressive, asymmetric and present a variety of characteristic clinical patterns. It is important to measure the size of the optic disc.
- Special attention should be paid to the shape and contour of neuroretinal rim. Localized narrowing of the inferior or superior rim that does not extend to the rim should arouse suspicion. If the rim extends to the edge of the disc for a clock hour, it is called a notch, typical of glaucomatous damage.
- Pallor of the rim outside the area of loss or out of proportion to the "cupping" is suggestive of other neurological causes.
- Peripapillary choroidal atrophy is a soft sign of glaucomatous damage. It is significant, if associated with other signs, or if it increases in size.

It is essential to record the appearance of the nerve head in such a way that will accurately reveal subtle glaucomatous changes over the course of follow-up evaluation.

Examination techniques. Careful assessment of disc changes can be made by direct ophthalmoscopy, slit-lamp biomicroscopy using a +90/78/60 D lens, Hruby lens or Goldmann contact lens and indirect ophthalmoscopy.

Recording and documentation techniques include:

- Serial drawings
- Photography and photogrammetry
- Structural changes, such as nerve fibre layer loss and rim notches often precede perimetric loss and can be measured in glaucoma suspects to determine initial risk and appropriate follow-up. Confocal scanning laser tomography (CSLT), i.e. Heidelberg

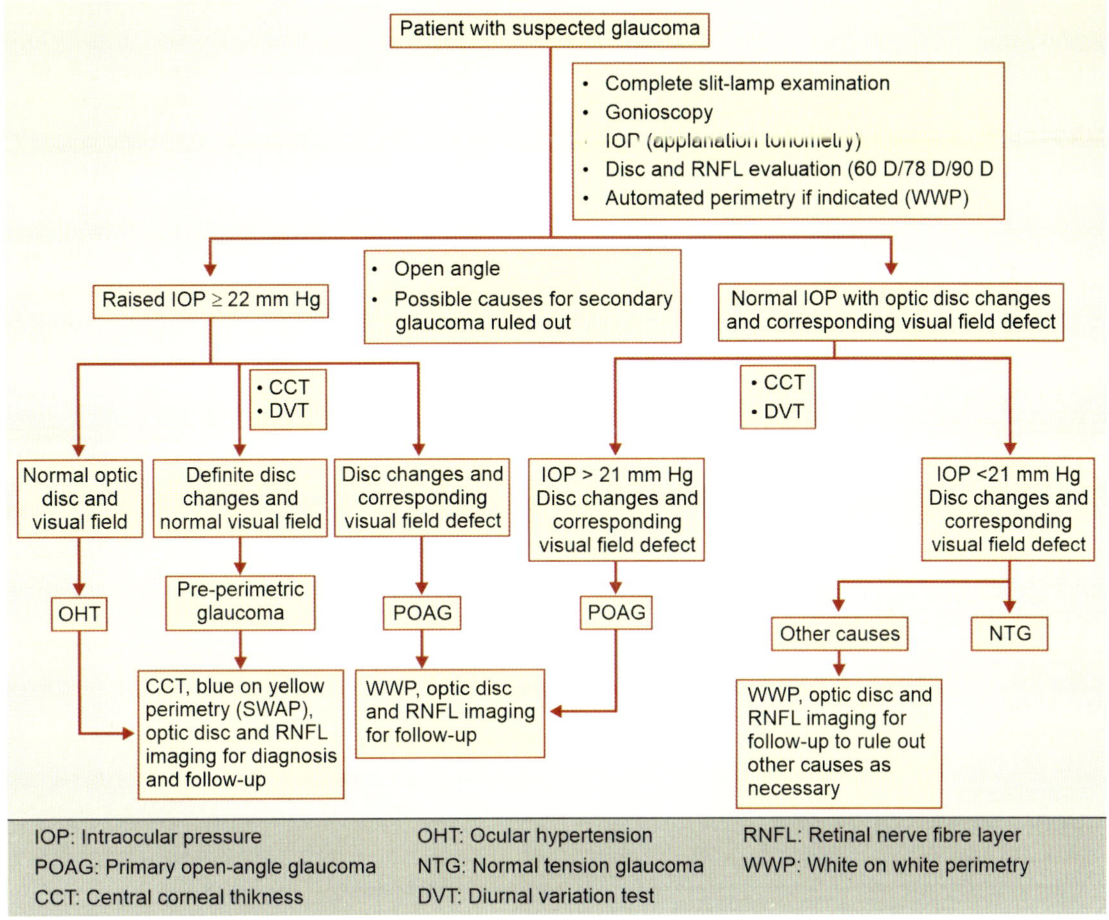

Fig. 5.1 *Flowchart for work-up for a patient with ocular hypertension and glaucoma suspect*

retinal tomograph (HRT) is an accurate and sensitive method for this purpose.

- Other advanced imaging techniques include optical coherence tomography (OCT) and scanning laser polarimetry, i.e. nerve fibre analyser (NFA).

Glaucomatous changes in the optic disc can be described as early changes, advanced changes and glaucomatous optic atrophy.

For detail of optic nerve head evaluation, *see* Chapters 8 and 9.

4. VISUAL FIELD EXAMINATION

- Visual field defects in glaucoma are initially observed in Bjerrum's area (10–30° from fixation point) and correlate well with optic disc changes.
- Visual field examination defines state of the optic nerve function and defines visual impairment.
- Visual fields must never be interpreted in isolation. The field should be correlated with structural changes in the optic disc and NFL.
- Many options exist today for testing visual field function/sensitivity. Automated visual field tests (using Humphrey Field Analyser/ Octopus) are more commonly used.
- Visual field examination should be performed when glaucoma is suspect. In cases of glaucoma, on therapy the follow-up visual field testing should be performed as per recommended guidelines.

Psychophysical tests other than visual fields include:

- Colour vision testing
- High pass resolution perimetry
- Motion detection perimetry

New techniques of perimetry, like blue on yellow and FDT may help in detecting glaucoma damage earlier than standard white on white perimetry.

5. OPTIC NERVE BLOOD FLOW

Assessment (using devices, such as HRF—Heidelberg retina flowmeter) has gained importance in recent years especially in patients with normotensive glaucoma.

6. ELECTROPHYSIOLOGICAL TESTS

Such as multiple visual evoked potential, multifocal ERG are also recommended for early detection of glaucoma.

VEP protocols: Flash VEP, pattern reversal VEP (PRVEP) and Multifocal VEP

- *Flash VEP*: Ganglion cell damage is reflected by prolonged P100 latency and reduced P1 amplitude. Amplitude reduction correlates with vertical C: D ratio. Confounder-Amplitudes reduction occurs in systemic vascular disease too.

  Note: Latency prolongation is more marked for flash VEP than PRVEP
- *Pattern reversal VEP:* Responses of PRVEP are less variable than flash VEP, however, since amplitudes are higher, response estimations are more reliable. Negative correlation is seen between MD values on perimetry, location and severity of scotomas with that of p100 latency.
- *Short duration transients (SD-tVEP)* with high and low contrast stimuli technique isolate magnocellular ganglions (selectively damaged earlier in glaucoma), document linear increase in latency with increasing disease severity and higher rate of glaucoma progression.
- *Multifocal VEP*: Both implicit time and amplitude in central area used to diagnose and prognosticate glaucoma especially in unreliable or unconfirmed visual field defect (VFD). Strong correlation has been documented between the quadrantic inter-eye relative asymmetry coefficients (RAC) and Humphrey quadrant threshold scores in asymmetric glaucoma.

7. GENETIC TESTING IN GLAUCOMA

It is also gaining importance. It is recommended that genetic testing can help to customize the glaucoma treatment protocols which is called *personalised medicine.*

Therefore, it is recommended to perform a comprehensive eye examination for every patient with the objective of detecting this potentially sight-threatening disease, glaucoma.

SUMMARY OF GLAUCOMA EVALUATION

Figure 5.1 summarizes the work-up for a glaucoma suspect.

SUGGESTED READING

1. Jonas JB, Budde WM, Panda-Jonas S. Ophthalmoscopic evaluation of the optic nerve head. Surv Ophthalmol 1999;43:293–320.
2. Sommer A. Glaucoma risk factors observed in the Baltimore Eye Survey. Curr Opin Ophthalmol 1996;7:93–98.
3. Thomas R, Parikh RS. How to assess a patient for glaucoma. Community Eye Health 2006;19:36–37.

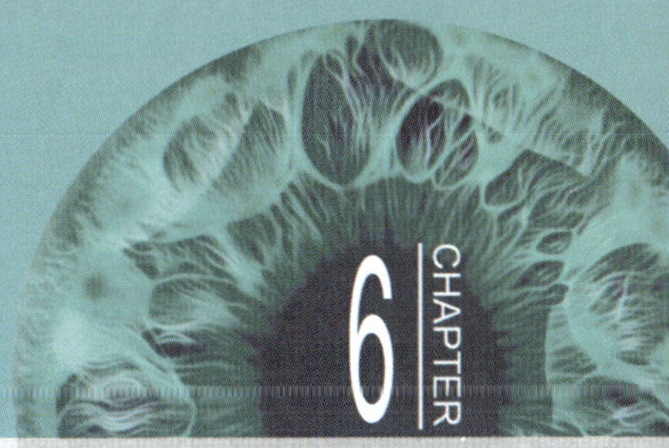

TONOMETRY

INTRODUCTION

MANOMETRY

Manometry is the only direct measure of IOP. In this method, a needle is introduced either into the anterior chamber or into the vitreous, which is then connected with a suitable mercury or water manometer to measure the IOP (Fig. 6.1).

Disadvantages

- Not a practical method for routine in human beings.
- Needs general anaesthesia which has its other effects on the IOP.
- Introduction of the needle produces breakdown of blood–aqueous barrier and release of prostaglandins which alter the IOP.

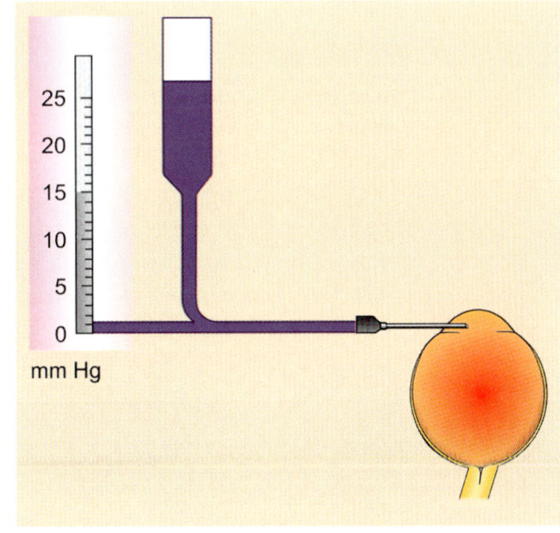

Fig. 6.1 *Manometry*

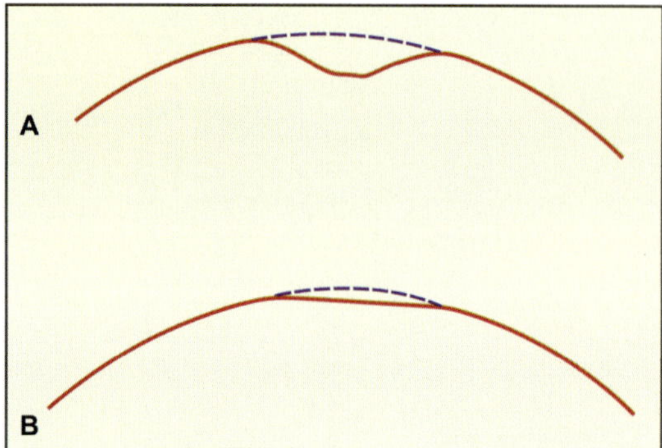

Fig. 6.2 *Corneal deformation created by (A) indentation tonometers (a truncated cone) and (B) applanation tonometers (simple flattening)*

Uses. Manometer is of the greatest and perhaps of the only use for a continuous measurements over time and recording the changes in IOP induced by physiological and pharmacological manipulations in the experiment research work on animal eyes.

TONOMETRY

Tonometry is an indirect method of measuring the intraocular pressure (IOP) with the help of specially designed instruments known as tonometers. Tonometry has been over 180 years long journey. In late 19th century, Donders designed the first instrument which displaced intraocular fluid by contact with the sclera. The first commonly used mechanical tonometer designed by Schiotz in early 1990's soon became the new gold standard.

All clinical tonometers measure the IOP by relating a deformation of the globe to the force responsible for the deformation. They are broadly of two types, differing according to the shape of the deformation (Fig. 6.2): the indentation or impression tonometers (truncated cone) and the applanation tonometers (simple flattening).

INDENTATION (IMPRESSION) TONOMETRY

Indentation (impression) tonometry is based on the fundamental fact that a plunger will indent soft eye more than a hard eye. The indentation tonometer in current use is that of Schiotz who devised it in 1905 and continued to refine it through 1927. Because of its simplicity, reliability, low price and relative accuracy, it is the most widely used tonometer in the world.

BASIC CONCEPT AND THEORY OF INDENTATION TONOMETRY

As the tonometer is placed on the cornea (Fig. 6.3), the different forces come into play: W, the weight of the tonometer, acts over an area A and indents the cornea displacing a volume V_c. The tensile force T set up in the outer coats of the eye at everywhere tangentially to the corneal surface, with a component opposing W, so that an additional force T is added to the original baseline or resting intraocular pressure (P_0) which is artificially raised to a new value (P_t). Thus, the scale reading of the tonometer actually measures the artificially raised IOP (P_t) (Fig. 6.3).

SCHIOTZ TONOMETER

A Schiotz tonometer consists of the following parts (Fig. 6.4):

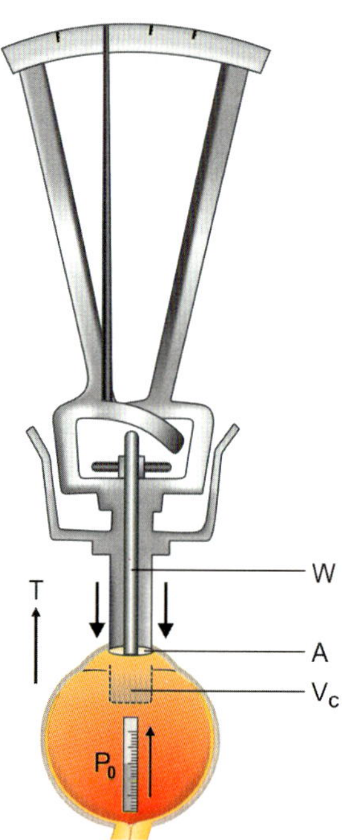

Fig. 6.3 *Basic principle of indentation tonometry*

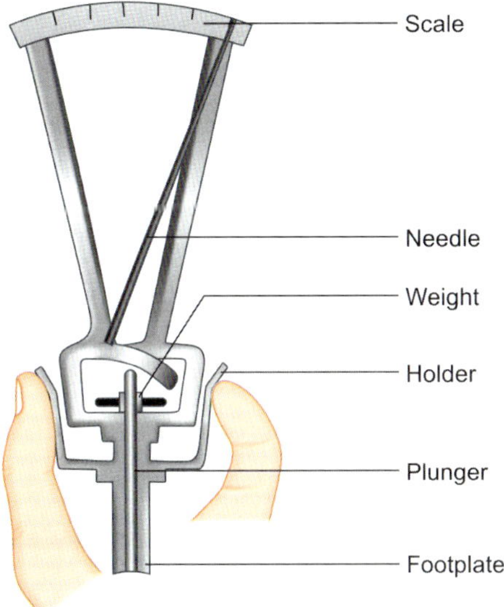

Fig. 6.4 *Schiotz tonometer*

- *Handle* for holding the instrument in vertical position on the cornea
- *Footplate* which rests on the cornea
- *Plunger* which moves freely within a shaft in the footplate
- A bent *lever* whose short arm rests on the upper end of the plunger and a long arm which acts as a pointer needle. The degree to which the plunger indents the cornea is indicated by the movement of this needle on a scale
- *Weights:* 5.5 g weight is permanently fixed to the plunger, which can be increased by extra weight to 7.5, 10 and 15 g.

Technique of Schiotz tonometry

After anaesthetising the cornea with 2–4% topical xylocaine, patient is made to lie supine on a couch and instructed to fix at a target on the ceiling. The examiner separates the lids with left hand and gently rests the footplate of the tonometer vertically on the centre of cornea. The reading on scale is recorded as soon as the needle becomes steady (Fig. 6.5).

It is customary to start with 5.5 g weight. However, if the scale reading is less than 3, additional weight should be added to the plunger to make it 7.5 g or 10 g as indicated; since with Schiotz tonometer the greatest

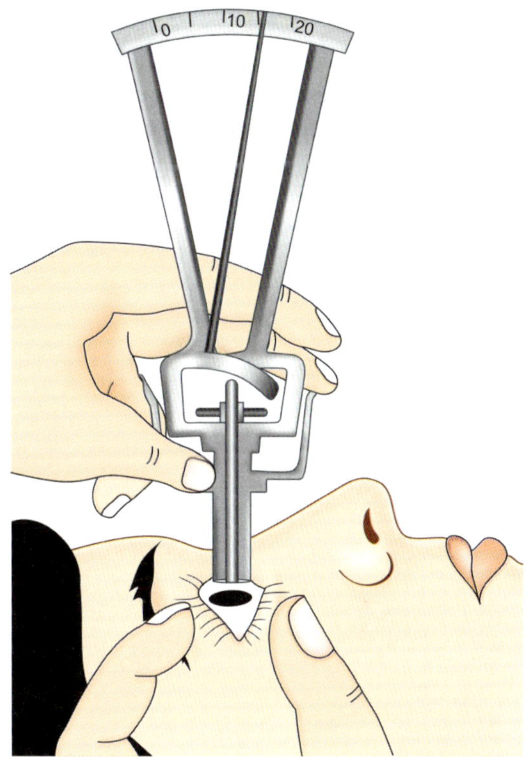

Fig. 6.5 *Technique of Schiotz tonometry*

accuracy is attained when the deflection of the lever is between 3 and 4.

Conversion of scale reading to baseline IOP

The conversion of P_t (pressure with the tonometer on the eye) to P_0 (baseline/resting intraocular pressure) is obtained from the conversion tables developed by Friedenwald. The calibration was carried by experiments in cadaveric eyes connected with a manometer through a cannula. The scale readings of the tonometer with different weights were recorded for different levels of IOP set in the manometer. The observations were plotted on a semilog scale, which serve as Friedenwald nomogram (Fig. 6.6). The original conversion tables, referred to as the 1948 tables were calculated using an average K of 0.0245. Friedenwald later revised the average K to a value of 0.0215, on which he based a new set of table known as Friedenwald Table (1955) (Table 6.1). Subsequent studies indicate that the 1948 tables agree more closely

Table 6.1 *Friedenwald (1955) Table for Schiotz tonometry*

Schiotz scale reading	*IOP (mm Hg) with different plunger body weights*			
	5.5 g	7.5 g	10 g	15 g
3.0	24.4	35.8	50.6	81.8
3.5	22.4	33.0	46.9	76.2
4.0	20.6	30.4	43.4	71.0
4.5	18.9	28.0	40.2	66.2
5.0	17.3	25.8	37.2	61.8
5.5	15.9	23.8	34.4	57.6
4.0	20.6	30.4	43.4	71.0
4.5	18.9	28.0	40.2	66.2
5.0	17.3	25.8	37.2	61.8
5.5	15.9	23.8	34.4	57.6
6.0	14.6	21.9	31.8	53.6
6.5	13.4	20.1	29.4	49.9
7.0	12.2	18.5	27.2	46.5
7.5	11.2	17.0	25.1	43.2
8.0	10.2	15.6	23.1	40.2
8.5	9.4	14.3	21.3	38.1
9.0	8.5	13.1	19.6	34.6
9.5	7.8	12.0	18.0	32.0
10.0	7.1	10.9	16.5	29.6

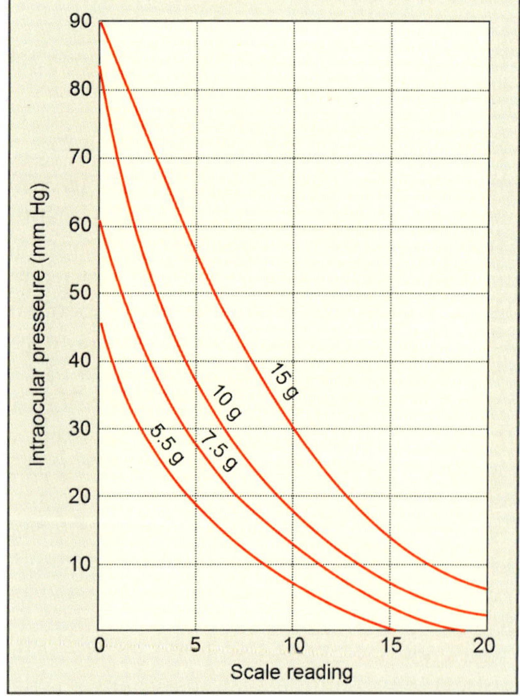

Fig. 6.6 *Friedenwald 1955 nomogram for Schiotz tonometer*

with measurements by Goldmann applanation tonometry.

Errors of indentation tonometry

1. ***Errors inherent in the instrument.*** These may be in the form of difference in the weight of different parts of the tonometer, difference in the size and shape and curvature of the footplate, friction arising in the working of plunger and differences in the smoothness of gliding movement of the pointer on the scale. The American Academy of Ophthalmology and Otolaryngology has established a committee on tonometer standardization, which has got rigid criteria for Schiotz tonometers.

2. ***Errors due to contraction of extraocular muscles.*** When a tonometer is placed on the eye, always there occurs some reflex contraction of the extraocular muscles, which tends to increase the intraocular pressure.

3. ***Errors due to accommodation.*** When the tonometer is brought near to the eye, there is a tendency to look at the tonometer and thus inadvertently accommodation comes into play.

The contraction of ciliary muscle in accommodation also increases the facility of aqueous outflow by pulling on the trabeculae and thus causes some lowering of IOP.

4. ***Errors due to ocular rigidity.*** Conversion tables of Schiotz tonometer are based on an average coefficient of ocular rigidity (K). However, the ocular rigidity may differ significantly in certain eyes and thus false values of IOP are obtained. Thus, the deduction of IOP from tonometric readings will be higher in an eye with a higher ocular rigidity and lower in an eye with an abnormal low ocular rigidity. Factors affecting ocular rigidity are described in the section of ocular rigidity.

5. ***Errors due to variation in corneal curvature and thickness.*** Either a steeper or thicker cornea will cause a greater displacement of fluid during indentation tonometry which leads to a falsely high IOP readings. Thus, errors may arise in cases of microphthalmos, buphthalmos, and high myopia and corneal scars.

6. ***Errors in scale reading.*** An error of one scale reading on either side may occur during observations. Thus, an actual IOP of 17.3 mm Hg (scale reading 5) may be noted as 14.6 mm Hg (scale reading 6) or 20.6 mm Hg (scale reading 4).

7. ***Blood volume alteration.*** The variable expulsion of intraocular blood during indentation tonometry may also influence the IOP measurement.

8. ***Moses effect.*** At low scale readings, the cornea may mould into the space between the plunger and hole, pushing the plunger up and leading to falsely high pressure readings.

9. ***Repeated measurements*** lower the IOP.

Conclusion. Thus, from the above, it is quite clear that the results of indentation tonometry are never absolutely accurate. An error to the tune of ± 2 mm Hg in normal range of IOP and of ± 4 mm Hg in higher range of IOP has been reported.

Sterilization of Schiotz tonometer

Dissemble between each use and the barrel is cleaned with two pipe cleaners, the first soaked in alcohol and the second dry. The footplate is cleaned with alcohol swab. All surfaces must be dried before reassembling.

Electronic Schiotz tonometer

It provides a continuous recording of IOP that is used for tonography. The scale is also magnified which makes it easier to detect small changes in IOP. It is limited to experimental studies in the present era.

APPLANATION TONOMETRY

The concept of applanation tonometry is based on *Imbert-Fick law* which states that the pressure inside a sphere (P) is equal to the force (W) required to flatten its surface divided by the area of flattening (A), i.e. P = W/A (Fig. 6.7).

Therefore, one can determine the pressure by measuring either the force necessary to flatten a fixed area or by measuring the area flattened by a fixed force. Applanation tonometers have been designed using both the principles.

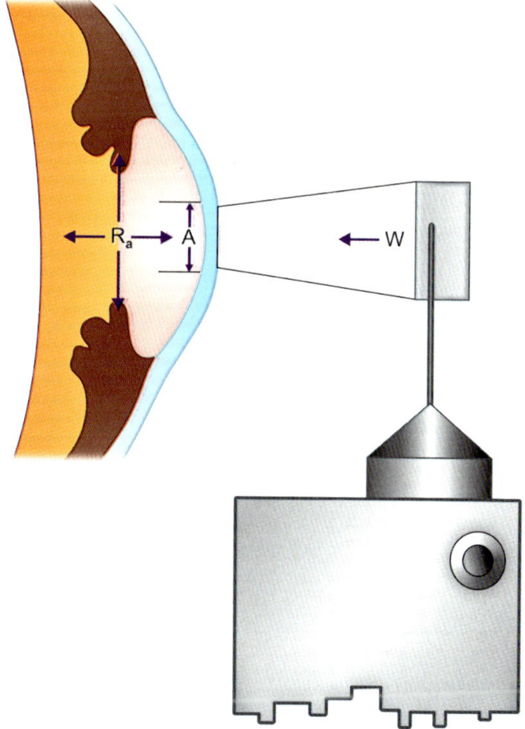

Fig. 6.7 *Imbert-Fick law: W= PA; Modified Imbert-Fick law: W+S= PA1 + B*

I. VARIABLE AREA (FIXED FORCE) APPLANATION TONOMETERS

This type of tonometer measures the area of the cornea that is flattened by a known force.

Maklakov tonometer

Introduced in 1885, it consisted of a dumb-bell-shaped metal cylinder with flat end plates of polished glass on either end with diameter of 10 mm. A set of four such instruments was available, weighing 5, 7.5, 10 and 15 g.

Technique

A thin coat of the dye is smeared on the anaesthetised cornea with the patient supine, the flat bottom of the tonometer allowed to rest on the cornea. In this way, the dye from the flattened part of cornea is transferred to the tonometer bottom, which allows the measurement of the area flattened by a fixed force. The IOP is then read from the conversion tables.

Presently, this tonometer is not much popular.

Other variable area applanation tonometers

Other variable area applanation tonometers developed are:

- ***Applanometer:*** Ceramic end plates
- ***Tonomat:*** Disposable end plates
- ***Halberg tonometer:*** Transparent end plate for direct reading
- ***Barraquer tonometer:*** Plastic tonometer for use in operating room
- ***Ocular tension indicator:*** Uses Goldmann prisms and standard weight, for screening (measures above or below 21 mm Hg)
- ***Glaucotest:*** Screening tonometer with multiple end plates for selecting different cut-off pressures.

II. VARIABLE FORCE (FIXED AREA) APPLANATION TONOMETERS

This type of tonometer measures the force that is required to applanate a standard area of the corneal surface.

Fick in 1888 devised the first fixed area applanation tonometer. However, it was Goldmann who in 1954 modernized this concept and developed a tonometer which has revolutionized the use of applanation tonometry all over the world. This method of tonometry is far more accurate than indentation tonometry since in this technique a very tiny area of the cornea is applanated so the ocular rigidity does not interfere with the readings.

Some of the fixed area applanation tonometers are described below.

Goldmann applanation tonometer (GAT)

Currently, Goldmann applanation tonometer (GAT) is the most popular and accurate tonometer. It is mounted on the end of a lever hinged on a standard slit-lamp.

Technique

After anaesthetising the cornea with a drop of 2% xylocaine and staining the tear film with fluorescein, patient is made to sit in front of a slit-lamp. The cornea and biprisms are illuminated with cobalt blue light from the slit-lamp. The examiner views through the centre of a plastic biprism, which is used to applanate the cornea. Biprism is then advanced until it just touches the apex of cornea (Fig. 6.8). At this

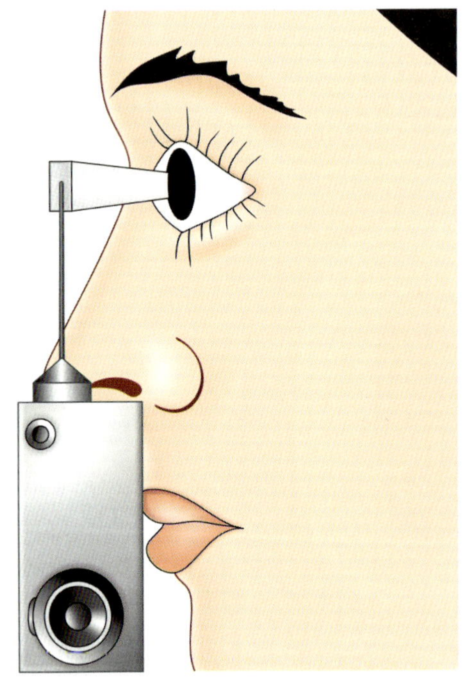

Fig. 6.8 *Technique of applanation tonometry*

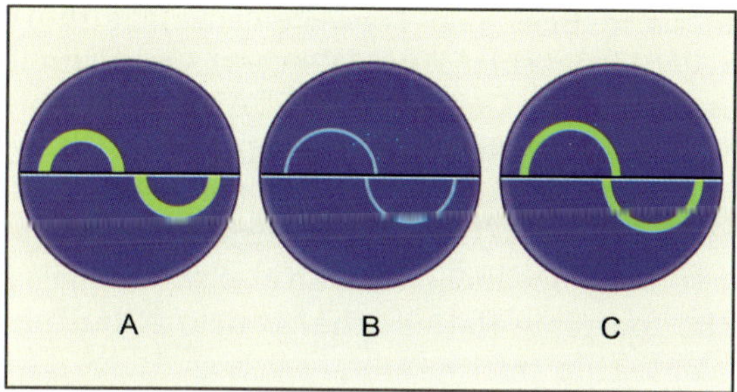

Fig. 6.9 *Goldmann applanation mires showing end point of applanation tonometry: (A) too small mires; (B) too large mires; (C) end point*

point, two fluorescent semicircles are viewed through the prism. Then, the applanation force against cornea is adjusted until the inner edges of the two semicircles just touch (Fig. 6.9). This is the end point. The prisms are caliberated in such a way that inner margins of semicircles touch when 3.06 mm of cornea is applanated. The intraocular pressure is determined by multiplying the dial reading with ten to obtain IOP in mm Hg.

Sources of error

1. ***Fluorescein concentration*** affects the thickness of the mires leading to overestimation (with thick mires) or underestimation (with thin mires) of IOP.

2. ***Inappropriate vertical alignment*** gives higher IOP readings.

3. ***Central corneal thickness.*** There is underestimation of IOP in thin corneas and overestimation in thick corneas.

4. ***Corneal curvature.*** For every 3D increase in corneal curvature, IOP rises approximately by 1 mm Hg as more fluid is displaced under steeper corneas causing increase in ocular rigidity.

5. ***Corneal astigmatism.*** With the rule (WTR) astigmatism underestimates while against the rule (ATR) astigmatism overestimates the IOP. To minimize this, tonometer biprism should be rotated so that axis of least corneal curvature is opposite the red mark on the biprism. This results in a separation of 43° and an applanation of an area of approximately 7.35 mm^2. The other method is to obtain measurements in both vertical and horizontal meridians and average these readings.

6. ***Irregular corneal surface*** leads to distortion of mires.

Effect of central corneal thickness

Variations in central corneal thickness (CCT) change the resistance of the cornea to indentation so that this is no longer balanced entirely by the tear film surface tension thus affecting the accuracy of IOP measurement. A thinner cornea (physiological variation, pathological or post-PRK/LASIK) would require less force to applanate it, leading to underestimation of IOP and vice versa.

Goldmann applanation tonometer was designed to give accurate reading when the CCT was 520 μ. There occurs a change in applanation readings of 0.7 mm Hg per 10 μ. Thus, a correction factor, as described by Dredsner (Table 6.2), is required to get accurate IOP levels with applanation tonometry.

Sterilization

Methods used to sterilize applanation tonometer biprisms include:

- Soaking applanation tip for 5–15 minutes in diluted sodium hypochlorite, hydrogen peroxide 3% or isopropyl alcohol 70%, or by wiping with alcohol, hydrogen peroxide, povidone iodine or 1 : 1000 merthiolate are some easy and handy methods to sterilize the biprism of applanation tonometer.
- Ten minutes of rinsing in running tap water.

Table 6.2 *Dredsner correction table for IOP measured using GAT*

Corneal thickness (in μ)	*Correction factor (in mm Hg)*
460–485	+3
486–512	+2
513–536	+1
537–562	0
563–587	–1
588–612	–2
613–637	–3
638–662	–4
663–687	–5

- Soap and water wash
- Disposable film covers for tips
- Exposure to UV light

Hand-held Tonometers

1. ***Perkin's applanation tonometer*** (Fig. 6.10). It is a hand-held tonometer utilizing the same biprism as in the Goldmann applanation tonometer. It is small, easy to carry and does not require slit-lamp. The light source is powered by a battery and the force is varied manually. A counterbalance makes it possible to use the instrument in either the vertical or horizontal position. It is not used commonly now.
2. ***Draeger applanation tonometer.*** Similar to the Perkin's tonometer, but uses a different biprism and has an electric motor that varies the force.

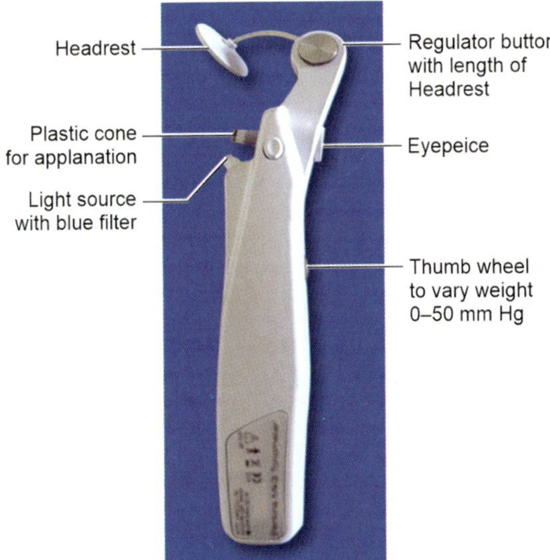

Fig. 6.10 *Perkin's hand-held applanation tonometer*

3. ***Tono-Pen.*** The Tono-Pen and the more recent Tono-Pen Avia (Reichert Ophthalmic Instruments, Depew, NY, USA) are portable lightweight battery-powered devices, which use the principles of applanation and indentation (Fig. 6.11A–C). The tonopen instrument is with a strain gauge that creates an electrical signal as the footplate flattens the cornea. A built-in single-chip microprocessor senses the proper force curves and averages 4 to 10 readings to give a final digital readout. It also provides the percentage of variability between the lowest and highest acceptable readings from 5 to 20%.

Numerous studies have reported the usefulness of these devices in clinics in comparison with GAT, but the repeatability coefficients for intra-session repeated measurement have been shown to be quite high (±4.3 mm Hg). Clinical studies have shown that Tono-Pen can be significantly affected by CCT. This tonometry, however, seems to provide better accuracy in edematous corneas in comparison with GAT and dynamic contour tonometry. It is important to note that different tonometers cannot be used interchangeably.

Advantages of Tono-pen

- Used in cases of corneal epithelial irregularities.
- Measurement of IOP over bandage contact lens.
- Useful in oedematous and scarred corneas.
- Useful in patients with nystagmus and head tremors.
- Used in operation theatre
- Portable

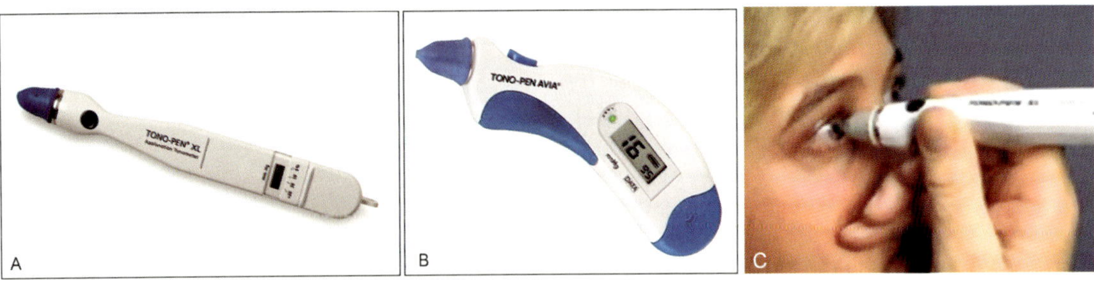

Fig. 6.11 *A, Tono-Pen; B, Tono-Pen Avia; C, Technique to Tono-pen tonometry*

4. ***iCARE or rebound tonometer***. iCARE or Rebound tonometer (Fig. 6.12) consists of a pair of coils coaxial with the probe shaft, a solenoid coil and a sensing coil. A lightweight probe is propelled towards the cornea by the solenoid and the sensing coil monitors the movement. The speed immediately before impact, the deceleration during impact and the ratio of these parameters are correlated to the IOP.

Does not require anaesthesia and can be used in children. Disposable tips enable it to be used in situations of high risk of infection.

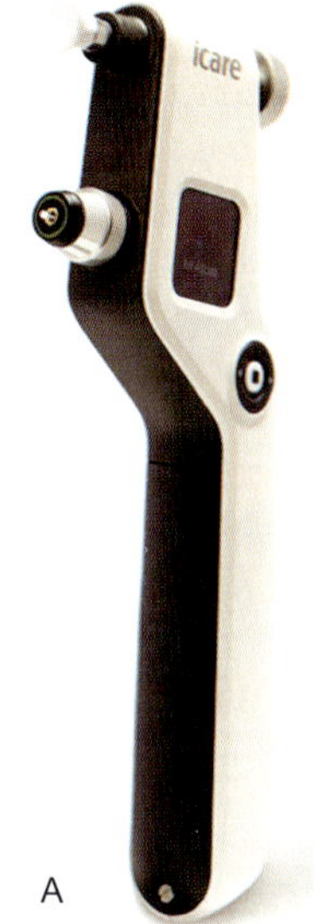

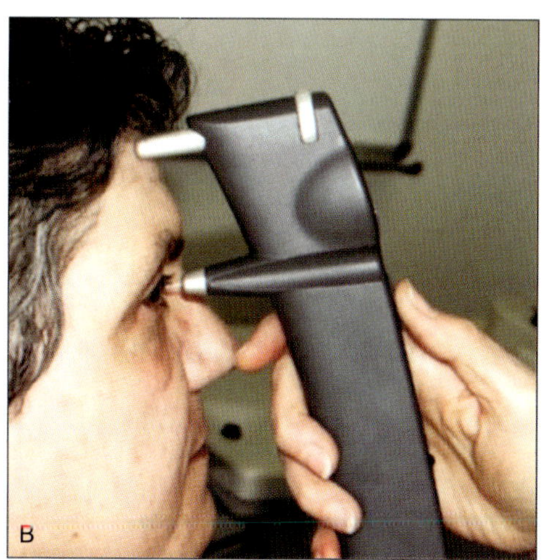

Fig. 6.12 *iCARE or rebound tonometers (A) and technique (B)*

It tends to overestimate IOP compared to GAT.

The iCare PRO version released in 2011 uses a shorter probe, which can also be used to measure IOP in a supine position. The most recent versions of this instrument, which are updated versions of the iCare PRO with a long probe (iCare IC100 and IC200) (Fig. 6.13A,B), provide new features, such as a red or green light to show if the position of the probe is correct, in addition to providing the possibility of measuring IOP in a supine position.

A simplified version [iCare One, replaced at first by the iCare Home and, recently, by the iCare Home2 (Fig. 6.14A–C)], which can autonomously be used by patients, has recently been introduced for at-home auto-tonometry. It can be helpful for detecting IOP peaks, especially in suspect glaucoma and in normal tension glaucoma subjects, when IOP measurements appear to be normal during office hours.

Numerous studies have compared the different versions of iCare with GAT and other non-conventional tonometers. When compared to gold standard GAT, clinical results report a good correlation of tonometry readings, with r values greater than 0.8 for low-to-moderate GAT readings. A recent study showed agreement between GAT readings and iCare to be good, with a <2 mm Hg mean difference for all ranges of IOP. For IOP >23 mm Hg, rebound tonometry tends to underestimate IOP compared to GAT, showing readings that are significantly lower.

Considering that rebound tonometry may be less traumatic on the cornea compared to GAT,

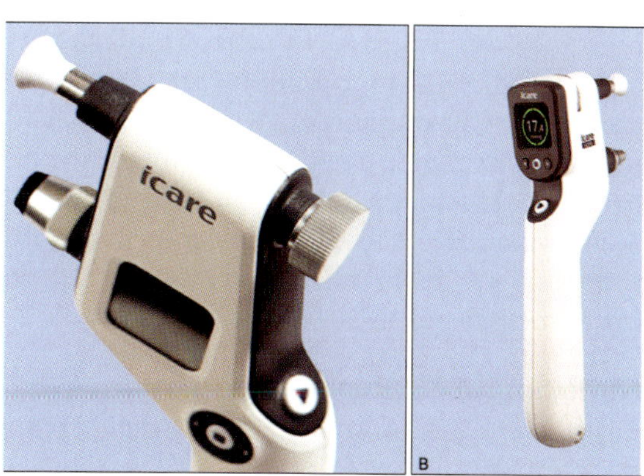

Fig. 6.13 A, *iCare 100;* B, *iCare 200 version*

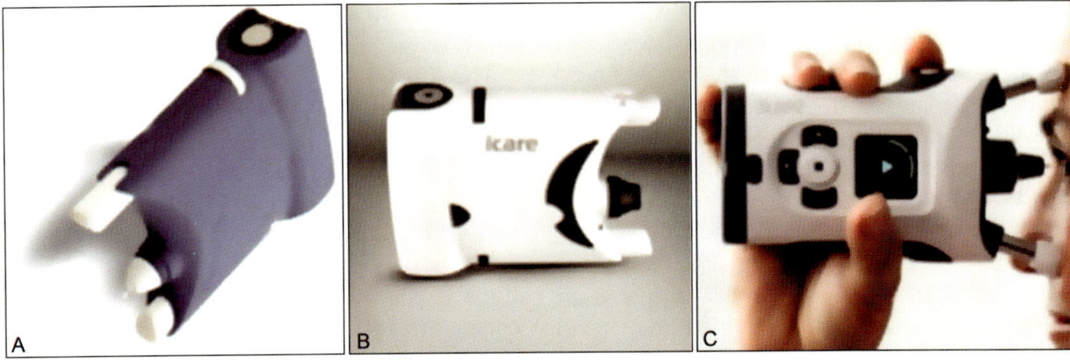

Fig. 6.14 *A, iCare One; B, iCare Home; C, iCare Home 2*

it could offer a better alternative in post-operative patients to provide information regarding IOP. It is important to note that GAT measurements tend to be lower than iCare for post-operative patients with corneal edema. The agreement between iCare and GAT has been reported to be acceptable in lamellar keratoplasty subjects; yet, it has been reported to be poor for patients with penetrating keratoplasty. Rebound tonometry surely cannot replace GAT. However, it may prove to be clinically useful in post-operative eyes with fragile anterior segments, or eyes with increased risk of infection, in which GAT is impractical or not indicated.

SmartLens for tonometry

It has a contact lens that incorporates an electronic pressure sensor, which is able to measure IOP and ocular pulse amplitude continuously by applanation of the central cornea. There is a Myler membrane covered hole at the centre of the lens. The cavity behind the membrane is filled with silicone oil and is connected with a piezoelectric pressure transducer. The measurement of IOP is achieved by the transmission of pressure through the oil to the transducer when the applanation membrane is displaced during its contact with the cornea. It is being used mainly in experimental studies.

Proview-pressue phosphene tonometer

It is a patient self-monitoring device that utilizes a psychophysical technique based on entopic phenomenon of pressure phosphenes.

Implantable IOP sensors

- ***IOP-IOL probe.*** A sensor incorporated in the haptics of an IOL for continuous monitoring of IOP.
- ***Contact lens sensor.*** It correlates the spherical deformation of eyeball with the changes in IOP.
- ***Choroid-IOP sensor.*** Sensor lies in contact with choroid.

NON-CONTACT TONOMETRY

Non-contact tonometry (NCT) was first designed by Zeiss and developed by Grolman in 1972. Several models have been proposed in the past few decades that use a pulse of air to flatten the cornea without the need for touching the eye (Fig. 6.15A and B); such models, therefore, do not require anesthesia or fluorescein drops. In the **Pulsair tonometer**, a light beam is used in combination with a sensor that stops the production of air and measures the force used at the moment of corneal flattening.

Numerous studies have examined the differences in IOP measured with various types of NCT instruments and other non-conventional tonometers compared to GAT. Demirci, et al. showed that IOP measurements with NCT were significantly higher than those obtained with both GAT and rebound tonometry, with significant differences ($p < 0.001$) in all age groups. A recent study confirmed that NCT tends to overestimate IOP GAT measurements in patients with IOP >16 mm Hg, which was more evident when IOP >20 mm Hg, showing a decrease in accuracy at higher values.

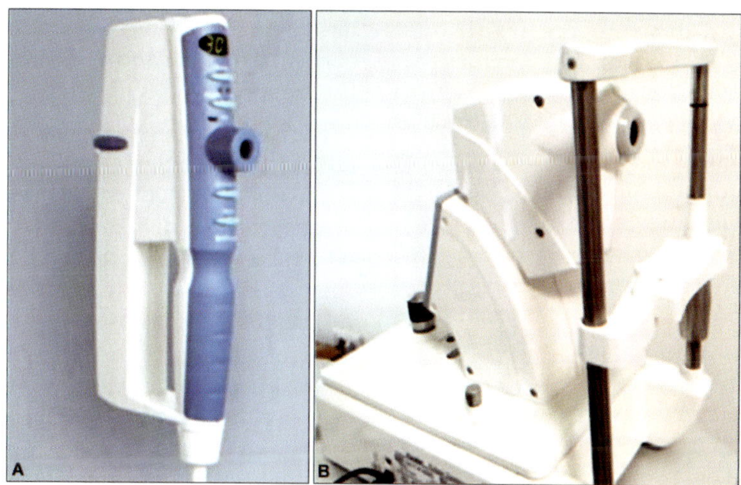

Fig. 6.15 *Pulsair EasyEye handheld: A, and Pulsair desktop; B, non-contact tonometers*

Early studies in 1989 based on the comparisons with GAT, showed that up to 70% of NCT measurements fell within ±3 mm Hg of readings taken with GAT. When using a screening criteria of IOP >21 mm Hg, NCT showed a sensitivity of 85% and a specificity of 95%.

Similar to GAT and other instruments, NCT is influenced by corneal parameters. Kyei, et al. showed a significant association between CCT and NCT, which is greater than that reported with GAT. These finding were confirmed in a recent study, which concluded that GAT measurements are not equivalent and cannot be interchanged with those obtained by NCT.

The pros of NCT are mostly based on the ease of use, non-contact nature and portability of several devices. Measurements can be taken by non-medical staff and patient compliance is relatively good. In most cases NCT does not require slit-lamp positioning; thus, it is easily used in cases with elderly individuals, children, disabled patients and patients with limited collaboration. NCT can be considered for patients that may not tolerate topical anesthetics, patients with limited collaboration or those at greater risk of infection.

The disadvantages of NCT include the fact that NCT is less accurate when IOP >20 mm Hg. Studies have shown that NCT results depend on the instrument brand, unit and model of the device used. Comparison studies between three NTC devices showed that, when taking GAT as the gold standard and aiming to detect IOP >21 mm Hg, sensitivities greatly differed from 40%, 48% and 80%, which showed that NCT readings are device dependent and that devices require regular calibration. Although NCT offers a non-contact mode of measuring that limits the risk of infection due to contaminated drops or Goldmann prisms, the risk of air-borne infection could be greater considering the air-puff nature, which should be considered in the midst of the recent COVID era.

NCT could be helpful in a day-to-day clinical setting that involves dealing mostly with normal patients undergoing routine checkups. This type of tonometry can be ideal as a screening tool, which can easily be performed by non-medical staff. Although studies have shown that NCT tends to overestimate GAT measurements, NCT can prove to be useful for post-operative patients with lid edema, limited collaboration, ocular pain, discomfort and increased tear film meniscus size, which are all factors that influence proper GAT measurements. NCT can be a useful screening tool, but should never replace or be interchanged with GAT, especially in the management of patients with risk factors, ocular hypertension, suspect patients and glaucoma.

Other types of non-contact tonometers, with new interesting features, have recently been introduced. In addition to the traditional tonometers, these devices show IOP values that take CCT and corneal biomechanics into account, claiming to provide more accurate IOP measurements.

Ocular Response Analyzer (Reichert Technologies, Depew, NY, USA) or ORA, developed in 2005 by Luce, et al., is a non-contact air-puff tonometer that provides an optical electrical device to measure the deformation of the cornea caused by the impact of the air (Fig. 6.16).

The force of the air makes the cornea move in an inward fashion in a first applanation state, causing it to take on a slight concave shape, to then move outward in a further applanation state, and finally to take on a normal configuration state. The electro-optical applanation detection system registers the curvature of the cornea in a diameter of 3 mm in the center for 20 msec. The two inward and outward applanation events, which are delayed by the viscoelastic corneal damping, allow for the calculations of two different IOP values based on the applanation principle. The instruments provide an average of these two pressure measurements and supply the so-called Goldmann-correlated IOP value (IOPg); the corneal hysteresis (CH) parameter is based on the difference between these two measurements of pressure. The instrument also provides a corneal-compensated IOP (IOPcc), which is

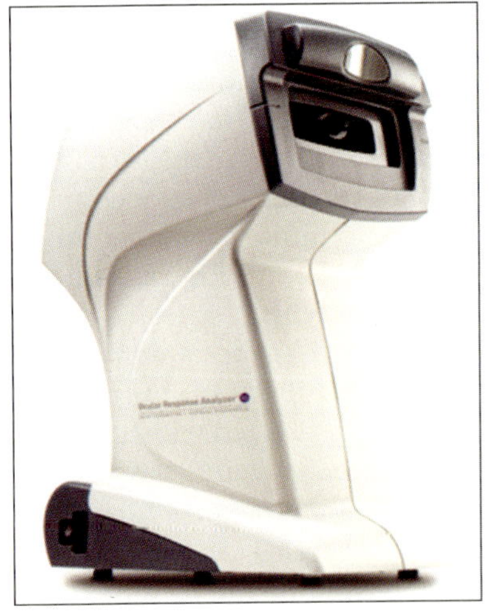

Fig. 6.16 *Ocular Response Analyzer (ORA) mod.G3*

based on the biomechanical properties of the cornea (elasticity and viscosity), to compensate for the measured IOP values.

The Reichert ORA measures corneal resistance factor (the viscoelastic properties of the cornea) and corneal hysteresis (the ability of the cornea to absorb and dissipate energy)-the latter of which has been reported to be an independent risk factor for both the development and progression of glaucoma.

Corneal hysteresis is the ability of the cornea to absorb and dissipate applied forces based on its viscoelastic and elasticity properties. ORA was designed to theoretically improve IOP accuracy, allowing clinicians to account for the variability in corneal biomechanical properties seen among patients. Corneal hysteresis has been demonstrated to contribute to glaucoma progression risk, with lower values imparting a greater risk of glaucoma progression. Like GAT, ORA is a desktop instrument and thus cannot be used on supine patients. Although the corneal compensation parameters have been developed to provide IOP measurements less affected by corneal factors, studies have shown overestimated ORA measurements in eyes with high levels of IOP. Further clinical studies are needed to assess the clinical use of ORA in glaucoma management.

The IOP value is a calculated value and not the true IOP, therefore, prone for errors.

Less influenced by the corneal resistance and thickness, ORA is useful in post-LASIK IOP measurement and in those having INTACS.

Pros and cons to the ORA is a relatively expensive device, but it is easy to handle, and topical anesthesia and fluorescein are not needed. In comparison with GAT, ORA has been demonstrated to significantly overestimate the IOP values, especially at high IOP levels. Several authors have demonstrated that the IOPcc is less affected by corneal properties and may better reflect the true IOP after refractive surgery of the cornea when compared to GAT IOP values.

Recent studies have shown that the ORA IOPcc values were superior to the GAT IOP measurements in predicting rates of glaucoma progression. The CH parameter has been associated with other parameters of damage due to glaucoma, such as high cup-to-disc ratio and defects in the visual field. Several studies have shown a low CH value to be an independent predictor of functional damage occurrence or progression in the visual field in patients affected by ocular hypertension or glaucoma. Moreover, the CH value can help in detecting patients with pathologies of the cornea such as keratoconus. It may also be a useful parameter for patients at risk of developing corneal ectasia after refractive LASIK surgery.

Corvis ST (Oculus, Wezlar, Germany), It is a novel non-contact instrument, released in 2011, based on the system that causes indentation of the cornea by a jet of air. The tonometer has a built-in Scheimpflug ultra-high-speed device (Fig. 6.17).

This instrument provides IOP measurements based on the indentation principle, in addition to pachymetry taken by on optical device and other biomechanical parameters of the cornea obtained by registering the surface deformation due to an applied air pulse, similar to an ORA device. A Scheimpflug camera visualizes an 8.5 mm diameter of the center of the surface of the cornea and precisely records the corneal deformation induced by the air-jet and its return to its normal shape with a high resolution and more than 4300 frames per second. A biomechanically corrected IOP value (bIOP), which takes the individual corneal deformation parameters into account, is also provided by the device.

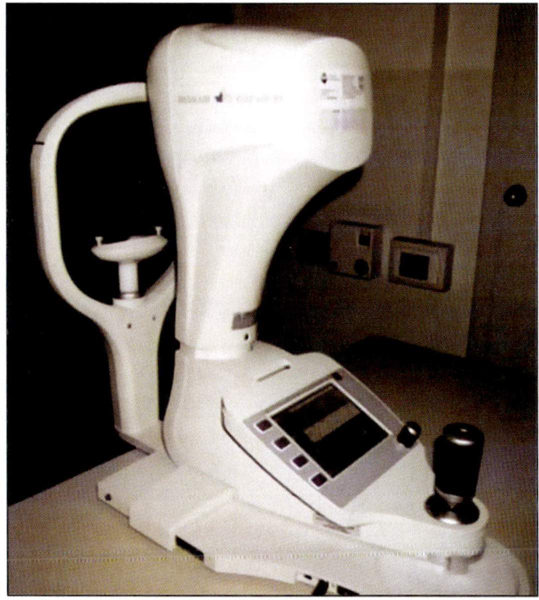

Fig. 6.17 *Corvis tonometer*

The Corvis ST precision for the CCT and IOP values has been shown to be excellent; however, it is moderate for the corneal deformation parameters. Previous studies demonstrated that Corvis ST tends to underestimate IOP readings obtained with GAT. The Corvis ST biomechanically corrected IOP values (bIOP) have been shown to be less influenced by the CCT and corneal biomechanics and to be more effective in measuring the IOP in subjects who underwent refractive surgery. Moreover, the Corvis ST corneal deformation parameters have been shown to be effective in discriminating between normal and keratoconic eyes.

PNEUMOTONOMETERS

Pneumotonometers are devices based on the applanation principle, which use a different technology: the tonometer probe consists of a hollow central tube flanked by a side exhaust, and the sensor is air pressure, which is dependent on the resistance of the exhaust. During the cornea applanation, the pressure within the central tubes increases to match the force generated by the IOP. A pneumatic electronic transducer converts the air pressure to a tracer on a strip of paper (Fig. 6.18).

In several studies, pneumotonometry proved to be quite accurate and reliable in glaucoma screening and showed a greater reliability compared to GAT after PRK and LASIK. Pneumotonometers such as the Pulsatile Ocular

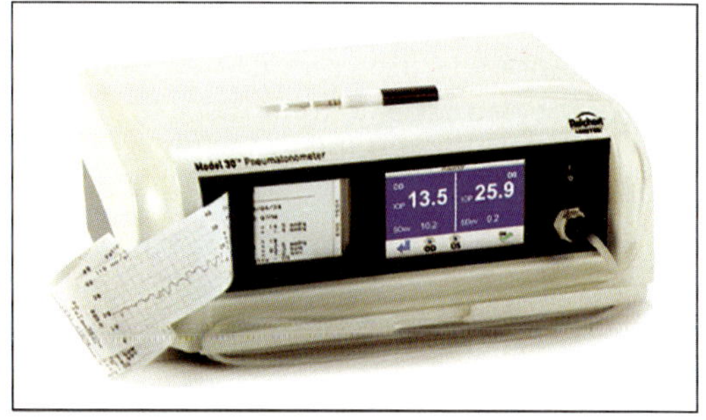

Fig. 6.18 *Pneumotonometer*

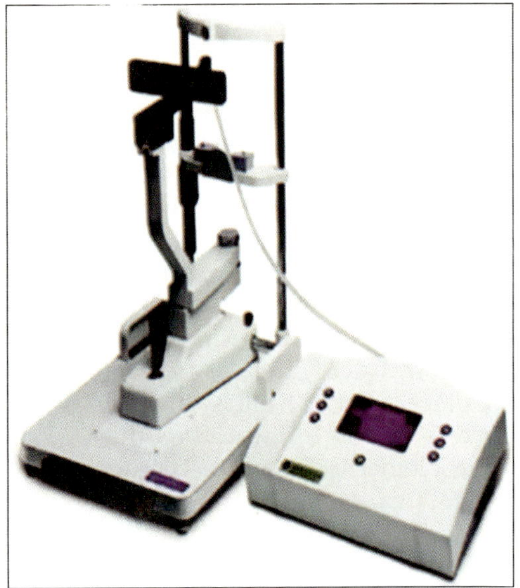

Fig. 6.19 *Langham ocular blood flow pneumotonometer*

Blood Flow (OBF, Fig. 6.19) have been used in the past to measure the pulse fluctuation and thereby give indirect information regarding the ocular blood pulse. OBF measurements, however, appear to be more influenced by CCT and more variable than GAT readings, with a significant overestimation. The clinical usefulness of this instrument in clinics still remains controversial.

MISCELLANEOUS ADVANCEMENTS IN TONOMETERS

PASCAL DYNAMIC CONTOUR TONOMETER

It is a newer applanation tonometer (Fig. 6.20) that uses principle of contour-matching to measure IOP instead of applanation to eliminate the systemic errors inherent in previous tonometers.

It uses a miniature pressure sensor embedded within a tonometer tip contour-matched to the shape of the cornea. The tonometer tip rests on the cornea with a constant appositional force of one gram. When the sensor is subjected to a change in pressure, the electrical resistance is altered and the Pascal's computer calculates a change in pressure in concordance with the change in resistance.

It repeatedly samples IOP 100 times per second in addition to ocular pulse amplitude and the systemic pulse rate and provides a digital output of the IOP and a graphic output of the ocular pressure pulse. A complete measurement cycle requires about eight seconds of contact time. Audio feedback helps the clinician to ensure proper contact with the cornea.

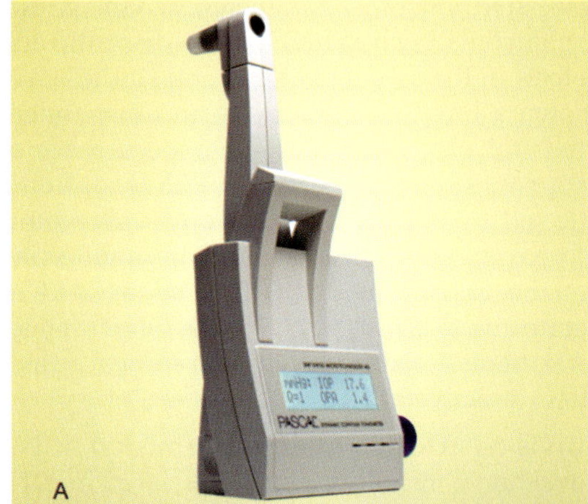

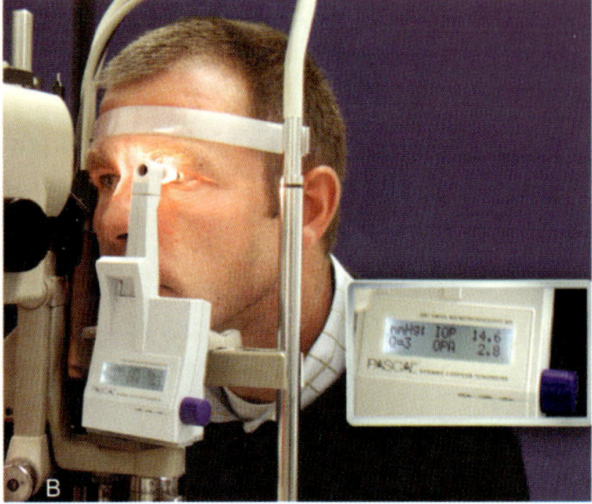

Fig. 6.20 *Pascal dynamic contour tonometer*

DIATOM TRANSPALPEBRAL TONOMETER

It is a hand-held device using a free falling thin rod on the stretched upper eyelid. It is based on processing the rod acceleration time resulting from its free fall from the constant height and the interaction with eye through the eyelid.

It requires no contact with the cornea, therefore, sterilization of the device and anaesthesia are not required. It is of use especially in children, those with corneal pathology, or those who have had corneal surgery.

TONOMETRY IN SPECIAL SITUATIONS

Tonometry in some special situations (Table 6.3) is as below.

Tonometry on irregular corneas

Pneumatic tonometers provide the most accurate result in eyes with diseased or irregular corneas. There is overestimation of IOP with Tono-Pen in such patients.

Other tonometers which can also be used are:

- Non-contact tonometers
- MacKay-Marg tonometer, and
- Tono-Pen

Tonometry over soft contact lens

Pneumotonometer and Tono-Pen measure IOP through bandage contact lenses with reasonable accuracy.

Tonometry in presence of intraocular gases

In eyes after pars plana vitrectomy and gas fluid exchange, there occurs alteration in scleral rigidity rendering indentation tonometry unsatisfactory. Pneumatic tonometers underestimate Goldmann IOP measurement. Tono-Pen measurements are comparable.

Tonometry in shallow anterior chamber

There is much variability in IOP measurements with GAT, pneumotonometer and Tono-Pen.

Tonometry in eyes with keratoprosthesis

Due to rigid surface of keratoprosthesis, it is impossible to measure IOP with indentation or applanation tonometers. Digital IOP assessment is the only applicable method in such eyes.

OCULAR RIGIDITY

Ocular or scleral rigidity is an expression of the stretchability of the eye in response to an increase in the intraocular pressure. The stretchability of any substance depends upon its inherent elasticity plus its thickness and a time-dependent variable called viscoelasticity. Viscoelasticity refers to the change in elasticity that occur over time. Like most viscoelastic systems, the sclera will stretch proportionately more with initial elevations of intraocular pressure, and as the pressure increases, the resistance to further stretching also increases. Therefore, small increase in the intraocular volume at a low pressure causes a small increase in IOP, wherein similar small volume changes at high IOP will cause a much large increase in IOP. This property of sclera, labelled as ocular rigidity, seems an unfortunate term because most persons associate the word rigidity with resistance to bending rather than resistance to stretching. Therefore, the term scleral distensibility would be preferable to scleral rigidity.

FACTORS AFFECTING OCULAR RIGIDITY

Friedenwald denoted the coefficient of scleral rigidity by the word 'E'. He calculated it on cadaveric eyes and found the average value of 'E' to be 0.0215. The Schiotz scale reading intraocular pressure (P_0) conversion table of Friedenwald has been calibrated using average value of ocular rigidity coefficient, assuming that it should work in most of the individuals. But, in practice, variation of ocular rigidity above or below the average value is not so uncommon among different patients. Thus, a high ocular rigidity will cause a falsely high IOP and a low 'E' value will lead to a falsely low reading:

Table 6.3. *Tonometry in special situations*

1. Irregular corneas	Pneumatic tonometer, Mackay Marg, Tono-Pen, DCT
2. Over soft contact lenses	Pneumatic tonometer and TonoPen
3. In Gas-Filled eyes	Pneumatic tonometer and TonoPen
4. Post LASIK status	DCT, ORA
5. Children/screening programs	Perkins, NCT, I- Care
6. In patients having INTACS	ORA
7. In shallow anterior chamber	GAT, pneumotonometer

However, in clinical practice, ocular rigidity measurements for individual patients are not made as often as they should be; this introduces significant errors and makes dependence on the scleral rigidity hazardous.

Conditions influencing ocular rigidity

1. ***Refractive errors.*** Higher values are reported in hypermetropes and lower than the normal in myopes.
2. ***Elevated IOP.*** E-value is decreased with increase in the IOP; this may explain the lower 'E' during water drinking provocative test. However, in long-standing glaucoma, 'E' has been found to be increased.
3. ***Drugs.*** Miotics, especially strong cholinesterase inhibitors, are said to reduce 'E'. Vasodilation may also diminish 'E', while vasoconstriction causes an increase.
4. ***Surgery.*** Ocular rigidity is reduced following retinal detachment surgery, or the intravitreal injection of compressible gas leading to a falsely low IOP estimation with indentation tonometry.
5. ***Age.*** Reports vary widely regarding the correlation of 'E' value and advancing age.

DETERMINATION OF OCULAR RIGIDITY

The technique of determining ocular rigidity is based on Friedenwald's concept of differential tonometry. To determine ocular rigidity, tonometric readings are obtained with any two weights (say 5.5 and 10 g). (A more accurate method is to use the applanation tonometry value as P_0 and one Schiotz reading.) The intraocular pressure in an eye with average normal ocular rigidity will be the same whatever weight is used. But if the rigidity is high then the 10 g weight will show a higher TOP and if the rigidity is low, the IOP with 10 g will be lower than that determined by 5.5 g weight.

In cases with abnormal ocular rigidity, a correction for it has to be done using the Friedenwald nomogram (Fig. 6.21), which consists of the following:

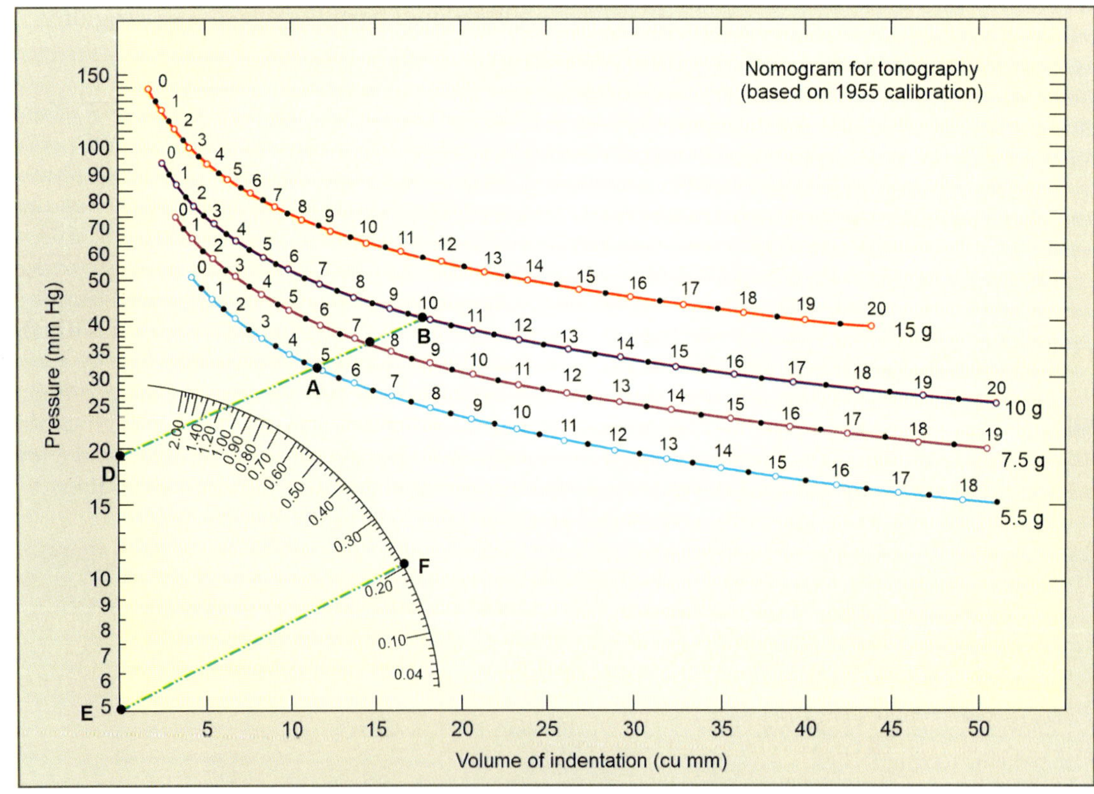

Fig. 6.21 *Scleral rigidity from Friedenwald nomogram (for details see text)*

- There are four slanting curves showing scale readings with 5.5, 7.5, 10 and 15 g weights.
- The ordinate (left margin) of the nomogram shows the IOP in mm Hg.
- The abscissa (lower margin) of the nomogram shows the value of indentation in cu mm.
- The semicircular scale at the lower left hand corner shows the coefficient of ocular rigidity.

How to use Friedenwald nomogram

Plot the result of differential tonometry on the nomogram. In Fig. 6.16, the point A represents the scale reading with 5.5 and B with 10 g weight during differential tonometry. The line joining A and B if extended to the left intersects the ordinate (left margin) at the point D which shows the actual value of intraocular pressure (P_0). Draw another line EF extended through lower left hand corner and parallel to the line DAB. Read scleral rigidity where the line EF crosses the semicircular scale. Normal average coefficient of ocular rigidity is 0.0215.

SUGGESTED READING

1. Comparison of intraocular pressure measured by Pascal dynamic contour tonometry and Goldmann applanation tonometry. Eye 2006; 20:191–98.
2. Development of a completely encapsulated intraocular pressure sensor. Ophthalmic Res 2000;32(6):278–84.
3. Effect of corneal parameters on measurements using the pulsatile ocular blood flow tonograph and Goldmann applanation tonometer. Br J Ophthalmol 2004;88(4):518–22.
4. First steps toward invasive intraocular pressure monitoring with a sensing contact lens. Invest Ophthalmol Vis Sci 2004;45(9):3113–17.

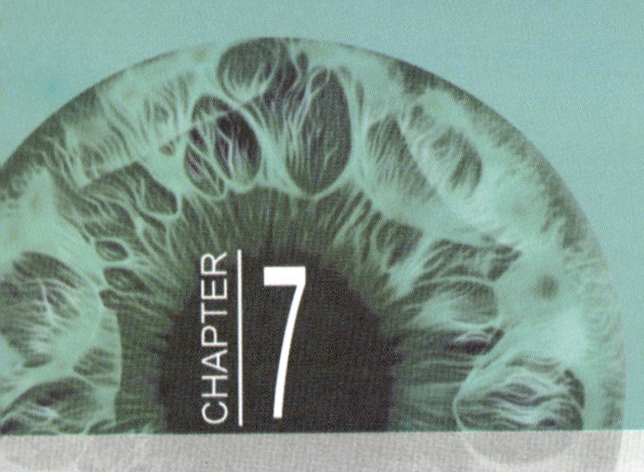

CHAPTER 7 GONIOSCOPY

PRINCIPLE AND INDICATIONS

Principle

Indications

- Diagnostic
- Therapeutic

TECHNIQUES OF GONIOSCOPY

Direct gonioscopy

- Procedure
- Advantages and disadvantages

Indirect gonioscopy

- Commercially available gonioprism
- Procedure

Functional techniques

- Advantages and disadvantages

GONIOSCOPIC VIEW AND GRADING OF ANGLE

- Gonioscopic view of angle structures
- Grading system for the angle
- Biometric gonioscopy

CLINICAL USES AND LIMITATIONS

- Clinical uses
- Critical questions to be answered during gonioscopy
- Limitations and artefacts

PRINCIPLE AND INDICATIONS

The term gonioscopy, derived from the Greek words gō'nē (angle) and ŏs'k-pē (view), was coined by Trantas in 1907. It is a clinical technique that is used to examine structures in the anterior chamber angle. Gonioscopic assessment is essential for diagnosing the type of glaucoma and for planning the appropriate therapy. In fact, without reasonable proficiency in the technique of gonioscopy, anybody should be able to manage glaucomas.

PRINCIPLE OF GONIOSCOPY

A direct view of the angle of anterior chamber is not normally possible with the slit-lamp because of overhanging opaque scleral shelf and the fact that light which emanates from the angle is reflected back into the eye by the cornea owing to phenomenon of total internal reflection.

The total internal reflection at the cornea occurs because the angle of incidence of the rays from the anterior chamber angle structures is greater than the critical angle of the cornea–air interface, which is approximately 46° (Fig. 7.1). The solution to this problem is to eliminate cornea optically. Gonioscopic contact lenses where refractive index is similar to that of cornea eliminate the optical effect of the front corneal surface. Therefore, light rays from the anterior chamber angle enter the contact lens and are made to pass through the new contact lens–air

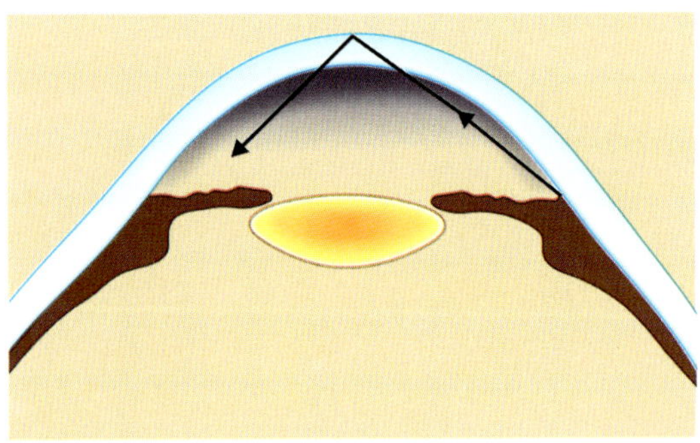

Fig. 7.1 *The angle of incidence of light rays originating from the angle structures is greater than the critical angle of the cornea–air interface, resulting in total internal reflection*

interface by one of the following two basic designs:

1. Direct gonioscopes. In these, the curve of the contact lens (goniolens) is such that the critical angle is not reached and the light rays are refracted at the contact lens–air interface (Fig. 7.2).

2. Indirect gonioscopes. In these, the light rays are reflected by a mirror in the contact lens (gonioprism) and leave the lens nearly at right angle to the contact lens–air interface (Fig. 7.3).

INDICATIONS

Diagnosis and management of glaucoma essentially needs good gonioscopic knowledge. It helps in viewing the trabecular meshwork and determining the cause for elevated intraocular pressure. The indications of gonioscopy can be divided into diagnostic and therapeutic ones.

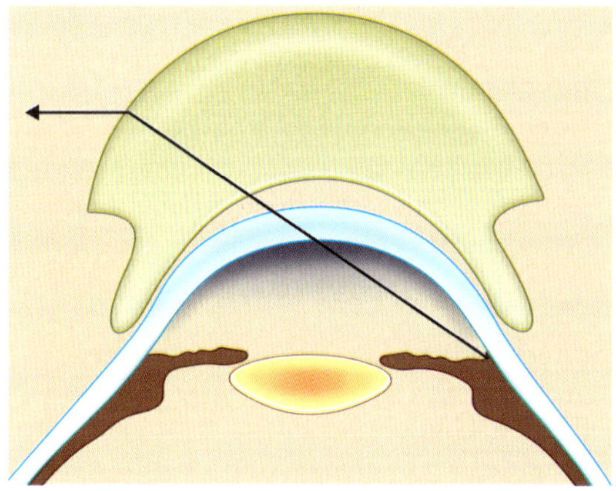

Fig. 7.2 *Schematic drawing of optics of a direct gonioscope*

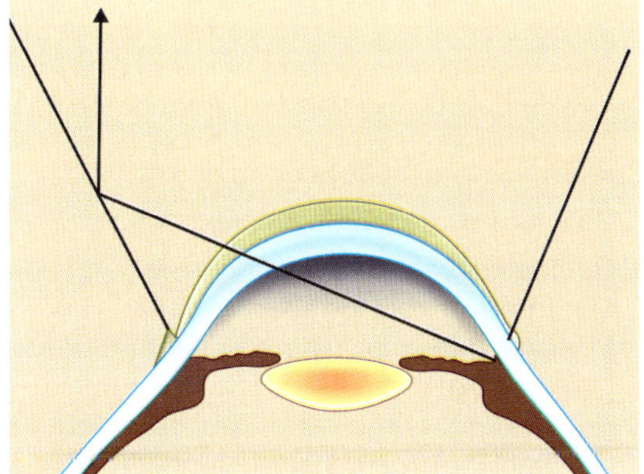

Fig. 7.3 *Schematic drawing of optics of an indirect gonioscope*

Diagnostic indications

- Classification of glaucoma—open angle or closed angle
- Assessment of the anterior chamber angle recess and risk of angle closure
- Identification of plateau iris
- Look for presence and extent of neovascularization of angle
- Assessment of abnormal angle pigmentation
- Identification of the abnormal pigmentation in pigmentary glaucoma
- Visualization of pseudoexfoliative material in the angle
- Look for post-traumatic angle recession, cyclodialysis
- Rule out foreign body in the angle after open-globe injury
- Neoplastic invasion into angle structures (ciliary body tumour)
- Diagnosis of blood in the Schlemm's canal (raised EVP)
- Look for Copper deposition on Descemet's membrane (KF ring)
- Evaluation of trabeculectomy fistula
- Visualization of glaucoma drainage devices
- Diagnosing anterior insertion of iris in developmental glaucoma
- Visualization of congenital anomalies—aniridia, iris processes.

Therapeutic indications

- Laser trabeculoplasty/goniophotocoagulation
- Goniotomy/gonioplasty/trabectome surgery
- Reopening of a blocked trabeculectomy opening
- Nd:YAG laser after deep sclerectomy
- Laser of suture tied around tube of a glaucoma drainage device
- Indentation gonioscopy to break an acute attack of angle-closure
- Insertion of microsurgical implants into Schlemm's canal.

TECHNIQUES OF GONIOSCOPY

As mentioned earlier, gonioscopy is of two types:
- Direct gonioscopy, and
- Indirect gonioscopy

DIRECT GONIOSCOPY

It is performed with a steep convex lens, which permits light from the angle to exit the eye closer to the perpendicular at the lens–air interface. These lenses are used with a portable slit-lamp or an operating microscope. Direct gonioscopy is useful but fairly impractical for routine use. Various types of direct goniolenses are given:

1. *Koeppe goniolens* is the most commonly used for diagnostic direct gonioscopy.
2. *Huskins-Barkan's lens* is a prototype surgical goniolens used for goniotomy.
3. *Swan Jacob's lens* is also used for surgical purpose.
4. *Richardson–Shaffer's goniolens* is basically a small Koeppe lens used for infants.
5. *Worth goniolens.* It anchors to cornea by partial vacuum.
6. *Sieback goniolens.* It is a tiny goniolens which floats on the cornea.

Procedure

Cornea is first anaesthetized with 4% xylocaine instilled topically. The ideal position for direct gonioscopy is the patient lying supine with the examiner sitting on the side of the eye to be examined. With the patient looking up, lower lip of goniolens is inserted below the lower lid. Now the patient is asked to look down and upper lip is placed beneath upper eyelid. Now with patient's head turned towards the examiner, the nasal lip of goniolens is slightly raised and normal saline drops are used for irrigation. This way all the air bubbles also rise on the top and are removed. Now gonioscopy is performed with the patient looking to the ceiling. A systematic approach is to be followed: Nasal angle–superior–temporal than inferior angle.

Advantages

- Greater flexibility because position of observer can be changed.
- Panoramic view is obtained so one part of angle could be compared with the other.
- Angle becomes deep in supine position so it is easy to see the angle.
- Detailed examination of minor structures is possible because the observer can change his or her height to look deeper into anterior chamber.
- Causes lesser distortion of anterior chamber.
- Can be used in sedated/anaesthetized patients as in infants.
- Provides a straight view rather than inverted view.
- Using two lenses, both eyes can be examined simultaneously.
- Can be used for surgical procedures, like goniotomy.

Disadvantages

- Inconvenient
- Annoying light reflexes from cornea
- Time-consuming
- Benefits of slit-lamp (like variable light and better clarity) are not available.

INDIRECT GONIOSCOPY

Indirect gonioscopy uses mirrors or prisms to overcome the problem of total internal reflection. Gonioprisms have an angled mirror through which light rays from anterior chamber angle are reflected so that they emerge perpendicular to the lens–air interface. Moreover, it uses the slit-lamp's illumination and magnification system to its advantage. And if we are examining all our patients on the slit-lamp—as indeed we should be—it makes sense to use an indirect gonioscope at the same time.

Commercially available gonioprisms

I. Gonioprisms requiring coupling agents

1. ***Goldmann three-mirror gonioprism*** (Fig. 7.4A). The three mirrors are used as below:
   - *Mirror having inclination of 59°* and domed upper border is used for gonioscopy. Goldmann goniomirror has broad area of contact (approximately 12 mm) with cornea and under pressure may artificially close the angle.

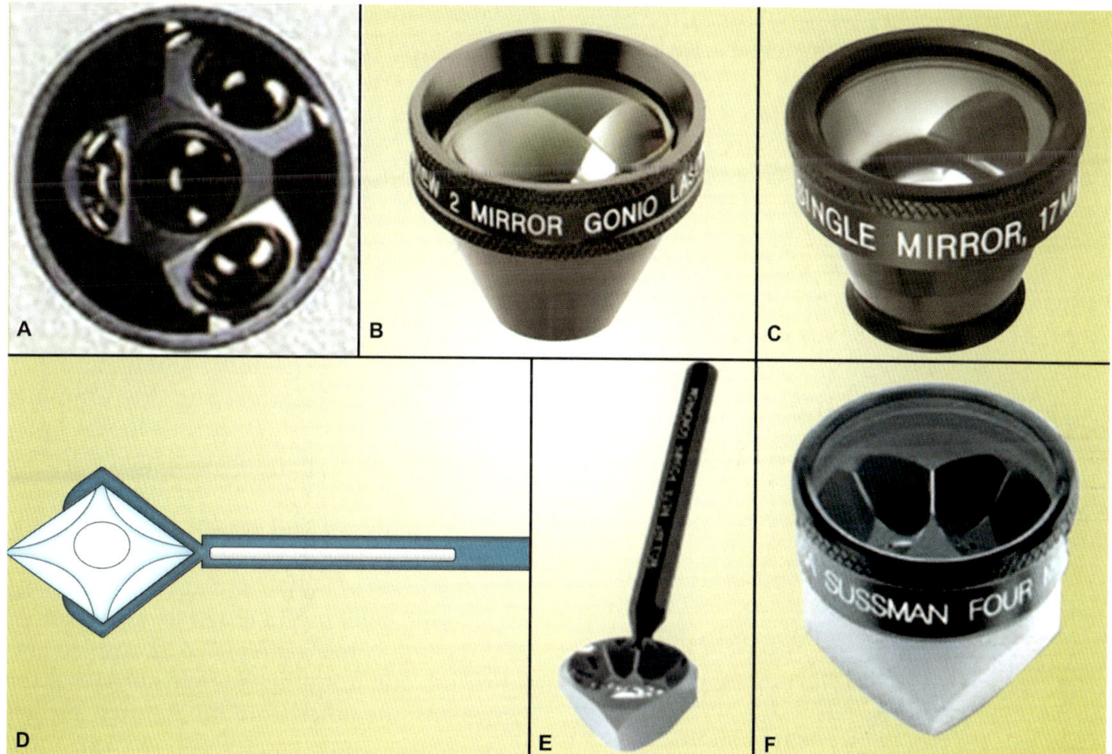

Figs 7.4A to F Various types of gonioscopes: (A) Goldmann three-mirror gonioprism; (B) Goldmann two-mirror gonioprism; (C) Goldmann single-mirror gonioprism; (D) Zeiss four-mirror gonioprism; (E) Posner gonioprism; (F) Sussman lens

- *Mirror inclined at 67°* is used to examine pars plana area of ciliary body.
- *Mirror having inclination of 73°* is used to examine ora serrata area of the peripheral fundus.

2. ***Goldmann two-mirror gonioprism*** (Fig. 7.4B). Both the mirrors are inclined at 62°. It needs to be rotated once to examine the whole angle.

3. ***Goldmann single-mirror gonioprism*** (Fig. 7.4C). The mirror is inclined at 62°. It is a prototype diagnostic gonioprism. It is to be rotated three times to examine the whole angle.

Advantages of Goldmann gonioprisms

(i) Easy to use, (ii) excellent view, (iii) stabilizes the globe and, therefore, can be used in argon laser trabeculoplasty, (iv) peripheral retina can be seen, (v) Goldmann two-mirror gives best in situ view of the angle.

Disadvantages of Goldmann gonioprisms

(i) Curvature of lens is more than that of cornea so a coupling material is required. It blurs vision and fundus; therefore, field charting, direct and indirect ophthalmoscopy cannot be done immediately after its use. (ii) Only one mirror is there for gonioscopy so it needs to be rotated by 360°. (iii) It cannot be used for indentation gonioscopy. (iv) Broad area of contact with cornea is there in case of Goldmann three-mirror and underpressure, it can lead to artefactual closure of angle.

4. ***Allen Thorpe gonioprism.*** It has got four prisms instead of mirrors and allows examination of the whole angle without rotating the prisms.

II. Gonioprisms not requiring coupling agents

1. ***Zeiss four-mirror gonioprism*** (Fig. 7.4D) has four identical mirrors angled at 64° which allow examination of the four quadrants without rotation of the lens. By turning only 11° through lens, the smaller areas in between the mirrors can be visualized. Because the lens has small area (9 mm) of contact with the cornea, the angle is deepened by pushing the lens backwards.

Advantages of Zeiss four-mirror gonioprism

(i) Coupling material is not required, (ii) easy to perform when mastered, (iii) all the four quadrants are visible at the same time so no need to rotate the gonioprism; a rotation of just 11° covers the area between the mirrors, (iv) indentation gonioscopy can be performed, (v) as coupling material is not used, visualization of fundus and photography is possible.

Disadvantages of Zeiss four-mirror gonioprism

(i) Difficult to master, (ii) does not stabilize the globe, (iii) may open the angle artefactually, if pressure is applied.

2. ***Posner gonioprism*** (Fig. 7.4E). It is similar to Zeiss gonioprism but is made of plastic instead of glass and also has fixed rather than detachable handle.

3. ***Sussman lens*** (Fig. 7.4F). It is also similar to Zeiss lens except that it has no handle.

4. ***Tokel gonioprism.*** It is a single-mirror gonioprism and has got a wider field of view.

Procedures of indirect gonioscopy

(1) The eye is anaesthetized with the topical anaesthetic agent. Coupling fluid is poured into the well of the gonioscope. (2) The patient who is sitting on the slit-lamp is asked to look down. (3) The thumb of one hand is used to retract the upper lid. (4) The lower edge of the gonioscope is placed on the lower lid and the gonioscope is tipped on to the cornea in one smooth manoeuvre. In the event of difficulty in keeping the gonioscope in place, a solution like hydroxy-propyl methylcellulose 2.5% may be used. This is thick and a little messy, so once one is more experienced, one can use the less viscous hydroxypropyl methylcellulose 0.7%. (5) Slit-lamp beam is focused on the mirror that shows the angle diametrically opposite to it. Image in indirect goniomirrors is inverted, but not laterally reversed. Three types of illuminations are used: diffuse, sclerotic scatter and direct focal illumination. By using all these, various subtle findings can be elicited.

Essential steps of gonioscopy

Gonioscopy should be performed for all glaucoma patients at diagnosis and during follow-up (at least yearly).

It is best performed in a dark room with minimal slit-lamp illumination and beam height (preferably 1 mm) aimed at the angle, taking care that the slit-beam never crosses the pupil and the patient maintains gaze in the primary position. If the angle structures are not visualized, a bright wide slit is used initially at low magnification to identify the angle and then changed to a short narrow slit. The examiner should wait for at least 60 seconds for the light-induced change in pupillary diameter before commenting on the angle detail.

Identifying the corneal wedge (Fig. 7.5) is the key step in defining the angle structures. By using a thin slit of light inclined 15–20° from the angle of the oculars and sharp focus, projected on to the iridocorneal angle, two light reflections are noted, one from the external surface of the cornea and the other from the internal surface of the cornea. These two reflections meet at the end of Descemet's membrane, the beginning of Schwalbe's line. At this landmark, the external and internal reflections of the three-dimensional parallele- piped of light merge into a two-dimensional single line with a brighter luminance, which extends in a perpendicular direction across the trabecular meshwork. However, identifying the corneal wedge may be difficult in some cases. By gently sliding the gonioscopy lens in the direction of the mirror being used, the examiner gains a better view of the cornea and the corneal wedge. Locating the wedge is easiest in the superior and inferior angles as it is easy to generate a vertical slit. Hence, the inferior and superior angle should be viewed first and then the temporal–nasal angle.

Then the observer should see if the posterior pigmented (functional) part of the trabecular meshwork is visible or not.

- *It is visible in open-angles (Fig. 7.6).*
- *If the posterior part of the trabecular meshwork is not visible,* it indicates that there may be irido-trabecular contact (angle-closure, Fig. 7.7) and further manipulation/indentation has to be

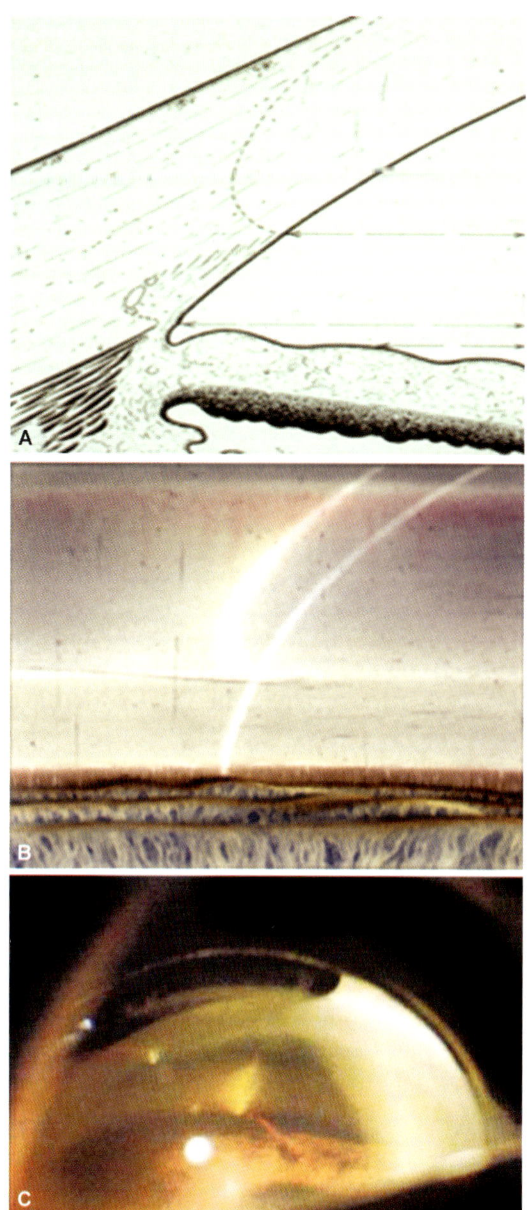

Fig. 7.5 *Corneal wedge: (A) Diagrammatic depiction; (B) as seen on the slit-lamp; and (C) as seen through the gonioscope*

done to view the angle and distinguish between appositional versus synaechial closure.

Functional techniques of gonioscopy

Gonioscopy is performed on a patient in order to answer at least two questions:

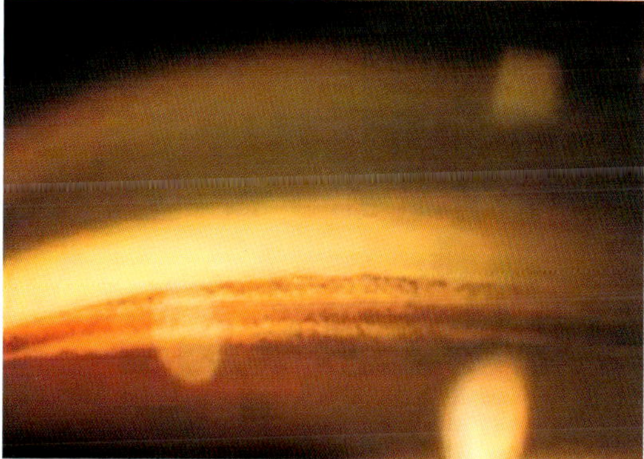

Fig. 7.6 *Open-angle with view of iris, ciliary body, scleral spur and trabecular meshwork*

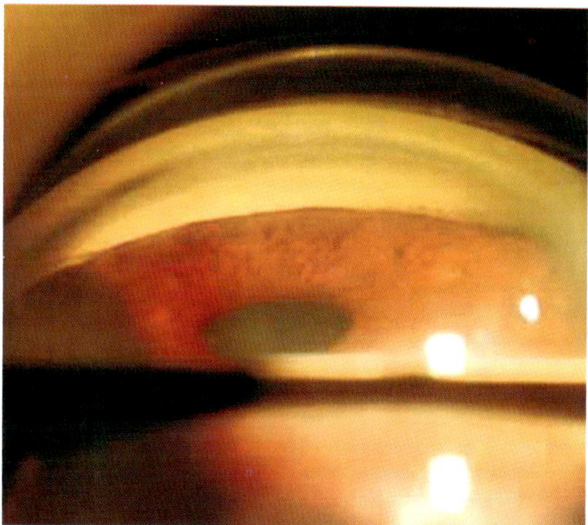

Fig. 7.7 *Closed-angle with no structure visible between iris and corneal periphery*

- Is the angle occludable?
- Are there any abnormalities in the angle?
- There are other questions, such as grading, of the angle.

To answer the above questions, gonioscopy is done by three functional techniques:

- Gonioscopy in situ,
- Manipulative gonioscopy, and
- Indentation gonioscopy.

1. *Gonioscopy in situ.* To answer the first question, the testing conditions must be appropriate; what we want is an in situ view of the angle. The act of placing any lens on the eye disturbs the angle, but we can routinely use a two-mirror lens to obtain as much of an in situ view as possible. The patient is asked to look straight ahead with the lens on the eye. The room lights are then dimmed; the illumination and the height of the slit-beam are decreased so that it does not impinge on the pupil and cause pupillary constriction (with attendant artefactual opening of the angle). The angle is then observed in situ to assess its occludability.

When no angle structure is directly visible on routine gonioscopy in situ, the closure of the angle can be due to three reasons:

- Optical or apparent closure (due to steep iris configuration)
- Appositional closure
- Synaechial closure

Having assessed occludability, we look for any other abnormality in the angle. To do this, we increase the room and slit-lamp illumination, and allow the light to impinge on the pupil, thereby opening up the angle.

2. *Manipulative gonioscopy.* On routine gonioscopy in situ, the angle structures may not be identified in eyes with a steep iris configuration and a narrow angle. To visualize the angle in eyes with a steep iris configuration, the examiner has to use a special manoeuvre to look over the iris. This technique of manipulating the goniolens to visualize over a steep iris (over the hill view) is known as dynamic or manipulative gonioscopy. This can be achieved in Goldmann type of lenses by simply asking the patient to look in the direction of the mirror or moving the mirror towards the angle being viewed (Figs 7.8A to D). This procedure is called *manipulation* (as opposed to indentation). This allows us to look for peripheral anterior synaechiae.

3. *Indentation gonioscopy.* If manipulation does not reveal the angle, it can be achieved by *indentation* using an indentation lens. Sussman four-mirror lens is preferred for indentation, since it is held in the hand while Zeiss four-mirror and Posner lenses have to be held by handle. Indentation gonioscopy requires more of patient's cooperation. The indentation lens

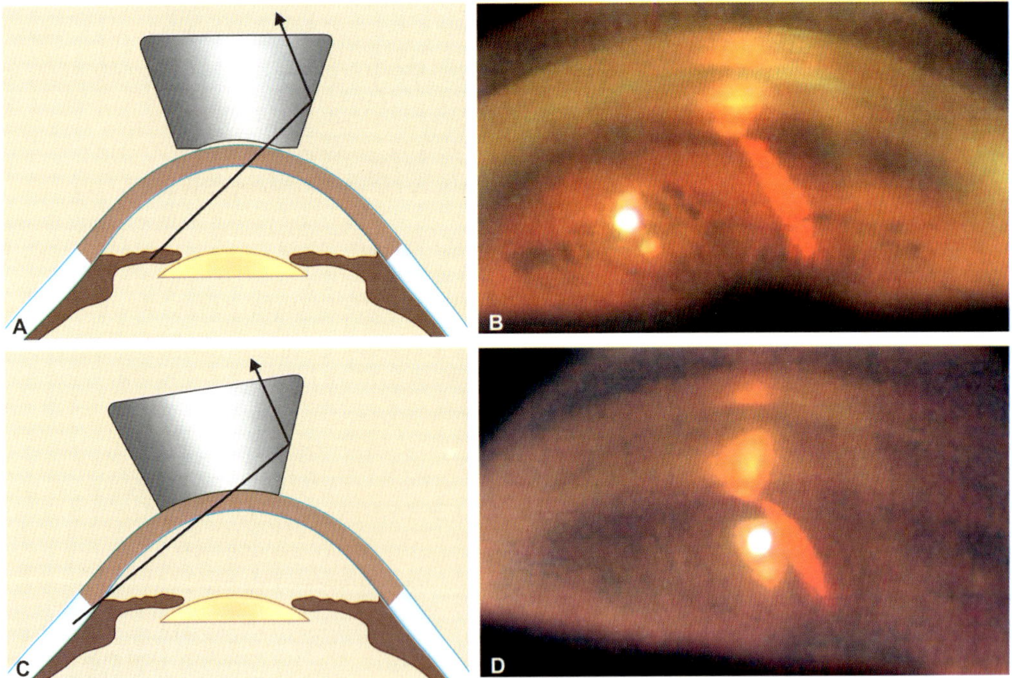

Fig. 7.8 *Gonioscopy in situ versus manipulative gonioscopy in steep iris configuration: (A) Schematic diagram to show how steep iris does not allow view of the angle on gonioscopy in situ and (B) gonioscopy view, shows narrow-angle recess; (C) Schematic diagram to show how manipulation of the gonioscope allows the view of angle recess, and (D) the gonioscopic view shows open-angle recess*

has to be continuously held just in opposition to the cornea without any pressure. It helps us to differentiate between angle closure due to synaechiae from appositional closure. Indentation deepens appositionally closed angle because of aqueous being pushed in the angle (Fig. 7.9).

Besides specific indentation lenses, Goldmann two-mirror lens can also be used. Another reason for using Goldmann two-mirror lens is that it is about half the price of an indentation lens. Although it would be nice to have both, but if one can afford only one lens, one can certainly manage very well with a two-mirror lens alone, which is useful 95% of the time.

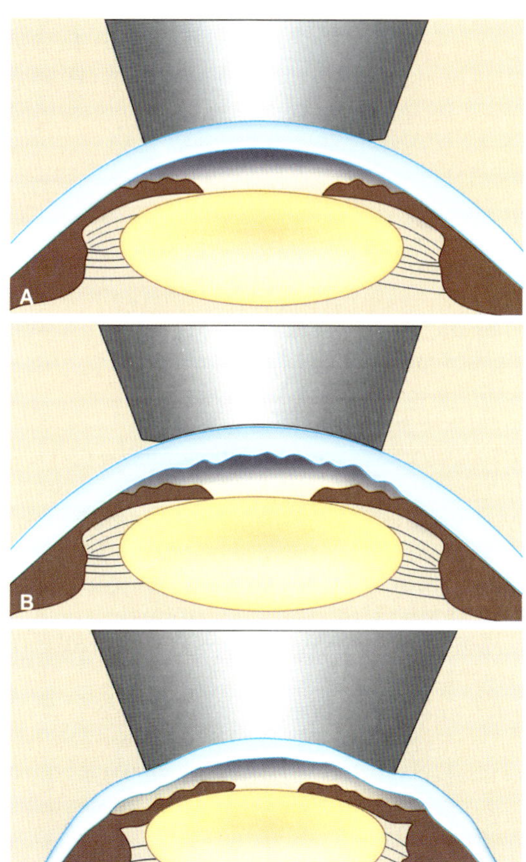

Figs 7.9A to C *Schematic diagram to depict how indentation opens the angle recess: (A) closed angle without indentation; (B) on indentation, the aqueous is pushed into the angle and the angle recess is opened in oppositional closure; (C) In synaechial angle closure, the angle recess is not opened on indentation*

Advantages and disadvantages of indirect gonioscopy

Advantages

- Easier to learn.
- Faster to perform.
- Requires less instrumentation and space.
- Slit-lamp provides better optics and lighting.
- Corneal wedge can be used to localize angle structures.
- Indentation gonioscopy can also be done.
- Magnified stereoscopic view of optic disc can also be obtained.

Disadvantages

- Comparison is not possible.
- Limited positioning of light rays.
- Difficult to perform in horizontal meridian.
- Mirror image seen, so confusing.
- Excessive pressure may open or close the angle artefactually.
- Exaggerates the degree of angle closure.

DISINFECTION OF GONIOSCOPIC LENSES

The American Academy of Ophthalmology issued guidelines for cleaning gonioscopic lens—keeping in mind the presence of HIV and other infectious agents in tears.

- After removing the lens from the patient's eye, it should be immediately rinsed with clean cold water. Mild soap or detergent is then used to clean the surface followed by rinsing with cold clean water and drying with a non-linting cloth.
- For disinfection, glutaraldehyde or bleaching powder is used. The lens is soaked in 2% glutaraldehyde for at least 20 minutes or a 10% bleach solution (1 part bleach to 9 parts water) for 10 minutes.
- The lens is then thoroughly rinsed with clean cold water and dried. It can also be wiped for 10 seconds with a sterile swab soaked in 70% isopropyl alcohol or cleaned with 1 : 1000 merthiolate solution.
- Sterilization follows disinfection which is achieved by ethylene oxide exposure (ETO) at 56°C (130°F) for one hour.
- Glass lenses can be autoclaved, when require.

Note. Formalin and phenol have been found to damage lenses.

GONIOSCOPIC VIEW AND GRADING OF ANGLE

GONIOSCOPIC VIEW OF ANGLE STRUCTURES

While performing gonioscopy, one can identify the structures from anterior to posterior or vice versa. *Angle structures* seen from anterior to posterior are (Fig. 7.10A):

1. *Schwalbe's line.* It is the peripheral termination of the cornea where the Descemet's membrane ends. It is marked only by a slight change in colour from trabecular meshwork or by a faint white line. It can be best identified by locating the *corneal wedge*. A thin slit of light slightly inclined from the oculars is projected on to the cornea. In the angle, two separate corneal reflections are perceived; one illuminates the inner and the other illuminates outer aspect of the cornea. In addition to the inner and outer parts of the cornea, the lines also illuminate the opaque scleral face. The portion between the two lines is called the corneal wedge; the corneal wedge intersects at and identifies Schwalbe's line.

Schwalbe's line is an important landmark in identifying the gonioscopic anatomy in confusing angles. It is easy to make a mistake while doing gonioscopy in eyes with closed angles, hazy corneas and pigmentation anterior to Schwalbe's line. Such a false angle can be mistaken for an open-angle. Therefore, one should stress on identifying the Schwalbe's line first and then identifying the structures from anterior to posterior.

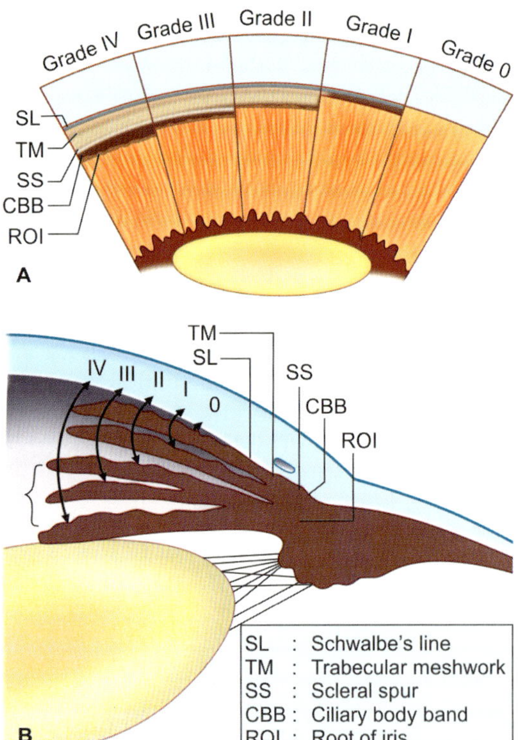

Fig. 7.10 *Diagrammatic depiction of various angle structures as seen in different grades of angle width (Shaffer's grading system): (A) Diagrammatic depiction of gonioscopic view; (B) Configuration of the angle in cross-section of the anterior chamber*

2. *Trabecular meshwork.* It lies between the scleral spur and Schwalbe's line. It has an anterior non-pigmented trabecular meshwork and a posterior pigmented trabecular meshwork. It is non-pigmented and smooth in infants but becomes coarse and pigmented with age.

3. *Scleral spur.* It appears as thin, white or light grey band (yellowish in elderly) just below the trabeculum. It is a fairly consistent landmark. Argon laser burns, if applied posterior to it, may have increased inflammatory response with concomitant increased intraocular pressure and peripheral anterior synaechiae.

4. *Ciliary body band.* It is light grey or dark brown, just posterior to the scleral spur. Width of the ciliary body band varies (narrow in hypermetropes, wide in myopes or aphakics).

5. *Root of iris.* Iris contour is slightly convex or flat. Colour varies in different individuals. Radial markings and crypts are present. Peripherally, concentric contraction rolls are present.

6. *Other structures* that may be visible:

- *Iris processes*. These are normal variants that should have disappeared in the normal course of development. They appear as fine strands extending from iris to the scleral spur. Unlike peripheral anterior synaechiae, iris processes follow the concavity of the angle, do not inhibit the movement of iris during indentation gonioscopy and do not obstruct the flow of aqueous.
- *Blood vessels*. Blood vessels may be present normally and are branches of the major circle

of iris. Unlike neovascularization, they are either arranged radially or form loops.

- *Schlemm's canal*. It lies deep in the posterior portion of trabecular meshwork and, therefore, is not visible generally. It can be made visible by filling it with blood. This could be done either by compressing ipsilateral jugular vein or by pressure from Goldmann's lens.

GRADING SYSTEMS FOR THE ANGLE OF ANTERIOR CHAMBER

Several grading systems have been devised to quantify the findings and for future reference:

I. Scheie's grading

Scheie gave his gonioscopic classification of the anterior chamber angle, based on the extent of visible angle structures as:

- *Wide open*. All structures visible.
- *Grade-I narrow*. Hard to see over iris root into recess.
- *Grade-II narrow*. Ciliary body band obscured.
- *Grade-III narrow*. Posterior trabeculum obscured.
- *Grade-IV narrow* (closed). Only Schwalbe's line visible.

II. Shaffer's grading

In this system, an estimation of the angle width is achieved by observing the amount of separation between the two imaginary lines, constructed tangential to the inner surface of the trabeculum and the anterior iris surface. This grading system also provides a method of comparing the widths of the different chamber angles. The system assigns a numerical grade (0–4) to each angle with associated anatomical description, the angle width in degrees and implied clinical interpretation is as below (Table 7.1 and Fig. 7.10).

1. *Grade IV* (35–45°) is the widest angle characteristic of myopia and aphakia in which the ciliary body can be visualized with ease. It is incapable of closure.
2. *Grade III* (20–35°) is an open angle in which at least the scleral spur can be identified. It is incapable of closure.
3. *Grade II* (20°) is a moderately narrow angle in which only the trabeculum can be identified. Angle closure is possible but unlikely.
4. *Grade I* (10°) is a very narrow angle in which only Schwalbe's line and perhaps also the top of the trabeculum can be identified. Angle closure is not inevitable, although the risk is high.
5. *A slit angle* is one in which there is no obvious iridocorneal contact but no angle structures can be identified. This angle has the greatest danger of imminent closure.
6. *Grade 0* (0°) is a closed angle resulting from iridocorneal contact; it is recognized by the inability to identify the apex of the corneal wedge (Fig. 7.11).

III. RP Centre gonioscopic grading

It has been described by Dr Rajendra Prasad Centre for Ophthalmic Sciences, AIIMS, New Delhi, and is based on indirect gonioscopic findings. There is a good interobserver agreement of this system.

Grade 0: No dipping of the beam

Grade 1: Dipping of the beam

Table 7.1 *Shaffer's system of grading the angle width*

Grade	*Angle width*	*Configuration closure*	*Chances on gonioscopy*	*Structures visible*
IV	35–45°	Wide open	Nil	From Schwalbe's line to ciliary body
III	20–35°	Open angle	Nil	From Schwalbe's line to scleral spur
II	20°	Moderately narrow	Possible	From Schwalbe's line to trabecular meshwork
I	10°	Very narrow	High	Schwalbe's line only
0	0°	Closed	Closed	None of the angle structures visible

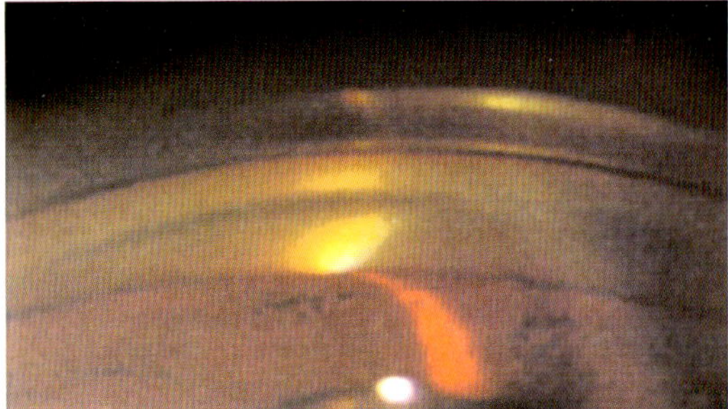

Fig. 7.11 *Gonioscopic photograph revealing grade 0—angle closure*

Grade 2: Schwalbe's line and anterior one-third of the trabecular meshwork visualized

Grade 3: Middle one-third of trabecular meshwork visualized

Grade 4: Posterior one-third of trabecular meshwork visualized

Grade 5: Scleral spur visualized

Grade 6: Ciliary body band visualized

Note. *Grade 3 and less are considered narrow. Grade 2 and less are considered closed.* The above classification can easily be modified to state the structures seen. This has the advantage that it does not have to be committed to memory; the angle is graded according to the structure seen without converting it into a numerical representation, thus decreasing the chance of interobserver variability.

IV. Modified gonioscopic grading

N: No dipping of the beam

D: Dipping of the beam

SL: Schwalbe's line and anterior one-third of trabecular meshwork seen

TM: Middle one-third of trabecular meshwork visualized

SC: Posterior one-third of trabecular meshwork (location of Schlemm's canal) visualized

SS: Scleral spur visualized

CB: Ciliary body band visualized

Whatever the classification used (or not used), in addition to the grading, the ophthalmologist should make a forced choice decision as to whether the angles are occludable or not, based on the type of entry into the angle (narrow or wide) and the angle structures visible.

SCHEMATIC DRAWING OF GONIOSCOPIC FINDINGS

Gonioscopy involves various systems of classifying the anterior chamber angle but they stop short of giving information about other pathologies seen. Becker came out with a scheme of representing the gonioscopic findings which involves (Fig. 7.12):

- Drawing a dark circle, depicting scleral spur
- Drawing three lighter circles outside that for the trabecular meshwork
- Drawing three circles inside it, depicting various levels of insertion of the iris
- Drawing the pupil in the centre
- Each eye is examined quadrant-wise—going clockwise, starting from the inferior angle because it usually is the widest and helps in orientation. Colour coding of findings simplifies the interpretation and provides all the information at one glance. For colour coding of gonioscopic findings, refer to Table 7.2.

Gonioscopic findings could be simplified to drawing only three circles as shown in Fig. 7.13.

These methods of standardized representation reduce the need for writing down every finding.

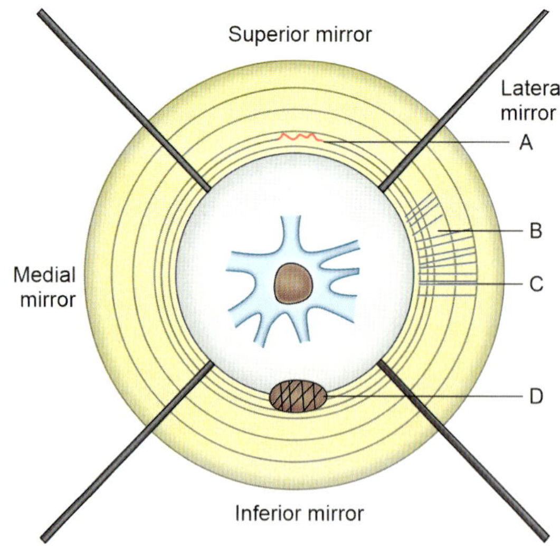

Fig. 7.12 *Schematic drawing of gonioscopic findings: (A) neovascularization; (B) peripheral anterior synaechiae; (C) level of insertion of iris; (D) peripheral iridectomy*

Table 7.2 *Colour codes for gonioscopic findings*

Findings	*Colour*
Iris	Drawn in colour of the eye, e.g. blue and brown
Iris pathology, e.g.	
Iridectomy	Black, cross-hatched
Blood vessels	Red
Synaechiae	Orange
Membranes	Yellow
Pigment	Black
Depigmentation	Purple
Angle recession	Brown, cross-hatched

They also help in better communication of facts between ophthalmologists. They also make follow-up quicker because the ophthalmologist does not have to refer to voluminous notes each time the patient comes for follow-up.

BIOMETRIC GONIOSCOPY

This is a new method for objective measurement of the anterior chamber angle, proposed by Congdon, et al. *Ophthalmology* 1999;106:2161–67.

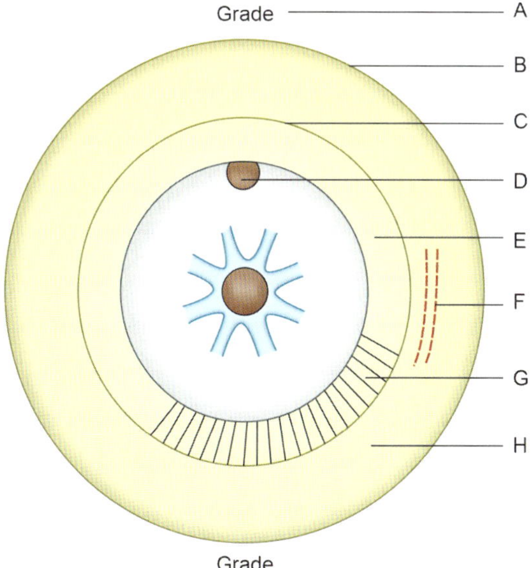

Fig. 7.13 *Modified method of representing gonioscopic findings: (A) grading of angle, (B) Schwalbe's line; (C) scleral spur; (D) peripheral iridectomy; (E) angle recess; (F) position of Schlemm's canal; (G) peripheral anterior synaechiae; (H) trabecular meshwork*

In this method, gonioscopic measurements are performed with the help of a special reticule. The anterior chamber angle is viewed under the following conditions on a Haag-Streit 900 BM slit-lamp: Ambient lighting from a small side lamp is used to provide only an indirect illumination with a total magnification of 16°, power of 6 W, middle filter setting and a slit-lamp beam of 4 mm length and 1 mm width. The reticule is mounted on a slit-lamp 10° ocular and ruled in 0.1 mm units, which is used to measure the distance between the insertion of the iris and the Schwalbe's line. Measurements are recorded separately in the superior, inferior, nasal and temporal quadrants. If the angle is closed, a measurement of 0 is recorded while an occludable angle is defined as one with an average measurement of 0.25 mm or less for the four quadrants.

This method correlates well with other measures of the anterior chamber angle like conventional gonioscopy and Scheimpflug photography, shows a much higher degree of interobserver reliability than conventional gonioscopy and can be readily learned and performed by an inexperienced observer. Hence, it offers a definite advantage over conventional gonioscopy, which is purely a subjective technique and has a long learning curve.

CLINICAL USES AND LIMITATIONS

CLINICAL USES OF GONIOSCOPY

Some of the many uses of gonioscopy are listed below:

- *To make the crucial differentiation* between primary open-angle glaucoma and primary angle-closure glaucoma.
- *To diagnose and provide a prognosis* for the congenital glaucomas.
- *To diagnose secondary glaucomas*, especially subtle angle recession, uveitic glaucoma and that due to early neovascularization, and iridocorneal endothelial syndromes. The black pigment balls are quite characteristic of the resolved hyphaema. This sign may be the only indicator of past trauma.

- *To diagnose conditions, like tumours* of the anterior segment, ciliary body cysts, intraocular foreign body and for early detection of Kayser-Fleischer ring.
- *To diagnose unusual causes of glaucoma*, e.g. a haptic of a posterior chamber lens protruding through the peripheral iridectomy and resting in the angle of anterior chamber. The resultant pseudophakic pigmentary glaucoma can only be diagnosed by gonioscopy.
- *Gonioscopy for treatment.* To perform argon laser trabeculoplasty, laser iridoplasty, laser cyclophotocoagulation. Gonioscopy is also necessary for follow-up on patients who have undergone peripheral iridotomy, trabeculectomy. It now becomes obvious that in addition to the patient care and academic purposes, learning gonioscopy has the potential to more than pay for the cost of gonioscopes.
- *Indentation gonioscopy can be used to break* an attack of acute angle-closure glaucoma.

CRITICAL QUESTIONS TO BE ANSWERED DURING GONIOSCOPY

1. ***What are the angle structures visible?*** The angle configuration depends on the posterior most angle structure visible in primary position without manipulation. If you are able to see the scleral spur in such circumstance, then angle is considered to be open.

2. ***Does the iris touch the trabecular meshwork?*** Irido-trabecular contact can be in the form of appositional/synaechial contact. Peripheral anterior synaechiae (Fig. 7.14) represent non-reversible contact. If peripheral anterior synaechiae are present, the extent of same should be specified to know its effect on the trabecular outflow.

3. ***Is there evidence of previous irido-TM contact?*** Coarse and blotchy pigment clumps (Fig. 7.15) in the angle are suggestive of previous irido-trabecular contact.

4. ***Is iridotrabecular contact—reversible?*** Irido-trabecular contact can be synaechial or appositional. Indentation gonioscopy with Zeiss type lenses (Posner, Sussman) is the "Gold Standard" for detecting angle closure and differentiating appositional from synaechial closure. When no angle structure is directly visible before indentation, four things can happen on indentation (Figs 7.16A to D).

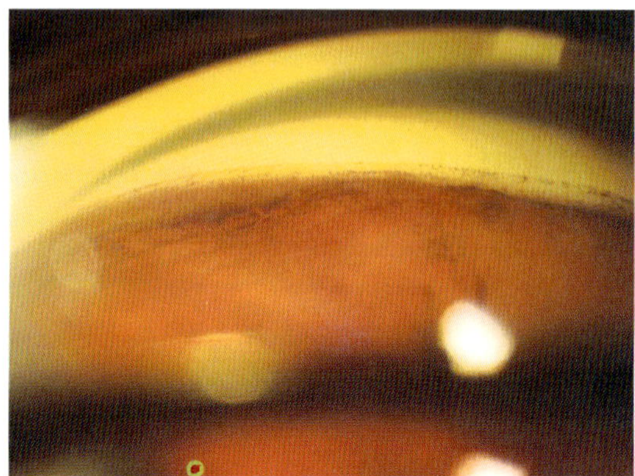

Fig. 7.14 *Peripheral anterior synaechiae*

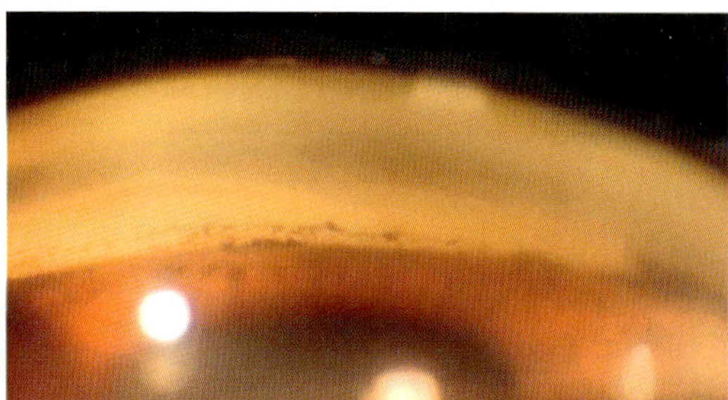

Fig. 7.15 *Pigment clumps in angle forming pseudotrabecular meshwork in angle-closure glaucoma*

- The iris moves peripherally backwards, assumes a concave configuration and the angle recess widens. This represents an appositional closure with a suspicion of a relative pupillary block.
- The iris moves peripherally backwards, but the periphery of the iris bulges out and does not assume a concave configuration. This represents an anteriorly displaced ciliary body and iris root, typically seen in plateau iris.
- The angle widens but iris strands remain attached to the outer wall of the angle. This represents organic synaechial closure of the angle.
- The iris moves only slightly and evenly backward, but retains a convex profile. This can occur due to an anteriorly displaced lens or a large diameter (thick) lens.

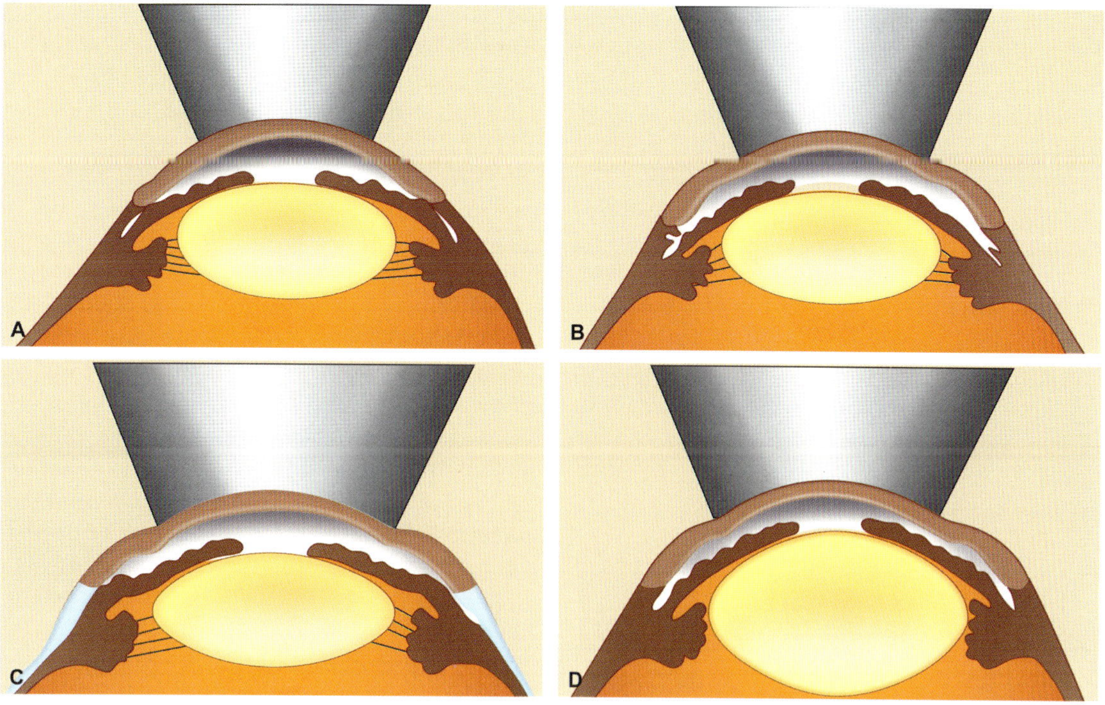

Fig. 7.16 *Indentation gonioscopy: (A) In an apparently closed angle; (B) Angle opens up in a case with appositional closure; (C) Indentation reveals synaechial closure; (D) Thick lens does not allow the chamber to deepen or the iris to move backwards*

5. ***What is the amount of angle pigmentation?*** Pigmentation in the angle can be in terms of:

- Pigmentation of trabecular meshwork—mild, moderate or heavy (Fig. 7.17)
- Pigmentation clumps as in uveitic, post-traumatic glaucomas
- Abnormal pigmentation anterior to trabecular meshwork
- Coarse, blotchy pigments in angle-closure glaucoma.

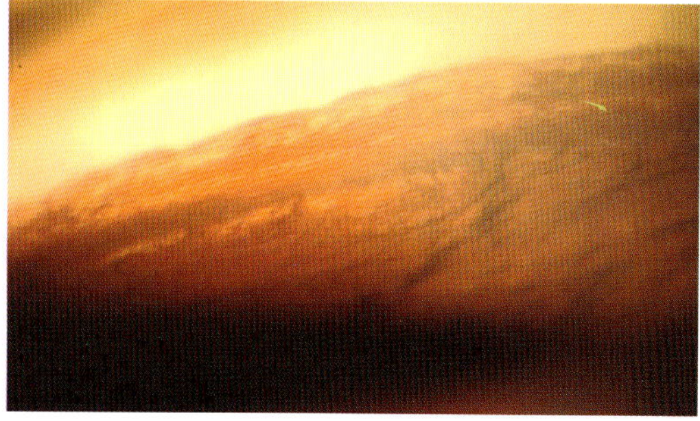

Fig. 7.17 *Dense and even angle pigmentation in pigment dispersion syndrome*

6. ***What is the type of iris configuration and angle recess?*** Iris configuration can vary from convex, regular to concave. Angle recess is the angle between a line tangential to the trabecular meshwork and a line tangential to the iris surface about one-third from periphery. It is usually narrow than 20° in angle-closure glaucoma.

7. ***Is there any new vessels crossing scleral spur?*** Angle neovascularization iris (NVI) is characterized by single vascular trunks which cross the scleral spur and arborize irregularly in irregular fashion (Fig. 7.18).

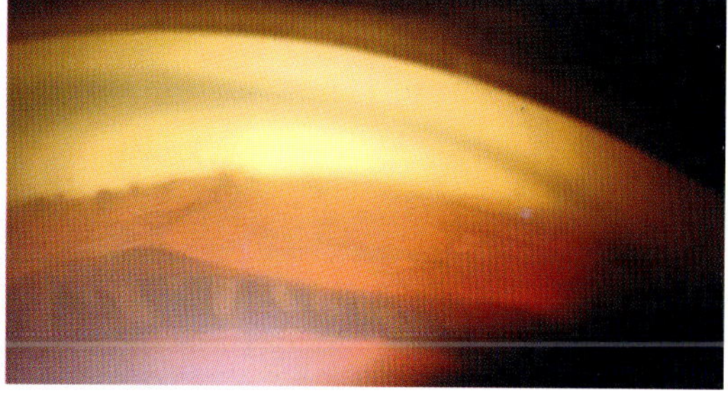

Fig. 7.18 *Neovascularization of iris with secondary angle closure*

8. ***Is there any prominent iris processes, anterior Schwalbe's line?*** Prominent, anteriorly placed Schwalbe's line can be seen in Axenfeld-Rieger syndrome. It can be a normal variant as well. Prominent iris processes are usually seen in juvenile open-angle glaucoma (Fig. 7.19).

9. ***How to differentiate peripheral anterior synaechiae from iris processes?*** Peripheral anterior synaechiae are broader, irregular, tent-shaped and bridge the recess instead of following it. They obscure the underlying angle details and are associated with anterior pigmentation. Iris processes, instead, are brown, lacy, finger-like fine extensions of the peripheral iris which follow the angle concavity.

Fig. 7.19 *Prominent iris processes*

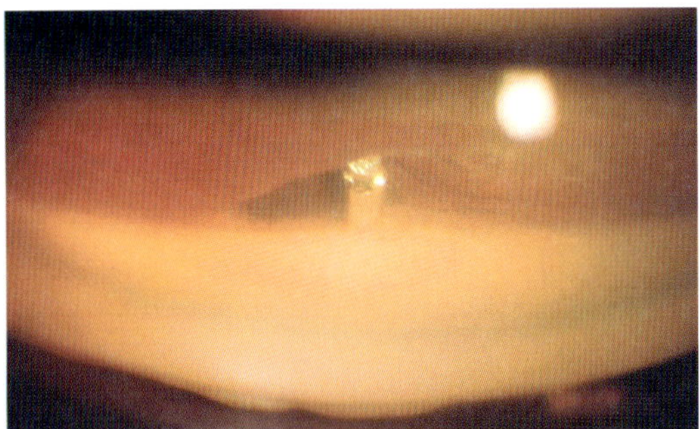

Fig. 7.20 *ExPRESS shunt in the angle with tip touching the iris*

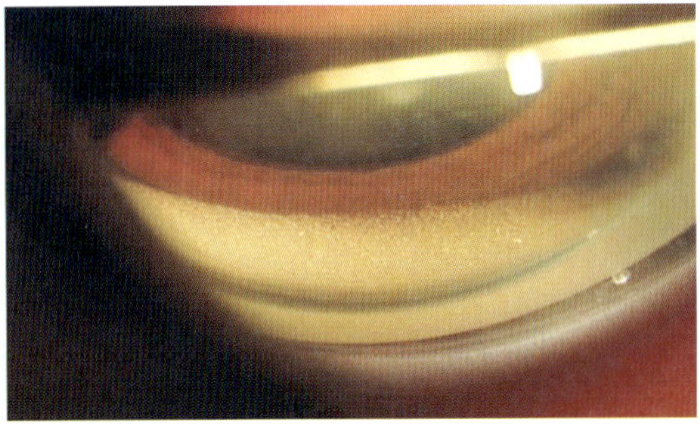

Fig. 7.21 *Silicone oil globules in post-vitrectomy glaucoma*

10. ***Patency of trabeculectomy ostium, view new microimplants?*** Gonioscopy can be used to assess the fistula created during filtering glaucoma surgery and it can also aid in visualizing new microimplants, such as Ex PRESS shunt (Fig. 7.20).

11. ***What do I see in post-vitrectomy secondary glaucoma patients?*** Emulsified oil globules can be seen with increased pigmentation of angle in such patients (Fig. 7.21).

12. ***What should be seen in post-traumatic patients?*** Gonioscopy is a must in unilateral glaucoma patients and it can show: Hyphaema (Fig. 7.22), synaechiae, increased pigmentation, cyclodialysis (Fig. 7.23), iridodialysis, angle recession (Fig. 7.24) and fibrosis of angle.

LIMITATIONS AND ARTEFACTS

Limitations of gonioscopy

- Gonioscopy is a contact investigation which causes discomfort to the patient.
- It can transmit a conjunctival infection to the patient.
- Gonioscopy should not be performed in suspected open-globe injury or early in the course of closed-globe injury with hyphaema as pressure can precipitate re-bleed.
- Gonioscopy is difficult in cases of acute angle closure with corneal oedema and eyes with corneal opacification.
- Excessive pressure while using Goldmann type of lens may artefactually close the angles and while using corneal type of gonioscopes it may give an open-angle appearance in narrow recess angle configuration.
- Use of slit-lamp illumination while doing gonioscopy leads to pupillary constriction and opens up/changes the angle configuration.
- Gonioscopy cannot objectively quantitate the angle parameters and there is a wide inter-observer variability.
- Gonioscopy is not useful to identify pathologies behind the iris.

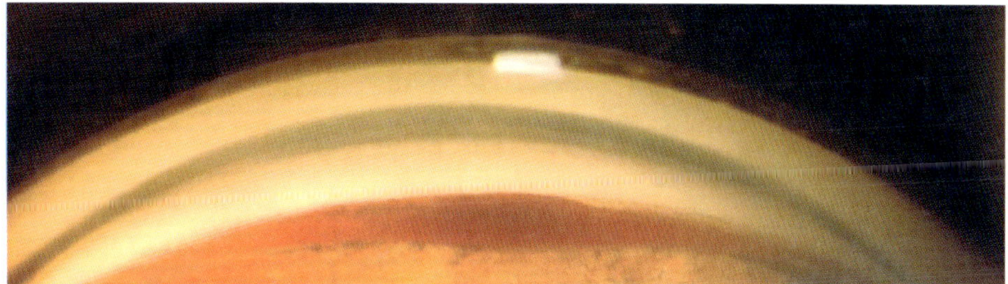

Fig. 7.22 *Post-traumatic hyphaema*

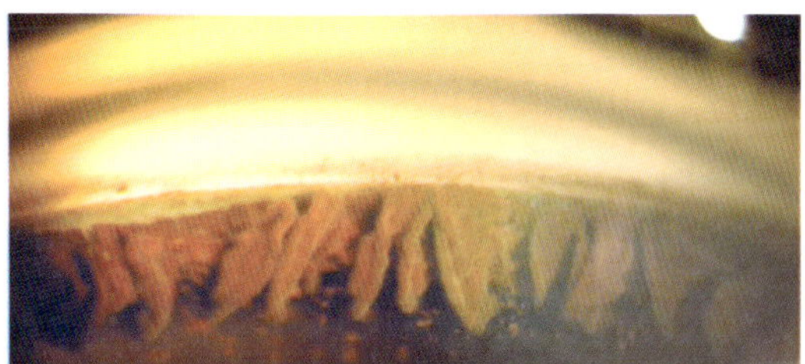

Fig. 7.23 *Cyclodialysis cleft with ciliary processes visible in a closed-globe injury with disinjection of iris from ciliary body*

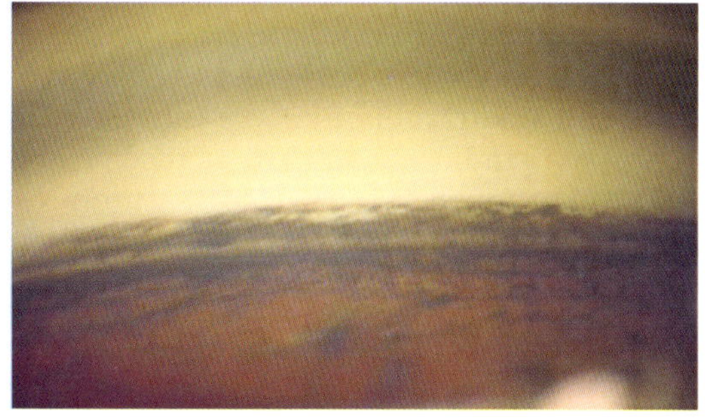

Fig. 7.24 *Angle recession*

- Indentation gonioscopy can lead to formation of corneal folds, distorting the view of angle structures and may cause corneal epithelial injury.
- It has a long learning curve requiring regular practice on a large number of patients.

Artefacts

- Excessive pressure artefactually opens an angle while using Goldmann's four-mirror or closes the angle while using Goldmann's single-mirror.
- Residues on lens because of oily secretion or methylcellulose may give rise to artefacts.
- Mirror in Goldmann's goniomirrors is closer to the centre of cornea; therefore, angle recess is better seen, which could give erroneous impression of open angle in case of narrow angle glaucoma.

SUGGESTED READING

1. Fisch BM. Gonioscopy and the Glaucomas. Boston: Butterworth-Heineman, 1993.
2. Gonioscopy: A text and atlas. Tanuj Dada. Jaypee Publications, 2014.
3. Gorin G, Posner A. Slit Lamp Gonioscopy. Baltimore: Williams & Wilkins Company, 1967.
4. Kanski JJ, McAllister JA. Glaucoma: A Color Manual of Diagnosis and Treatment. Oxford: Butterworth-Heineman, 1989.
5. Prokopich CL, Flanagan JG: Gonioscopy: evaluation of the anterior chamber angle. Part 1. Ophthal. Physiol. Opt 1996;16(2):S39–42.
6. Rubin ML: Optics for Clinicians, 2nd edition. Gainsesville, FL. Triad Scientific Publishing, 1974;56.
7. Salzmann M. Die Ophthalmoskopie der Kammerbucht. Z Augenheilk 1914;31:1.
8. Trantas AL 'ophthalmoscopie de l' angleirido-corneen (gonioscopie). Conclusions a entirer pour la nature du canal de Schlemm Arch Ophthalmol (Paris) 1918;36:257.
9. Vargas E, Drance SM. Anterior chamber depth in angle closure glaucoma: Clinical methods of depth determination in people with and without the disease. Arch Ophthalmol 1973; 90(6): 438–45.

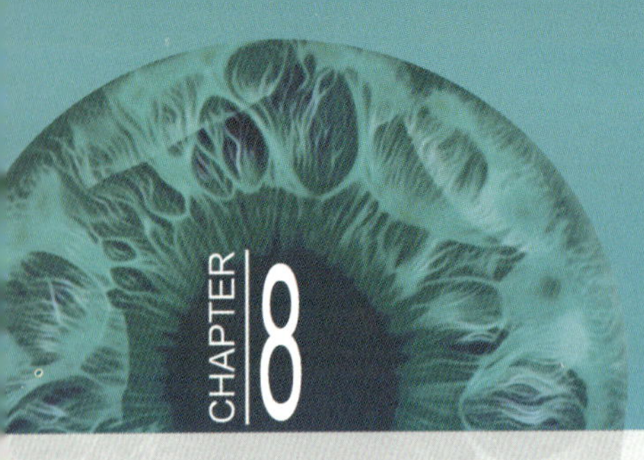

EVALUATION OF OPTIC NERVE HEAD

INTRODUCTION

Glaucoma is defined as a chronic optic neuropathy, typically causing structural damage in the optic disc, usually accompanied by or leading to corresponding functional changes in the visual field. Though intraocular pressure (IOP) assessment and perimetry aid in diagnosis of glaucoma, individually neither of these are enough by themselves. Raised intraocular pressure (IOP) is the only treatable causal risk factor for glaucoma but neither sufficient nor necessary for the diagnosis.

Damage to the RGC axons within the lamina cribrosa is the central pathophysiology underlying visual loss due to glaucoma. Despite the availability of sophisticated imaging devices, clinical optic disc evaluation has proved to be indispensable in clinical practice and has been shown to be valuable for evaluating change. Glaucoma diagnosis is essentially diagnosing glaucomatous optic neuropathy (GON).

An estimated 12 million people are affected by glaucoma in India, the majority of whom (90%) are undiagnosed. By 2020, this number is expected to be 16 million. The major element of glaucoma strategy is case detection, i.e. to at least detect and manage the "obvious" and clear-cut glaucoma cases with established functional loss. To achieve this, a clinician must be proficient at examining the optic nerve head and be able to diagnose even subtle changes, ranging from early changes to glaucomatous optic atrophy.

TECHNIQUES FOR DISC EVALUATION

Glaucoma affects the surface contour of the optic nerve head. Surface changes are best appreciated with a stereoscopic view. Therefore, the initial examination, and follow-up examination for surface changes, should be made through the pupil when it is at least 4 mm in diameter. Interim examination, for disc haemorrhages, can also be performed through an undilated pupil. Stereoscopic examination of the posterior pole is best performed with the following techniques:

I. ***Indirect fundus-lens technique.*** With enough magnification at the slit-lamp, the 60D, 78D and 90D fundus lenses provide high magnification stereoscopic view and have an advantage in identifying many subtle alterations in the ONH, such as discrepancies between the cup size based on colour criteria and contour criteria.

A +90D lens provides a wide field of view but less magnification in comparison to a +60D, which provides a narrower field of view but × 1.15 × magnification. It is this magnification and depth of field that makes the +60D lens an excellent choice for examining the optic disc. A +78D lens lies between these lenses with properties of both.

II. ***Direct fundus-lens technique*** involves examination with central part of Goldmann and Zeiss four-mirror at the slit-lamp. The direct fundus lens examination is very useful for ONH and retinal nerve fibre layer (RNFL) examination and can give additional information, such as RNFL defects and disc haemorrhages. Three-dimensional information using parallax movements is possible.

OPTIC DISC CHANGES IN GLAUCOMA

Evaluation of glaucomatous optic disc changes requires assessment and understanding of the morphology and pathology affecting the optic nerve head. Normally, the size and location of optic cup and pallor are the same. However, this is not always the case, especially in disease states. Thus, these two parameters should not be thought of as being synonymous.

- Neural rim is the tissue between the cup and disc margins and it represents the location of the bulk of the axons. Normally, it is seen as orange-red colour because of the associated capillaries.
- *Retinal vessels* ride up the nasal wall of the cup, often kinking at the cup margin before crossing the neural rim to the retina.

Complete optic nerve head evaluation includes eight intrapapillary and four peripapillary features (Table 8.1).

INTRAPAPILLARY CHANGES

Optic disc size

- ***Optic disc size is independent*** of age after first decade and refractive error less than ± 5.0D provides only little variation in size estimation.
- ***Normally mean area*** of the optic nerve head ranges from 2.1 to 2.8 mm^2.
- ***Estimation of optic nerve head size can be done by direct ophthalmoscope.*** 5 degree aperture of the Welch Allyn direct ophthalmoscope in an emmetropic eye equals and area of 1.7 mm^2 thereby providing rough estimation of optic nerve head size.
- ***Another method to evaluate the disc*** is by direct measurement of horizontal and vertical diameters of the optic nerve head on slit-lamp and the obtained values are corrected with a correction on 1.26 (diameter × 1.26).
- ***Optic disc diameter*** (mm) = (X/H) × D × C
  - X = height of beam as measured by the millimetre rule (mm)
  - H = height setting on the beam height indicator when checking with the millimetre rule (mm)
  - D = diameter of disc as measured by the beam height indicator (mm)
  - C = correction factor based on high plus lens power
- ***Corrective factor for different lenses*** are for Volk 90.0D × 1.5, 78D × 1.3, 60D × 1.

Table 8.1 *Intrapapillary and peripapillary features for glaucomatous disc evaluation*

8 Intrapapillary features	*4 Peripapillary features*
2 aspects of optic disc: Size; shape	Optic disc haemorrhage
2 aspects of NRR: Size; shape	RNFL assessment
3 aspects of cup: Size; shape; C/D ratio	Arteriolar diameter
Position of central retinal vascular trunk	Parapapillary choroidal atrophy

- ***Optic disc size correlates with*** a variety of morphological and clinical features:
- ***Small discs*** are associated with small cups (Fig. 8.1), ONH drusen, pseudopapilloedema, and non-arteritic anterior ischaemic optic neuropathy.
- ***Intermediate disc*** size is associated with arteritic anterior ischaemic optic neuropathy, central retinal vein occlusion, and the most common forms of glaucoma—POAG, juvenile open-angle glaucoma, age-related ('senile sclerotic') open-angle glaucoma, and pseudo-exfoliation glaucoma.
- ***Large discs*** have a greater neuroretinal rim area more axonal fibres, larger size and number of laminar pores thereby less susceptible to damage when compared to small disc and is associated with large cups (Fig. 8.2), morning glory syndrome, congenital optic nerve pit.

Optic disc shape

- Optic disc shape is independent of age, sex, body weight, and height.
- Normal optic disc is oval and has a vertical dimension 7–10% larger than the horizontal dimension.
- Corneal astigmatism affects the shape of the disc as seen in high degree of astigmatism.
- Myopia of more than 12D is associated with increase in ovality of disc.

Neuroretinal rim shape

- Neural retinal rim (NRR) changes in glaucoma is what leads to subsequent changes in the cup and thereby loss of visual field.
- Cup-to-disc ratio provides only an indirect assessment of the amount of neural tissue in the optic nerve head and thereby may be misleading, because a larger diameter of the nerve head may be associated with a thinner neural rim width and larger cup size despite a stable number of axons.
- Normally, the NRR follows the ISNT rule: The neural rim of the normal optic nerve head is typically broadest in the inferior quadrant, followed by the superior and then the nasal rims, with the temporal rim being the thinnest.
- As glaucoma progresses, the NRR is diffusely lost in all sectors. Its diminution can predict for subsequent visual field loss. Infero-temporal and superotemporal regions are the earliest to be lost, followed by the temporal sector, and lastly the nasal rim.
- NRR area is most import predictor of optic nerve head status. NRR pallor can also act indicator to identify, non-glaucomatous optic atrophy which manifests with neither with enlargement of the optic cup nor with a decrease in the NRR area—but rather with increased NRR pallor and attenuation of the peripapillary retinal vessels.

Fig. 8.1 *Small disc with small cup*

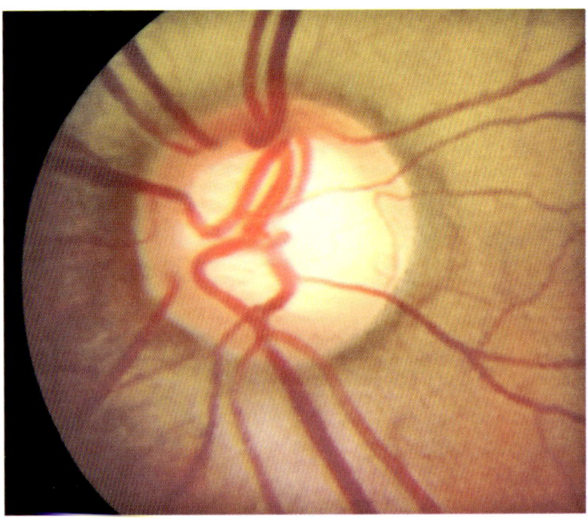

Fig. 8.2 *Large disc with large cup*

- Also of clinical interest is the observation that the sector of the NRR farthest from the central trunk of retinal vessels may be affected by rim loss earlier than other sectors.

Cup–disc ratio

- *Normally*, there is vertically oval disc and has a horizontally oval cup with cup disc ratios (CDR) larger horizontally. Seven per cent of normal people have a reversed cup disc ratio.
- *There is symmetric enlargement* of the physiologic cup in glaucoma, but usually some portion of the rim erodes more rapidly than the rest. Figure 8.3 shows a glaucomatous disc with 0.9 cupping.
- *In myopic eyes* and discs with age-related open-angle glaucoma, the cup tends to be shallow, especially temporally.
- *Contour cup vs. colour cup.* To assess the width of the NRR, the edge of the cup has to be clearly delineated, most people equate the central pallor of the disc, with cup, but in some glaucomatous discs, there is a discrepancy between the extent of central pallor (colour cup) and the site at which the vessels change their contour (contour cup).
- *NRR thinning* can be localized and appear as a notch, or less frequently, as a pit at the disc rim.
- *An acquired pit of the optic nerve* (APON) is a discrete, focal area of depression within the optic cup at the level of the lamina cribrosa. APONs occur more frequently unilaterally, inferotemporally in 70–80% cases (superotemporally in rest) and in patients with normal-tension glaucoma (NTG). They often correspond to a deep, sharp-margined scotoma approaching or involving fixation.
- *When notches are present* both inferiorly and superiorly, the cup becomes vertically oval. In glaucoma, the vertical cup always enlarges faster.
- *Cup deepening is characterized by:*
  - *Overpass cupping,* i.e. blood vessel crossing over an area of NRR loss prior to sinking in and taking on the bayonet appearance.
  - *Laminar dot appearance,* i.e. exposure of the lamina cribrosa

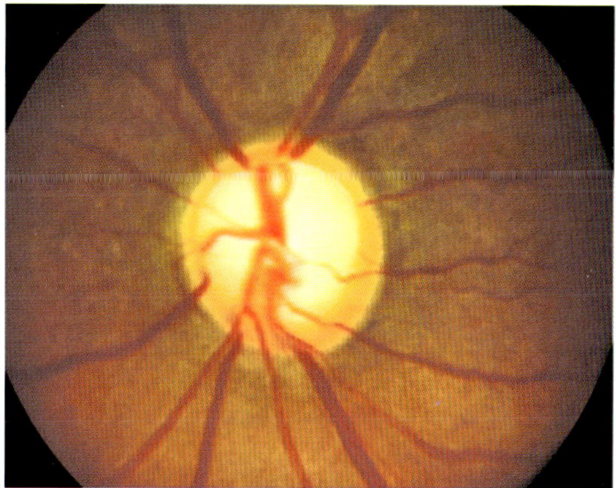

Fig. 8.3 *Advanced GON with a C : D ratio of 0.9*

- *Disadvantages of the CDR system* for diagnosing and quantifying glaucoma are the variation in cup sizes in the population and more importantly, the fact that the discs do not grow concentrically and eccentric cups may display localized notching. There may be significant intra- and inter-observer error in this method. Therefore, disc damage likelihood score system (Fig. 8.4) was created by Dr George Spaeth.

Disc damage likelihood score

Disc damage likelihood score (DDLS) relies on the optic nerve head as a direct indicator of disease. The DDLS is based on the radial width of the neuroretinal rim measured at its thinnest point. The unit of measurement is the rim/disc ratio—that is, the radial width of the rim compared to the diameter of the disc in the same axis.

When there is no rim remaining the rim/disc ratio is 0. The circumferential extent of rim absence (0 rim/disc ratio) is measured in degrees. Caution must be taken to differentiate the actual absence of rim from sloping of the rim, e.g. can occur temporally in some patients with myopia. A sloping rim is not an absent rim. Because rim width is a function of disc size, disc size must be evaluated before attributing a DDLS stage. This is done with a 60D or a 90D lens with appropriate corrective factors. Because the scale divides glaucomatous progression into 10 stages, it is better able to monitor disease progression than methods with fewer stages,

New DDLS stage	Narrowest width of rim (rim/disc ratio)			
	For small disc <1.50 mm	For average size disc 1.50–2.00 mm	For large disc >2.00 mm	Old DDLS stage
1	0.5 or more	0.4 or more	0.3 or more	0a
2	0.4 to 0.49	0.3 to 0.39	0.2 to 0.29	0b
3	0.3 to 0.39	0.2 to 0.29	0.1 to 0.19	1
4	0.2 to 0.29	0.1 to 0.19	Less than 0.1	2
5	0.1 to 0.19	Less than 0.1	0 for less than 45°	3
6	Less than 0.1	0 for less than 45°	0 for 46° to 90°	4
7	0 for less than 45°	0 for 46° to 90°	0 for 91° to 180°	5
8	0 for 46° to 90°	0 for 91° to 180°	0 for 181° to 270°	6
9	0 for 91° to 180°	0 for 181° to 270°	0 for more than 270°	7a
10	0 for more than 180°	0 for more than 270°		7b

Fig. 8.4 *Disc damage likelihood score*

such as the algorithm described by Hodapp-Parrish-Anderson.

Position of central retinal vessels and branches

- Rim sector farthest from the major trunk of the central retinal vessels is susceptible to damage.
- Normally, the retinal vessels pass perpendicularly through the disc tissue to reach the retina. These vessels travel vertically along the cup wall and then horizontally on the retinal surface, the change in course is seen as a bend in the vessel.
- Outward shifting of the bend is associated with thinning of neuroretinal rim. They tend to get nasalised as the glaucomatous changes advance. In early stages, there orientation is vertical bearing of circumlinear vessels common in glaucomatous cups. It may be seen normally as well.

PERIPAPILLARY DISC CHANGES

With the advancement of glaucoma, the following changes occur in the juxtapapillary region: Optic disc haemorrhage, changes in the RNFL; variations in the diameter of retinal arterioles; and patterns of peripapillary choroidal atrophy.

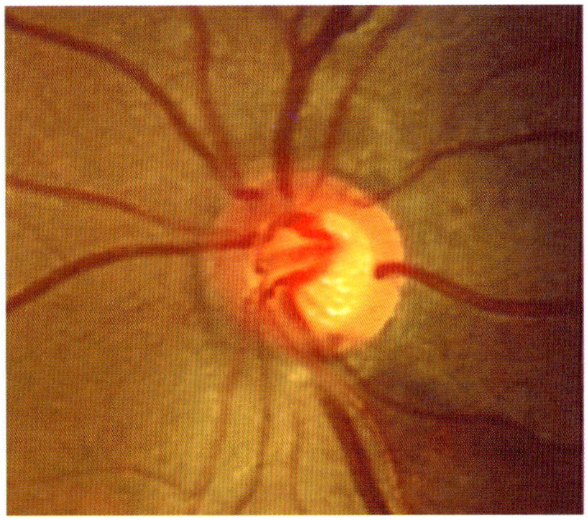

Fig. 8.5 *Optic disc haemorrhage*

Optic disc haemorrhages

- Located within the neuroretinal rim the disc haemorrhages are usually flame-shaped haemorrhages but can sometimes be blot haemorrhages (Fig. 8.5).
- They are usually seen extending across the disc rim into the retina, but they may occur deep in the disc tissue. As they appear in areas

of preserved NRR, they are not usually seen in advanced cases of cupping in which little rim remains.
- They may last up to 35 weeks from the time of presentation.
- Non-glaucomatous factors, such as aspirin use and diabetes, are also associated with such haemorrhages.
- Normotensive glaucomas have a predilection for optic disc haemorrhage.
- They may very rarely be found in non-glaucomatous eyes (about 1%).
- *Major studies:* EMGT, OHTS, and collaborative normal tension glaucoma study (CNTGS) indicated that disc haemorrhages were strongly associated with progression.

Curiosities

- *OHTS.* Majority of eyes with disc haemorrhages have not converted to glaucoma.
- *EMGT.* While disc haemorrhages were predictive of progression, IOP-reducing treatment was unrelated to the presence or frequency of disc haemorrhages. Disc haemorrhages were equally common in both the treated and untreated groups of patients. The results may suggest that disc haemorrhages cannot be considered an indication of insufficient IOP-lowering treatment, and that glaucoma progression in eyes with disc haemorrhages cannot be totally halted by IOP reduction. The results also suggest that disc haemorrhages do not occur in all patients with glaucoma.
- *CNTGS.* While disc haemorrhages predicted progression, treating eyes with disc haemorrhages did not benefit the patient or affect the clinical course of the disease.

Nerve fibre layer defects

- *RNFL evaluation* is best done by a red-free direct ophthalmoscopy or a wide-angle camera with either blue or green filters. Serial photographs can assess ongoing glaucomatous changes.
- *In healthy eyes*, the RNFL appears slightly opaque with radially oriented striations, which has been likened to "horsehair" (Fig. 8.6). Fibres of RNFL follow an arcuate pattern above and below the macula and are typically brighter at the superior and inferior arcuate bundles than the temporal and nasal bundles.

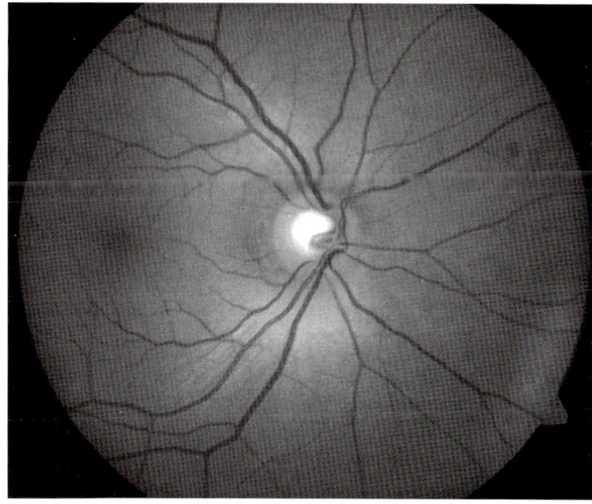

Fig. 8.6 *Red-free photograph showing radial striations of RNFL in a healthy disc*

- *RNFL defects* usually precede the appearance of functional changes in the fields. RNFL defects can be—localized wedge defects and diffuse loss which alone or in combination of both in glaucoma patients.
- *Localized loss* is more easily and consistently recognized, but is less common. The nerve fibres are seen most easily in the retinal area adjacent to the superior and inferior temporal aspects of the disc (superior and inferior Bjerrum's area), where the RNFL is thickest, more obvious in moderately dark fundi as in young and becomes increasingly difficult to see in patients with media opacities or lighter fundus pigmentation as for older patients. Localized loss may occur along with diffuse or generalized loss.
- *Diffuse loss* is more difficult to assess. In cases where RNFL is poorly visible, vessels and vascular reflexes can help differentiate a normal patient from a thinned or generally atrophic RNFL in a patient with disease. If the retinal vessel reflexes are bright and sharp and smaller branches are easily visualized, generalized atrophy may be present.

Diameter of retinal arterioles

- As disease progresses, there is progressive loss of the axonal mass and so demands for peripapillary perfusion decreases. This leads to diffuse narrowing of the retinal vessels on the ONH.

- Narrowing of the retinal vessels is a nonspecific indicator of optic atrophy, seen both with descending atrophy and non-arteritic anterior ischaemic optic neuropathy. Such narrowing increases with age but is significantly pronounced in proportion to the degree of optic atrophy.

Peripapillary choroidal atrophy

Normal optic nerve head may be surrounded by zones that vary in width, circumference, and pigmentation. A scleral lip, which appears commonly as a thin, even, white rim that marks the disc margin, usually for the full 360°, represents an anterior extension of sclera between the choroid and optic nerve head. There are two zones described in conjunction with glaucoma:

Beta zone: This zone is broader, irregular and incomplete area of depigmentation.

- An area of depigmentation is caused by retraction of retinal pigment epithelium from the disc margin, with a thinning or absence of choroid next to the disc, thereby exposing underneath sclera (Fig. 8.7).
- It is commonly seen with a tilted scleral canal, as in myopia.
- When zone beta completely surrounds the ONH, it is called the *halo glaucomatous*.
- It also prognosticates the risk of glaucomatous damage in ocular hypertension.

Alpha zone. It is a peripapillary crescent of increased pigmentation that may represent a malposition of the embryonic fold with a double layer or irregularity of retinal pigment epithelium. It is located outside beta zone but may be seen adjacent to the disc, if the zone beta is absent.

DIAGNOSTIC CLUES

To summarize, clues for diagnosing glaucoma are:

- Neuroretinal rim tissue that does not respect the "ISNT" rule
- Associated notching of the rim, verticalization of the optic cup with baring of a circumlinear vessel
- Vessel bayoneting at the optic rim (indicating bean-pot cupping) and nasalization of vessels
- Disc haemorrhage (Drance haemorrhage) and
- Abnormally large peripapillary atrophy
- Laminar dot sign is seen in advanced glaucoma.

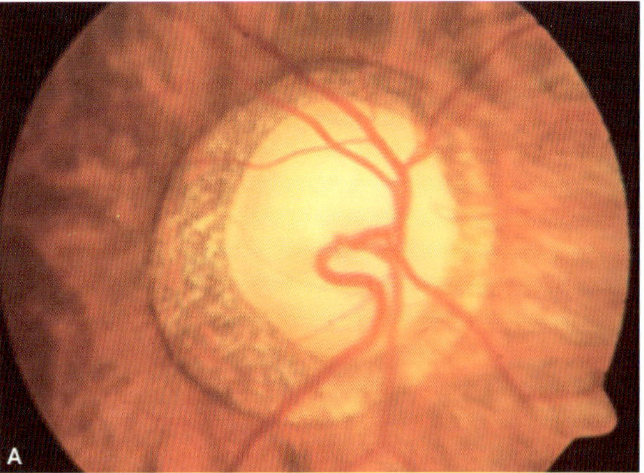

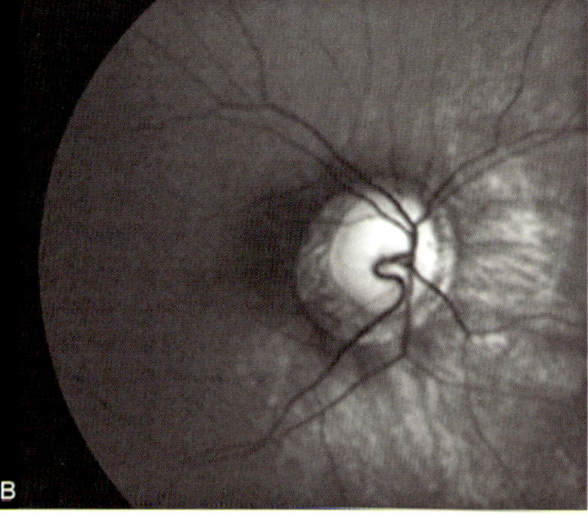

Figs 8.7A and B *Glaucomatous optic discs with diffuse thinning of NRR with corresponding total atrophy of the retinal pigment epithelium and choriocapillaris, designated beta zone*

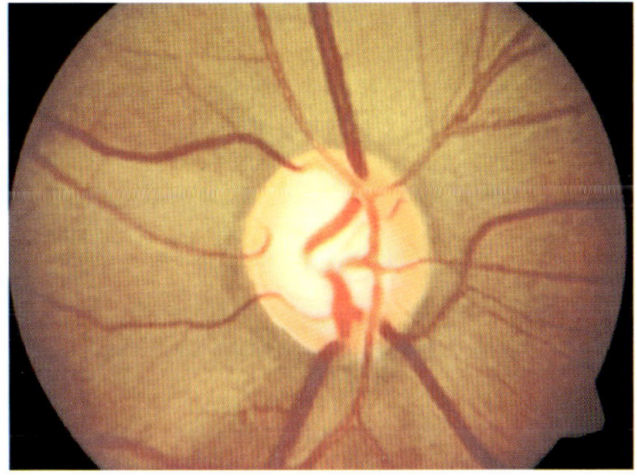

Fig. 8.8 *Focal ischaemic glaucomatous optic disc*

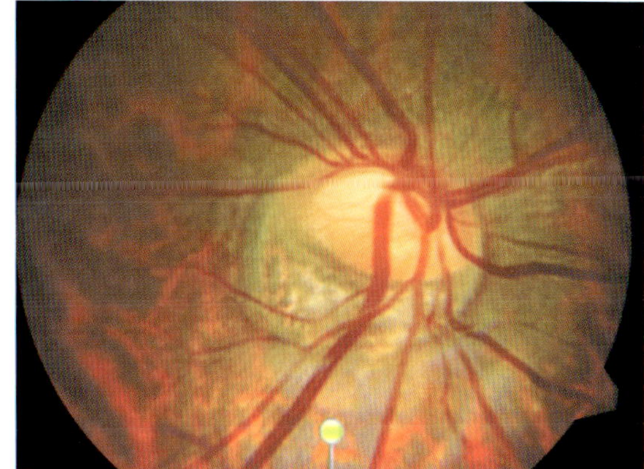

Fig. 8.9 *Myopic glaucomatous optic disc*

PATTERNS OF OPTIC DISC CHANGES AND SUBTYPES OF GLAUCOMATOUS DISCS

Focal glaucomatous optic disc

In this, there is localized NRR loss at inferior or superior pole just temporal to midline (Fig. 8.8). Such disc changes are commonly associated with migraine and vasospasm. Clinical associations for this disc appearance include a higher frequency among women, scotomas near fixation in the superior visual field, and smaller disc size than other glaucomatous disc types. It may be associated with localized field defects with early threat to fixation.

Myopic glaucomatous optic disc

These discs tend to occur in younger male patients. Myopic glaucomatous discs are usually tilted or obliquely implanted (Fig. 8.9). It has a shallow appearance and is usually associated with the presence of temporal crescent. Additional features of glaucomatous damage, such as notching, are often present.

Senile sclerotic (atrophic glaucomatous) optic disc

It is shallow, saucerized cup and a gently sloping NRR, variable peripapillary atrophy and peripheral visual field loss (Fig. 8.10). As the concentric cupping progresses, the neural rim may nevertheless retain a pale but almost normal colour. The clinical appreciation of such colour/cup discrepancy is important and often explains why visual field loss appears to be greater than the optic disc changes. The clinical associations for this disc appearance include a higher frequency in older patient group. Hypertension and cardiovascular disease is more common.

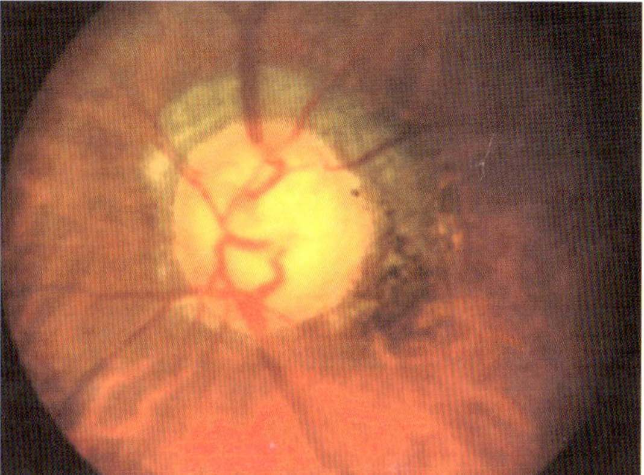

Fig. 8.10 *Senile sclerotic glaucomatous optic disc*

Concentrically enlarging optic discs

These discs have uniform NRR thinning (Fig. 8.11) and are frequently associated with diffuse visual field loss. At presentation, IOP is often significantly elevated.

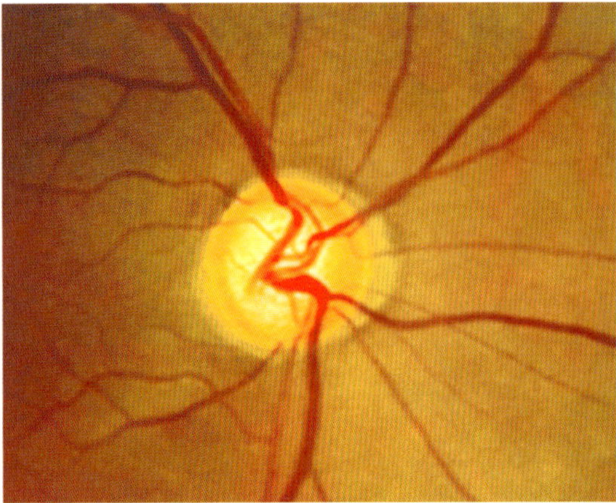

Fig. 8.11 *Concentrically enlarging optic disc*

DIFFERENTIAL DIAGNOSIS AND CONCLUSION

DIFFERENTIAL DIAGNOSIS OF OPTIC DISC CUPPING

Other types of optic neuropathies have been reported to cause cupping of the optic nerve, mimicking that found in glaucoma, include:

- Arteritic anterior ischaemic optic neuropathy (A-AION)
- Non-arteritic anterior ischaemic optic neuropathy (NA-AION)
- Posterior ischaemic optic neuropathy (PION)
- Intracranial tumours
- Optic neuritis
- Dominant optic atrophy
- Methanol toxicity
- Shock optic neuropathy
- Leber hereditary optic neuropathy

CONCLUSION

Patients remain undetected till the late stages of glaucoma due to the asymptomatic nature of the disease combined with the diagnostic dilemma of glaucoma. Diagnosis of end-stage glaucoma straightforward but time delay in diagnosis makes blindness inevitable. So judicially diagnosing glaucoma in earlier stage by careful evaluation of early glaucomatous changes in the optic nerve head can alter the course of the disease and change the prognosis. It is best, if we can detect cases at a stage of early optic neuropathy and there is reasonable certainly that treating the particular patient will help prevent visual impairment due to glaucoma.

SUGGESTED READING

1. Brown GC. Differential diagnosis of the glaucomatous optic disc. In: Varma R, Spaeth GL, Parker KW, editors. The optic nerve in glaucoma, Philadelphia, Lippincott-Raven, 1993.
2. Drance SM, Begg IS. Sector haemorrhage: A probable acute disc change in chronic simple glaucoma. Can J Ophthalmol 1970;5:137–41.
3. Gross PG, Drance SM. Comparison of a simple ophthalmoscopic and planimetric measurement of glaucomatous neuroretinal rim areas, J Glaucoma 1995;4:314.
4. Jonas JB, Gusek GC, Naumann GO. Optic disc, cup and neuroretinal rim size, configuration and correlations in normal eyes. Invest Ophthalmol Vis Sci 1988;29:1151.
5. Jonas JB, Fernandez MC. Shape of the neuroretinal rim and position of the central retinal vessels in glaucoma, Br J Ophthalmol 1994;78:99.
6. Papastathopoulos KI, Jonas JB. Focal narrowing of retinal arterioles in optic nerve atrophy. Ophthalmology 1995;102:1706.
7. Quigley HA, Broman AT. The number of people with glaucoma worldwide in 2010 and 2020.Br J Ophthalmol 2006;90:262–67.
8. Quigley HA, Miller NR, George T. Clinical evaluation of nerve fiber layer atrophy as an indicator of glaucomatous optic nerve damage: Arch Ophthalmol 1980;98:1564.
9. Schwartz B. Optic disc changes in ocular hypertension. Surv Ophthalmol 1980;25:148–54.
10. Schwartz B, Reinstein NM, Lieberman DM. Pallor of the optic disc: Quantitative photographic evaluation. Arch Ophthalmol 1973;89:278–86.
11. Tsai CS, Ritch R, Shin DH, et al. Age-related decline of disc rim area in visually normal subjects. Ophthalmology 1992;99:29–35.
12. Varma R, et al. Positional changes in the vasculature of the optic disc in glaucoma. Am J Ophthalmol 1987;104:457.

IMAGING IN GLAUCOMA

CHAPTER 9

INTRODUCTION

Establishing functional and structural damage of optic nerve head forms an integral part of glaucoma management. Perimetry is a well-established modality monitoring the functional status in patients of glaucoma. Stereometric examination of optic disc and evaluation of optic disc photograph are subjective methods of assessment of the structural status of optic disc. In the last decade, various objective methods of *in vivo* imaging, namely time domain optical coherence tomography (TD OCT), confocal scanning laser ophthalmoscopy (CSLO), and scanning laser polarimetry (SLP), have been introduced in clinical practice. The recent development of spectral domain optical coherence tomography (SDOCT) has added another dimension of studying the ganglion cell complex. It is perceived that structural damage precedes functional damage in glaucoma. By the time white on white perimetry shows some defect, about 40–45% of ganglion cells have been damaged, hence the importance of imaging the optic disc and retinal nerve fibre layer. The technologies are new and evolving, it should be interpreted cautiously. The purpose of this section is to provide the basic understanding of these devices, so that they can be utilized appropriately in the diagnosis as well as follow-up of glaucoma patients.

POSTERIOR SEGMENT OPTICAL COHERENCE TOMOGRAPHY IN GLAUCOMA

Tomography is imaging by sectioning or "slicing" through tissue. In ophthalmology, optical coherence tomography (OCT) represents this technique. OCT can image the anterior segment (cornea and anterior chamber) (Fig. 9.1A) and posterior segment (vitreous and retina) (Fig. 9.1 B), but focussing limitations cannot effectively image both anterior and posterior chambers simultaneously.

Time domain technology was the first wave of OCT technology represented in clinical use by the Zeiss Stratus OCT. This is the proprietary design of the Carl Zeiss Company.

Spectral domain/Fourier domain is the second wave of OCT technology developed by many companies, with many spectral domain OCT machines coming on the market at about the same time.

PRINCIPLE

The principle of OCT imaging is based on the measurement of delay in back reflected light from various tissue structures. The OCT utilizes an infrared diode light source (wavelength of 830 or 1310 nm) and a Michelson-type interferometer that detects differential light back scattering from the tissue microstructures. The amplitudes and delays in tissue reflections are scanned by the reference mirror and the interferometric signal is simultaneously recorded. The OCT's false-colour images denote the regions with strongest reflection with red and white colours and the regions with weakest reflection with blue and black.

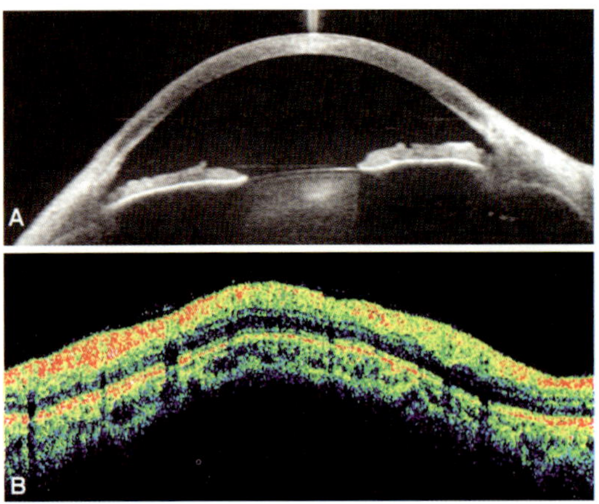

Fig. 9.1 *OCT: (A) Anterior segment; (B) Posterior segment*

STRATUS OCT SCAN OF POSTERIOR SEGMENT IN GLAUCOMA

INDICATIONS

OCT can be used for both detection and progression of glaucoma. It is particularly important in the setting of suspicious optic discs but normal visual fields which may be the stage of "pre-perimetric glaucoma" undetected on standard achromatic perimetry.

INDICATIONS FOR OCT IMAGING IN GLAUCOMA

- Ocular hypertension (OHT).
- Mild and moderate glaucoma, especially in patients who are unable to perform reliable visual fields.
- Assessing progression in OHT, mild and moderate glaucoma patients.

SCREENING PROTOCOL

The Stratus OCT enables scanning three regions for glaucoma detection—peripapillary retinal nerve fibre layer (RNFL), the macular region and the optic nerve head.

1. *RNFL measurements.* With the OCT are able to differentiate glaucomatous from normal subjects with good sensitivity and specificity. The RNFL thickness in the inferior region and the mean RNFL thickness are reported to have the best performance to discriminate healthy eyes from eyes with early to moderate glaucoma.

2. *Optic nerve head (ONH) analysis.* The utility for the topographic evaluation of the optic nerve head with the OCT for glaucoma diagnosis and monitoring still needs to be further evaluated. As the automatic algorithm for detection of the disc margin is based upon the determination of the ends of the RPE/choriocapillaris layer, it is possible that disc margin evaluation may be influenced by changes in these layers, such as in progressive peripapillary atrophy in glaucoma. Another source of error may be that the ONH measurements are obtained from six linear scans, each is composed of 128 sampling points in a radial spoke-like pattern with mathematical interpolation to fill in the gaps.

Nevertheless, recent reports have demonstrated good discriminating ability of (albeit different) ONH parameters. One study showed the rim area and horizontal integrated rim width as the best ONH parameters, while the other found the cup-disc area ratio as the best ONH discriminator.

3. ***Macular thickness.*** The mean macular thickness of glaucomatous eyes has been shown to be significantly lower than that of normal control eyes. In addition, a significant correlation between OCT macular thickness and visual field mean defect in glaucomatous eyes had been demonstrated. However, the ability of these measurements to discriminate glaucomatous form normal eyes is less than that of RNFL measurements.

READING A PRINTOUT

- ***Patient details:*** Confirm that you have the right patient. Age is important as comparison is with age matched normative data base.
- ***Signal strength value*** [Image Quality Information]

  This appears above the RNFL circle scan image. Signal strength ranges from 0 (Minimum) to 10 (Maximum). When values are less than 6, it is below the acceptable threshold and this data must not be considered for progression analysis. Remember, Garbage In, Garbage Out.
- ***Refractive error adjustment:*** Cirrus SD-OCT has the facility of internal fixation focus adjustment for refractive errors from –20.0 D to +20.0 D.
- ***Blink/saccades:*** The newer SD-OCT machines have a built-in eye tracker which uses blood vessel registration or iris tracking and can compensate for eye movement.
- ***Media opacities:*** The en face scanning laser ophthalmoscope (SLO) image must always be examined to ensure the absence of a media opacity within the circumpapillary scan area, such as a posterior vitreous detachment (PVD). Areas in which the data is missing due to an opacity are represented in black.
- ***Key parameters:*** Compared to normative database for RNFL analysis and various disc parameters. When disc area is less than 1.3 mm^2 or greater than 2.5 mm^2, Cup: Disc ratio and Cup: disc volume are shown in grey color.
- ***RNFL thickness map:*** RNFL Thickness Maps derive from pixel average thickness measurements and report thickness using a color pattern, where cool colors (blues, greens) represent thinner areas and warm colors (yellows, reds) represent thicker areas. The maps exclude the optic disc, which appears solid blue.

  A typically normal map shows an hourglass shape of yellow and red colors around the disc.
- ***RNFL deviation map:*** It has an enface fundus image and shows the machine-derived boundary of the cup and the disc and the calculation circle placement for the NFL. Deviation from normal maps are derived from superpixel average thickness measurements and report the results of a statistical comparison against the normal thickness range for each superpixel.

  These maps apply the yellow and red colors (not the green) of the age-matched normative data to superpixels whose average thickness falls in the yellow and red normal distribution percentiles.

  The localized RNFL defect may be missed in circumpapillary RNFL measurement due to the outward distribution of defect. It is important to carefully assess this map as small localized defects may be seen on this map.
  - RNFL TSNIT Graph

    TSNIT Thickness Profiles (TSNIT stands for Temporal, Superior, Nasal, Inferior, and Temporal) display thickness at each A-scan location along the calculation circle and include as a backdrop the white-green-yellow-red color code based on the age-matched RNFL normative data.
  - *Extracted horizontal and vertical tomograms:* Horizontal and vertical B-scans of optic disc confirm the cup configuration and identify

artifacts related to the NRR measurements. Look for quality of image and segmentation errors in RNFL circular tomogram, e.g., those caused by an epiretinal membrane or diabetic retinopathy changes.

GLAUCOMA ANALYSIS PROTOCOLS

Most frequently used glaucoma analysis protocols include:

- RNFL thickness (single eye)
- RNFL thickness average (OU)
- RNFL thickness serial analysis (OU)
- Optic nerve head (single eye), and
- Guided progression analysis

RNFL thickness protocol

The RNFL thickness is the most frequently used scan protocol. Advantages of imaging the RNFL for glaucoma are:

- RNFL thickness is lost as the glaucomatous disease state progresses
- The status of the RNFL thickness can be followed serially from visit to visit, and
- RNFL thickness of the patient can be compared to the range of thickness derived from a "normal" population.

RNFL thickness protocols include:

RNFL thickness (single eye). This is a peripapillary scan protocol (Fig. 9.2). The 3.4 mm diameter circular scan has been found to be optimum for RNFL measurement. The scan circle is centred at the optic disc. Graphs of RNFL thickness are shown along scans made around the optic disc. The normal scan appearance is of "double hump" pattern indicative of increased RNFL thickness at superior and inferior poles.

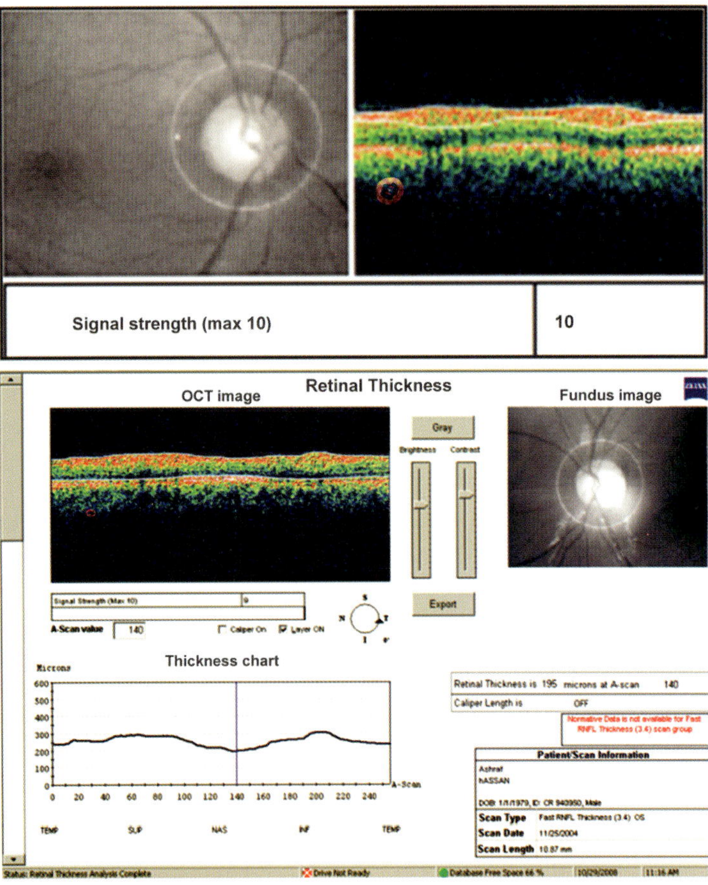

Fig. 9.2 *RNFL thickness (single eye)*

RNFL thickness average (OU). This analysis protocol shows retinal nerve fibre thickness representing the right and left eye around the optic disc (Fig. 9.3). One map shows RNFL thickness using a colour code, and the other shows average RNFL thickness in microns. The Stratus OCT has incorporated normative age-matched RNFL thickness data. The software displays graphs that are colour-coded according to the probability of the RNFL thickness measured in the particular patient being normal when compared to age-matched controls.

RNFL thickness serial analysis (OU). This analysis protocol allows the comparison of RNFL thickness over time. It utilizes circle scans around the optic disc to analyze the changes in RNFL thickness from one exam visit to the next. The RNFL thickness graphs of up to 4 visits are superimposed on the same chart and each visit is colour-coded (Fig. 9.4).

Optic nerve head analysis (single eye)

The algorithm detects and measures all features of the disc anatomy based on the anatomical markers (disc reference points) on each side of the disc where the RPE ends (Fig. 9.5).

The output chart enables measurement of the optic disc, optic cup, neuroretinal rim and cup/disc ratios using these measurements (Fig. 9.5).

- Cirrus acquires ONH data by defining the edge of the optic disc as the termination of Bruch's membrane and then finds the shortest perpendicular distance to Internal Limiting Membrane (ILM) viz., minimum band distance, to define the inner cup margin in each slice in a spiral around the optic disc cube data until a center is located. This allows the

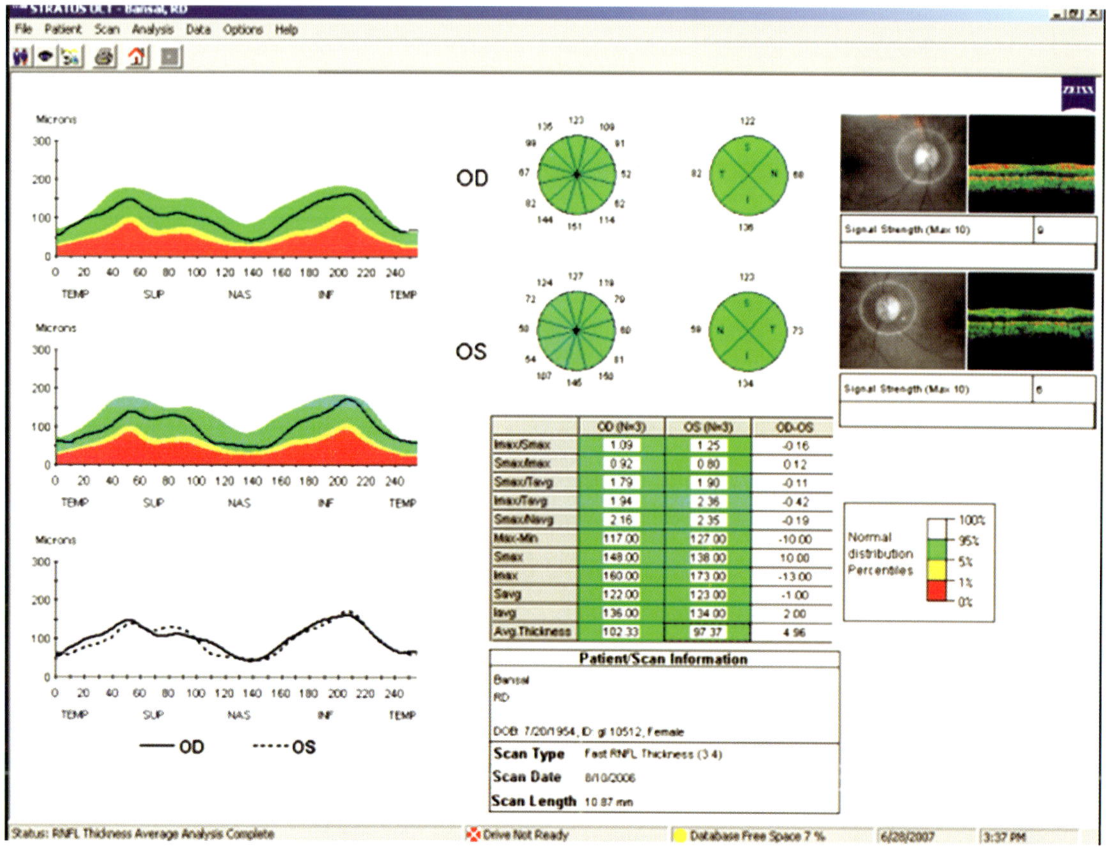

	OD (N=3)	OS (N=3)	OD-OS
Imax/Smax	1.09	1.25	-0.16
Smax/Imax	0.92	0.80	0.12
Smax/Tavg	1.79	1.90	-0.11
Imax/Tavg	1.94	2.36	-0.42
Smax/Navg	2.16	2.35	-0.19
Max-Min	117.00	127.00	-10.00
Smax	148.00	138.00	10.00
Imax	160.00	173.00	-13.00
Savg	122.00	123.00	-1.00
Iavg	136.00	134.00	2.00
Avg.Thickness	102.33	97.37	4.96

Fig. 9.3 *RNFL thickness average analysis (both eyes)*

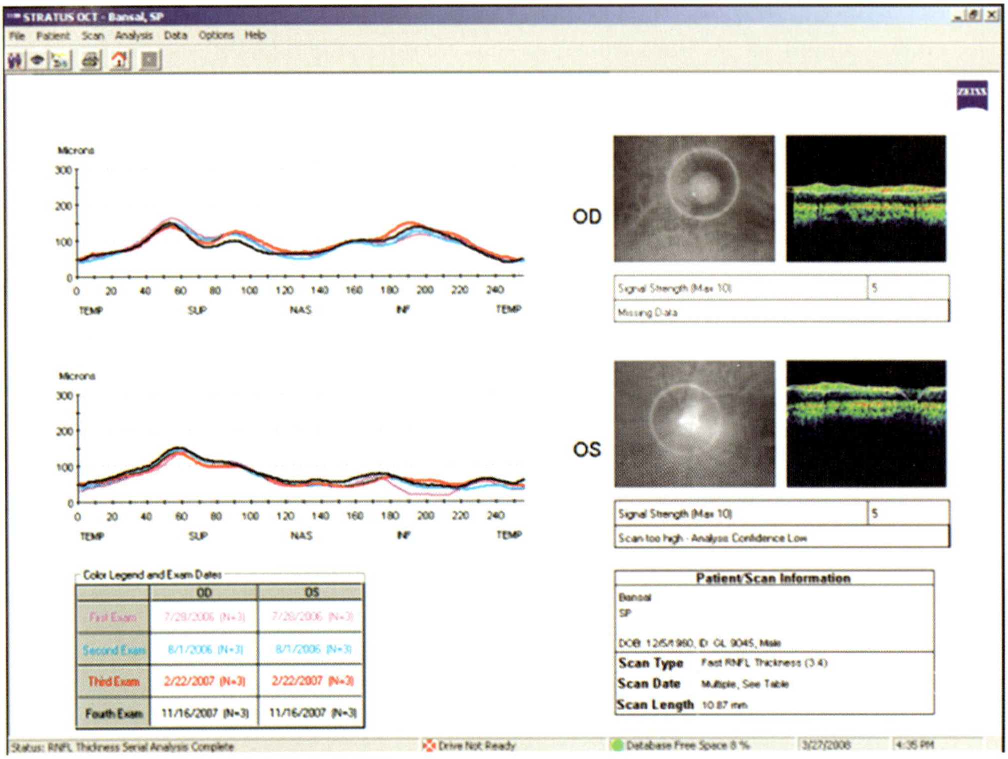

STRATUS OCT - Bansal, SP

File Patient Scan Analysis Data Options Help

Microns

300 200 100 0

0 20 40 60 80 100 120 140 160 180 200 220 240

TEMP SUP NAS INF TEMP

OD

Signal Strength (Max 10) 5

Missing Data

Microns

300 200 100 0

0 20 40 60 80 100 120 140 160 180 200 220 240

TEMP SUP NAS INF TEMP

OS

Signal Strength (Max 10) 5

Scan too high - Analysis Confidence Low

Color Legend and Exam Dates

	OD	OS
First Exam	7/28/2006 (N=3)	7/28/2006 (N=3)
Second Exam	8/1/2006 (N=3)	8/1/2006 (N=3)
Third Exam	2/22/2007 (N=3)	2/22/2007 (N=3)
Fourth Exam	11/16/2007 (N=3)	11/16/2007 (N=3)

Patient/Scan Information

Bansal

SP

DOB: 12/5/1960, ID: GL 9045, Male

Scan Type Fast RNFL Thickness (3.4)

Scan Date Multiple, See Table

Scan Length 10.87 mm

Status: RNFL Thickness Serial Analysis Complete   Drive Not Ready   Database Free Space 8 %   3/27/2008   4:35 PM

Fig. 9.4 *RNFL thickness serial analysis*

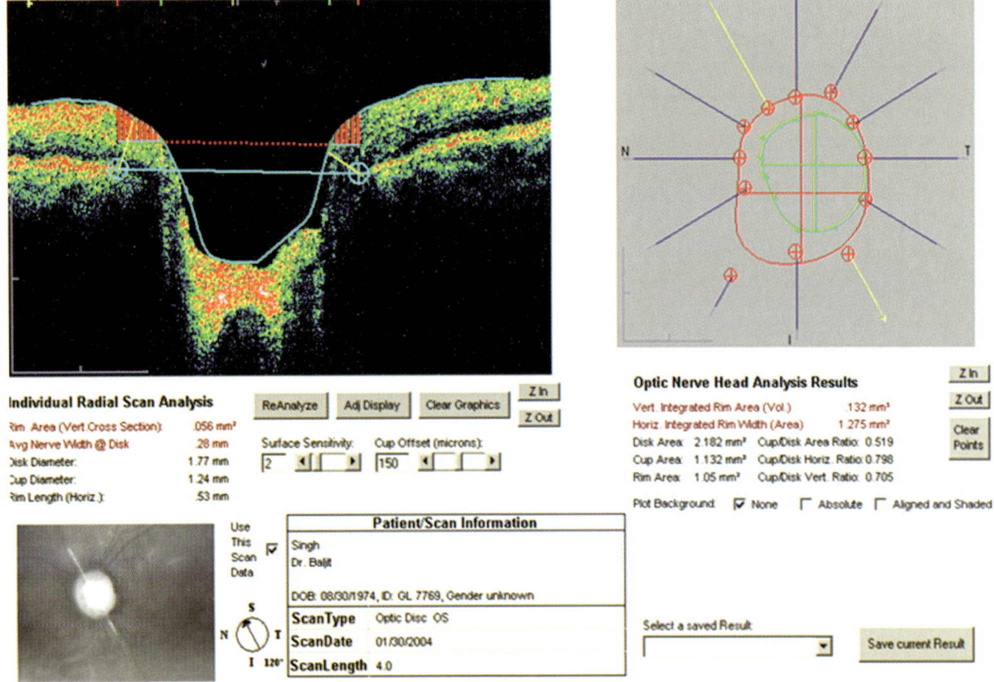

Fig. 9.5 *Optic nerve head analysis (single eye)*

3.4 mm RNFL circle to always be centered in the same place within the cube.

- ONH diameters >4.0 mm can falsely affect the accuracy of RNFL analysis results. A diagnostic capability study with SD-OCT of glaucoma and age-matched healthy controls reported that these ONH parameters can discriminate between healthy and eyes with mild glaucoma like RNFL thickness.

Guided progression analysis

Recent introduction to the guided progression analysis (GPA) protocol, the advanced serial analysis on the Stratus OCT, has enhanced the clinicians ability to detect progression, since it compares the change detected over time to the variability of the measurements seen in a patient with glaucoma of the same stage (Fig. 9.6A).

SD-OCT glaucoma progression algorithms (Fig. 9.6B) measure RNFL changes based on either event-based or trend-based analysis.

- *Event-based analysis:* It identifies a gradual change over time that eventually crosses a threshold or an acute event that exceeds a threshold value. This approach is susceptible to the effect of outliers that can be falsely labeled as progression.
- *Trend-based analysis:* This detects progression by evaluating the slope of measured parameter over time. Trend analysis is less sensitive to measurement variability and identifies a rate of progression that may be extrapolated for time-to-event predictions. This approach requires several tests before the analysis can be considered as reliable.

CIRRUS OCT takes two baseline scans for progression analysis, unlike spectralis which uses only one baseline scan.

TECHNIQUE OF STRATUS OCT SCANNING

Technique of OCT scanning for different protocols includes following steps:

1. *Initial preparation.* The initial preparation for scan acquisition is common for all protocols. The patient details are entered (or selected from the patient menu, if it is a follow-up scan). The height of the Stratus OCT desktop and chin-rest is adjusted to bring the forehead-rest level with the patient's forehead. The height of the chin cup is so adjusted so that the eyes align with the

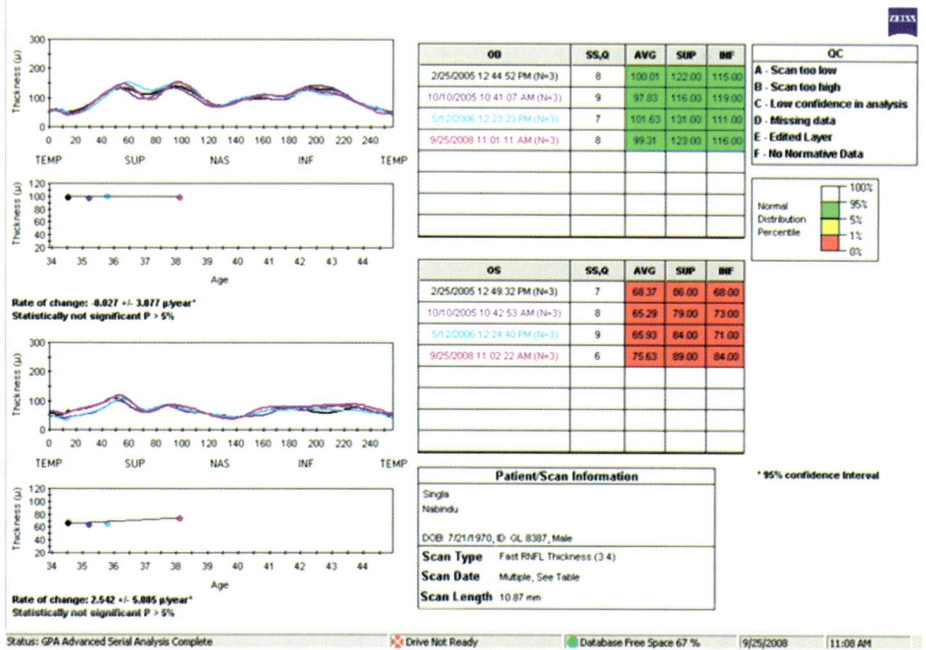

Fig. 9.6A *GPA advanced serial analysis*

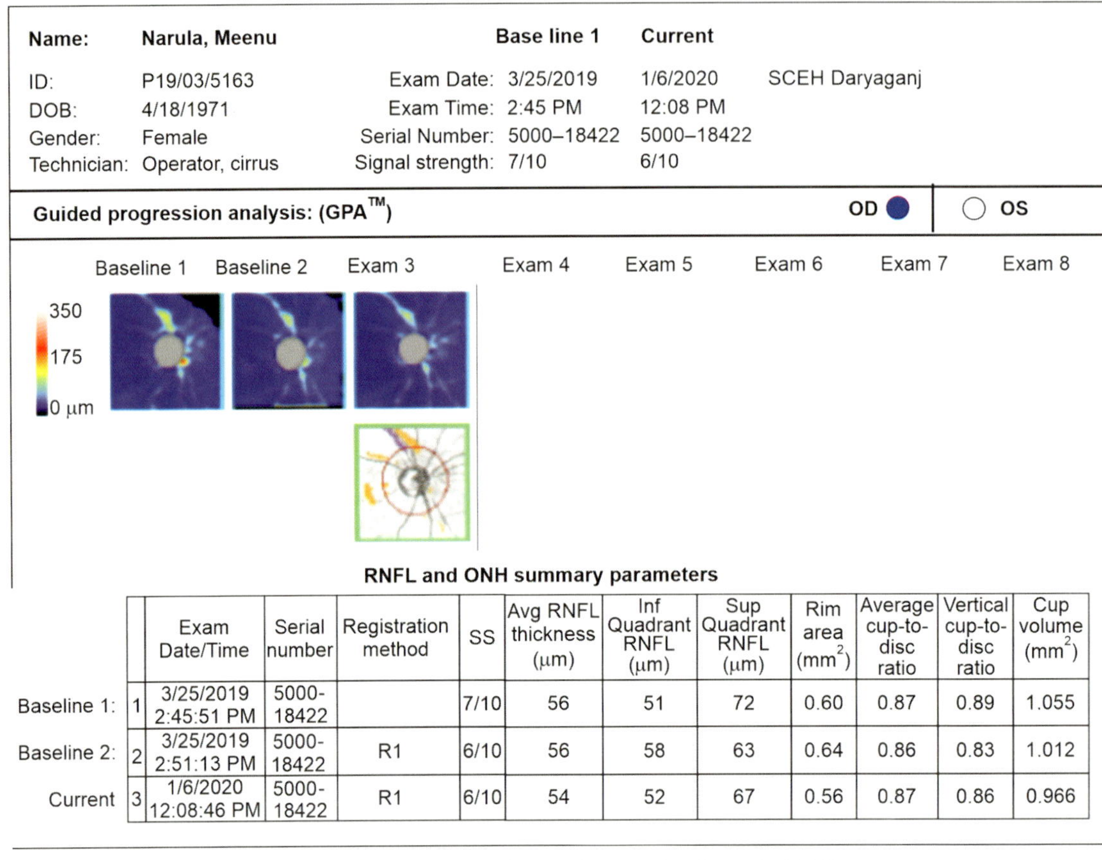

Name:	Narula, Meenu		Base line 1	Current
ID:	P19/03/5163	Exam Date:	3/25/2019	1/6/2020 SCEH Daryaganj
DOB:	4/18/1971	Exam Time:	2:45 PM	12:08 PM
Gender:	Female	Serial Number:	5000–18422	5000–18422
Technician:	Operator, cirrus	Signal strength:	7/10	6/10

Guided progression analysis: (GPA™) OD ● ○ OS

RNFL and ONH summary parameters

		Exam Date/Time	Serial number	Registration method	SS	Avg RNFL thickness (μm)	Inf Quadrant RNFL (μm)	Sup Quadrant RNFL (μm)	Rim area (mm^2)	Average cup-to-disc ratio	Vertical cup-to-disc ratio	Cup volume (mm^2)
Baseline 1:	1	3/25/2019 2:45:51 PM	5000-18422		7/10	56	51	72	0.60	0.87	0.89	1.055
Baseline 2:	2	3/25/2019 2:51:13 PM	5000-18422	R1	6/10	56	58	63	0.64	0.86	0.83	1.012
Current	3	1/6/2020 12:08:46 PM	5000-18422	R1	6/10	54	52	67	0.56	0.87	0.86	0.966

Fig. 9.6B *Cirrus OCT-Guided Progression Analysis [GPA]*

alignment markers on the side of the patient head mount.

2. ***Scan acquisition.*** From the main window (Fig. 9.7), the glaucoma tab (A) is selected. This would open up a window with the glaucoma protocols (B) displayed. The desired scan protocol is selected by "double clicking" on it.

This activates the scan acquisition window (Fig. 9.8), from which video and scan parameters can be adjusted from a single interface, enabling the acquisition of high quality scans.

In this window, the scan image is seen on the left of the screen (A), and the video image is seen on the right (B).

3. ***Scan placement.*** The scanner activates by default in the scan alignment mode, in which the scanner traces an aiming pattern which is seen on the video monitor. This is useful for scan placement on the desired position on the optic disc or retina.

- *Scan placement for RNFL protocols.* These are circle scans centred in the middle of the optic disc (Fig. 9.9A).
- *Optic nerve head protocols.* These are line scans arranged like spokes of a wheel, the centre of which should be in the middle of the optic disc (Fig. 9.9B).

Once the video image is satisfactory, and a scan image is placed satisfactorily, the scan mode button is clicked to display the scan acquisition mode. Here the scanner traces the actual scan pattern to be used more slowly. The scan is frozen with or without the flash, using the freeze with flash or freeze without flash buttons. If the quality of the scan image frozen on screen is satisfactory, it is saved using the save button. (If not entirely satisfied, one can click the cancel button and return to the scan acquisition mode to acquire another scan.)

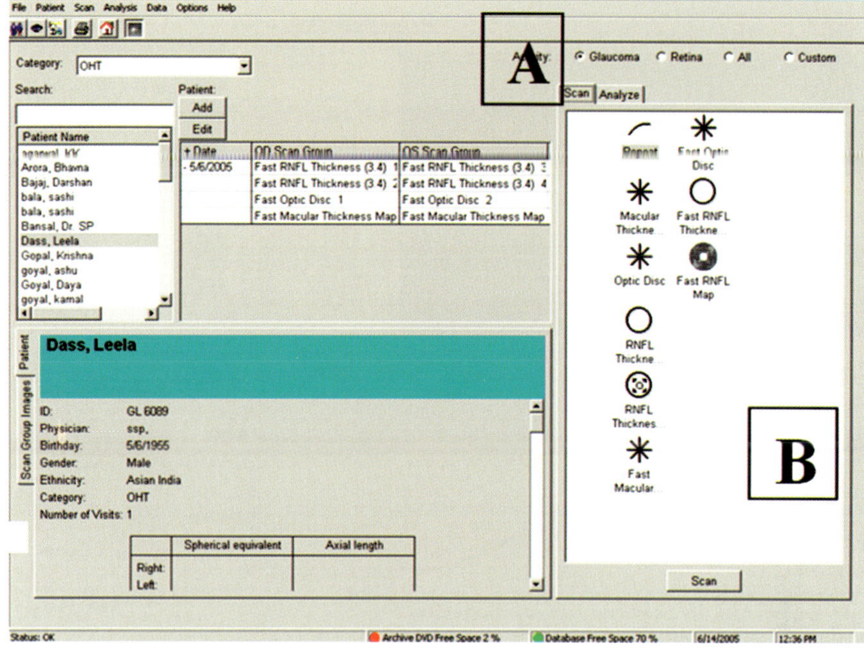

Fig. 9.7 *Main window*

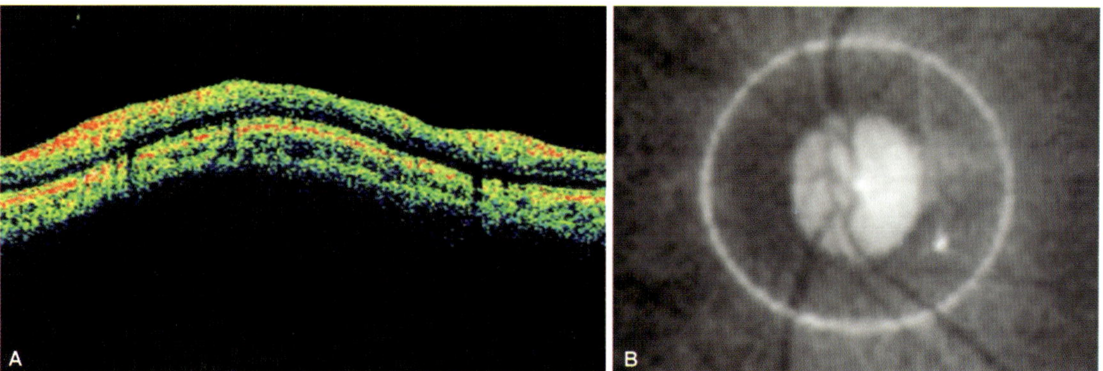

Fig. 9.8 *Scan acquisition window*

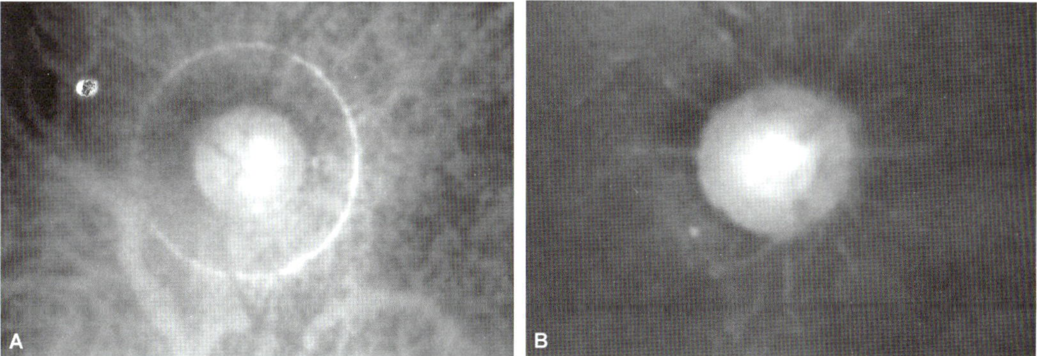

Fig. 9.9 *(A) RNFL scan placement around optic disc; (B) ONH scan placement on optic disc*

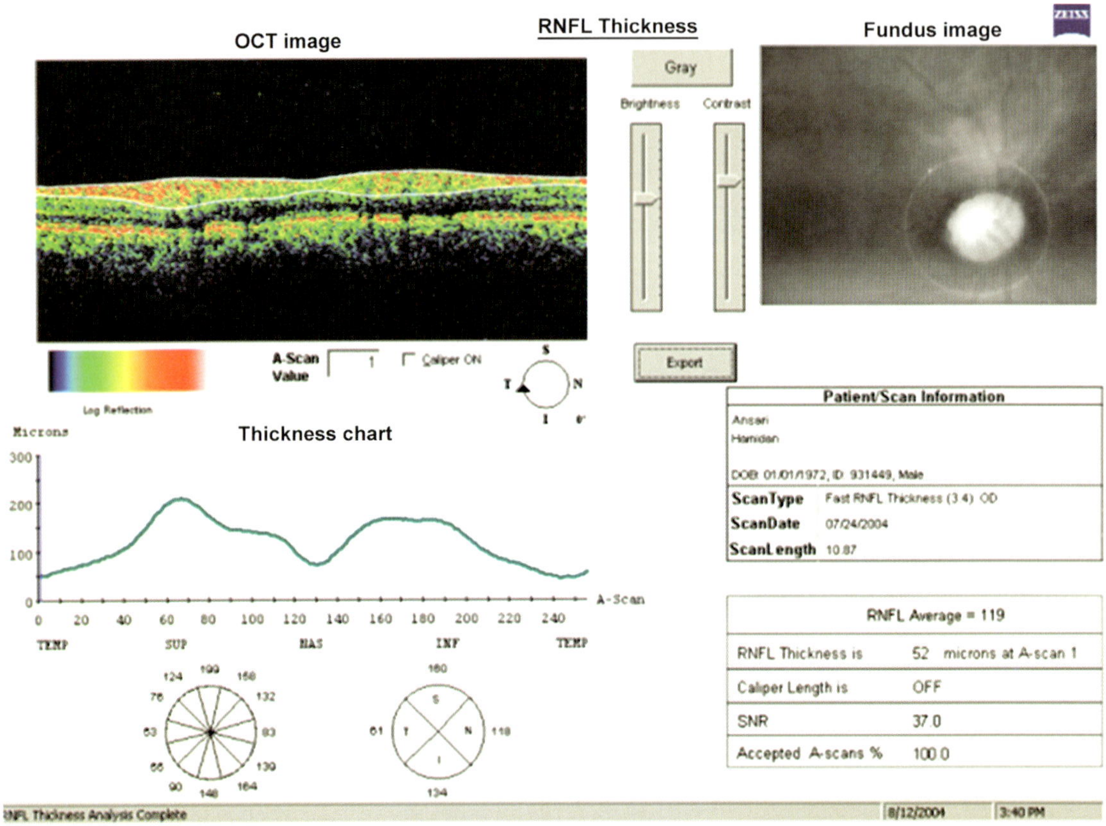

OCT image

RNFL Thickness

Fundus image

Gray

Brightness Contrast

Export

A-Scan Value 1 Caliper ON

Log Reflection

Thickness chart

Microns

300 200 100 0

0 20 40 60 80 100 120 140 160 180 200 220 240 A-Scan

TEMP SUP NAS INF TEMP

Patient/Scan Information	
Ansari Hamidan DOB: 01/01/1972, ID: 931449, Male	
ScanType	Fast RNFL Thickness (3.4) OD
ScanDate	07/24/2004
ScanLength	10.87

RNFL Average = 119	
RNFL Thickness is	52 microns at A-scan 1
Caliper Length is	OFF
SNR	37.0
Accepted A-scans %	100.0

RNFL Thickness Analysis Complete 8/12/2004 3:40 PM

Fig. 9.10 *Decentred scan*

LIMITATIONS OF TIME DOMAIN TECHNOLOGY WHEN USED FOR RNFL THICKNESS ANALYSIS

Three major sources of error while using the Stratus OCT for RNFL thickness measurement are: motion artifacts, failure to identify the upper and lower borders of the RNFL on low signal to noise ratio scans, and lack of registration.

1. *Motion artifacts.* OCT scan acquisition takes just short of 2 seconds because the reference arm is moving. It is difficult for an eye with good fixation to remain motionless for this time. In eyes with decreased vision due to pathology, eye movement increases dramatically due to which the eye continues to move even after the operator centres the scan circle. This results in a decentered scan (Fig. 9.10).

2. *Failure to identify the borders of the RNFL on low signal to noise ratio (SNR) scans.* Boundaries of RNFL are identifiable because they are more highly reflective than the bordering structures (Fig. 9.11). RNFL thickness is measured as the vertical distance between the two lines. There are measurement errors when the software fails to identify the upper and lower boundaries accurately. A poor scan may be due to optical opacities or operator error (Fig. 9.12). There is reduced signal-to-noise ratio and this prevents the software from making a proper identification and tracing.

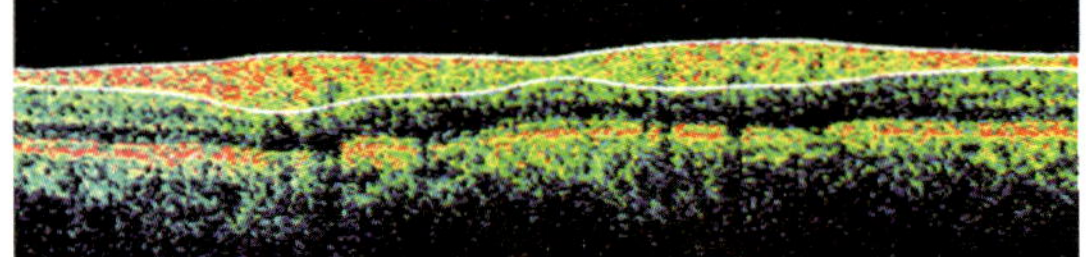

Fig. 9.11 *Good SNR scan with RNFL boundaries clearly visible*

3. *Lack of registration.* When performing serial scans over time, it is important to scan in the exact same position around the optic nerve head. With the Zeiss Stratus OCT 3, it is difficult to

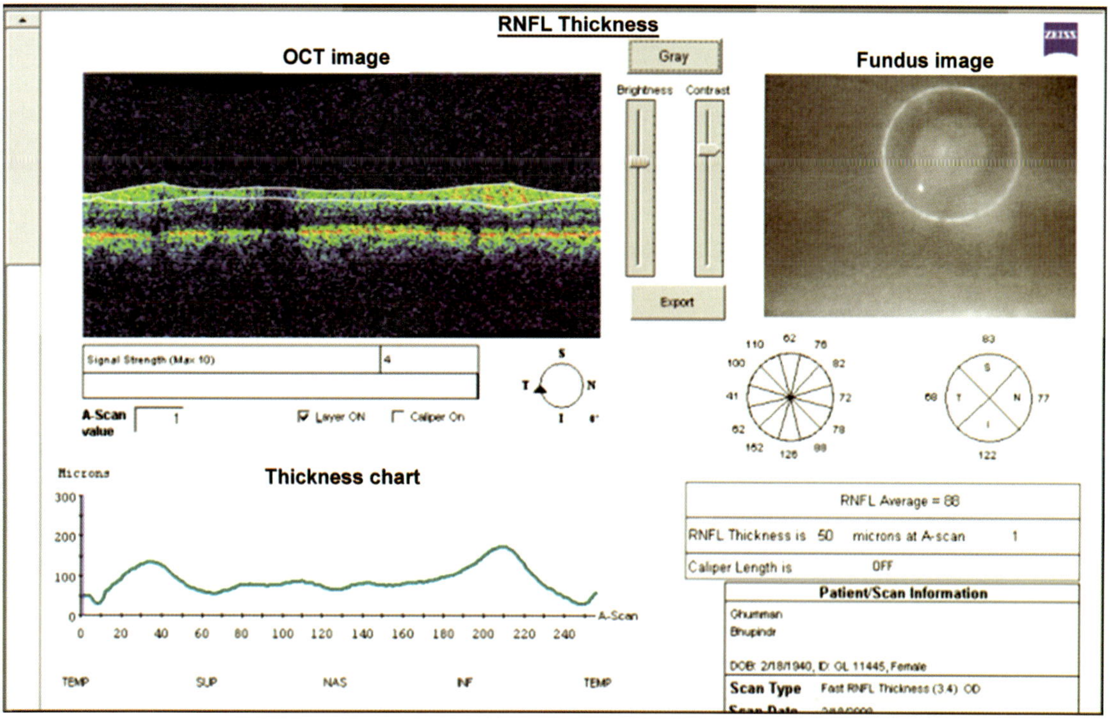

Fig. 9.12 *Poor SNR scan with RNFL boundaries not visualized, resulting in erroneous thin RNFL measurement visible*

register the scanning circle with anatomical landmarks in order to keep the positioning the same.

Theoretically, one can use a "landmark" (Fig. 9.13) to mark a certain characteristic, such as a bend in the blood vessel, but practically the operator must be relied upon to centre the circle visually as best as he or she can.

RNFL SCANNING USING STRATUS® VERSUS CIRRUS™ OCT

Table 9.1 and Fig. 9.14 sum-up the RNFL scanning using Stratus® versus Cirrus™ OCT machine.

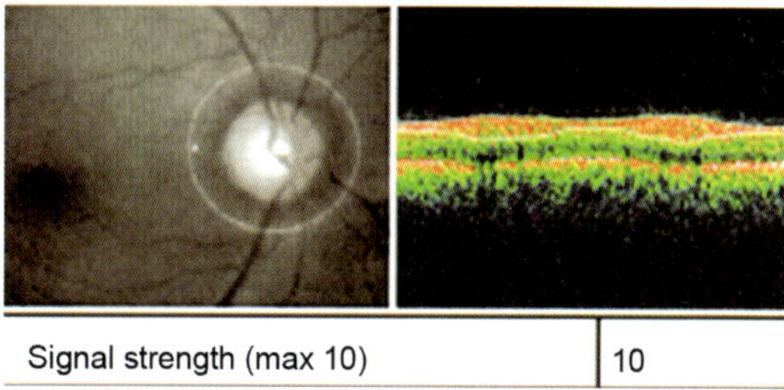

Fig. 9.13 *White dot as landmark to mark seen circle position*

SPECTRAL DOMAIN OCT IN GLAUCOMA

- SD-OCT obtains a 3-dimensional cube of data of the scanned region

Table 9.1 *Sum-up of RNFL scanning using the Stratus® and Cirrus™ OCT*

	Stratus®	*Cirrus™*
Scan protocol	Fast RNFL	Optic disc scan (200 × 200)
Scans	256 scans × 3 circles	512 scans extracted circle × 1
Laser source wavelength	820 nm	840 nm
A-scan speed	400 per sec	27,000 per sec
Axial resolution	8–10 microns	5 microns (better coherence)
Transverse resolution	20 microns	15 microns

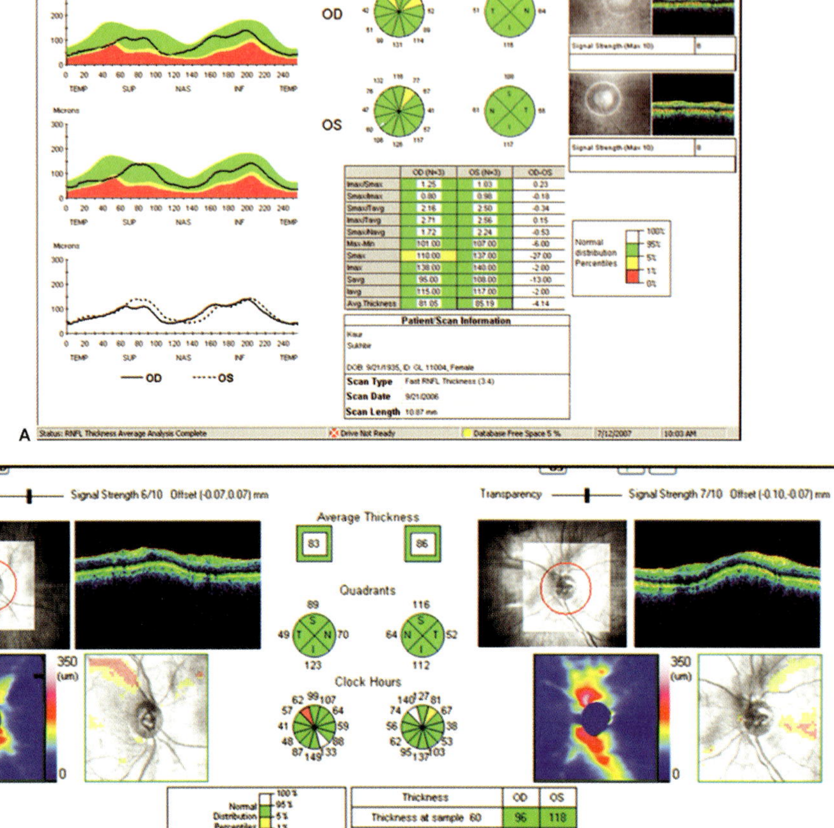

Fig. 9.14 *Patient with superotemporal RNFL defect imaged with the Stratus OCT (A) and Cirrus OCT (B)*

- Most used SD-OCT devices are Cirrus HD OCT [Carl Zeiss Meditec, Dublin, CA, USA], RTVue-100 [Optovue Inc., Fermont, CA, USA], Spectralis OCT [Heidelberg Engineering, Heidelberg, Germany] and Topcon 3D-OCT2000 [Topcon Corporation, Tokyo, Japan].
- Each machine differs in its different glaucoma scan patterns, software algorithms, display outputs and therefore the results are not interchangeable (Table 9.2).

Glaucoma analysis protocol by Cirrus™

The scan protocol used is the optic disc cube 200 × 200. It generates a cube of data through a 6 mm square grid. The machine acquires a series of 200 horizontal scan lines each is composed of 200 A-scans. A 3.4 mm circle of RNFL thickness extracted in this cube (Fig. 9.15A). It comprises 512 axial scans—equal to that of a regular Stratus RNFL scan.

Table 9.2 *Basic differences between the common SDOCT machines*

	RTVue	*Cirrus*	*Spectralis*
Principle	Superluminescent diode scan–840 nm	Superluminescent diode scan—840 nm	CSLO and SD OCT scanners (870 nm wavelength)
Motion artifacts	Higher	Reduced	Minimal-real time eye tracking system-adjusts for eye movements
A scans	26,000/sec	27,000/sec	40,000/sec
Axial resolution	5 microns	5 microns	3.9 microns
RNFL thickness	Circle of 3.45 mm diameter manually centered around the optic disc	Circle of 3.45 mm diameter automatically centered around the optic disc	Circle of 3.45 mm diameter automatically centered around the optic disc
Macular scan	GCC-RNFL+ GCL+IPL	GCA- GCL+IPL	
Signal strength	>30	>6	>15

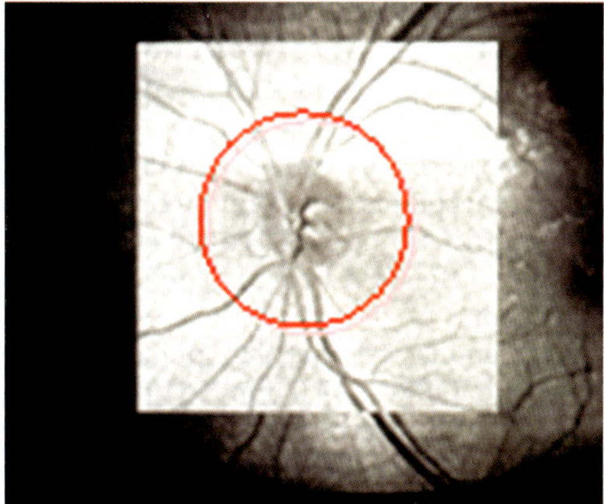

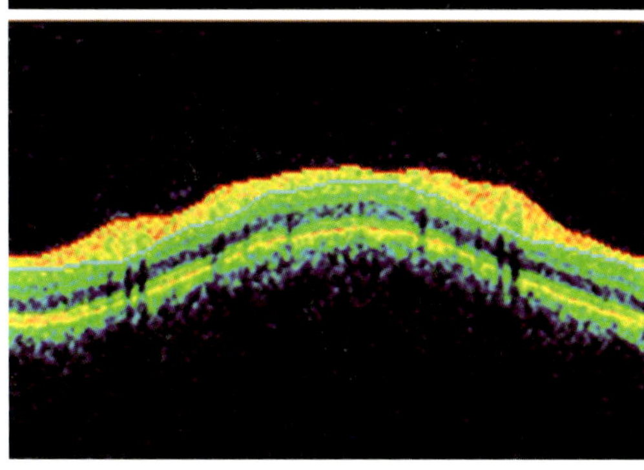

Fig. 9.15A *Optic disc cube 200 × 200*

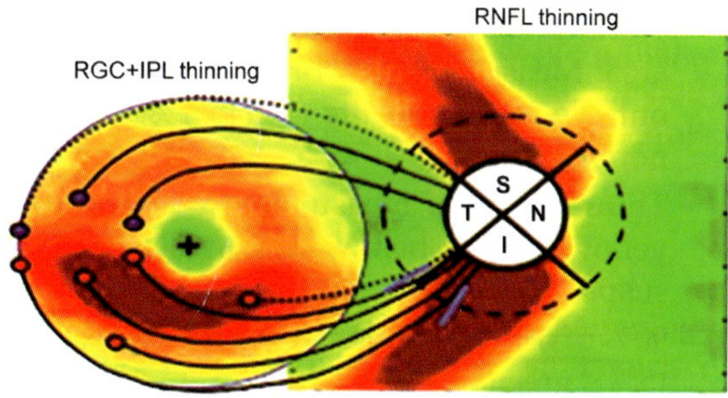

Fig. 9.15B *Macular mapping*

Macular thickness parameters in OCT for glaucoma diagnosis

SD-OCT segmentation algorithms have enabled quantification of individual layers in the macular region that are particularly impacted by glaucomatous damage, specifically, macular RNFL (mRNFL), ganglion cell layer with inner plexiform layer (GCIPL in Cirrus OCT) and ganglion cell complex (GCC = mRNFL + GCIPL in Optovue), whereas spectralis measures the total macular thickness (Fig. 9.15B). For this scan, the horizontal tomogram must pass through fovea.

Indications of RNFL scanning by spectral domain OCT for glaucoma

It is useful as a baseline and follow-up tool for objective RNFL assessment in ocular hypertensives (OHT) and glaucoma suspects with discs suspicious for glaucoma. In patients with glaucoma, it can be used as an adjunct to visual fields when it is very difficult to assess progression. It may also be useful in glaucoma patients with macular pathology and poor fixation where visual fields may not be possible.

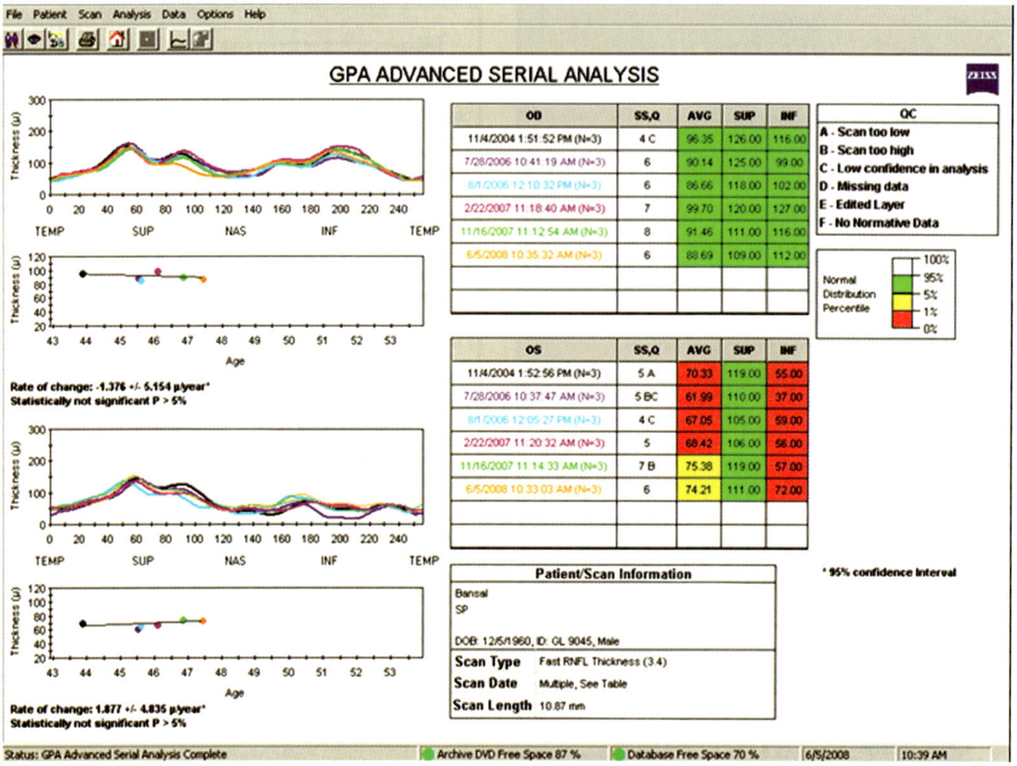

File Patient Scan Analysis Data Options Help

GPA ADVANCED SERIAL ANALYSIS

OD	SS,Q	AVG	SUP	INF
11/4/2004 1:51:52 PM (N=3)	4 C	96.35	126.00	116.00
7/28/2006 10:41:19 AM (N=3)	6	90.14	125.00	99.00
8/1/2006 12:10:32 PM (N=3)	6	86.66	118.00	102.00
2/22/2007 11:18:40 AM (N=3)	7	99.70	120.00	127.00
11/16/2007 11:12:54 AM (N=3)	8	91.46	111.00	116.00
6/5/2008 10:35:32 AM (N=3)	6	88.69	109.00	112.00

OS	SS,Q	AVG	SUP	INF
11/4/2004 1:52:56 PM (N=3)	5 A	70.33	119.00	55.00
7/28/2006 10:37:47 AM (N=3)	5 BC	61.99	110.00	37.00
8/1/2006 12:05:27 PM (N=3)	4 C	67.05	105.00	59.00
2/22/2007 11:20:32 AM (N=3)	5	68.42	106.00	56.00
11/16/2007 11:14:33 AM (N=3)	7 B	75.38	119.00	57.00
6/5/2008 10:33:03 AM (N=3)	6	74.21	111.00	72.00

QC
A - Scan too low
B - Scan too high
C - Low confidence in analysis
D - Missing data
E - Edited Layer
F - No Normative Data

Normal Distribution Percentile: 100%, 95%, 5%, 1%, 0%

Thickness (µ) 0–300; 0 20 40 60 80 100 120 140 160 180 200 220 240; TEMP SUP NAS INF TEMP

Thickness (µ) 20–120; Age 43–53

Rate of change: -1.376 +/- 5.154 µ/year*
Statistically not significant P > 5%

Rate of change: 1.877 +/- 4.836 µ/year*
Statistically not significant P > 5%

* 95% confidence interval

Patient/Scan Information
Bansal
SP
DOB: 12/5/1960, ID: GL 9045, Male
Scan Type: Fast RNFL Thickness (3.4)
Scan Date: Multiple, See Table
Scan Length: 10.87 mm

Status: GPA Advanced Serial Analysis Complete | Archive DVD Free Space 87 % | Database Free Space 70 % | 6/5/2008 | 10:39 AM

Fig. 9.19 *GPA on OCT showing no change in RNFL thickness*

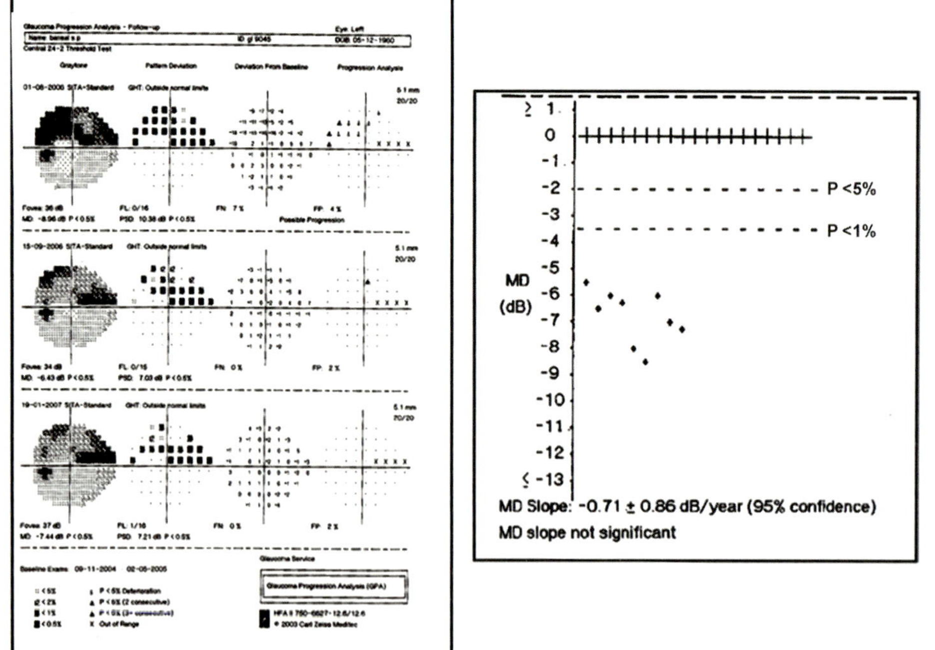

Fig. 9.20 *MD slope after repeat visual fields*

glaucoma, just as much as a normal OCT does not mean absence of disease.

The following examples will illustrate how the OCT can be misleading.

1. Abnormal OCT not glaucoma by default

If one just looks at the optic discs (Fig. 9.21) and OCT images (Fig. 9.22) of this 64-year-old woman, one would be justified in making a diagnosis of glaucoma in the right eye.

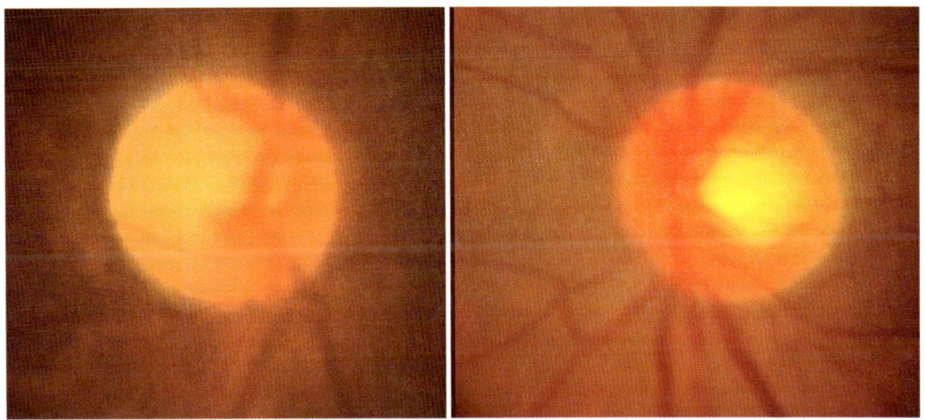

Fig. 9.21 *Optic disc photographs suggestive of glaucoma*

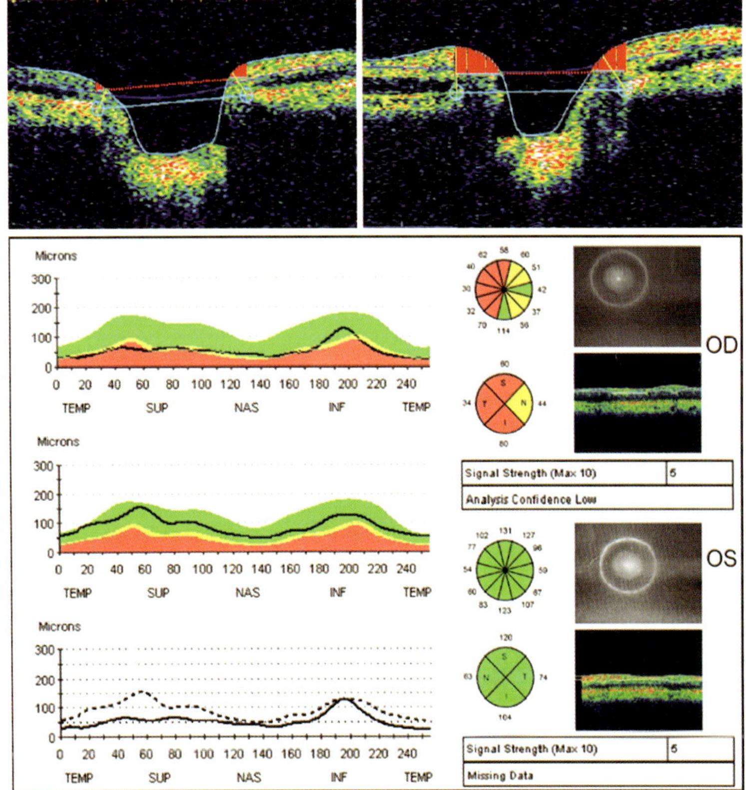

Fig. 9.22 *ONH and RNFL thickness on OCT of the same patient whose optic disc photographs are shown in Fig. 9.21*

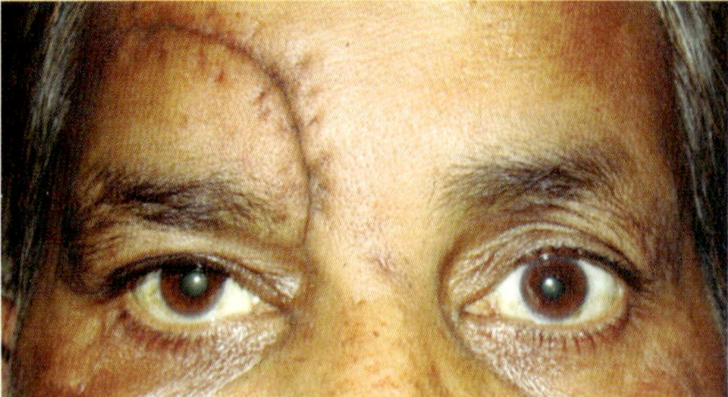

Fig. 9.23 *Large scar of trauma to right side of the head of a patient with traumatic optic neuropathy whose fundus photographs (Fig. 9.21) and OCT findings (Fig. 9.22) are suggestive of glaucoma*

There is superior neuroretinal rim thinning clinically. The OCT shows flattening of the normal RNFL hump superiorly and corresponding loss of rim in the optic disc cross-sectional scan images.

However, clinical examination reveals a relative afferent pupillary defect in the right eye, and a large scar of trauma to the right side of the head (Fig. 9.23). This makes a diagnosis of traumatic optic neuropathy which has resulted in RNFL loss. Any RNFL loss would show up as an abnormality on the OCT, but it does not necessarily mean that it is due to glaucoma.

2. Normal OCT does not mean it's not glaucoma

This 60-year-old woman presented with complaints of intermittent headache. The IOP was 16 and 18 mm Hg. The right eye optic disc was normal, while the left eye showed an inferotemporal notch with disc haemorrhage (Fig. 9.24) and RNFL defect.

There were corresponding visual field defects in the left eye (Fig. 9.25).

Despite clinically fulfilling a diagnosis of glaucoma, all RNFL measurements on the OCT were flagged green and looked normal (Fig. 9.26).

Conclusion

OCT is a very useful adjunct in glaucoma management and probably has a greater role in objectively following up patients. The new generation spectral domain OCT looks like having overcome some of the limitations of the older time-domain technology. Nevertheless, as for any other investigative modality, it is never

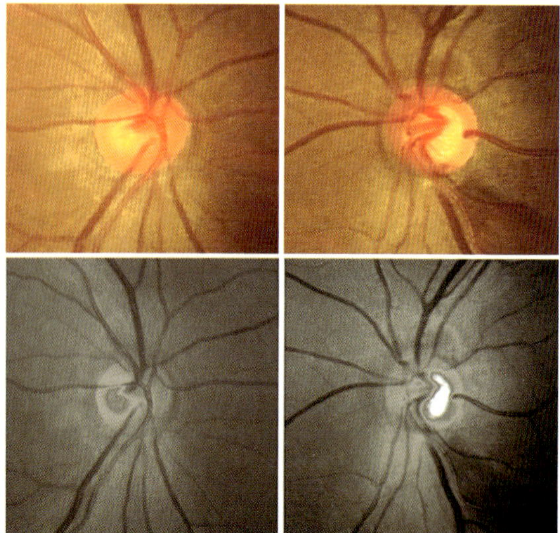

Fig. 9.24 *Optic discs of the patient*

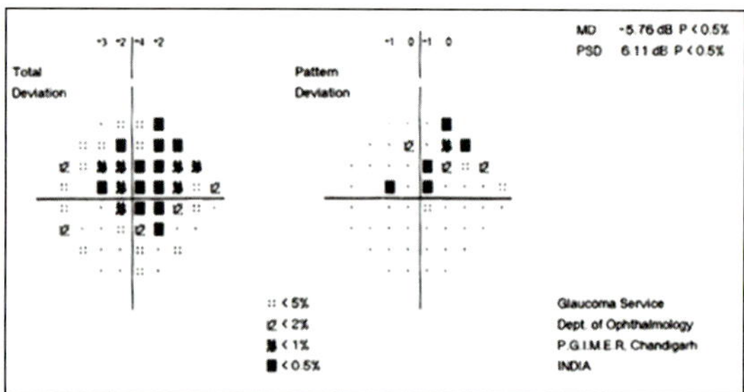

Fig. 9.25 *Visual field defect*

to be used in isolation without understanding the clinical setting in which the test was performed.

CONFOCAL SCANNING LASER OPHTHALMOSCOPY

The confocal scanning laser ophthalmoscopy (CSLO) commercially available for optic disc imaging is the Heidelberg retina tomograph (HRT), whose latest version is HRT III (Fig. 9.27). The data of older versions (HRT and HRT II) are compatible with HRT III and are transferable.

IMAGE ACQUISITION

It uses a focused diode laser beam of 670 micron to scan over the area of the fundus to be imaged. A pinhole, or confocal aperture, is placed in front

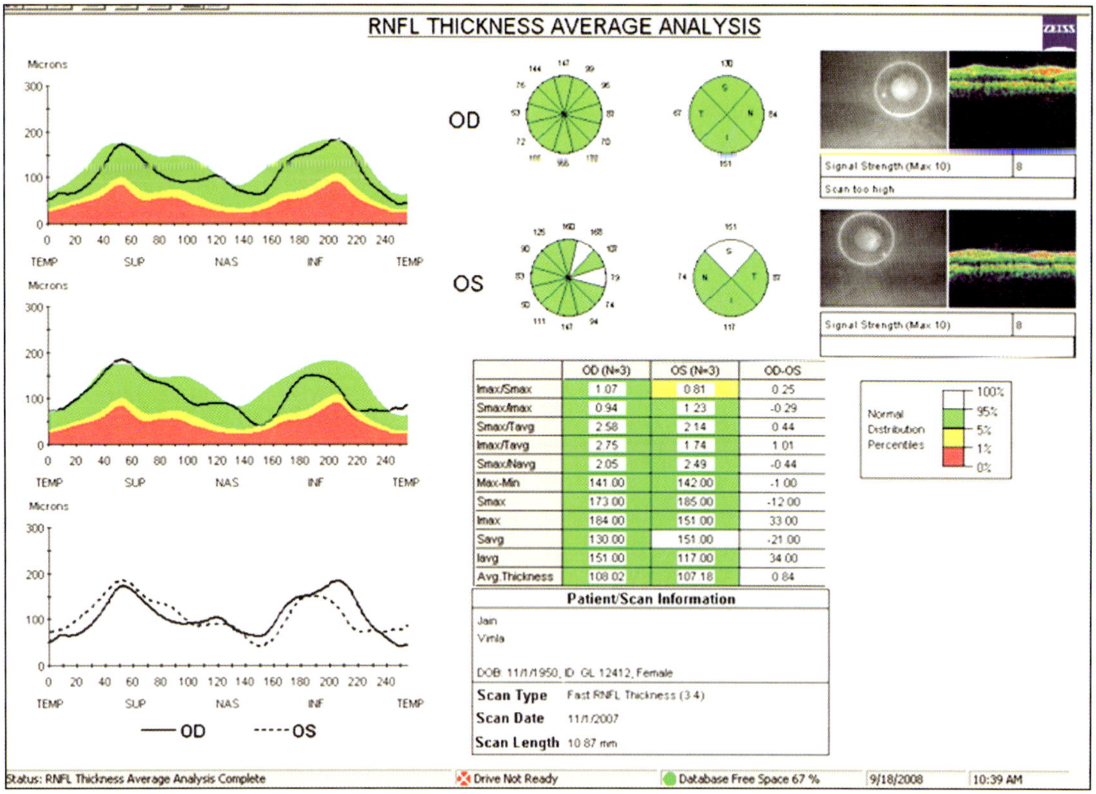

RNFL THICKNESS AVERAGE ANALYSIS
ZEISS
Microns
TEMP SUP NAS INF TEMP
OD
OS
Signal Strength (Max 10) 8
Scan too high
Signal Strength (Max 10) 8
OD (N=3) OS (N=3) OD-OS
Imax/Smax 1.07 0.81 0.25
Smax/Imax 0.94 1.23 -0.29
Smax/Tavg 2.58 2.14 0.44
Imax/Tavg 2.75 1.74 1.01
Smax/Navg 2.05 2.49 -0.44
Max-Min 141.00 142.00 -1.00
Smax 173.00 185.00 -12.00
Imax 184.00 151.00 33.00
Savg 130.00 151.00 -21.00
Iavg 151.00 117.00 34.00
Avg.Thickness 108.02 107.18 0.84
Normal Distribution Percentiles
100% 95% 5% 1% 0%
Patient/Scan Information
Jain
Vimla
DOB: 11/1/1950, ID: GL 12412, Female
Scan Type Fast RNFL Thickness (3.4)
Scan Date 11/1/2007
Scan Length 10.87 mm
Status: RNFL Thickness Average Analysis Complete
Drive Not Ready
Database Free Space 67 %
9/18/2008
10:39 AM

Fig. 9.26 *Normal RNFL thickness on OCT in a patient whose optic discs (Fig. 9.24) and visual field defect (Fig. 9.25) are suggestive of glaucoma*

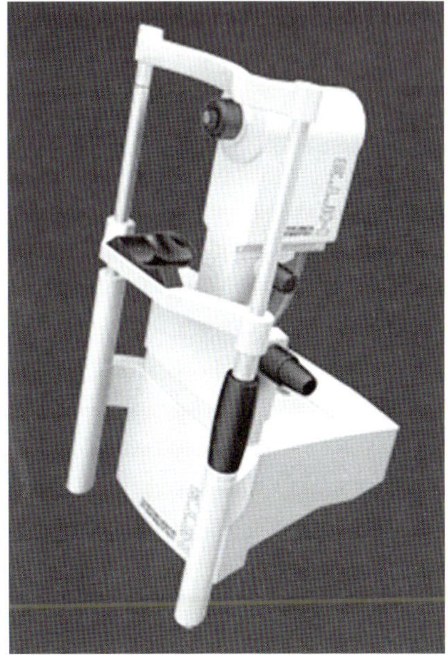

Fig. 9.27 *HRT III (Courtesy: Heidelberg Engineering)*

of the photo detector to eliminate scattered light. The aperture is conjugate to the laser focus, and the resulting image is said to be 'confocal'. This allows much higher axial and lateral resolution than that achieved with conventional light microscopy, such as with a fundus camera. Volume of tissue from which reflected light at that instant is accepted by the confocal aperture is called a voxel, the size of voxel is inversely proportional to resolution of the image. It acquires high resolution images, both perpendicular to the optic axis (x- and y-axis) and along the optic axis (z-axis). Oscillating mirrors in the HRT device redirect the laser beam to the x- and y-axis, along a plane of focus that is perpendicular to the optic axis (z-axis). A bi-dimensional image (15 × 15°) is obtained at each focal plane. As the device changes the focal plane, other bi-dimensional images of the optic nerve are obtained. Each one represents an optical section of the optic nerve. A total of 64 sections, each done with 1/16 mm of depth interval, are obtained and used to create a three-dimensional image of the optic nerve. These 64 sections are equivalent to a depth of 4 mm.

Once the image is taken, the operator delineates the optic nerve contour line over the reflectance or topography image. The operator places points at the external edge of the disc border and the machine draws a 'best-fit' ellipse linking these points together. Heidelberg retina tomography proceeds to define the 'reference plane' based on the disc contour drawn by the operator.

The reference plane is located 50 microns posterior to the mean height along a 6° arc of the contour line at the temporal inferior sector. Structures above the reference plane and within the contour line are considered to be rim. Anything below the reference plane is considered cup. Computation of stereometric parameters, classification of the eye and comparison to previous examinations are then done by the HRT. Classification of the eye is done with Moorefield's regression analysis or other discriminating method in HRT II, or with neural network analysis in HRT III.

The latest software available, HRT III, can provide ONH stereometric analysis without manual delineation of the disc margin by the operator. After a three-dimensional model of the ONH is constructed, five optic nerve parameters are calculated and then analyzed with an artificial intelligence classifier, the relevance vector machine (RVM). From this analysis, a glaucoma probability score (GPS) is created. Adjustments are made to the parameters to account for differences in age and disc size by both versions of HRT. However, HRT III is equipped with a larger and more diverse normative database than its predecessor. There are several printout formats currently available: Initial report, follow-up report and 'OU report,' among others. Discussed below are the different components of HRT printout.

COMPONENTS OF HRT REPORT

Interpretation of HRT III report printout (Fig. 9.28) is as below:

1. *Patient data.* Name, sex, date of birth, patient ID, and date of exam are provided here.

2. *Topography image.* This is the colour-coded representation of disc. Darker colour represents superficial areas while lighter colour represents deeper areas. Colours, like green and blue, indicate neuroretinal rim tissue (above the reference plane) while red indicates the cup (area below the reference plane). Blue indicates sloping rim.

3. *Reflectance image.* It is also a colour representation image where brighter areas representing highest reflectance, like the cup and is similar to a photograph. The reflectance image is overlaid with Moorfields analysis.

4. *Retinal surface height variation graph.* It consists of green and red lines where green line representing the retinal height and a red line representing the reference. It graphically represents the retinal height along the contour line and of the thickness of the nerve fibre layer. It appears as "double hump" where hills or 'humps' correspond to the superior and inferior nerve fibre layers, which are normally thicker than the rest of the areas. Left to right the graph depicts: the thicknesses of the temporal (T); temporal-superior (TS); nasal-superior (NS); nasal (N); nasal-inferior (NI); temporal-inferior (TI); and temporal (T) sectors.

5. *Vertical and horizontal interactive analysis.* It depicts optic nerve retinal surface height in horizontal and vertical cross-sections. A non-smooth or jagged trace represents a better quality scan. Observation of the trace can provide information of the disc steepness, presence of sloping, etc.

6. *Stereometric analysis.* HRT II provides a list of 14 nerve parameters. They are: disc, cup and rim area, cup and rim volume, cup/disc area ratio, linear cup/disc ratio, mean cup depth, maximum cup depth, cup shape measure, height variation contour, mean retinal nerve fibre layer (RNFL) thickness, RNFL cross-sectional area and reference height. To the right of the stereometric parameters, a column specifies ± one standard deviation from the mean of the normative database for each of the parameters. HRT III only provides values for 6 stereometric parameters in the 'OU printout'. These are: cup/disc area ratio, cup shape measure, rim area and volume, height variation

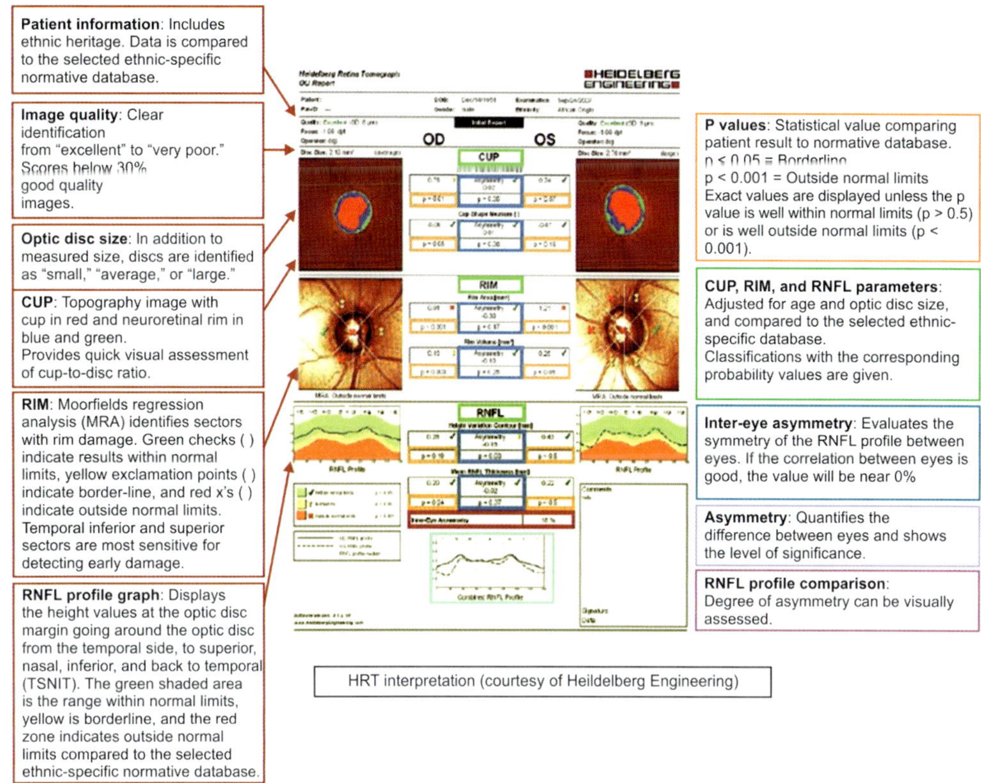

Fig. 9.28 *Interpretation of HRT III printout (Courtesy: Heidelberg Engineering)*

contour and mean RNFL thickness. Each value is designated as within normal limits, borderline or outside normal limits after comparing to the normative database.

7. ***Moorfields regression analysis (MRA).*** The MRA is based on a normative database of 112 Caucasian subjects with refractive error ±6D and disc size within the range of 1.2–2.8 mm. The ratio values of these subjects represents the value obtained in 50% of the normal subjects studied. In this way, outside normal limits (red x) represents the rim area of any segment (global assessment or any of the 6 sectors) is below the 99.9% prediction interval, that is, 99.9% of 'normals' have a higher rim area/disc area value than that of the nerve being classified as outside normal limits (ONL). Borderline (yellow checkmark) represents the rim area between the 95 and 99.9% prediction lines. Green checkmark (within normal limits) appears when rim areas fall above the 95% prediction level.

The Moorfields analysis graph is shown in the printout, indicating the predicted intervals on which the nerve classification is based. Green colour represents the rim and red represents the cup. Seven different columns representing all sectors are shown and classified as within normal limits (WNL), borderline (BL) or ONL. Moorfields classification is shown over the reflectance image as a green checkmark, yellow exclamation point, or a red 'x'. The Moorfields classification of the nerve is written at the bottom of the graph. Disc is classified on the basis of the worst classified sector in Moorfields regression. Moorfields regression analysis can discriminate glaucomatous nerves from normals with 84.3% sensitivity and 96.3% specificity. It tends to overestimate rim area in small optic nerves and to underestimate rim area in large nerves. So on either extreme of disc size range, care should be taken when analyzing these scans.

8. ***Glaucoma probability score (GPS).*** A new addition in the HRT III generation allows calculation of the GPS. A three-dimensional model of the ONH and peripapillary RNFL is constructed by using five parameters: cup size, cup depth, rim steepness, and horizontal and vertical RNFL. The complete three-dimensional model is then subjected to analysis by an artificial intelligence classifier, the relevance vector machine (RVM), that compares it to a predetermined normal and glaucoma model and then derives the probability of glaucoma for the scanned eye:

- Probability <28% is within normal limits (WNL)
- Probability between 28 and 64% in borderline (BL)
- Probability >64% is outside normal limits (ONL).

EVALUATING SCAN QUALITY

The value of any data lies on identification of good quality scan. Good quality indicators are even luminance and sharp borders of the topography and reflectance images, as well as good centration of the disc. The standard deviation (SD) measures, variability of the same pixel values among three different scans. The average light intensity for each point is what is used for the RNFL height measurement. The manufacturer has suggested not analyzing scans with an SD value greater than 40. It is important to point out that SD should not be the only parameter to use when assessing quality. A poor quality scan can still have a low SD value, if there is small or no variability among the three scans. The manufacturer's classification of scans by SD values is:

- 10: Excellent
- 11–20: Very good
- 21–30: Good
- 31–40: Acceptable
- 41–50: Poor
- 50: Very poor.

Looking at cross-sections can also help determine the degree of noise in the obtained images. The contour cross-sectional trace should be soft and not 'jagged'.

STRENGTHS AND LIMITATIONS OF HRT

HRT machines have stood the test of time and HRT III machine (the latest version) is backward compatible. The data from the previous models can be transferred to the newer models so that the progression over time can be evaluated: The most important aspect of the structural imaging systems. The sensitivity and specificity for both MRA and GPS are in the same range of around 83% sensitivity and 87% specificity. However, both the systems of analysis are dependent on the disc size for sensitivity and specificity. Small discs show lower sensitivity and higher specificity as compared to larger discs which show higher sensitivity and lower specificity. The measurements are based on the contour line and standard reference plane. It is considered as a major limitation. Some of the eyes show variable HRT measurements based on intraocular pressure, is another limitation. We should remember that we should never rely too much on the diagnostic abilities of these devices and only judicious use should be incorporated in the management of glaucoma.

Progression analysis

In the print out of progression analysis, the top row is topography image and the second row is the corresponding reflectance image of the serial scans performed on different dates. The follow-up reflectance images show superimposed red areas (significantly depressed from baseline) and green areas (significantly elevated from baseline). When at least four scans have been performed on one patient, an additional third row significance map appears, which starts flagging significance level, if the same area is showing similar change in at least three consecutive scans. This gives a fairly good idea about progression based on event-based analysis.

Tread analysis

This has multiple stereometric parameters. When multiple tests have been performed, all stereometric parameters combined can be studied either globally or sector-wise. Similarly, any isolated stereometric parameter also can be studied either globally or in a particular sector.

The starting point on trend line is 0 and if it moves downward and reaches up to 1.0, it is a definitive trend of deterioration.

HRT SCANS OF NORMAL AND GLAUCOMATOUS DISCS

Figures 9.29 to 9.32 show representative cases with normal disc, early, moderate and advanced glaucomatous changes, respectively.

SCANNING LASER POLARIMETRY (GDx)

INTRODUCTION

Scanning laser polarimetry is used to measure peripapillary RNFL thickness. The principle utilized in this technology is of birefringence. Birefringent intraocular tissues are the cornea, lens and the retina. In the retina, microtubules in retinal ganglion cell axons which are arranged parallel cause change in the polarization of light passing through them. This change in the polarization of light is known as retardation, and this can be measured. The retardation caused by the RNFL is linearly related to the thickness of RNFL. Glaucoma Diagnostics (GDx Carl Zeiss Meditec; Jena, Germany, and Dublin, California) (Fig. 9.33) utilize this technology. Different birefringence patterns are detected when the RNFL is healthy versus atrophied from glaucoma.

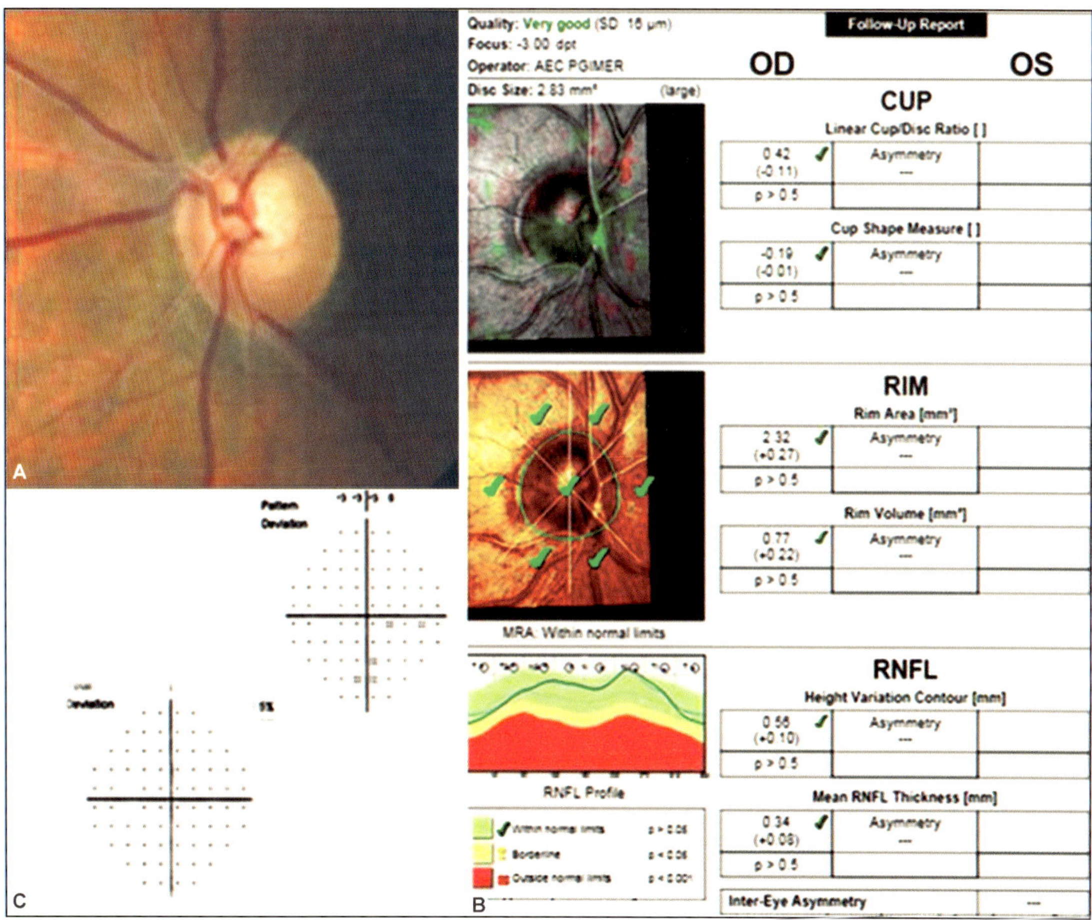

Fig. 9.29 *Normal disc: (A) Colour photograph of a right optic nerve; (B) Corresponding image from an HRT II showing thinning of RNFL. Red colour shows areas of neuroretinal rim thickness less than normative database; (C) Field changes correlating disc changes on total and pattern deviation plot*

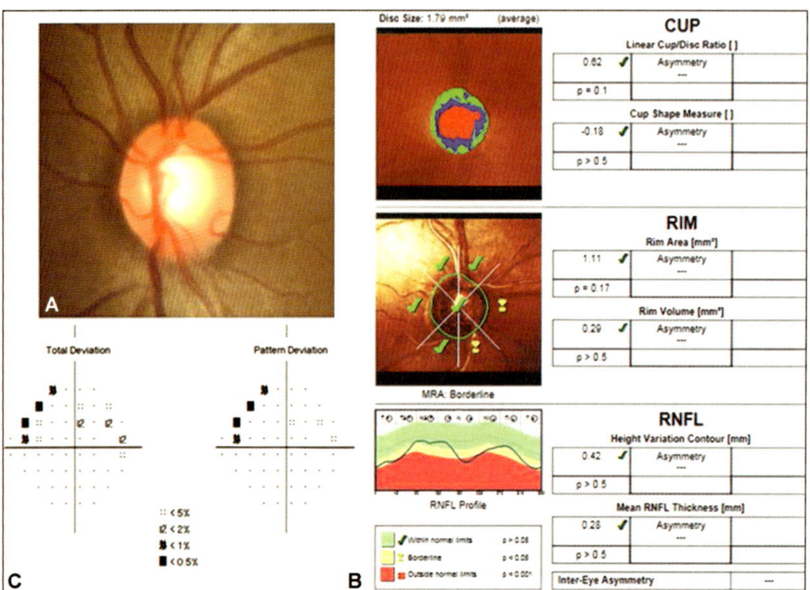

Fig. 9.30 *Early glaucomatous change: (A) Colour photograph of a right optic nerve; (B) Corresponding image from an HRT II showing thinning of RNFL. Red colour shows areas of neuroretinal rim thickness less than normative database; (C) Field changes correlating disc changes on total and pattern deviation plot*

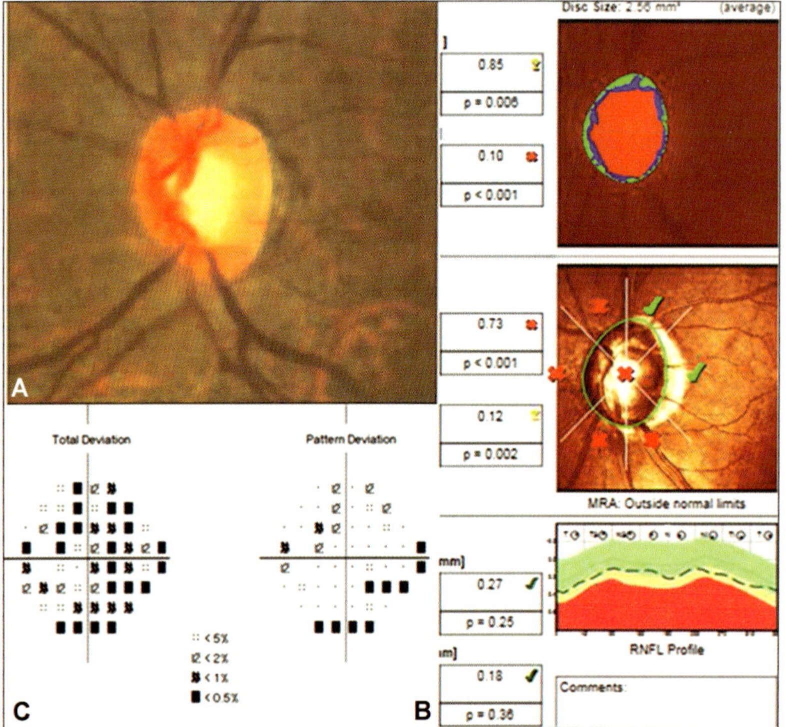

Fig. 9.31 *Moderate glaucomatous change: (A) Colour photograph of a right optic nerve; (B) Corresponding image from an HRT II showing thinning of RNFL. Red colour shows areas of neuroretinal rim thickness less than normative database; (C) Field changes correlating disc changes on total and pattern deviation plot*

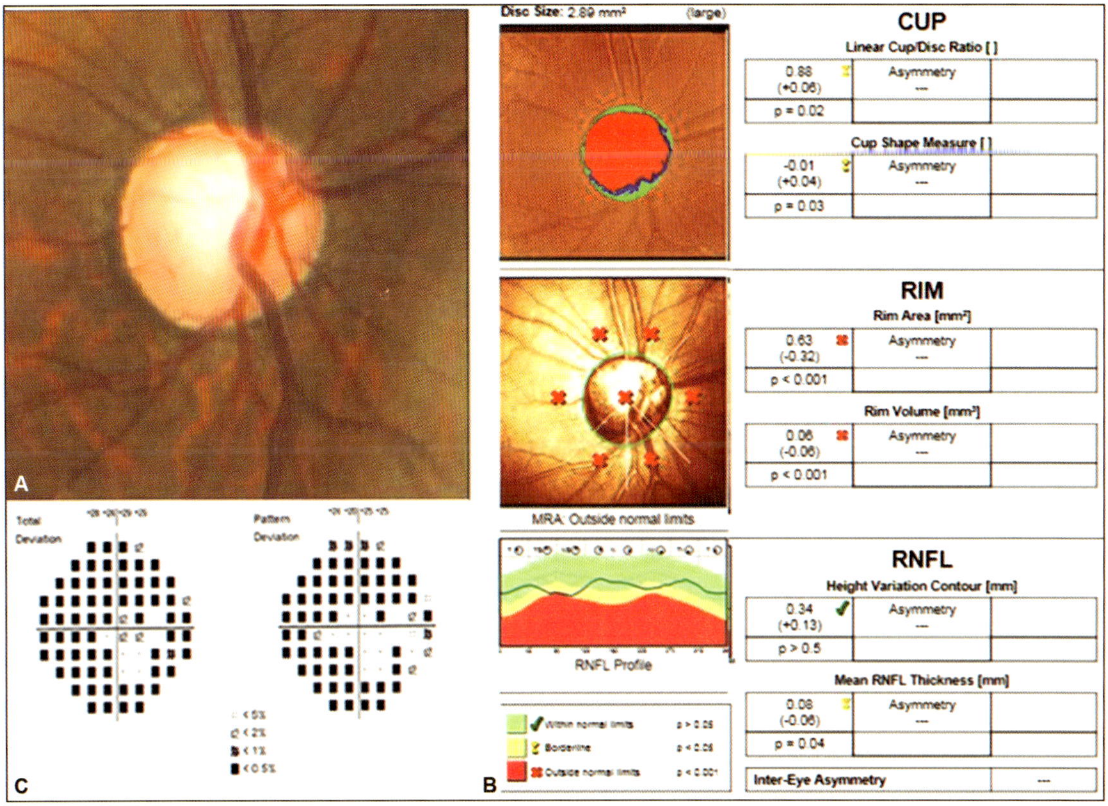

Fig. 9.32 *Advance glaucomatous damage: (A) Colour photograph of a right optic nerve; (B) Corresponding image from an HRT II showing thinning of RNFL in all quadrants. Red colour shows areas of neuroretinal rim thickness less than normative database; (C) Advanced visual field changes on total and pattern deviation plot*

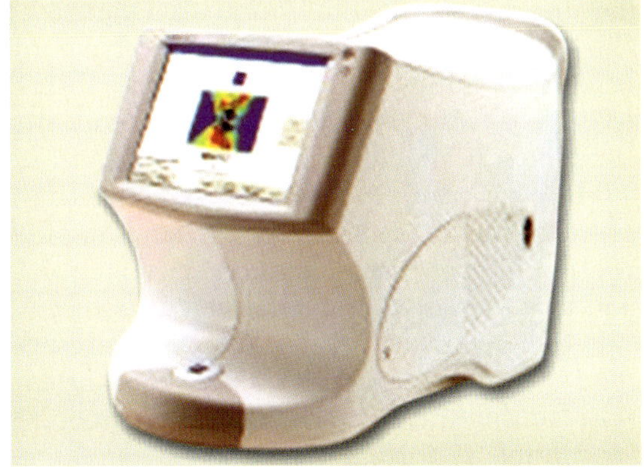

Fig. 9.33 *GDx PRO (Courtesy: Carl Zeiss Inc.)*

IMAGE ACQUISITION

This device also uses a polarized diode laser (780 nm) to fixed scan circle of 3.2 mm diameter centred on the optic disc. Images with abnormal definition of the blood vessel borders or the optic nerve indicate eye movement leads to erroneous acquisition. Data acquired from the scanned area are displayed as a 256 × 256 pixel colour-coded grid which displays a "heat map" of RNFL thickness, with hotter colours representing greater retardation that is thicker RNFL values. In a normal RNFL thickness map, bright yellow and red indicates thicker RNFL and is seen in the superior and inferior sectors, while green and blue indicates thinner RNFL and is seen in the nasal and temporal sectors. A statistical deviation map and a TSINT graph are included in the printout.

The new generation has the GDx variable corneal compensator (GDx VCC) and GDx enhanced corneal compensator (ECC). GDx VCC provides individual customized compensation of anterior segment birefringence using retardation measurements obtained from the macula.

GDx ECC performed significantly better than GDx VCC in glaucoma detection in patients with more severe atypical retardation patterns.

It is based on the form birefringence shown by Henle's fibre layer of fovea as it is known to be uniform (form birefringence is an optical property where light refracts differently in perpendicular planes due to the molecular organization of a material). Scanning laser polarimetry of the macula without VCC gives rise to a non-uniform pattern at the fovea due to birefringence of the cornea. It is seen as hourglass pattern and it indicates the axis and magnitude of the uncorrected cornea birefringence.

COMPONENTS OF THE GDx REPORT

1. ***Patient data.*** It consists of patient's name, date of birth, gender and ethnicity which are given at the top of the printout.

2. ***Quality score.*** An ideal quality score ranges from 7 to 10.

3. ***Reflectivity image.*** It is located at the top of the report display. It is a image of the posterior pole that measures 20° × 20°. 16000 or more data points are acquired to construct this image. This image provides information about the quality of the scan. The ellipse is centred over the ONH in this image. The ellipse size is defaulted to a small setting can be changed by changing the calculation circle thereby changing the size of the ellipse. The calculation circle is the area located between the two concentric circles, one which measures the temporal-superior-nasal-inferior-temporal (TSNIT) and other that measures nerve fibre indicator (NFI) parameters. One can measure beyond a large peripapillary atrophy area by resizing the calculation circle and ellipse.

4. ***RNFL thickness map or retardation image.*** This is a colour-coded map depicting the different thicknesses of peripapillary RNFL. Hot colours, like red and yellow, mean high retardation or thicker RNFL and cool colours, like blue and green, mean low retardation or thinner areas. A typical scan is of a vertical bow-tie pattern that is the one with thicker RNFL superiorly and inferiorly.

5. ***TSNIT graph or (RNFL profile plots).*** Located at the bottom of the report display. It measures RNFL thickness values around the measurement annulus in relation to the normal range of thickness values (normative data of over 500 eyes). This graph demonstrates the patient's RNFL thickness as a black line drawn over a shaded area of normality. The green and purple shaded areas indicate the normal range of values for the left and right eyes, respectively.

6. ***TSNIT symmetry graph.*** This graph with right and left eye plots superimposed on each other.

7. ***TSNIT comparison graph and serial analysis graph.*** It compares two or more scans of the same eye obtained on different visits of the patient. They are not a part of the regular printout.

8. ***Deviation from normal map.*** This map compares RNFL thickness of patient the values derived from the normative database. Colour-coded squares are used to indicate the amount of deviation from normal at each given location. A colour legend defining statistical significance of deviation from normal is seen at the bottom.

9. ***TSNIT parameters.*** These are computed automatically from the calculation circle data and are compared to the normative database. They are also colour-coded on the basis of different p values. The parameters are: TSNIT average (average thickness values within the calculation circle), superior average (average of pixels in superior 120° of the calculation circle), inferior average (same as above, but along the inferior 120° of the calculation circle), TSNIT standard deviation and inter-eye asymmetry. Inter-eye symmetry values near 1.0 represent good symmetry, and values near 0 represent poor symmetry. A GDx VCC scan may be considered abnormal, if the TSNIT average, superior average, inferior average, TSNIT standard deviation, and inter-eye symmetry have $p < 1\%$. A GDx VCC scan may be considered borderline, if these same parameters fall outside normal at the $p < 5\%$ level.

10. ***Nerve fibre indicator (NFI).*** The NFI is an indicator of the likelihood that an eye has glaucoma. It is a proprietary value, consensus regarding the definition of an abnormal scan has not been established. Data within and outside the calculation circle are used to generate the NFI value. It ranges from 0 to 100. The higher NFI reflects towards patient being glaucomatous.

GDx offers the following as a guideline on the NFI interpretation:

- <30: Low likelihood of glaucoma
- 30–50: Glaucoma suspect
- >50: High likelihood of glaucoma.

Recently, software has been introduced in the GDx VCC to assess serial images for the identification of progression (GDx Review with Guided Progression Analysis (GPA)™, Carl Zeiss Meditec, Dublin, CA, USA). The analysis software requires an external computer linked to the GDx VCC. To assess and confirm RNFL progression requires detection of change on three consecutive follow-up images which is compared to an average of two high quality baseline scans. Three algorithms are used to evaluate statistically significant progression and changes are colour-coded: Red demonstrates likely reduction in RNFL thickness, yellow indicates possible reduction, and purple indicates possible increase in RNFL thickness. Narrow focal RNFL change may be detected using the image progression map.

QUALITY ASSESSMENT

Proper focusing and illumination of the retinal area being scanned is necessary.

The ONH must be inside a black square when scan is being acquired. Motion artifacts may occur, if the eye moves too much, and that can decrease the quality of the scan. These are sometimes noticed as black rectangles at the edges of the scans or lines along the vessels. The ellipse must be centred over the ONH. Centration is usually more important than adequate size. A typical scan identified by the thicker bundles along the vertical axis, where the RNFL is thicker (vertical bow-tie). An atypical scan is one where the overall thickness is increased, where the thickness axis is tilted or where the thickness is along radial lines through the periphery of the scan. An objective way to evaluate atypical scans is with a support vector machine, which assigns a typical scan score.

STRENGTHS AND LIMITATIONS

GDx allows for rapid and simple imaging of peripapillary RNFL. Good interactive features to assess for quality of the image are included in the software. Pupillary dilation is not required. Macular pathology was a hindrance in assessing the GDxVCC but now alternative strategies for corneal compensation in eyes with macular pathology have been described. In general, the reported sensitivity and specificity of scanning laser polarimetry to detect glaucoma is above 80%.

Figures 9.34 to 9.37 show representative cases with normal disc, early, moderate and advanced glaucomatous changes, respectively on HRT, OCT and perimetry.

ULTRASOUND BIOMICROSCOPY

INTRODUCTION

Ultrasound biomicroscopy (UBM) is an imaging technique that uses high frequency ultrasound to produce images of the eye at near microscopic resolution.

Ultrasound biomicroscopy was introduced in the late 1980s by Pavlin et al. It was originally designed to have a field of view of 2 × 2 mm and a frequency of 100 Mega Hertz (MHz). With it the first views of enucleated eyes were obtained. Details of the angle of the eye, the cornea, the sclera, the iris and the ciliary body were visualized with impressive clarity. However, despite good resolution, there was the drawback of non-appreciation of deeper structures. To overcome this problem, the next design incorporated transducers ranging from 50–80 MHz with a field of view of 4 × 4 mm. This proved to be a useful compromise that allowed important structures of the anterior segment to be well visualized.

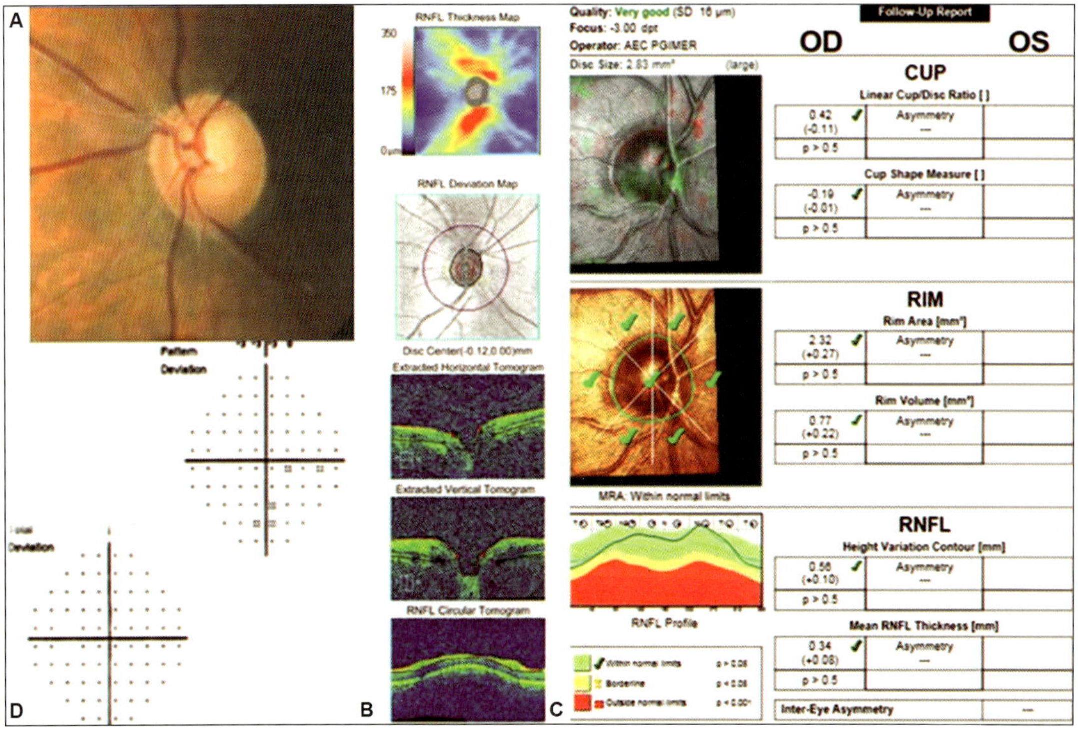

Fig. 9.34 *Normal disc: (A) Colour photograph of optic nerve; (B) OCT shows healthy RNFL; (C) corresponding image from an HRT II correlating OCT finding; (D) normal field changes on perimetry*

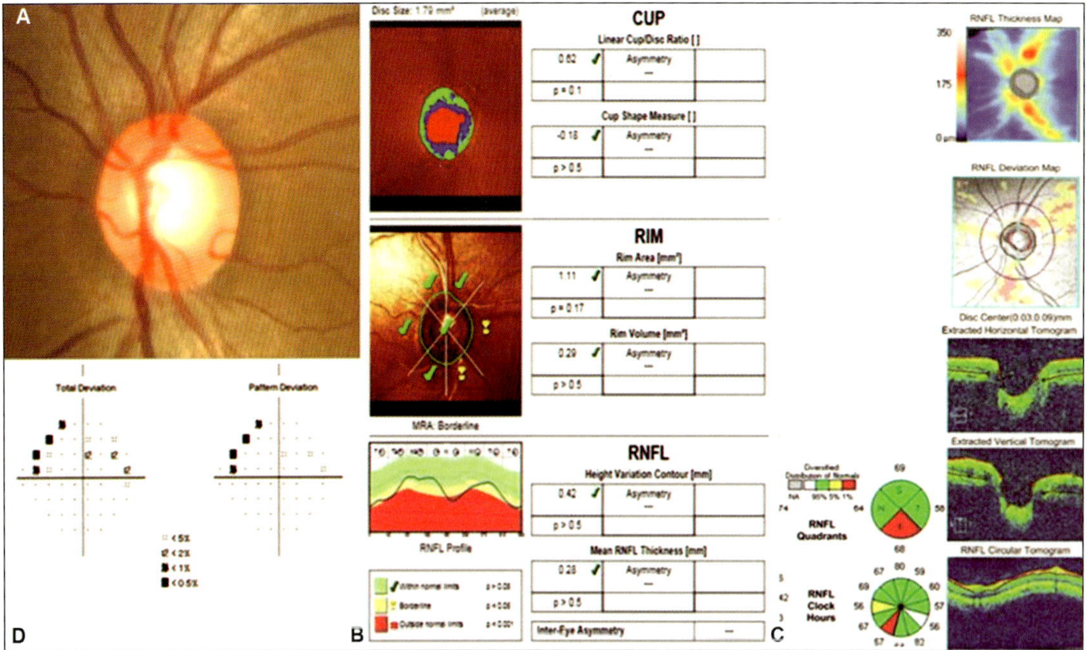

Fig. 9.35 *Early glaucomatous change: (A) Colour photograph of optic nerve showing slight inferior thinning of NRR; (B) HRT II MRA showing; (C) correlating RNFL thinning on OCT; (D) superior field changes on perimetry*

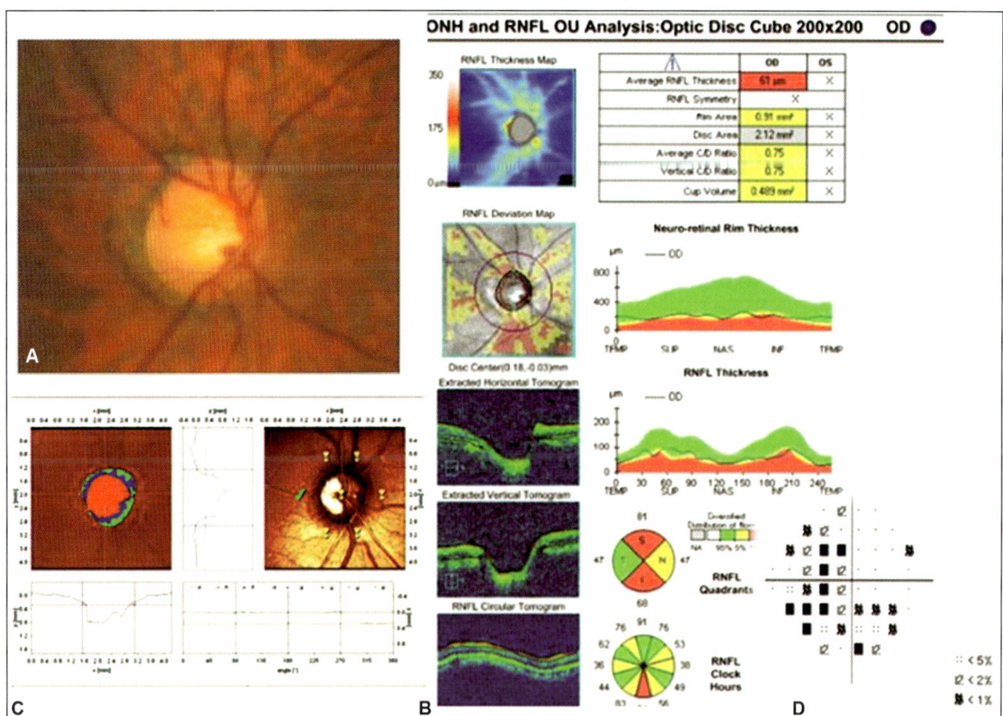

Fig. 9.36 *Moderate glaucomatous damage: (A) Colour photograph of optic nerve showing NRR loss superiorly, inferiorly and nasally; (B) Correlating RNFL loss on OCT; (C) Corresponding image from an HRT II showing borderline thinning in all quadrants except in temporal quadrant; (D) Associated field changes on perimetry*

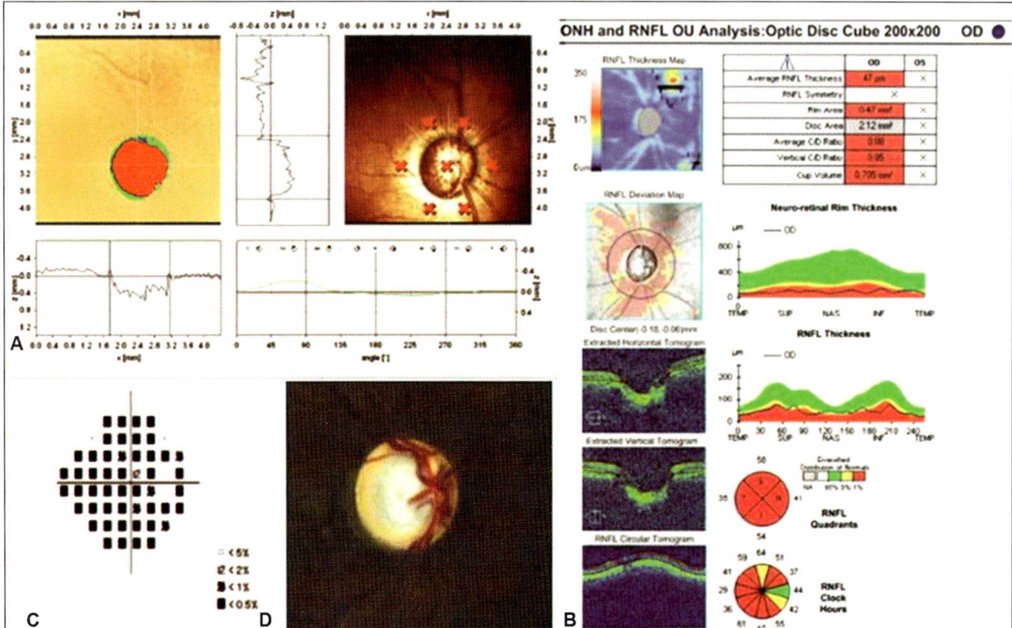

Fig. 9.37 *Advance glaucomatous changes: (A) HRT II MRA showing thinning of RNFL in all quadrants; (B) Correlating RNFL loss as seen on OCT; (C) Advanced visual field changes seen on perimetry; (D) Colour photograph of glaucomatous optic nerve head showing advanced loss of neuroretinal rim*

The UBM was brought into clinical use in 1990 using a water bath. Scanning was performed by placing the probe close to the area of interest and observing the resulting image on the screen. Fine movement of the probe was performed manually with reference to the screen image.

Today, the UBM is an important adjunct in the diagnosis and management of conditions involving the anterior segment of the eye usually not visualized through established clinical methods or conventional ophthalmic ultrasound. In addition, ultrasound biomicroscopy also provides a view of subsurface structures in their normal relationships without the distortion that occurs with preparation of histological specimens. It has also enhanced our knowledge regarding specific glaucoma types, such as angle closure glaucoma which may be caused by pupillary block or plateau iris syndrome, pigmentary glaucoma, lens-induced angle closure, iris cysts and tumours, ciliary body rotation due to effusion, and malignant glaucoma.

The present UBM machines typically have high frequency transducers (50–100 MHz), providing a lateral resolution of 50 μ and axial resolution of 25 μ. The tissue penetration is 4–5 mm.

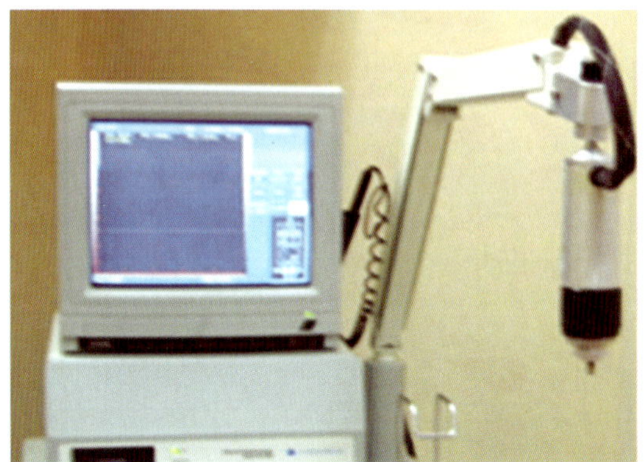

Fig. 9.38 *Paradigm P45 UBM machine*

IMAGE ACQUISITION

Images are acquired with the patient lying supine. Room illumination, fixation, and accommodative effort affect anterior segment anatomy and should be held constant, particularly when quantitative information is being gathered.

In the paradigm instruments UBM, the probe is suspended from a gantry arm to minimize motion artifacts (Figs 9.38 and 9.39). In the OTI (Ophthalmic Technologies, Toronto, Canada) device, the probe is small and light enough not to require a suspension arm (Fig. 9.39).

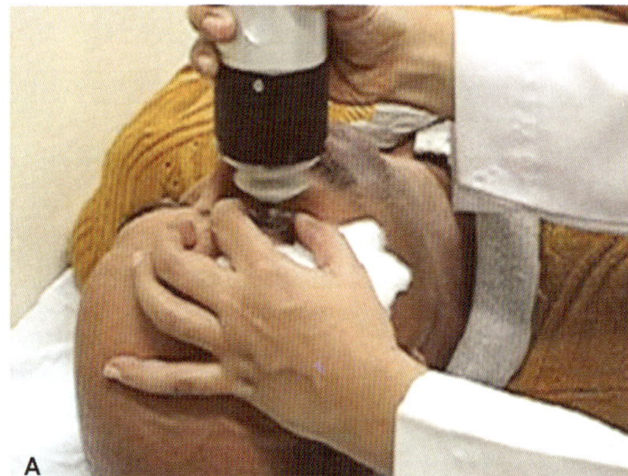

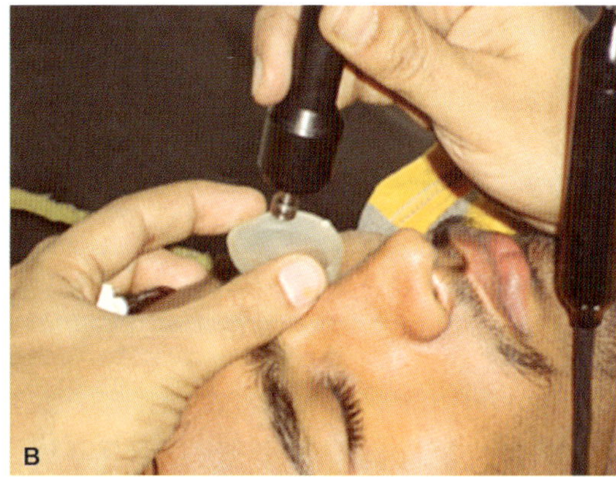

Fig. 9.39 *(A) Left: probe in position using paradigm UBM machine; (B) Right: probe in place using the OTI UBM machine*

Scanning is performed with the patient in the supine position under topical anesthesia. The room illumination and fixation is to be kept constant to prevent changes in accommodation and pupil size to any measurements being taken.

A plastic eye cup of the appropriate size (usually 20.0 mm) is inserted between the lids, holding methylcellulose or normal saline coupling medium (Fig. 9.39). Usually scanning is performed in radial cuts in the area of interest. This may be uncomfortable and may potentially distort the eye anatomy and angle configuration. The procedure is minimally invasive and may make it impractical for many clinical situations, such as perforating ocular injuries or infective corneal perforations. In addition, a highly skilled operator is needed to obtain high quality images, and the learning curve of the technique is fairly steep.

Also this is one technique where it is preferable and at times may be mandatory for the treating physician to do the procedure himself, since it is imperative to image precisely the area of interest. The high magnification renders general scanning of the eye of little use for both diagnosis and management.

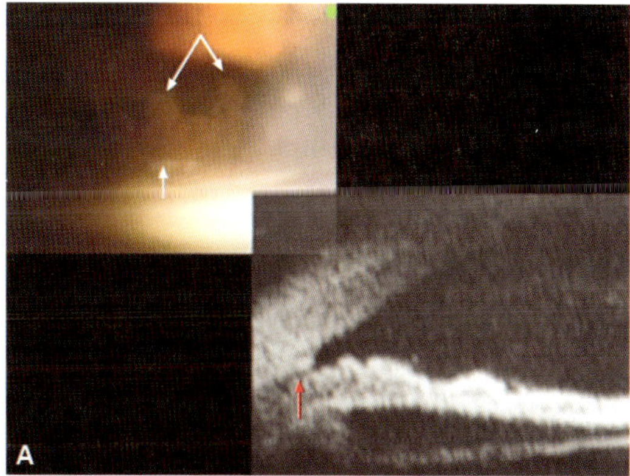

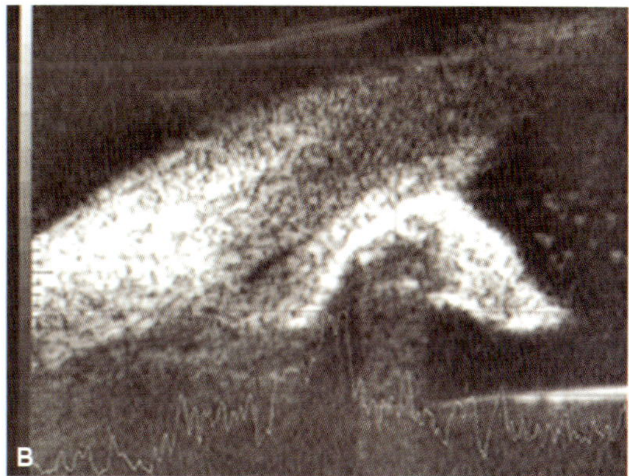

Fig. 9.40 *UBM showing: (A) Small cyclodialysis cleft; (B) Occult foreign body embedded in the posterior iris stroma. Note the back shadowing from foreign body (reproduced with permission from Kaushik S, Pandav SS. Ultrasound Biomicroscopy in glaucoma. In: Recent Advances in Ophthalmology. Nema HV, Ed. Delhi: Jaypee Highlight Medical Publishers Ltd. 2010: 98–110)*

CLINICAL APPLICATIONS IN GLAUCOMA

The applications of UBM in glaucoma are manifold and what follows are representative of the potential of this exciting investigative modality.

1. Trauma

Trauma can result in many derangements in the anterior segment stating from angle recession, iridodialysis, unexplained hypotony due to a cyclodialysis cleft or an occult intraocular foreign body. Many times, UBM is the only modality that is able to pick up these abnormalities (Fig. 9.40).

2. Primary angle closure

Commonly primary angle closure (PAC) occurs as a result of papillary block (Fig. 9.41). But non-pupillary block mechanisms, such as Plateau iris syndrome, can also cause PAC.

UBM helps in differentiating between the two and helps in taking the decision of an iridoplasty in case a laser iridotomy is insufficient to control the disease (Fig. 9.42).

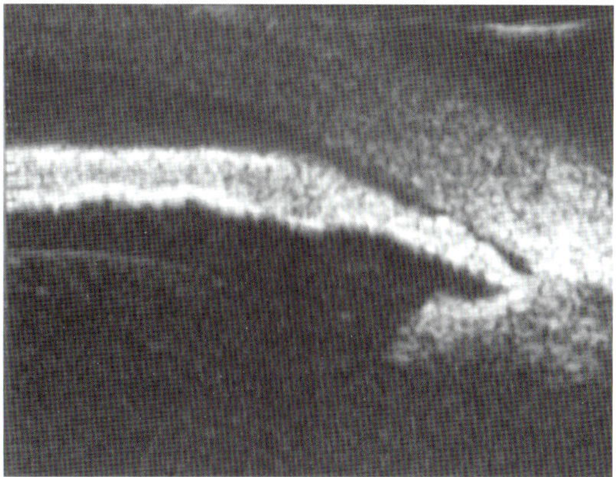

Fig. 9.41 *Pupillary block angle-closure. Note the wide ciliary sulcus and convex configuration of iris forming a bombe-like pattern and closing the angle*

3. Iris/ciliary body cysts

Sometimes iris or ciliary body cysts may close the angle in what can be termed a "pseudo-plateau iris" configuration. On gonioscopy, where is a trademark "bumpy" appearance of the preripheral iris and the UBM demonstrates the underlying cause (Fig. 9.43).

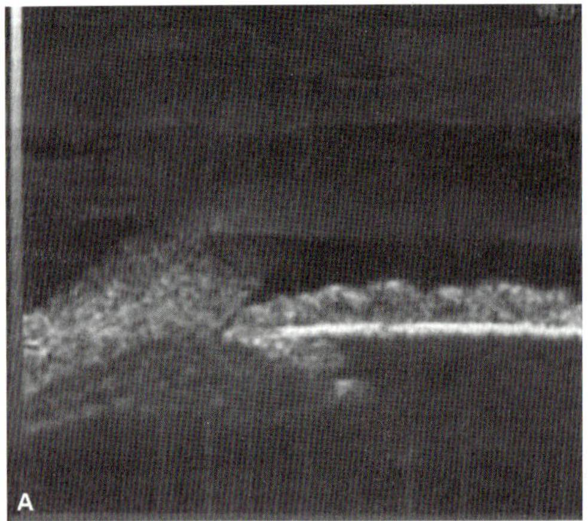

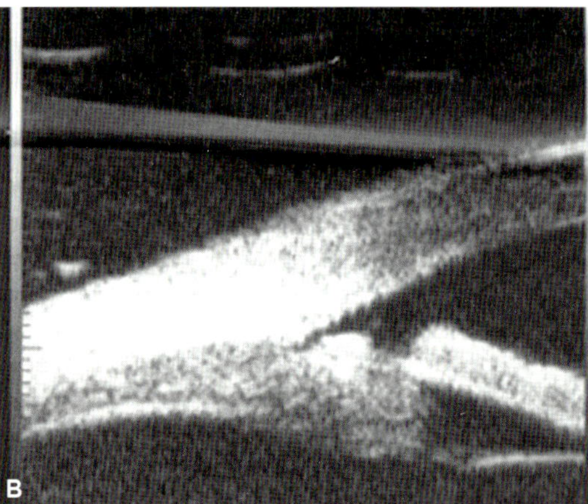

Fig. 9.42 *Plateau iris syndrome: (A) Note the ciliary processes pushing up the iris to close the angle. No ciliary sulcus is appreciable; (B) Patent laser iridotomy but angle is still closed. Prominent ciliary process is pushing up the iris and crowding the angle*

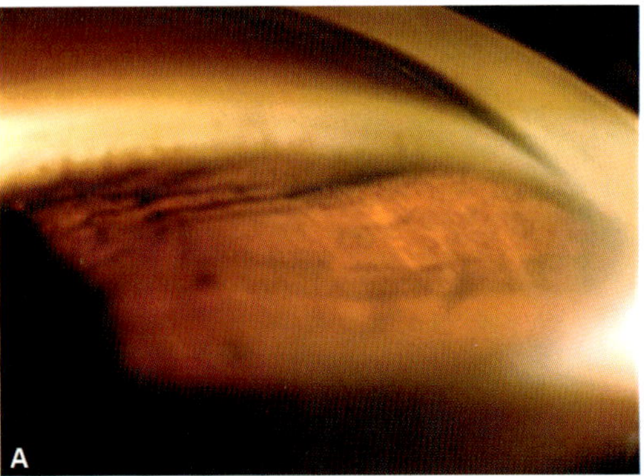

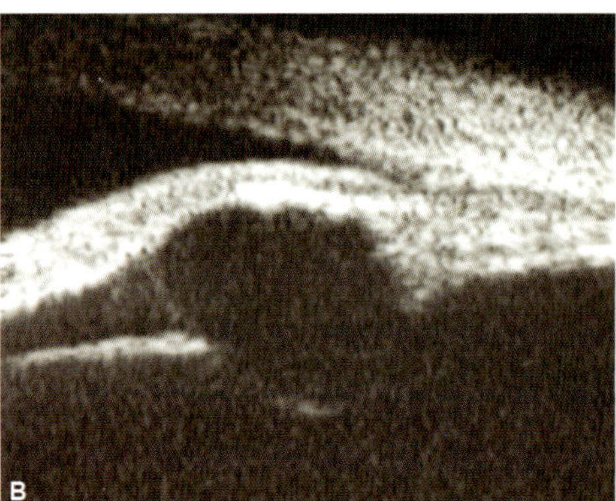

Fig. 9.43 *(A) Gonioscopy showing bumpy appearance of peripheral iris; (B) UBM picture reveals a large iridociliary cyst*

4. Pigment dispersion syndrome

UBM has helped in understanding the pathophysiology of pigment dispersion syndrome. The iris has a concave appearance, which causes the aqueous to dam anteriorly causing what is termed a "reverse papillary block". The posterior surface of the iris rubbing against the zonules causes release of pigment throughout the anterior segment. Laser iridotomy is beneficial in many cases (Fig. 9.44).

5. Pseudoexfoliation with angle closure

Though pseudoexfoliation is usually associated with an open-angle secondary glaucoma, it is not uncommon to see pseudoexfoliation with angle closure also. In such cases, it is very important to carefully look at the anterior chamber depth and examine the lens for phacodonesis. The zonules in this condition are weak and many times may be broken leading to the lens becoming more spherical and causing a secondary angle closure (Fig. 9.45).

6. Imaging failed trabeculectomy blebs

Trabeculectomy is the gold standard for glaucoma surgery. However, failure of the bleb after an interval of apparent success is a fairly common problem. Filtration surgery failure is most commonly due to fibrosis involving episcleral–tenon–conjunctival interface. The status of filtration under the scleral flap cannot be commented upon reliably by clinical

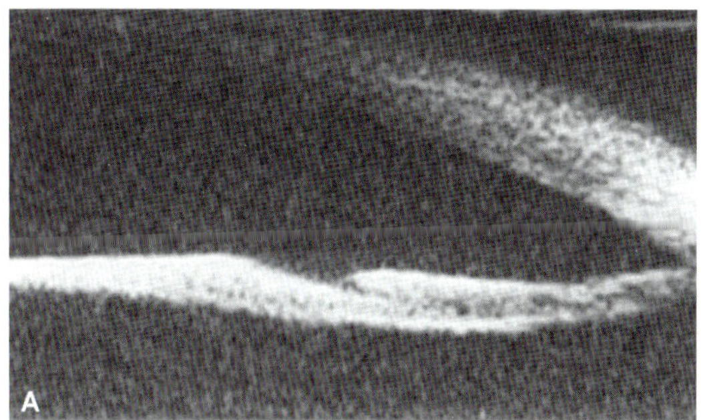

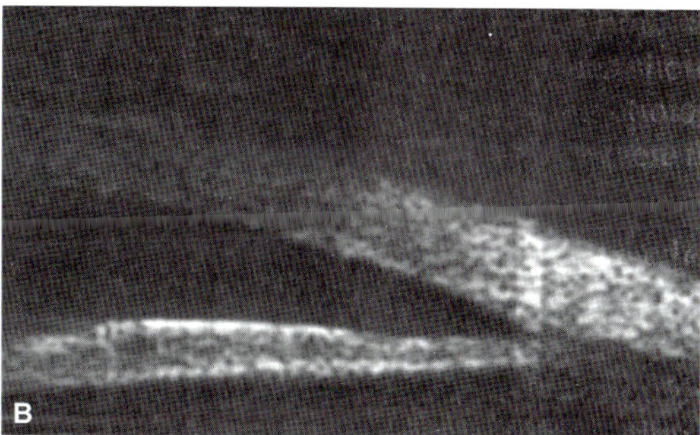

Fig. 9.44 *(A) Pigmentary glaucoma with concave iris configuration; (B) Same iris after laser iridotomy. Note the straightening of the iris*

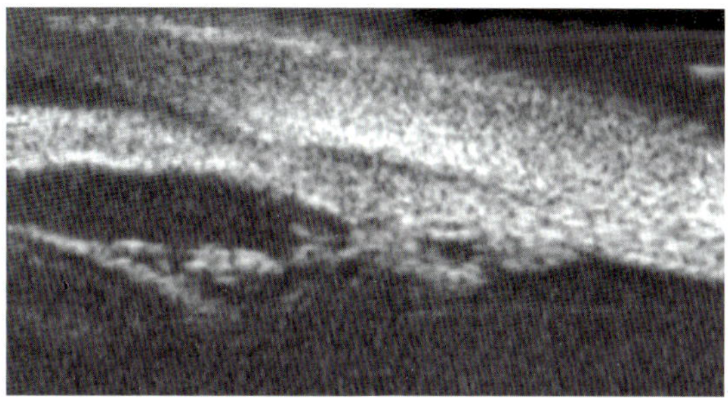

Fig. 9.45 *Pseudoexfoliation glaucoma with broken zonules. Note the pseudoexfoliative material on the zonular surface giving it a granular look. Also notice the secondary angle closure caused by forward movement of the spherical lens*

examination. Most reports of bleb needling describe disrupting the subtenon's scarred tissue without entry in the subscleral space or the eye, since it is essentially a blind procedure. However, unless there is aqueous flow under the scleral flap, disruption of episcleral-tenon scar tissue alone may not be effective. UBM is a useful tool for evaluation of the filtering bleb. It can visualize the internal sclerostomy opening, aqueous outflow route under the scleral flap and other bleb characteristics). It can also be used as a predictor for success of needling in scarred blebs (Fig. 9.46).

CONCLUSION

Ultrasound biomicroscopy technology is a very useful non-invasive quick and convenient tool in qualitative and quantitative assessment of the anterior segment. It has clarified concepts in the pathophysiology of diseases, such as pigment dispersion, plateau iris and pseudoexfoliation glaucoma. Limitations of limited resolution and poor tissue penetration remain. Future advancements including incorporation of Doppler technology may further enhance the utility of the device in quantitative assessment of the anterior segment.

ANTERIOR SEGMENT OPTICAL COHERENCE TOMOGRAPHY

INTRODUCTION

Anterior segment optical coherence tomography (ASOCT) is an imaging modality that provides both quantitative and qualitative information on the cornea, anterior chamber angle, iris and crystalline lens. Assessment of the anterior segment is an integral part of glaucoma examination. Traditionally, the anterior segment and iridocorneal angle are evaluated with the help of a slit-lamp, gonioscope and UBM. The advancement of technology, led to development of low coherence interferometry, upon which optical coherence tomography (OCT) is based. OCT provides multiple detailed cross-sectional images of the internal structures in biological tissues. Currently, two anterior segment OCT (AS-OCT) models are commercially available—the Visante OCT (Carl Zeiss Meditec, Dublin, CA, USA) and the slit-lamp OCT (SLOCT) (Heidelberg Engineering, GmbH, Dossenheim, Germany).

Ophthalmic OCT was initially developed for retinal imaging and used a near-infrared 800 nm superluminescent diode (SLD) as the light

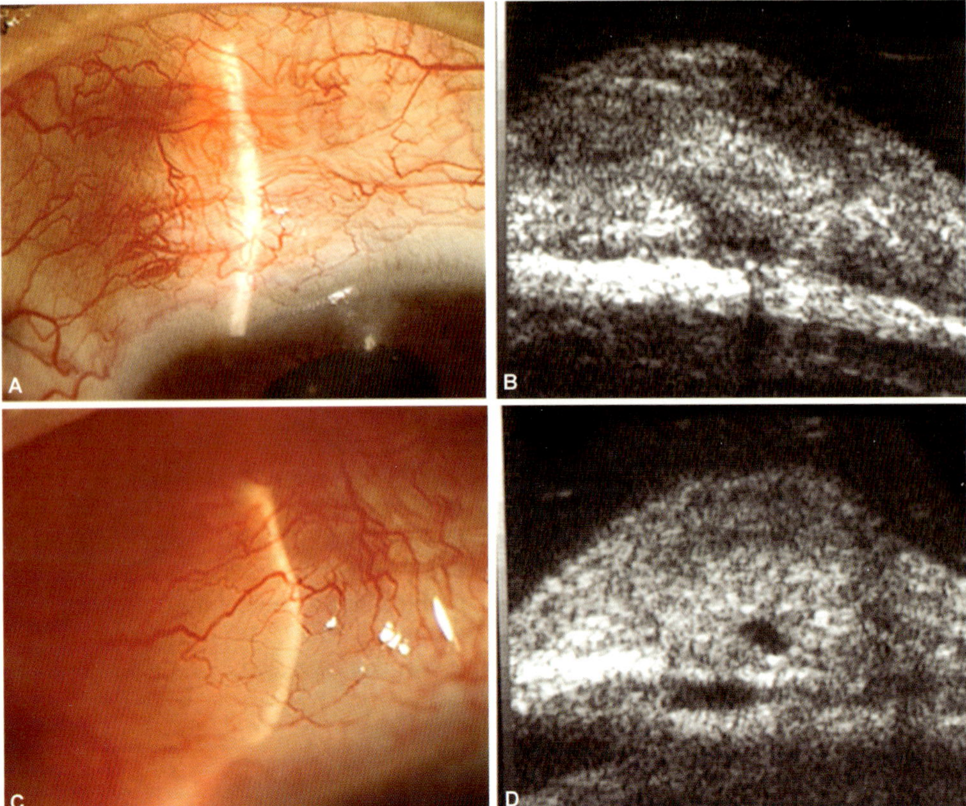

Fig. 9.46 *(A) Scarred trabeculectomy bleb; (B) UBM appearance of the same bleb showing high internal reflectivity with no aqueous spaces; (C) Same bleb after needling; (D) Note on UBM the spaces within the bleb after needling*

emitting source. This OCT model was subsequently applied to anterior segment imaging, capturing images of the cornea, anterior chamber angle, iris and crystalline lens.

With the improvements in speed and light penetration, the entire anterior segment can now be captured in one frame, in 0.125 seconds and in 18 µm resolution (Visante™ OCT User Manual, 2006).

APPLICATIONS OF AS-OCT IN GLAUCOMA

OCT allows fast imaging and can be used in patient who are non-compliant, younger age and in the immediate postoperative period where UBM may be difficult to perform.

1. ***Anterior chamber and angle.*** Gonioscopy differentiates between angle-closure and open-angle glaucoma. It is a contact based technique and has a learning curve and requires illumination. AS-OCT enables assessment of narrow or suspicious angle that may be occludable. OCT scans can be performed with light on or off and thereby give valuable information in regards to occludability of the angle. The most important parameters are the angle opening distance (AOD) and the trabecular–iris angle (TIA), angle recess area (ARA) and trabecular–iris space area (TISA). The ARA is, theoretically, a better measurement parameter than the AOD because it takes into account of the whole contour of the iris surface rather than measuring at a single point on the iris as is the case with the AOD. Other parameters assessed are anterior chamber depth (ACD). Anterior chamber volume (ACV) is another useful parameter for detecting individuals at risk of developing primary angle closure.

Newer parameter on ASOCT in angle closure glaucoma

Newer parameter on ASOCT in angle closure glaucoma, which have enhanced our understanding of diseases include:

i. ***Irido-trabecular contact (ITC).*** The extent of angle closure (contact between iris and angle wall anterior to SS) expressed as percentage ITC index has good diagnostic performance compared to gonioscopy for estimating the degree of angle-closure, and above all it is a non-contact, rapid method.

ii. ***Lens vault*** is calculated as perpendicular distance between a straight line joining SS on either side to anterior pole of the crystalline lens. It Indicates increased thickness and bulk of lens anterior to scleral spur plane, pushing peripheral iris against. Increased LV and not lens thickness is more relevant for angle closure. Cataract surgery has been shown to be superior to LPI in these cases

iii. ***Iris parameters:*** Iris thickness at 750 μm and 2000 μm from scleral spur (IT750 and IT2000) are significantly associated with narrow angles.

2. ***Imaging of filtering blebs.*** The noncontact nature of OCT imaging provides a much safer approach to examine the intrableb morphology in the early postoperative period, thereby offering a unique opportunity to study the healing and remodelling process inside the blebs longitudinally. Using ASOCT, four different patterns of intrableb morphology, including diffuse filtering blebs, cystic blebs, encapsulated blebs and flattened blebs were identified and found to be closely related to slit-lamp appearance and bleb function.

3. ***Trauma.*** In ocular trauma and in postoperative period, AS-OCT should be kept in mind for evaluating any trauma/postoperative-associated changes in ocular anatomy, e.g. cyclodialysis cleft.

4. ***Glaucoma drainage implants.*** The position, patency and course of drainage tubes can be ascertained using AS-OCT. ASOCT would be especially helpful in assessing the tube inserted into the ciliary sulcus. The anatomic relationships can be assessed, as can compression of the tube at the scleral entry site.

5. ***Evaluation of iris after iridotomy.*** Patency in doubtful cases can be confirmed on AS-OCT.

ADVANTAGES AND LIMITATIONS OF AS-OCT

Advantages of the AS-OCT

- High speed, non-invasive
- Can image in the immediate postoperative period
- Visante OCT can give us a limbus to limbus view.

Limitations of AS-OCT

- Limited role in opaque or cloudy media
- Ciliary body, retroiridal structures not visualized.

SUGGESTED READING

OPTICAL COHERENCE TOMOGRAPHY

1. Bowd C, Weinreb RN, Williams JM, et al. The retinal nerve fibre layer thickness in ocular hypertensive, normal, and glaucomatous eyes with optical coherence tomography. Arch Ophthalmol. 2000;118(1):22–26.
2. Budenz DL, Chang RT, Huang X, et al. Reproducibility of retinal nerve fibre thickness measurements using the stratus OCT in normal and glaucomatous eyes. Invest Ophthalmol Vis Sci 2005;46:2440–43.
3. Forooghian F, Cukras C, Meyerle CB, et al. Evaluation of time domain and spectral domain optical coherence tomography in the measurement of diabetic macular edema. Invest Ophthalmol Vis Sci 2008;49(10):4290–96.
4. Gyatsho J, Kaushik S, Pandav SS, et al. Retinal Nerve Fiber Layer Thickness in Normal, Ocular Hypertensive, and Glaucomatous Indian Eyes. An Optical Coherence Tomography. Study J Glaucoma 2008;17:122–27.
5. Lalezary M, Medeiros FA, Weinreb RN, et al. Baseline optical coherence tomography predicts the development of glaucomatous change in glaucoma suspects. Am J Ophthalmol 2006;142: 576–82.
6. Leitgeb RA, Schmetterer L, Hitzenberger CK, et al. Real-time measurement of *in vitro* flow by Fourier-domain colour Doppler optical coherence tomography. Opt Lett 2004;29:171–73.

7. Leung CK, Chan WM, Chong KK, et al. Comparative study of retinal nerve fibre layer measurement by Stratus OCT and GDx VCC. I: correlation analysis in glaucoma. Invest Ophthalmol Vis Sci 2005;46:3214–20.
8. Leung CK, Cheung CY, Weinreb RN, et al. Retinal nerve fibre layer imaging with spectral-domain optical coherence tomography: A variability and diagnostic performance study. Ophthalmology 2010;117(2):267–74.
9. Leung CK, Cheung CY. Evaluation of Retinal Nerve Fiber Layer Progression in Glaucoma: A Study on Optical Coherence Tomography Guided Progression Analysis. Invest Ophthalmol Vis Sci 2010;51:217–22.
10. Medeiros FA, Zangwill LM, Bowd C, et al. Evaluation of retinal nerve fibre layer, optic nerve head, and macular thickness measurements for glaucoma detection using optical coherence tomography. Am J Ophthalmol 2005;139:44–55.
11. Moreno-Montanes J, Olmo N, Alvarez A, et al. Cirrus High-Definition Optical Coherence Tomography Compared to Stratus Optical Coherence Tomography in Glaucoma Diagnosis. Invest Ophthalmol Vis Sci, 2009.
12. Schuman JS, Pedut-Kloizman T, Hertzmark E, et al. Reproducibility of nerve fibre layer thickness measurements using optical coherence tomography. Ophthalmology 1996;103: 1889–98.
13. Sony P, Sihota R, Tewari HK. Quantification of the retinal nerve fibre layer thickness in normal Indian eyes with optical coherence tomography. Indian J Ophthalmol 2004 Dec;52(4):303–09.
14. Sung KR, Kim DY, Park SB, et al. Comparison of retinal nerve fibre layer thickness measured by Cirrus HD and Stratus optical coherence tomography. Ophthalmology Jul 2009;116(7): 1264–70.
15. Vizzeri G, Weinreb RN, Gonzalez-Garcia AO. Agreement between Spectral-Domain and Time-Domain OCT for measuring RNFL thickness. Br J Ophthalmol. 2009 Jun;93(6):775–81.
16. Wollstein G, Ishikawa H, Wang J, et al. Comparison of three optical coherence tomography scanning areas for detection of glaucomatous damage. Am J Ophthalmol 2005;139:39–43.

CONFOCAL SCANNING LASER OPHTHALMOSCOPY

1. Hatch WV, et al. Interobserver agreement of Heidelberg retina tomography parameters, J Glaucoma 1999;8:232.
2. Mikelberg FS, Parfitt CM, Swindale NV. Ability of the Heidelberg retina tomograph to detect early glaucomatous visual field loss, J Glaucoma 1996;4:242.
3. Wollstein G, Garway-Heath DF, Hitchings RA. Identification of early glaucoma cases with the scanning laser ophthalmoscope, Ophthalmology 1998;105:1557.

SCANNING LASER POLARIMETRY

1. Garway-Heath, DF, Greaney MJ, et al. Correction for the erroneous compensation of anterior segment birefringence with the scanning laser polarimeter for glaucoma diagnosis. Invest Ophthalmol Vis Sci 2002;43:1465–74.
2. Huang XR. Knighton RW. Linear birefringenceof the retinal nerve fibre layer measured *in vitro* with a multispectral imaging micropolarimer. J Biomed Opt 2002;7:199–204.
3. Knighton RW, Huang XR. Analytical methods for scanning laser polarimetry. Optics Express 2002;10: 1179–89.
4. Knighton RW, Huang XR. Analytical model of scanning laser polarimetry for retinal nerve fiber layer assessment. Invest Ophthalmol Vis Sci 2002; 43:383–92.

ULTRASOUND BIOMICROSCOPY

1. Dada T, Gadia R, Sharma A, et al. Ultrasound biomicroscopy in glaucoma. Surv Ophthalmol 2011;56(5):433–50.
2. Kaushik S, Ichhpujani P, Ramaswamy A, et al. Occult Intraocular Foreign Body: Ultrasound biomicroscopy holds the key. Int Ophthalmol 2008;1:71–73.
3. Kaushik S, Tiwari A, Ichhpujani P, et al. The use of Ultrasound Biomicroscopy to predict the long-term outcome of sub-tenon needle revision of failed trabeculectomy blebs: A pilot study. Eur J Ophthalmol 2011 Nov;21(6):700–07.
4. Pavlin CJ, Foster FS. Ultrasound biomicroscopy. High-frequency ultrasound imaging of the eye at microscopic resolution. Radiol Clin North Am 1998; 36:1047–58.
5. Pavlin CJ, Foster FS. Ultrasoundbiomicroscopy of the eye. 1st edition, New York, springer-Verlag 1995;140–54.
6. Pavlin CJ, Harasiewicz K, Sherar MD, et al. Clinical use of ultrasound biomicroscopy. Ophthalmology 1991;98:287–95.
7. Pavlin CJ. Practical application of ultrasound biomicroscopy. Can J Ophthalmol 1995;30:225–29.

8. Sherar MD, Starkoski BG, Taylor WB, et al. A 100 MHz B-scan ultrasound back scatter microscope. Ultrasonic imaging 1989;11:95–105.

ANTERIOR SEGMENT OCT

1. Bechmann M, Thiel MJ, Neubauer AS, et al. Central corneal thickness measurement with a retinal optical coherence tomography device versus standard ultrasonic pachymetry. Cornea 2001;20:50–54.
2. Leung CK, Chan WM, Ko CY. Visualization of anterior chamber angle dynamics using optical coherence tomography. Ophthalmology 2005;112: 980–84.
3. Leung CK, Yick DW, Kwong YY, et al. Analysis of bleb morphology after trabeculectomy with Visante anterior segment optical coherence tomography. Br J Ophthalmol 2007;91:340–44.
4. Leung DY, Lam DK, Yeung BY, et al. Comparison between central corneal thickness measurements by ultrasound pachymetry and optical coherence tomography. Clin Experiment Ophthalmol 2006;34:751–54.
5. Madgula IM, Kotta S. Stratus optical coherence tomogram III: A novel, reliable and accurate way to measure corneal thickness. Indian J Ophthalmol 2007;55:301–03.
6. Wirbelauer C, Scholz C, Hoerauf H, et al. Corneal optical coherence tomography before and immediately after excimer laser photorefractive keratectomy. Am J Ophthalmol 2000;130:693–99.
7. Wong AC, Wong CC, Yuen NS, et al. Correlational study of central corneal thickness measurements on Hong Kong, Chinese, using optical coherence tomography, Orbscan and ultrasound pachymetry. Eye 2002;16:715–21.

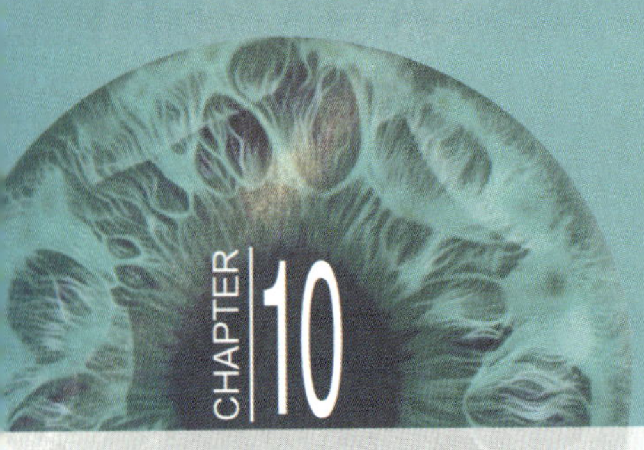

PERIMETRY AND OTHER PSYCHOPHYSICAL TESTS IN GLAUCOMA

PERIMETRY

VISUAL FIELDS: GENERAL CONSIDERATIONS

DEFINITION, LIMITS, AND ANALOGY

Definition

Visual field. Visual field refers to the sum total of visual perception for an eye fixed on a stationary object of regard with the head and body held fixed in position.

Field of gaze. The visual field is different from the "field of gaze", in which the eye is permitted to have freedom of rotational movement while the head and body are kept in a constant position.

Field of view. Here both the eye as well as the head can be moved.

Normal limits

- The normal human visual field (Fig. 10.1A) extends to approximately 60° nasally (toward the nose, or inward) from the vertical meridian in each eye, to 100° temporally (away from the nose, or outwards) from the vertical meridian, and approximately 60° above and 75° below the horizontal meridian.
- The macula corresponds to the central 13° of the visual field; the fovea to the central 3°.
- The normal visual field reaches 180° in the horizontal plane (160° for monocular vision) and 135° in the vertical plane.

Classic analogy

The visual field can be compared with a topographic map of an island. Traquair proposed the concept of "an island of vision surrounded by a sea of darkness". The height of the island correlates to the sensitivity of the retina. Vision perception is most sensitive at the fovea, and sensitivity decreases towards the periphery. In the "island of vision", a deep well represents the blind spot, roughly 15° temporal to the point of fixation. The blind spot is an

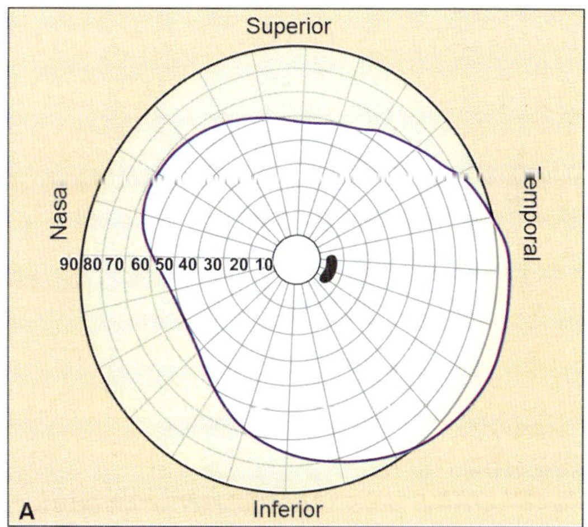

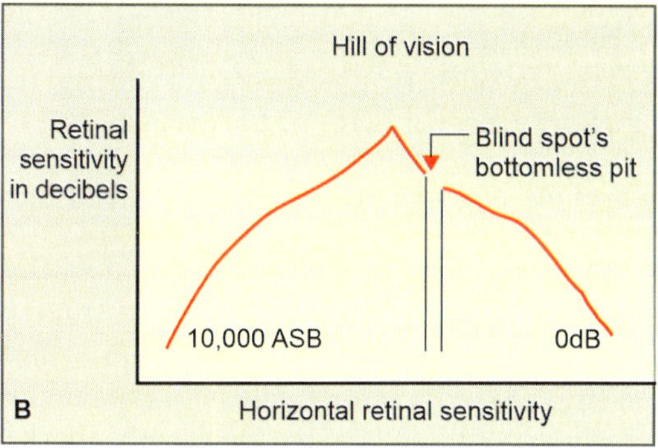

Fig. 10.1 *(A) Extent of normal visual field; (B) Traquir's normal hill of vision*

absolute visual field defect caused by the optic nerve head, which has no overlying retina (Fig. 10.1B).

CENTRAL VERSUS PERIPHERAL FIELDS

The visual field can be divided into central and peripheral fields:

- *Central field* includes an area from the fixation point to a circle 30° away. The central zone contains physiological blind spot on the temporal side.
- *Peripheral field* of vision refers to the rest of area beyond 30° to outer extent of field of vision.
- *Isopter*. Visual field, i.e. the three-dimensional hill of vision can be divided into many isopters depending upon the perception sensitivity. Thus, each isopter can be defined as a threshold line forming points of equal sensitivity on a visual field chart.
- *Scotoma* refers to an area of loss of vision totally (absolute scotoma) or partially (relative scotoma) in the visual field.

METHODS OF ASSESSMENT OF VISUAL FIELDS

Campimetry

This refers to examination of the visual field projected on to a flat surface, e.g. on a transparent screen or flat-panel monitor. It is best suited to examination of the central visual field, up to approximately 20° of eccentricity.

Perimetry

This refers to examination of the visual field performed with a hemispherical surface on to which the visual field is projected. The standard unit of measurement in the visual field is the differential light sensitivity (DLS). Basic principle underlying all forms of perimetry is same. The eye to be examined is positioned at the geometric centre of the hemisphere, such that all points on its inner surface are equidistant from the eye. The surface is uniformly illuminated and test objects are small spots of light that are projected on top of the adapting background.

Indications for perimetry

Indications for visual field testing include visual field deficits, vision loss, headache, and neurologic deficits.

Perimetry is typically the only clinical procedure that evaluates the status of the afferent visual pathways for locations outside the macular region. It is used especially for detection of glaucoma.

Once glaucoma has been diagnosed, it helps in the following:

- Progress of disease,
- Effectiveness of treatment, and
- To explain visual prognosis.

Types of perimetry

Kinetic perimetry. In this form, test objects used are fixed in size and brightness. They are moved from non-seeing areas into seeing portions of the visual field, the subject is asked to respond when the object first becomes visible.

Static perimetry. In this form, stationary test objects that vary in size and brightness, but never move are employed. Brightness of the test object at a point is gradually increased till the patient responds.

Basic differences between the two forms of perimetry are enlisted in Table 10.1 and shown in Fig. 10.2.

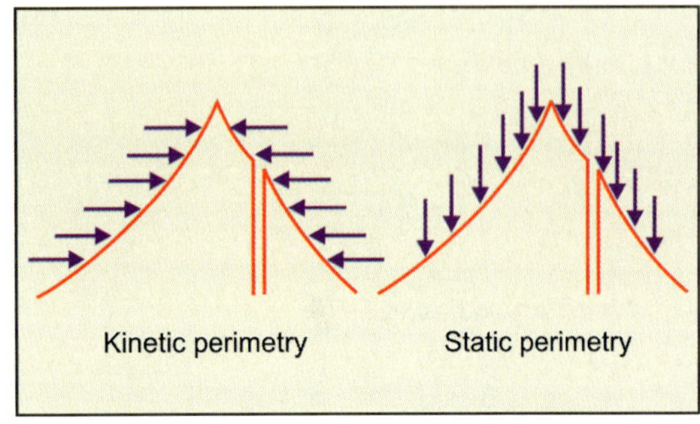

Fig. 10.2 *Kinetic versus static perimetry*

KINETIC PERIMETRY

Kinetic perimetry is still an indispensable diagnostic method in a number of clinical situations where the periphery needs to be tested or where automated static perimetry reaches its limits.

Types of kinetic perimetry

1. *Manual kinetic perimetry*

Prototype is Goldmann perimeter. In 2007, the production of the Goldmann perimeter ceased.

2. *Semiautomated kinetic perimetry*

Prototype is Octopus 101. Strong agreement has been shown with Goldmann perimetry for type and location of defect.

3. *Automated kinetic perimetry*

Prototype is Octopus 900. The Octopus 900 provides 90° full field projection perimetry with a range of 47 decibels and capable of performing both kinetic and static perimetry programmes (Fig. 10.3).

Indications include:

- Assessment of young children
- Patients with poor vision or severely restricted visual fields
- Patients with brain injury involving the posterior hemispheres of the brain.

Technique of automated perimetry is summarized below:

- Using the built-in telescope, the examiner tracks the patient's eye for good fixation. A moving stimulus is presented from a non-seeing area to a seeing area. It is repeated at various points around the clock and a mark is made as soon as the point is seen.
- These points are then joined by a line, an "isoptre". The process is repeated with a point of lesser luminescence and another isoptre is created. Thus, a number of isoptres are plotted so the end result is a chart of the maximal peripheral vision for decreasing level of brightness.

Table 10.1 *Differences between kinetic and static perimetry*

	Kinetic	*Static*
Stimulus presentation	From non-seeing to seeing	Can be presented from seeing to non-seeing or vice versa
Optimal stimulus speed	4°/sec	Independent of reaction time
Sensitivity for detection of shallow focal loss	Likely to be missed, especially if in periphery	More sensitive than kinetic
Time required for test	Dependent on patient reaction time	Manual static more time consuming than automated static

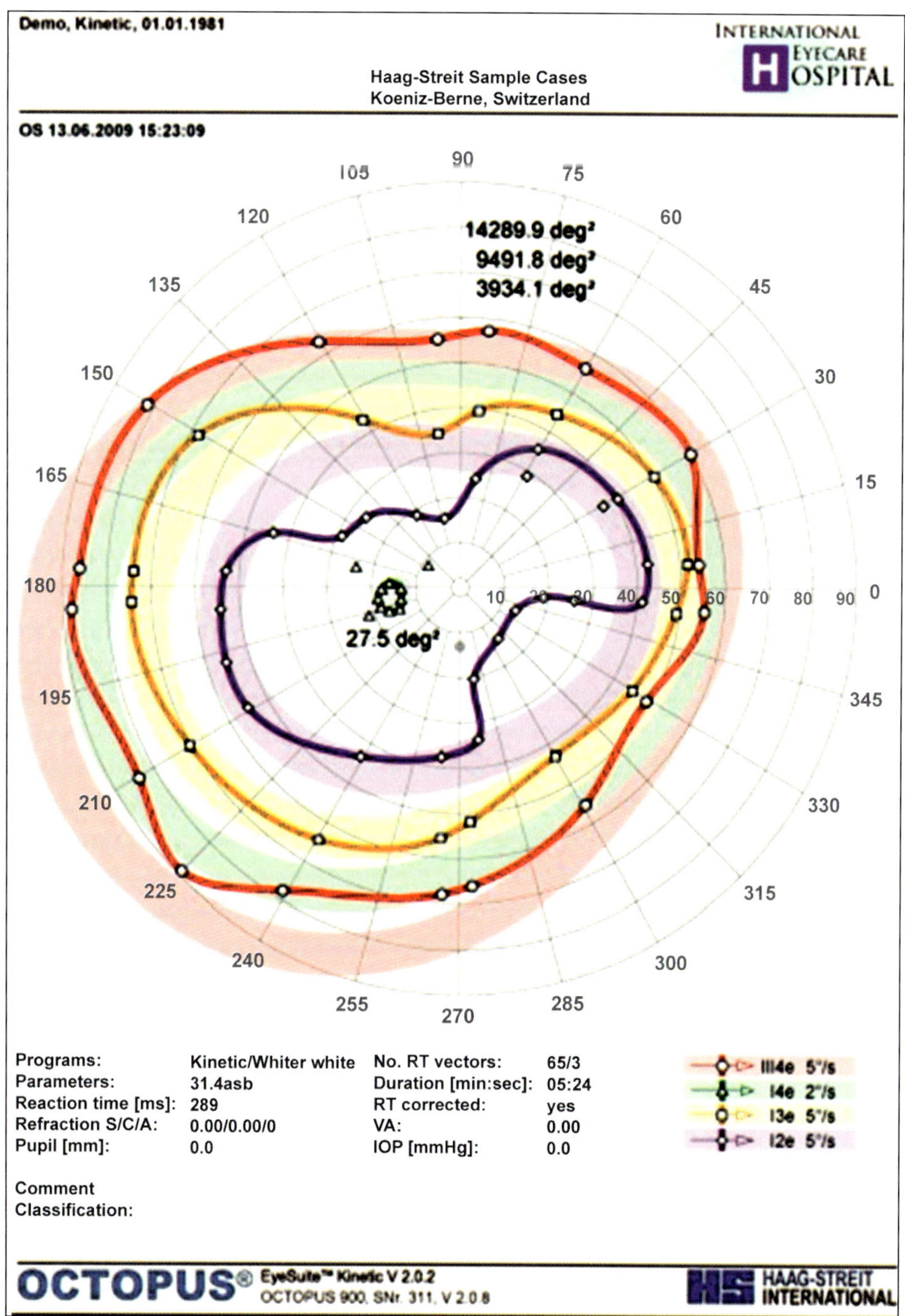

Fig. 10.3 *Octopus 900 kinetic perimetry*

- The results differ depending on photopic, mesopic, or scotopic background luminosity.
- For current Octopus kinetic perimetry, the visual field strategy currently utilised when screening with Octopus perimeter is a 5°/sec stimulus speed for peripheral and central visual field isopters using I4e and I2e targets along with a 3°/sec stimulus speed using I4e

target for blind spot mapping and further evaluation of field loss area. This is coupled with suprathreshold static assessment within the central visual field using the I4e target.

STATIC PERIMETRY

Static perimetry requires presenting a stimulus of a constant size of varying intensity at a fixed location to determine the threshold sensitivity at that locus. This technique is performed at every designated location in a preselected area and pattern, and a map of threshold sensitivities for a given field of vision is generated.

ADVANTAGES OF AUTOMATED STATIC PERIMETRY OVER MANUAL KINETIC PERIMETRY

- Test administration is more standardized and, therefore, more reproducible.
- Less input from a technician is required, minimizing testing variability.
- Reliability is improved with automated fixation monitoring and reduced examination time for static testing compared with manual static testing.
- Patient dependability may be quantitated and statistically assessed.

AUTOMATED PERIMETRY: TERMINOLOGIES AND VARIABLES

Luminous intensity

- Current standard unit of luminous intensity is candela/m² (cd/m²).
- Unit used in HFA is apostilb (asb), which is an European unit; Apostilb (asb) is a unit of brightness per unit area and is defined as 35^{-1} candela/m².
- Americans use millilambert instead of apostilb.
- 10,000 asb = 1 lambert or 3183 cd/m².
- 1 asb is the least intense stimulus that can be seen foveally.

Concepts of luminous intensity: Log

Basic mathematics of log tables:

- $10^1 = 10$
- $10^2 = 100$
- $10^3 = 1000$
- $10^4 = 10000$
- $10^5 = 100000$
- $10^6 = 1000000$
- $10,000 \times 100 = 1,000,000$ or $10^4 \times 10^2 = 10^6$ (Note: 4 + 2 = 6)

In considerations of luminosity, log scale (geometric progression) is used because sensation relates to factors rather than addition of intensity, e.g. if a patient has failed to see a 1000 asb stimulus, increasing intensity by 1 asb will not have any meaning as the difference would be very little to appreciate. However, if it is increased by 1/10 of a log factor, it will increase illumination by 25% and 3/10 of log factor will double the intensity.

Decibel

Decibel is not a unit of luminosity. It describes retinal sensitivity, i.e. less the light required to be perceived by retina at a particular point, more is the sensitivity of retina at that point. In a normal person, it is maximum at fovea. One dB is described as one-tenth of log unit. Maximum intensity of stimulus that HFA can produce is 10000 asb. Figure of 10000 can have a maximum log of 4 ($10000 = 10^4$). Since 1 dB is 1/10 of log, maximum possible sensitivity is 40 dB which is equivalent of 1 asb which is the minimum intensity of stimulus which can be perceived by a young trained observer and thus this 40 dB is the maximum possible foveal threshold in a HVF printout.

Automated perimeter variables

1. *Background illumination*. HFA uses 31.5 apostilb (asb) background illumination. Apostilb (asb) is a unit of brightness per unit area (and is defined as 35^{-1} candela/m²).

2. *Stimulus intensity*. HFA uses projected stimuli which can be varied in intensity over a range of more than 5% log units (51 decibels) between 0.08 and 10,000 asb. In decibel notation (dB), the value refers to retinal sensitivity rather than to stimulus intensity. Therefore, 0 dB corresponds to 10,000 asb and 51 dB to 0.08 asb (Fig. 10.4). In contrast to kinetic perimetry, the higher numbers indicate a logarithmic reduction in test object brightness, and hence greater sensitivity of vision (Fig. 10.4).

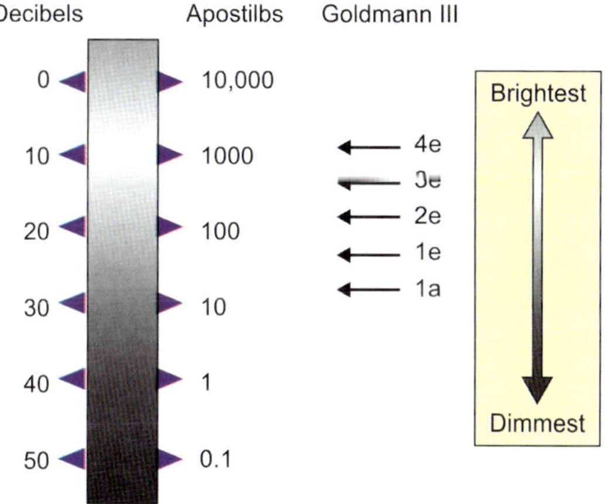

Fig. 10.4 *Stimulus intensity scales compared*

3. *Stimulus size.* HFA usually offers five sizes of stimuli corresponding to the Goldmann perimeter stimuli I through V. Unless otherwise instructed, the standard target size for automated perimetry is equivalent to Goldmann size III (4 mm^2) white target.

4. *Stimulus duration.* Stimulus duration should be shorter than the latency time for voluntary eye movements (about 0.25 seconds). HFA uses a stimulus duration of 0.2 sec while Octopus has 0.1 sec.

Concept of threshold, suprathreshold and infrathreshold

Threshold. Minimal intensity of light at which a stimulus is perceived by the visual system at a specific location in the field of vision. In statistical terms, it is the point on a frequency-of-seeing curve at which a stimulus is perceived 50% of the time.

Suprathreshold. Intensity of light at which stimuli are perceived greater than 95% of the time on the frequency-of-seeing curve, or any stimulus brighter than threshold.

Infrathreshold. Intensity of light at which stimuli are perceived with a frequency of less than 5%, or any stimulus weaker than threshold.

A threshold value is determined by presenting stimuli of gradually increasing and decreasing intensities, determining the dimmest stimulus presented that is seen and the brightest that is not seen, and either averaging these values or using the last seen or not-seen stimulus as the threshold value. Threshold sensitivity may vary with retinal adaptation (background illumination), stimulus colour and size, duration of stimulus presentation, and degree of stimulus movement.

TESTING STRATEGIES AND PATTERNS

Testing strategies

Two basic categories of testing strategies are offered by most instruments: suprathreshold screening and threshold testing.

Suprathreshold screening

This enables rapid discovery of gross field defects. A fixed stimulus that is presumed to be threshold at approximately 30° is used for the entire test area, without adjusting for decreased sensitivity as per the normal contour of the hill of vision. The tested points are recorded as either seen or not seen.

Indications for screening include:

- *Baseline testing* for a patient before ocular or neurosurgical operative procedures
- *Routine examination* for occupational licensing
- *Localization* of a postchiasmal neuro-ophthalmologic lesion.

Threshold testing

Threshold strategies report actual retinal sensitivities at each point tested in numeric form (dB). As in the screening strategies, the sensitivities are displayed in a pattern corresponding to that employed in the test. Along with actual values, a display of differences from expected values or depth of defect may be provided. If the actual values are within 4 to 5 dB of expected values, they are considered within the limits of normal variability and may be recorded as "normal".

Visual threshold is the physiologic ability to detect a stimulus under defined testing conditions. The normal threshold is defined as the mean threshold in normal people in a given age group at a given location in the visual field. It is against these values that the machine compares the patient's sensitivity. Thresholds are reported in decibels in a range of 0–50. Fifty decibel (dB) is the dimmest target the perimeter can project. 0 dB is the brightest illumination the perimeter can project. The lower the decibel value the lower the sensitivity; the higher the decibel value, the higher is the sensitivity.

Threshold testing provides more precise results than suprathreshold testing and is thus preferred by most clinicians, although it takes more time and the equipment often costs more.

Common threshold testing strategies

1. ***Full threshold testing.*** This testing modality involves performing the bracketing ("staircase") process at every point tested (4-2 on the Humphrey and 4-2-1 on the Octopus perimeter). A stimulus brighter than the patient's expected threshold is presented at a point. If the stimulus is seen, stimuli of successively reduced intensity are presented until the stimulus is not seen. Then stimuli of increasingly higher intensity are presented until one is seen. Most instruments use 4 dB increments until threshold is crossed for the first time. Subsequent changes in intensity are usually of 2 dB steps. A point somewhere between suprathreshold and infrathreshold is determined to be threshold for that point. Most perimeters bracket until threshold is crossed twice, from the supra-threshold and infrathreshold directions. Several points in the field are in the process of being thresholded at the same time.

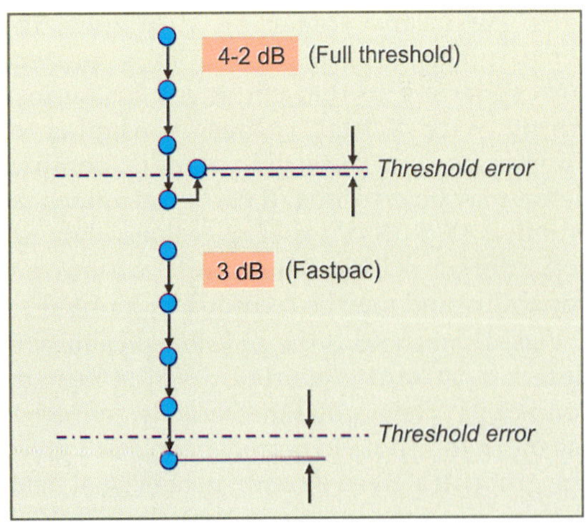

Fig. 10.5 *Bracketting in FASTPAC versus full threshold*

2. ***FASTPAC*** is a rapid thresholding strategy in the Humphrey Field Analyzer:

- This uses a 3 dB step size and estimates the threshold after only one crossing, but thresholds the four primary seed points in a similar manner to standard full-threshold testing (Fig. 10.5).
- Half of the points start at 1 dB brighter and the other half start at 2 dB dimmer than the predicted threshold values.
- After a single crossing, the threshold is estimated. Thresholds of locations that differ from expected values by 4 dB or more are then re-estimated.

Studies have shown that FASTPAC, underestimates mean deviation and pattern standard deviation when compared with the standard algorithm.

3. ***Swedish interactive thresholding algorithm (SITA).*** SITA strategy uses continuous estimation of threshold values and measurement errors throughout the test, using advanced visual field models and mathematical analyses performed in real-time. Models are initially based on prior visual fields. Staircase procedures are used to alter stimulus intensities at predetermined test point locations. Test time is further reduced by eliminating catch trials to determine the frequencies of false-positive answers and by using a more effective timing algorithm. The SITA Standard and SITA Fast strategies are available as software implemented on the Humphrey Field Analyzer II.

Threshold testing is preferred over screening strategies for patients in whom a defect is likely to be present (e.g. those with optic neuritis accompanied by reduced acuity, glaucoma patients with pathologic-appearing optic discs).

Testing Patterns

Basic testing patterns are chosen depending on the area of field to be tested and the density and distribution of points within. The options for areas to be tested include the central 30°, the peripheral 30° to 60° area, full 60°, central 10°, and central 5°. Special test configurations are also available, including glaucoma patterns (central 30° plus peripheral nasal step area and temporal periphery), peripheral nasal step area, temporal crescent region, and neurologic patterns for examining the vertical meridian.

Standard test programmes used with satic threshold strategy on the Humphrey Field Analyzer can be grouped as below:

A. *Central field tests*
- Central 30-2 test
- Central 24-2 test
- Central 10-2 test, and
- Macular test.

B. *Peripheral field tests*
- Peripheral 30/60-1
- Peripheral 30/60-2,
- Nasal step, and
- Temporal crescent

C. *Speciality tests*
- Neurological-20,
- Neurological-50,
- Central 10-12, and
- Macular test

D. *Custom tests*

HFA SINGLE PRINTOUT: EVALUATION

The standard HFA printout is obtained using a software called *Statpac printout*. For the purpose of evaluation, the Humphrey single field printout (Statpac printout) with central 30-2 test can be studied in eight parts I to VIII as described below (Fig. 10.6).

I. Patient data and test parameters: general information

At the top of printout page (part I) are printed:
- Patient's data [name, date of birth, eye (right/left), pupil size and visual acuity]
- Test parameters (test name, strategy, stimulus used, background).

For interpreting any field, first look at the general information for the following reasons: The data provided is about both the testing conditions and demographics. It helps to identify the patient. It is important to look at the test pattern and test strategy being used as tests using different test strategies may not be comparable.

- *Correct name and date of birth of the patient* not only identify the patient but are absolutely essential to enable comparison with normative data for the present field and also with future fields to detect change.
- *The date and time of testing* is given on top right. It is advisable to record the date in DD/MM/YYYY format as it is most familiar format in our country.
- *Eye being tested* should be confirmed as a wrongly entered eye would not allow fixation monitor tests and a wrong normogram for the eye would identify blind spot as scotoma.
- *Pupil size* is automatically detected in newer models. Fields may be carried out on a normal or a dilated pupil but not while it is dilating.
- *Visual acuity* of the patient and trial lens selection are given. Not using proper trial lens in cases obviously requiring the same may cause generalized depression of fields.
- *Stimulus size*, colour and background brightness should be noted as an improper stimulus size will misrepresent fields and certain STATPAC features may not be available for non-standard parameters.

  A larger stimulus size may be required in patients with poor vision or coloured stimuli may be used for certain retinal or optic nerve conditions.
- *Test duration*, if prolonged, indirectly indicates that the patient was taking too long as points were thresholded repeatedly which could be due to unreliable responses, fatigue or increased variability in defective fields. A SITA Standard test typically takes around 7 minutes.
- *Foveal threshold*. A look at the foveal threshold just under the test duration can yield useful information. A good foveal threshold but a poor visual acuity may indicate improper refraction while vice versa may indicate early foveal damage.

II. Reliability Indices

Patient reliability may be appraised by several parameters. These include the fixation losses, false-positive and -negative responses, and degree of response variability. During the examination, rest periods as well as additional

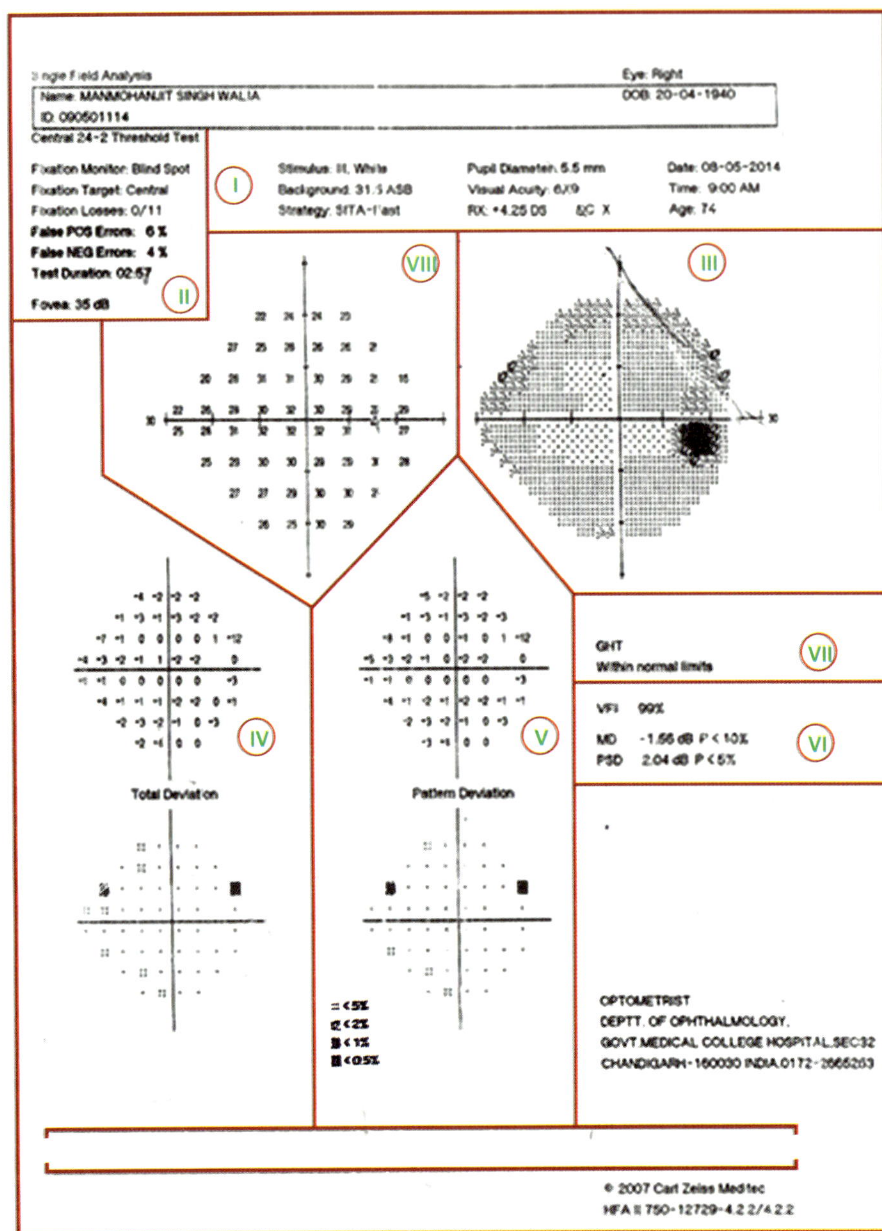

Fig. 10.6 *Normal Humphrey visual field printout*

instructions may be needed to ensure optimal reliability. In addition, if machine-determined parameters of reliability suggest that the patient performed poorly but fixation was observed to be of good quality, the field may be of more value than would have otherwise been determined.

1. *Fixation losses*

Methods to monitor fixation

i. *Blind-spot monitoring technique.* It is done by repeatedly representing the stimulus to blind spot and noting the response. Fixation losses are recorded as a fraction, with the number of losses of fixation in the numerator and the number of

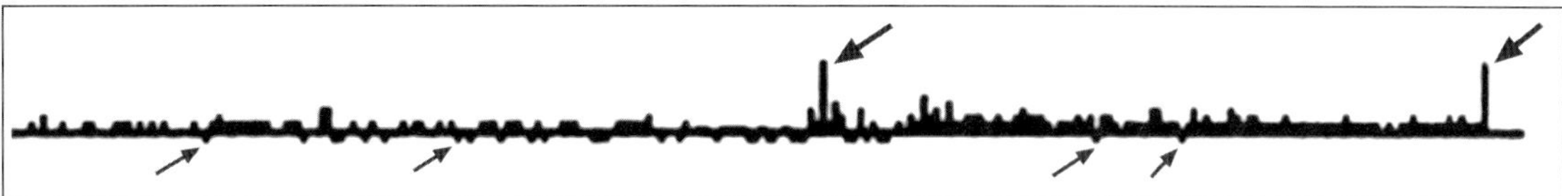

Fig. 10.7 Gaze tracking

blind-spot presentations in the denominator. It is also known as Heijl-Krakau method.

ii. *Sensor monitoring*. If eye movement sensors are used, an absolute number of fixation losses is recorded.

iii. *Manual monitoring* of fixation by the examiner.

iv. *Gaze tracker*. It is printed at the bottom of the test result (Fig. 10.7)

- Upward deviation going fully up indicates 10 degrees gaze error (fixation loss).
- Downward deviation indicates blinks (wherein the tracker could not measure fixation).
- An even smooth line, with minimal excursions implies good fixation.

Reliability status

Fixation losses when exceed 20% the test results are considered unreliable. If this arbitrary cutoff point be increased to 33%, which would decrease the number of fields deemed unreliable without significantly affecting the sensitivity or specificity of the test.

Pseudofixation losses may be seen from high refractive errors due to lens-induced shift in blind spot location.

2. False-positive and negative responses

False-positive response is recorded when a patient signals that a stimulus has been seen when one has not been presented, usually in response to an audible click rather than a visual stimulus. It gives an unusually white out graph (white scotoma).

False-negative response is registered when a patient fails to respond to the presentation of a stimulus at a given location that is significantly brighter than the previously determined threshold at that point (suprathreshold). It gives a clover leaf-like pattern of graph.

Reliability status

Examinations in which false responses of greater than 33% are registered have been considered unreliable. A higher rate of false-negative responses has been shown to occur in patients with glaucomatous field loss compared with normal.

Cut off values of reliability indices

The visual field examination is considered unreliable, if three or more of the following reliability indices have below mentioned values:

- Fixation losses ≥20%,
- False-positive error ≥33%,
- False-negative error ≥33%,
- Short-term fluctuation ≥4.0 dB,
- Total questions ≥400.

III. Grayscale

Grayscale simulation of the test data is depicted in part III of the printout (Fig. 10.6). Grayscale printout is generated by delegating different symbols to actual decibel values of threshold sensitivities, with a specific symbol representing a particular range of stimulus intensities. Darker areas indicate a lower differential light sensitivity and lighter areas indicate zones of higher sensitivity. The resultant printout assigns a retinal sensitivity to every area of field tested, but in reality only a limited number of points were actually thresholded. To allow for continuity, values of presumed retinal sensitivity are interposed to unassessed area of the field. It gives only a gross assessment of the field. The darker the printout, the worse is the field. The grayscale provides the field defects at a glance. However, in general we do not make a diagnosis based on the grayscale. The main emphasis on statistical help shows in part IV to VIII of the printout (threshold values).

IV. Total deviation plots

Total deviation plots provide the deviation of patient's threshold values from that of age corrected normal data. The two total deviation plots are numeric value plot and the probability plot (grayscale symbol plot).

Numeric value plot. Simple threshold sensitivities are measured in decibels and given in the numeric plot. Values above 40 dB are generally not expected and may be indicative of a trigger happy field. The actual numeric values may not be concentrated upon for day-to-day interpretation of field but only with specific purposes. In other words, numeric value plot represents the differences in decibels. SA zero value means that the patient has the expected threshold for that age. Positive numbers reflect points that are more sensitive than average for that age; whereas negative numbers reflect points that are depressed compared with the average.

Probability plot (grayscale symbol plot). In the lower part of part IV of the printout, the total deviation plot is represented graphically. The darker the graphic representation the more significant it is.

Note. In general, the total deviation plot is an indicator of the general depression and is not capable of revealing the hidden scotomas that may be present in the overall depressed field.

V. Pattern deviation plots

The two pattern deviation plots (numeric pattern deviation plot and probability pattern deviation plot) shown in part V of the printout are similar to total deviation plots except that here Statpac software has corrected the results for the changes caused by cataract, small pupil, etc.

VI. Global indices

Global indices are depicted in the part VI of the printout. Global indices refer to some calculations made by Statpac software to provide overall guidelines to help the practitioner to assess the field results as a whole rather than on point-to-point basis as shown in the total deviation and pattern deviation plots.

Below mentioned four global indices are provided with the full threshold programme

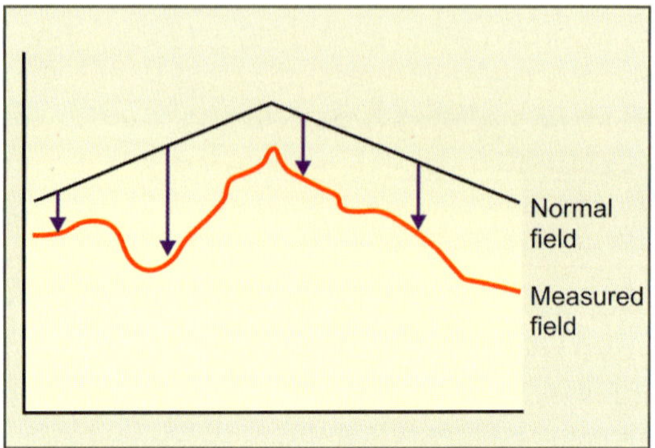

Fig. 10.8 *Total/mean deviation: Relative visual field sensitivity = Normal field sensitivity—Measured field sensitivity*

which summarize the status of visual fields at a glance. Principally, the global indices are used to monitor progression of glaucomatous damage rather than for initial diagnosis.

1. *Total deviation or mean deviation.* The mean sensitivity is an average value of threshold sensitivity for all points tested. The mean deviation is the difference between mean sensitivity obtained and that expected (Fig. 10.8). Mean deviation should be in the range of zero in normals. It is more affected by generalized decreases in sensitivities rather than by small, localized defects but is increased in the presence of any defect. Mean sensitivity may also be decreased by media opacities, significant pupil constriction, blur, and unreliability.

2. *Pattern standard deviation.* Pattern standard deviation reflects the regional non-uniformity of a visual field, or frequency of deviation of sensitivity values after adjusting for the mean defect of the entire field (Fig. 10.9). It is a

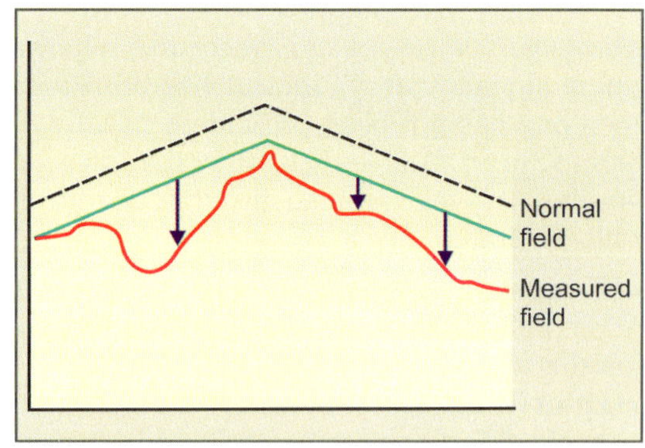

Fig. 10.9 *Pattern deviation: Individual visual field sensitivity*

measure of variability within the visual field, i.e. it measures the difference between a given point and adjacent points. A high value indicates an irregularity to the expected normal hill of vision, suggesting localized defects. Therefore, a normal value is in the range of zero. A low value is also found in a field with a diffuse but regular decrease in threshold sensitivities. It actually points out towards localized field loss and is most useful in identifying early defects. It loses its advantage in marked depression.

3. ***Short-term fluctuation (SF).*** It is a measure of the variability between two different evaluations of the same 10 points in the field. It is not available with SITA strategy. A high SF means either decreased reliability or an early finding indicative of glaucoma.

4. ***Corrected pattern standard deviation (CPSD).*** It is the PSD corrected for SF. It indicates the variability between adjacent points that may be due to disease rather than due to intra-test variability.

VII. Glaucoma Hemifield test (GHT)

Glaucoma Hemifield test compares 24-2 visual fields into 10 regions, with 5 inferior regions representing mirror images of 5 corresponding superior regions (Fig. 10.10). These clusters of points have been developed based on the anatomical distribution of the nerve fibres and are specific to the detection of glaucoma. Differences between corresponding superior and inferior zones are compared with the differences present in the population of normal controls. Possible test outcomes are:

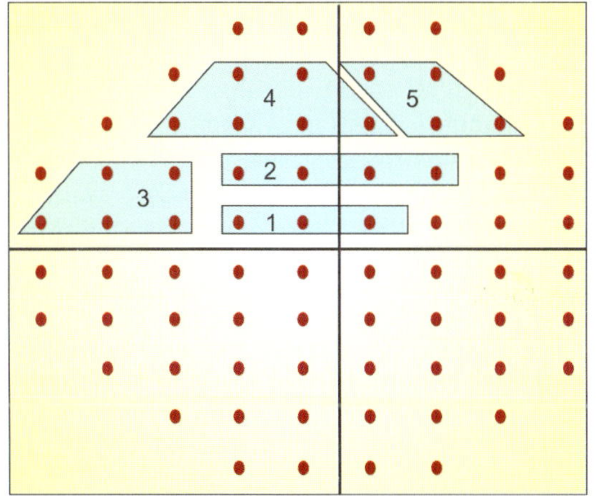

Fig. 10.10 *Glaucoma Hemifield test*

Outside normal limits. The GHT outside normal limits denotes that either the values between upper and lower clusters differ to an extent found in less than 1% of the population or any one pair of clusters is depressed to an extent that would be expected in less than 0.5% of the population. In other words, the GHT is described as "outside normal limits" when differences between a matched pair of corresponding zones exceeds the difference found in 99% of the normal population, or when both members of a pair of zones are more abnormal than 99.5% of the individuals with the normative population.

Borderline. The GHT is considered borderline when the difference between any one of the upper and lower mirror clusters is what might be expected in less than 3% of the population. In other words, the GHT is described as borderline when matched pairs of zones are abnormal at the 97th percentile within the normative database.

General reduction of sensitivity. VFs are described to have generalized reduction of sensitivity when both conditions for "outside normal limits" are not met, and the best region of the VF is depressed to a level at the 99.5th percentile within individuals of the normative database. In other words, GHT is considered to have generalized reduction sensitivity, if the best part of field is depressed to an extent expected in less than 0.5% of the population.

Abnormally high sensitivity. The GHT is described as having abnormally high sensitivity when the overall sensitivity in the affected region of the VF is better than 99.5% of individuals within the normative population. In other words, abnormally high sensitivity is labelled when the best part of the visual field is such as would be expected in less than 0.5% of the population.

Within normal limits. VFs are described as being within normal limits when none of the above conditions are met.

VIII. Actual threshold values

Actual threshold values are shown in part VIII of the printout may be inspected for any pattern or scotoma when clinical features are suspeciant and even if all the seven other parts of the printout are normal.

Scotoma by definition is the depressed part of the field as compared to the surrounding and not as compared to normal.

Sensitivity of the test is lost when the actual test threshold values are below 15 dB.

INTERPRETATION OF FIELD DEFECTS

Systematic approach to interpretation of glaucoma field defects on HFA

In assessing a visual field, particularly that of a glaucoma patient, a systematic approach is recommended.

Step I. Evaluate the field for diffuse or generalized changes when compared to normals or previous fields. Look at the level of overall sensitivities using mean deviation values. If a reduction is noted, look for confounding factors such as media opacities, pupil diameter, or blur.

Step II. After generalized defects, look for localized defects. Look for one or several contiguous loci at which threshold sensitivity is less than that at surrounding loci. Local areas of minimally decreased sensitivity may be within normal limits (one point reduced by 5 dB). The more severely the sensitivity is reduced, the more likely the area in question is pathologic. Several adjacent points of reduction may represent a true defect and deserve careful follow-up or additional testing.

Glaucomatous defects are more likely to occur in Bjerrum's area (10° to 20°), paracentral area (within 10°), and nasal step regions. When loci of reduced sensitivity are detected in these areas, they should arouse suspicion of glaucoma.

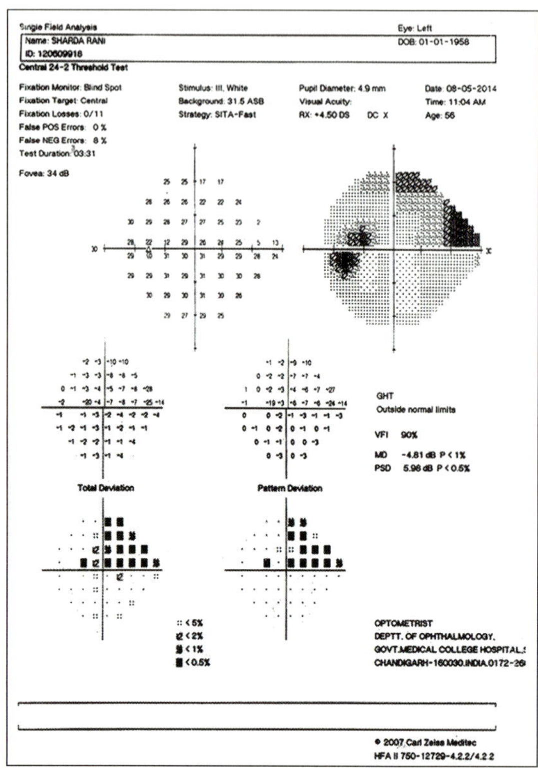

Fig. 10.11 *HVF SITA-FAST 24-2 showing early visual field defect in superior arcuate region*

Classify the defect as per Hodapp-Anderson-Parrish criterion (Table 10.2).

Classical examples of early visual field defect, advanced visual field defect and split fixation, are depicted in Figs 10.11 to 10.13 respectively.

Assessing the visual field progression in glaucoma

Important considerations

- Although structural damage appears first in glaucoma, evaluation of longitudinal series of visual fields to determine the progression of glaucoma remains one of the most commonly used method to detect early changes in the

Table 10.2 *Hodapp-Anderson-Parrish criterion*

Class	*MD*	*Pattern deviation significance*		*Sensitivity within five degrees*
Early	–6.00 to –12.00 dB	<18 locations	<10 locations	No location <15 dB
Moderate	< –12.00 dB	<37 locations	<20 locations	No location at 0 dB only one horizontal Hemifield <15 dB
Severe	< –12.00 dB	>37 locations	>20 locations	Any locations at 0 dB or <15 dB

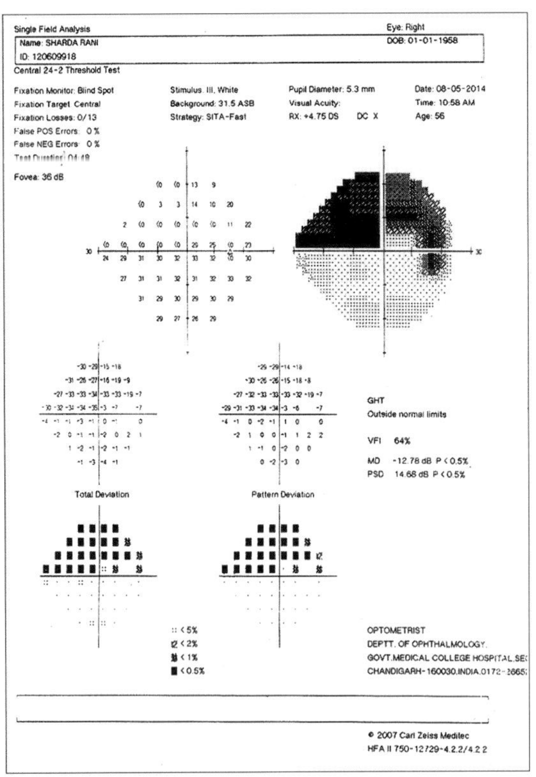

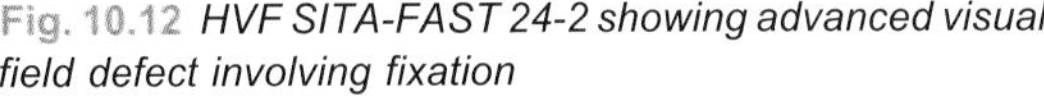

Fig. 10.12 *HVF SITA-FAST 24-2 showing advanced visual field defect involving fixation*

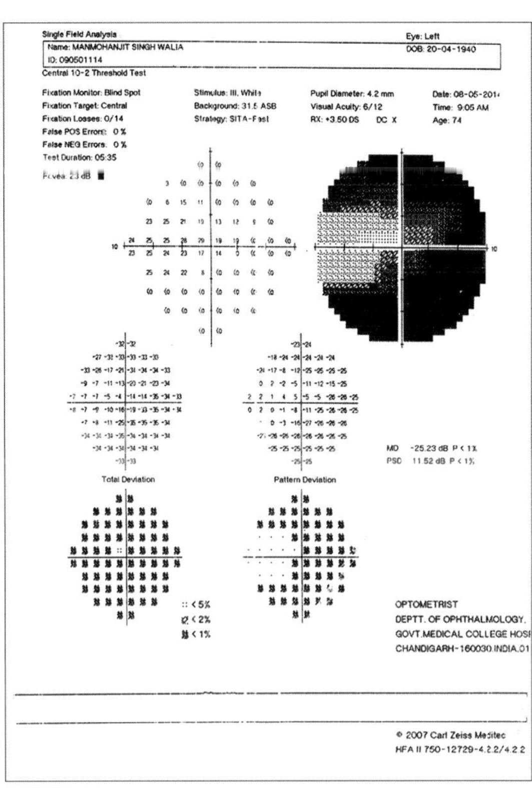

Fig. 10.13 *HVF SITA-FAST 10-2 showing split fixation*

function and indicates worsening of disease and an indication of intensification of treatment regime.

- The time required to detect progression and the pattern of progression are influenced by several factors including underlying rate and type of progression, degree of variability and frequency of examination.
- Whenever a change is detected in the visual fields, it is important to assess whether it is just a variability or true change from neuronal loss prior to jumping at any conclusion.

Note. Reliability indices should be regarded as the primary consideration whenever assessing the visual fields for progression.

Visual field progression: methods used for assessing

1. ***Subjective judgement*** by just looking at a series of visual field printouts. It is dependent upon the clinical expertise of the clinician and is reliable in expert hands.

2. ***Overview printout,*** in which up to 16 previously tested visual fields can be shown in a single printout without any statistical analysis.

3. ***Statistical methods*** which include detecting the changes in global indices, like mean deviation. If there is stable field, mean deviation is unlikely to change. However, in cases where there is localized progression in certain parts of the field, mean deviation may not show change and thus is unreliable.

4. ***Progression analysis software,*** like glaucoma progression analysis (GPA) in Humphrey and peritrend in Octopus, are now being widely used. These are capable of detecting changes in a part of field and individual locations. This compares a single visual field to the results of one or two earlier tests. In other words, a follow-up examination is compared to a baseline of a single or a mean of two or more previous tests. Progression is said to have occurred, if threshold sensitivity at a particular test location changes

more than the expected variability of the mean of previous tests. The glaucoma progression analysis software also classifies whether there is no progression, possible progression, or likely progression of visual field loss.

5. ***Visual field index (VFI)*** is a new measure that captures glaucoma progression. The VFI uses regression to offer a trend-based analysis of the speed by which visual field loss is occurring. The VFI generates a score from 0 (complete loss of field) to 100 (completely full field).

Note. Whenever a progression in field loss is suspected, before reaching a firm conclusion or recomending a change in therapy it is advisable to:

- Repeat the visual field examination, and
- Perform a coroborative optic nerve head and fundus evaluation.

Summary criteria for visual field progression

- *GPA* = Threshold deviation outside test–rest variability boundaries from baseline threshold deviation in ≥3 locations, over 3 consecutive VF
- *MD rate of change*: Significant regression slope with $p < 0.05$, of ≤0.5 db/y
- *VFI rate of change*: Sign regression slope $p < 0.05$, of ≤–1.8
- *AGIS*: Worsening of ≥ = 4 points vs baseline, sustained over 3 consecutive VF
- *CIGTS*: Worsening of > = points vs average of first 2 tests, over 3 consecutive VF
- *Pointwise linear regression (PLR)*: 3 points with significant regression
- *Pointwise linear progression (PoPLR):* Original VF sequence over 95th percentile vs distribution of randomly permutated series
- *Glaucoma rate index (GRI)* score <6

Non-glaucomatous visual field defects

I. ***Visual field defects caused by neurological diseases,*** such as:

- *Optic neuritis, tobacco–alcohol amblyopia, mechanical compression of optic nerve.* Central scotoma.
- *Anterior ischaemic optic neuropathy (AION)?* Non-arteritic ischaemic optic neuropathy (NAAION): Altitudinal defect? Arteritic—generally more extensive
- *Optic nerve head oedema.* Enlargement of blind spot
- *Optic nerve head drusen.* Arcuate defect
- *Optic nerve head coloboma*
- *Thyroid ophthalmopathy.* Variable defects
- *Optic chiasma.* Variable degree of bitemporal hemianopia
- *Post-chiasmal lesions.* Variable degree of homonymous hemianopia

II. ***Visual field defects caused by retinal diseases,*** such as:

- *Diabetic retinopathy.* Multifocal mottled
- *Retinal detachment.* Relative scotoma
- *Retinoschisis.* Absolute scotoma with sharp margins
- *Retinitis pigmentosa.* Circular defect to tunnel vision
- *Retinal vascular lesions.* Arterial absolute; venous variable.
- *BRVO.* Arcuate defect
- *Field defects related to lasered retina*

OCTOPUS PRINTOUT EVALUATION

Data representations in the Octopus printout are similar to those in the Humphrey printout (Fig. 10.14). Patient and examination data are at the top of the printout, followed by the value table (numeric scale) and the grayscale (which is coloured).

Numeric scale and grayscale are followed by a comparison table and a corrected comparison table (total deviation and pattern deviation). The probability plots for those tables follow.

Visual field indices (global indices) are at the bottom right hand side of the printout page.

Indices. Mean sensitivity (MS) which is the mean value of all test results, MD (mean defect) which is the same as mean deviation, LV (lost variance) which is the same as pattern standard deviation, and CLV (corrected lost variance), which is the same as corrected pattern standard deviation. The RF (reliability factor) is a score of patient's reliability (0 to 15%).

Bebie curve is a cumulative defect curve that allows ranking of VF defects (it looks only at the defects, not the field). In the presence of established glaucoma diagnosis, this is useful

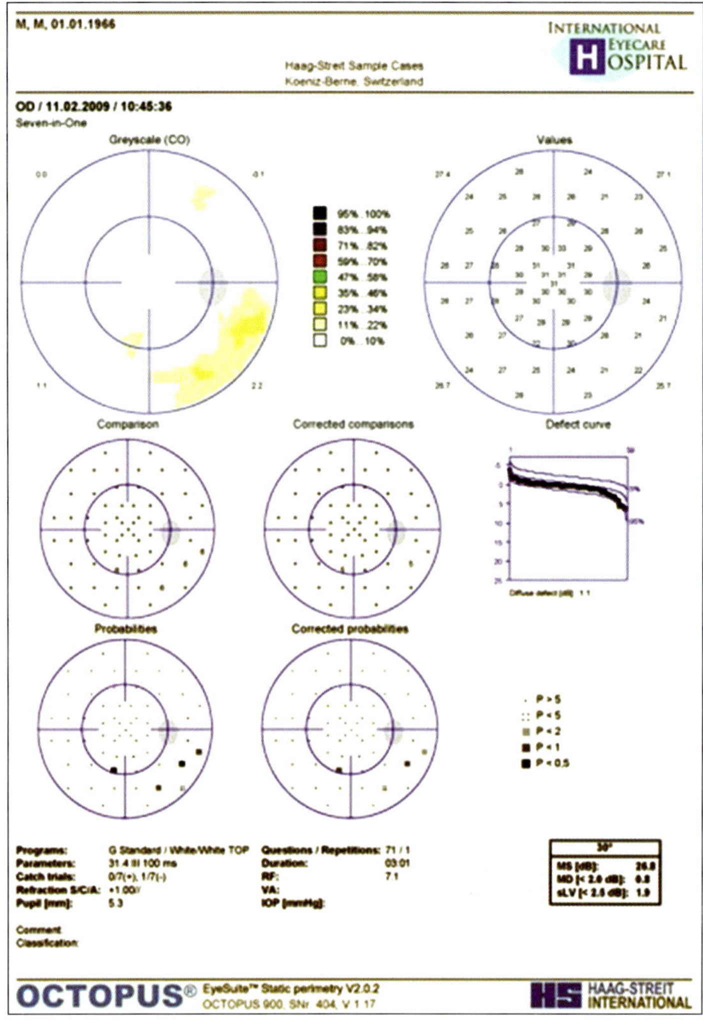

Fig. 10.14 *Octopus visual field printout (Source: www.haag-streit.com)*

to monitor the progression of both overall depression and localised defects.

Staging VF testing is a useful feature. It allows collecting examination results from points considered most important for glaucoma diagnosis in the first and second stages (80% of the test). This allows printing of these results and stopping the testing process, in case of patient fatigue. In all other perimeters, the entire testing process has to be completed before printing of the results.

Octopus criteria for a visual field defect

- MD greater than 2 dB
- LV greater than 6 dB
- At least 7 points with sensitivity decreased by ≥5 dB, 3 of them being contagious.

Octopus versus Humphrey's field analyzer terminologies

Table 10.3 briefly compares the Octopus versus Humphrey's field analyzer terminologies.

VISUAL FIELDS: FREQUENTLY ASKED QUESTIONS

Why is target presentation random in automated static perimetry?

The computer allows stimuli to be presented in a pseudorandom, unpredictable fashion. Patients do not know where the next stimulus will appear, so fixation is improved, thereby

Table 10.3 *Essential parameters: Humphrey's field analyzer (HFA) versus octopus automated perimeter*

Parameter	*HFA*	*Octopus*
Testing conditions		
Bowel type	Aspherical bowl	Direct projection
Background illumination	31.5 asb	31.4 asb
Stimulus size	Goldmann size I–V	Goldmann size III and V
Stimulus duration	200 ms	100 ms
Luminance for zero dB	10,000 asb	4800 asb
Testing strategies		
	Full threshold 4-2 bracketing	Normal 4-2-1 bracketing
	SITA fast	TOP (tendency oriented perimetry)
	SITA standard	Dynamic
Test programmes	30-2 (76 points)	G1
	24-2 (54 points)	G1x (59 points)
	10-2 (68 points in 10°)	M2x (45 points in 5°)
	Macula (10 points in 5°)	
Deviation plots	Total deviation	Comparison
	Pattern deviation	Corrected comparison
Global indices	Mean deviation	Mean defect
	Pattern standard deviation	Loss variance
	Corrected pattern standard deviation	Corrected loss variance
Cluster testing in Bjerrum's area	Glaucoma Hemifield test	Defect curve (Bebie curve)
Glaucoma progression software	Glaucoma progression analysis (GPA)	Peritrend

increasing the reliability of the test. Random presentations also increase the speed with which perimetry can be performed by bypassing the problem of local retinal adaptation, which requires a 2-second interval between stimuli, if adjacent locations are tested.

Concept of foveal threshold?

As one ascends the hill of vision toward the fovea, the sensitivity of the retina increases, dimmer targets will become visible, and the brightness of the target at threshold will decrease. Therefore, as retinal sensitivity increases, the differential light threshold measured in apostilbs decreases (HFA: 1 apostilb = 40 dB). The decibel scale is a relative scale created by the manufacturers of automated perimeters to measure the sensitivity of the island of vision. It is an inverted logarithmic scale. Zero decibel is set as the brightest stimulus that the perimeter can produce.

Why is fovea most sensitive?

The highest concentration of cones is in the fovea, and most of these cones project to their own ganglion cell. This one-to-one ratio between foveal cone and ganglion cell results in maximal resolution at the fovea.

Why is background illumination of HFA 31.5 asb?

It has been taken from Goldmann's calculation which suggested that 31.5 asb is the minimum intensity for photopic recording of visual fields. This is also the level of luminance to which eye can quickly adapt, can produce most reliable and stable response properties within and between subjects.

Anderson's and Patella's criteria for perimetric diagnosis of glaucoma?

1. Three or more contiguous non-edge points depressed <5% population and at least 1 point

depressed <1% population should be clustered in the arcuate area
2. PSD depressed <5% population
3. GHT-outside normal limits

Why is grayscale condemned by glaucoma specialists?

Grayscale gives gradations of darkness in fixed scale of 5 dB. Thus, a change of threshold from 21 to 22 dB will give same colour gradation as that from 16 to 24 dB. However, it has role in explaining the patient about damage and in cases with high false positive where white areas are seen. It does help us in understanding some artifacts, e.g. clover leaf pattern in a fatigued patient.

What does 24-2 mean?

A 24-2 test points 24° around the fovea. The second number refers to the testing protocol. The HVF has historically had two main testing protocols, 1 and 2. Protocol 1 tested points directly on the horizontal and vertical axes. Protocol 2 test points on either side of the horizontal and vertical axes. Since defects found right on the line can be difficult to interpret, everyone uses 2.

Why is 24-2 better than 30-2?

Humphrey programme 24-2 eliminates the most peripheral ring of test locations from programme 30-2, except in the nasal step region, and tests only the central 24°. This test is very useful because the peripheral ring of thresholds provides the least reliable data, and testing time can be shortened.

What is Visual Field Index (VFI)?

The VFI is a new global metric that represents the entire visual field as a single percentage of normal. It is based largely on the pattern deviation and weighs central points more than peripheral ones.

A full visual field has a VFI of 100% while a perimetrically-blind visual field has a VFI of 0% represents the percentage of useful vision a patient has left.

VFI takes the patient's age and the "velocity" of the change in visual field into account. The rate of change of the VFI over time characterizes the rate of progression, while a statistical analysis of this rate generates a p-value indicating whether or not the rate of change is significantly different from zero.

HFA software uses both event based and trend-based assessment of progression (visual field index/VFI).

- *For event-based-VF* sensitivities of current test are compared to prior tests and progression is established if a threshold is exceeded for a specific number of test locations. Within the individual data, magnitude of change over time to long-term variability is observed.
- *For trend-based analyses-* VF sensitivities of all tests available during follow-up are analyzed for significant change over time, employing a linear regression approach. It provides estimates of rates of VF progression over time, to differentiate fast progressor's (VFI).

What is the relevance of Guided progression analysis (GPA) and how to interpret it?

Guided progression analysis (GPA) software incorporated in Humphrey analyser II is analogous to Humphrey analyser I glaucoma change probability software. It assists in confirming glaucoma progression by analyzing visual field VF points accounting for pattern deviation, compared to glaucoma change probability (GCP) which used total deviation.

GPA: Uses EMGT's criteria by > = 3 points, with 5% worsening on > 3 consecutive VF + CNTG criteria of minimal 2 VF requirement for progression is utilized by GPA using average of first 2 reliable VF as base-line, compared to 3rd consecutive field.

Visual field requirement for driving?

'A minimum horizontal field of vision of 120° and no significant defect within 20° of fixation'.

How to interpret gaze tracker?

Upward deflection (gaze deviation); downward deflection (blink).

PRACTICAL PEARLS

- Test a patient's better-seeing eye first, especially if he or she has not undergone perimetry before.

- Foveal function should always be on. The foveal function helps clinicians to determine the etiology of visual field loss.
- Goldmann size III (about ½ degree in diameter) is generally used, but Goldmann size V (approximately 2 degrees in diameter) is available for patients with decreased visual acuity (<20/200) or other visual impairment.
- When examining the test results, you must hold the two printouts (right eye printout in your right hand facing your right eye, and left eye printout in your left hand facing your left eye), and examine them together.

OTHER PSYCHOPHYSICAL TESTS IN GLAUCOMA

INTRODUCTION

For the past several years, several different perimeters and test strategies have been developed, but none has had more studies and has been more used than standard white-on-white perimetry with the Humphrey Field Analyzer (HFA; Carl Zeiss Meditec, Dublin, CA, USA). Although SAP is still considered the gold standard, function-specific perimetry may offer advantages for early diagnosis.

Other tests have been developed in addition to traditional perimetry to detect early glaucomatous visual loss. Psychophysical tests are designed to isolate various retinal pathways. Psychophysical tests other than traditional perimetry include:

- Short wavelength automated perimetry
- Frequency doubling perimetry
- High-pass resolution (ring)
- Motion detection types of perimetry
- Pattern discrimination types of perimetry
- Contrast sensitivity (both spatial and temporal), and
- Colour vision

ANATOMICAL BASIS

At this point, it would help to understand the basic retinal anatomy and physiology. Retinal nerve fibres transmit signals from the retinal receptor cells by way of the optic nerve to the lateral geniculate body and ultimately to the visual cortex. These are broadly classified into the magnocellular (or M) cells, and the parvocellular (or P) cells.

P cells. The P cell pathway is responsible for high contrast, low temporal frequency (or static) stimulus detection.

M cells. The M cell pathway detects low-contrast; high temporal frequency (or motion) stimuli, and constitute approximately 10% of the total retinal nerve fibres. Non-linear M cells are a subset of the large diameter M cells, and are affected before any other cell type in glaucoma. Therefore, detection of this cell loss helps to identify RGC loss before it can be detected by traditional automated perimetry.

SHORT WAVELENGTH AUTOMATED PERIMETRY

Short wavelength automated perimetry (SWAD) is also known as blue on yellow perimetry as in this blue colour stimulus is presented on a yellow background. Blue colour saturates rods and yellow colour stimulates only the short wavelength system (SWS) cones, i.e the koniocellular pathway. It uses the same testing patterns as standard white on white perimetry, however, it is able to detect visual field changes earlier. Additionally, the size of defect in SWAP is larger and progression typically greater than standard automated perimetry. But it is more variable and is affected by the absorption properties of crystalline lenses.

FREQUENCY DOUBLING PERIMETRY (FDP)

Frequency doubling illusion. When a low spatial frequency sinusoidal grating with alternating wide light and dark bars (Fig. 10.15) undergoes high temporal-frequency counterphase flicker, (i.e. the black and white bands reverse to become white and black, respectively in a rapid sequence) the spatial frequency of the grating appears doubled. This phenomenon is called the frequency doubling illusion.

Selective testing of the magnocellular pathway by presenting alternate grating stimuli, therefore, may help in early detection of glaucomatous cell loss.

First and second generations of FDT instruments never achieved sufficiently widespread clinical use despite confirming this technology's potential.

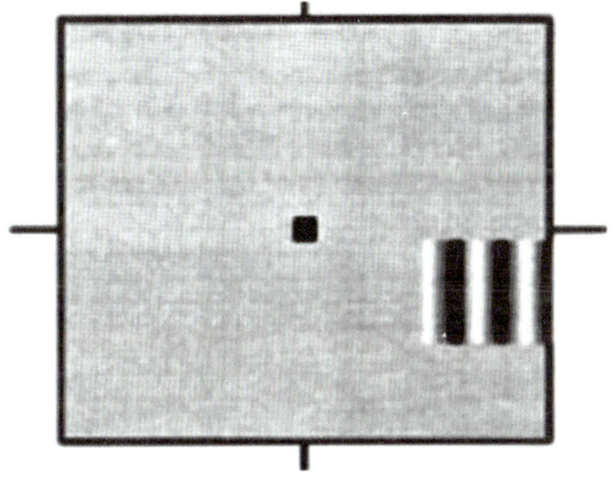

Fig. 10.15 *FDP target: Sinusoidal gratings consisting of alternate black and white bars*

Newer Humphrey matrix perimeter with Welch Allyn frequency-doubling technology from Carl-Zeiss Meditec has found its foothold into clinical practice.

Matrix offers three main testing algorithms for generating visual fields. One is a screening algorithm similar to SITA-Fast where parts of the visual field are not retested. In the new testing protocol, the FDT Matrix utilizes grating targets smaller than the original FDT to enable standard 24-2 and 30-2 test patterns, which look identical to those in SAP. It also can perform central 10-degree testing, which can be used to follow a patient with advanced glaucoma. It is a portable device and particularly useful in children.

MOTION DETECTION PERIMETRY (MDP)

Motion detection may be related to temporal contrast sensitivity—both seem to be modulated primarily by the M ganglion cells. Motion detection perimetry is a method that measures a subject's ability to detect a coherent shift in position of dots in a circular area against a background of non-moving dots (Fig. 10.16). Motion size threshold is the smallest detectable circular area in which the subject can detect motion. Subjects respond by touching a computer screen with a light pen where they detect motion stimuli. Their localization errors, as the number of pixels from target centre and reaction time, are then calculated.

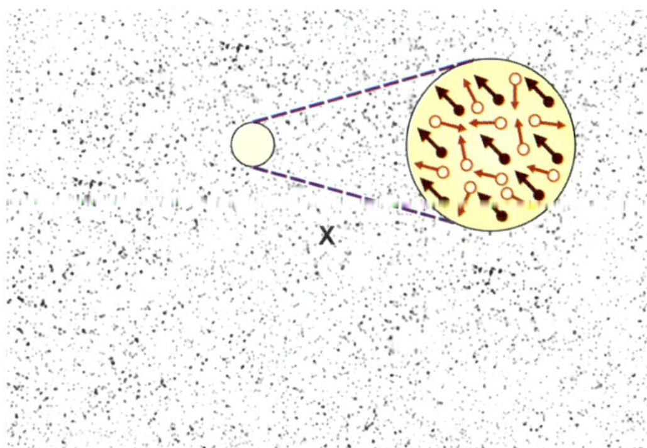

Fig. 10.16 *Motion perimetry video display. The small circle (left) represents a medium-sized random-dot motion perimetry target. A magnified view of the target (right) shows that 50% of the dots are moving in random directions (°) and 50% are moving coherently (•). X, fixation target*

FLICKER-DEFINED FORM PERIMETRY

Flicker-defined form (FDF) as a testing stimulus was conceived for preferential stimulation of the magnocellular projecting retinal ganglion cells (RGCs). This psychophysical approach was thought to have advantages for the early detection of glaucoma due to theories of reduced redundancy (selective testing) and/or selective damage to the magnocellular RGCs. FDF is now thought to measure early functional changes due to impaired higher order visual mechanisms required for complex and integrated neural processing involving both temporal and spatial vision. The Heidelberg Edge Perimeter (HEP; Heidelberg Engineering) has FDF stimulus for early detection of glaucomatous visual deficits. The flickering stimulus of the HEP creates an illusionary edge contour that the patient perceives as a circle against the mean luminance background (Fig. 10.17). This process aims to

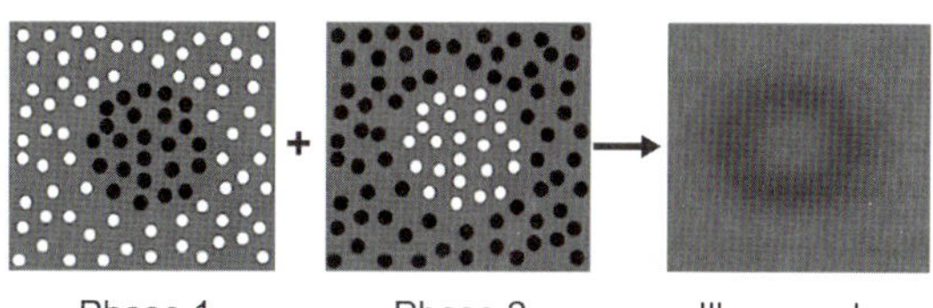

Fig. 10.17 *Phase reversal of randomly positioned black and white dots in flicker-defined form (FDF) perimetry. At high temporal frequencies, subjects cannot differentiate between the flickering dots but perceive an illusory circular edge contour*

facilitate better "test/retest" reliability by diminishing the degree of variability in patients' responses.

HIGH PASS RESOLUTION PERIMETRY (HPRP)

High pass resolution perimetry uses a series of ring stimuli varying in size that are displayed on a computer monitor at various locations within the central visual field. The stimuli resemble visual acuity optotypes, such as the Landolt C and consist of a dark ring surrounding a central circular white region (Fig. 10.18). HRP tests 50 locations inside the 30° central visual field.

The locations are distributed in a pattern reminiscent of normal isopters. This is calculated to facilitate both visual recognition of common field defect patterns and statistical analysis of results. The subject is asked to press the response button each time a stimulus is detected, and the programme performs a staircase procedure to increase and decrease target size until a detection threshold is achieved. Normal examination time is about 5 minutes. Being a resolution test, it is sensitive to media opacities.

Ophthimus (High Tech Vision, Malmö, Sweden) is the currently marketed high pass resolution perimeter.

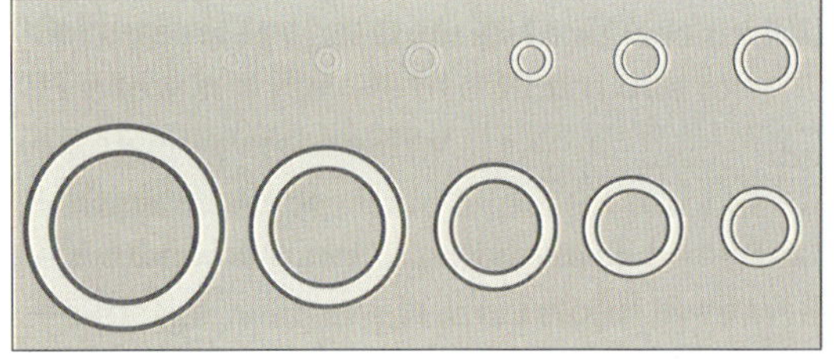

Fig. 10.18 *Ring stimuli of high pass resolution perimeter*

PULSAR PERIMETRY

Pulsar perimetry was developed in 2000 and the Pulsar T30W test utilizes a circular sinusoidal grating pattern that examines 66 areas of the central 30 degrees VF (Fig. 10.19). The stimulus consists of a circular sinusoidal 5 degrees diameter grating pattern that is presented for 500 msec (Fig. 10.20). The stimulus undergoes a counterphase pulse motion at 30 Hz, in which

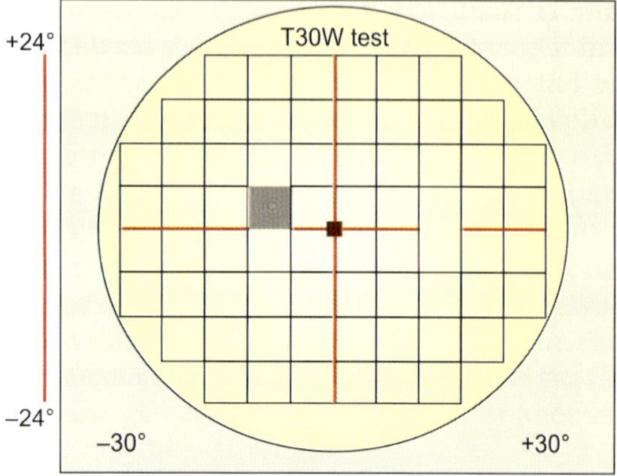

Fig. 10.19 *Size and distribution of the 66 test-areas in the central visual field in pulsar perimetry*

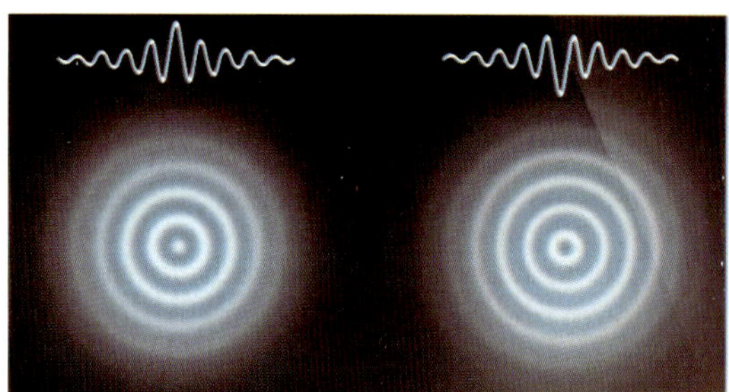

Fig. 10.20 *Pulsar stimulus*

both spatial resolution (SR, from 0.5 to 6.3 cyc/deg on a 12-step log scale) and contrast (C, from 3 to 100% on a 32-step log scale) are simultaneously modified. Threshold sensitivity based on tendency oriented perimetry (TOP) threshold strategy is expressed in spatial resolution contrast units (src). Pulsar has given promising preliminary results in the early detection of glaucomatous VF damage.

Pulsar and FDT use a similar counterphase flickering grating stimulus with high temporal frequency. The testing methods differ in that FDT uses a squared test target, while the circular stimulus used in Pulsar helps to keep the same level of contrast around the edges, in order to avoid stimulation of those cells that selectively respond to a given orientation. FDT uses fixed low spatial frequency and contrast is modified, whereas the Pulsar T30W test examines the contrast sensitivity function by measuring the contrast threshold resolution at several spatial frequencies. The instruments use different threshold strategies; MOBS in FDT and TOP in Pulsar.

OCTOPUS® 600 (Haag Streit Diagnostics) is the first perimeter combining both the Pulsar method for early diagnosis and standard white-on-white perimetry in one device.

SUGGESTED READING

1. Johnson CA, Adams AJ, Casson EJ, Brandt JD: Blue-on-Yellow perimetry can predict the development of glaucomatous visual field loss. Archives of Ophthalmology, 1993;111:645–50.
2. Johnson CA. Psychophysical factors that have been applied to clinical perimetry. Vision Res. 2013 Sep 20;90:25–31.
3. Johnson CA, Sample PA, Zangwill LM, Vasile CG, Cioffi GA, Liebmnn JR, Weinreb RN, Structure and function evaluation (SAFE) II. Comparison of optic disc and visual field characteristics. Am J Ophthalmol 2003;135:148–54.
4. Sample PA, Dannheim F, Artes PH, Dietzsch J, Henson D, Johnson CA, Ng M, Schiefer U, Wall M; IPS Standards Group. Imaging and Perimetry Society standards and guidelines. Optom Vis Sci. 2011 Jan;88(1):4–7.
5. Stamper RL. Psychophysical changes in glaucoma. Surv Ophthalmol. 1989;33:309–18.

CHAPTER 11

ELECTROPHYSIOLOGICAL TECHNIQUES IN GLAUCOMA

ELECTROPHYSIOLOGICAL TESTS IN GLAUCOMA

Glaucoma is characterized by significant loss of ganglion cells leading to visual disability. There is an inbuilt redundancy in the visual system which allows a large number of neurons to be lost without becoming manifest in standard tests of visual function. The techniques, like routine testing of intraocular pressure (IOP), automated perimetry and optic nerve fibre layer photography fail to detect early glaucomatous damage. Eyes with no clinically manifest visual field loss or change in the appearance of the optic nerve head may have lost about 30% of their axons. Therefore, early diagnosis of glaucoma remains a challenge to the clinician as early nerve damage can be detected only by a test that is sensitive to its dysfunction even before structural and functional changes occur. Electrophysiological evaluation is the answer in such a situation.

Visual input passes through various processes before reaching visual cortex. Various electrophysiological techniques exist for assessing the integrity of each such processing stage (Fig. 11.1) Various electrophysiological techniques useful in glaucoma are:

1. Pattern electroretinogram (PERG),
2. Photopic negative response,
3. S-cone visual evoked potential, and
4. Multifocal visual evoked potential (mfVEP).

PATTERN ELECTRORETINOGRAM

Pattern electroretinogram (PERG) is a direct indicator of ganglion cell function and thus a promising test to detect early glaucomatous damage.

Placement of electrodes. The retinal potential is recorded with the help of corneal electrodes like gold foil electrode or DTL.

Stimulus. Checkerboard pattern is used as stimulus which reverses its local luminance while keeping average luminance constant. The size of the checks should be between 0.8° and 16° to give accurate results.

Recordings and interpretation. Two types of responses are evoked depending upon the frequency of the checkerboard reversal. Reversal rate <4 rev/s produces a transient response and

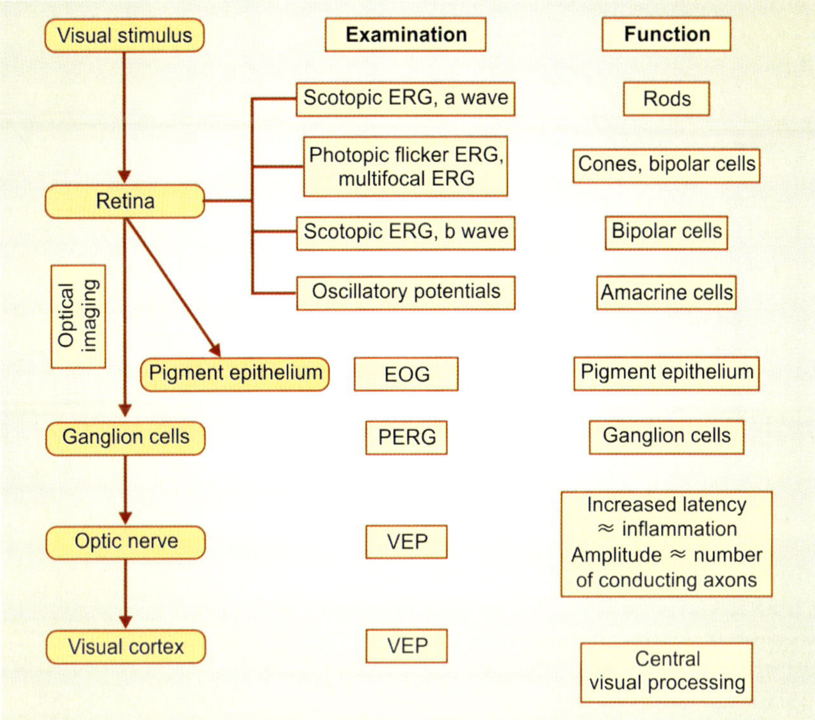

Fig. 11.1 *Electrophysiological techniques for evaluating visual pathways at different levels*

reversal rate >8 rev/s produces a steady state response.

Waveform of PERG as depicted in Fig. 11.2 shows the following components:

- *A small negative wave* the trough of which is obtained at around 35 ms (N35)
- *A large positive wave* the peak of which is obtained at around 45–60 ms (P50)
- *A large negative component* the trough of which lies at around 90–100 ms (N95).

The recordings from a normal individual, a patient with early glaucoma and a patient with advanced glaucoma are depicted in Fig. 11.3. The PERG to small check sizes (0.8°, centre column) is affected in early and late glaucoma, whereas the PERG to large stimulus checks (16°,

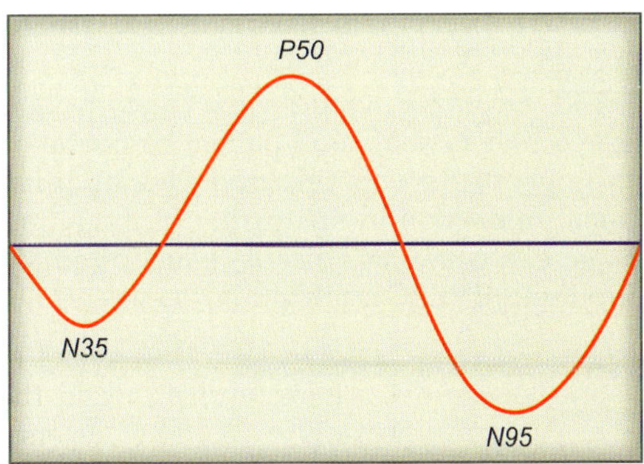

Fig. 11.2 *Normal waveform patterns of PERG*

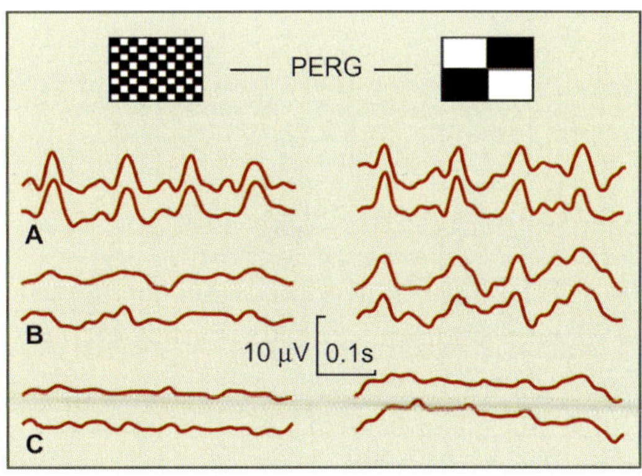

Fig. 11.3 *Waveform patterns in (A) normal, (B) early and (C) advanced glaucoma*

right column) is relatively normal in early glaucoma but markedly reduced in the advanced glaucoma.

$$\text{PERG ratio} = \frac{\text{PERG amplitude to } 0.8° \text{ checks}}{\text{PERG amplitude to } 16° \text{ checks}}$$

Figure 11.4 depicts amplitude variation with transient and steady-state stimulation in normal and glaucomatous eyes. The amplitude is markedly reduced in glaucomatous eyes after steady state stimulation. Figure 11.5 shows the scatter of a normal control population data from Porciatti and Ventura. There is a high correlation between the amplitudes to 0.8° and 16° check size in normals. In glaucoma, this correlation is decoupled: initially the 0.8° response is reduced, then later the 16° response. Consequently, an untreated or treatment-resistant glaucoma eye will likely follow the hypothetical curve indicated by the curved arrow in Fig. 11.5. A constant PERG ratio of 1 corresponds to the 45° line in this figure. For individual diagnosis, the lower and upper lines indicate the 5 and 95% confidence interval for the PERG ratio, respectively. PERGs from individual eyes that fall below the lower confidence line may be at risk of developing glaucoma

Another well-standardized paradigm to employ the PERG in glaucoma is called, "PERGLA" by the authors, Porciatti and Ventura. A main feature of their approach is the use of skin electrodes, which avoid the contact

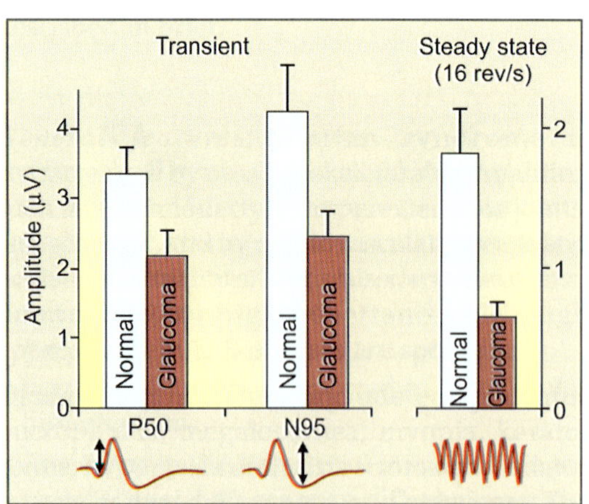

Fig. 11.4 *Depicts amplitude variation in PERG in transient versus steady state stimulation*

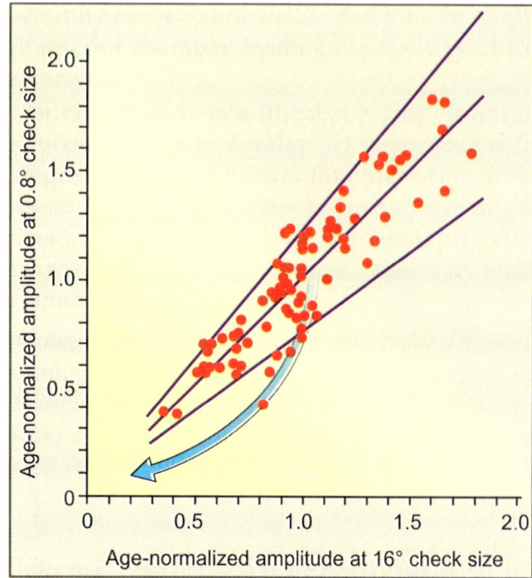

Fig. 11.5 *PERG amplitudes to two check sizes (0.8°/16°) in 85 normal eyes. A wide scatter of amplitude between individuals is seen. The mean course of disease is likely to follow the gray-dashed arrow. (Source: Bach M, Hoffmann MB.Optom Vis Sci 2008:85(6):386–95.)*

to the cornea. The use of a grating rather than a checkerboard is a minor difference, the dominant spatial frequency is very similar to a 0.8° checkerboard.

Role in glaucoma

- PERG is useful in early diagnosis of glaucoma as it picks up a panretinal damage mechanism, which affects the ganglion cells before reliable field damage is observed.
- It is highly specific in identifying those patients with elevated IOP in whom glaucoma damage is incipient before visual field changes occur.

PERG recording requires refractive correction, clear ocular media, good patient co-operation for proper placement of electrodes because even a small reduction in the quality of the retinal image can cause significant reduction in the amplitude of PERG leading to erroneous results.

PHOTOPIC NEGATIVE RESPONSE

Genesis

Flash ERG recorded under photopic conditions specified by International Society for Clinical

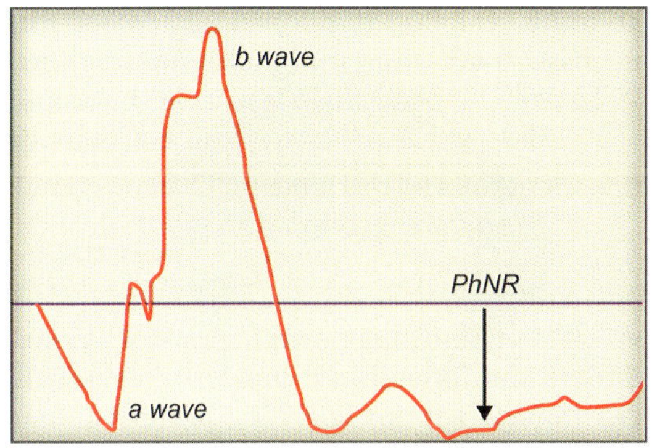

Fig. 11.6 *Photopic negative response*

Electrophysiology of Vision (ISCEV) identifies a new component named photopic negative response (PhNR)

- PhNR is the negative wave following the 'b' wave (Fig. 11.6)
- The amplitude of PhNR is measured from the baseline to the trough of the wave.

The photopic negative response is driven by retinal ganglion cells (RGCs). The function of RGCs is objectively evaluated by analysing the PhNR.

PhNR is selectively attenuated in eyes with optic nerve atrophy induced by trauma, compression, inflammation, gene mutation, and ischaemia.

Advantages of photopic negative response

- The main advantage of this test over PERG is that it can be recorded even in patients with poor co-operation and hazy ocular media. The only requirement is the presence of dilated pupils.
- Another advantage of the PhNR is that it can be recorded using a conventional ERG recording device.
- Furthermore, the PhNR is a component of the cone ERG, so a and b waves can be recorded simultaneously enabling the function of middle and outer retinal layers to be evaluated at the same time. This benefit is not available when assessing RGC function with the conventional means of the VEP or PERG.

S-CONE VISUAL EVOKED POTENTIALS

VEP recording after cone-specific flash stimulation using selective colour channels gives responses which are different for long, medium and short wavelength sensitive cones (L-, M-, S-cones). The S-cone responses have significantly different slopes for the first positive wave in glaucoma. This is not observed in the L- and M-cone responses. This S-cone pathway is affected in glaucoma before standard subjective perimetry. Recently a blue-on-yellow VEP method has been presented as a functional test of the blue-sensitive S-cone pathway. S-cone VEP is an evolving technique which may prove to be useful for early detection of glaucoma.

MULTIFOCAL VISUAL EVOKED POTENTIALS

Definition

The multifocal visual evoked potential (mfVEP), was developed by Baseler (1994) to provide a method for obtaining local visual evoked potential (VEP) responses from the visual field. It is an objective method for topographical assessment of visual function. The technique combines conventional VEP recording methods with a display that is subdivided into a number of regions thereby making it possible to record visual evoked potentials (VEPs) simultaneously from many regions of the visual field. The display covers about the same retinal area as the 24-2 Humphrey visual field (HVF). All visual field locations are stimulated in parallel with their individual stimulus sequence and due to the independence of the stimulus sequences, the responses for each visual field location can be extracted using mathematical algorithms (Fig. 11.7).

Visually evoked potentials elicited by flash stimuli can be recorded from many scalp locations in humans. Visual stimuli stimulate both primary visual cortices and secondary areas. Clinical VEPs are usually recorded from occipital scalp overlying the calcarine fissure. This is the closest location to primary visual cortex (Brodmann's area 17).

Technique

Placement of electrodes. There are two common systems of placing scalp electrodes, viz. 10–20 International system and Queen square system. Various laboratories use their own preferred methods of placement of electrodes to record

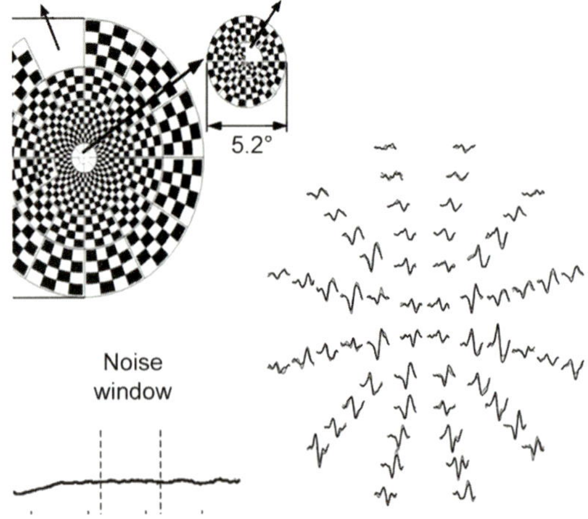

Fig. 11.7 *Typical multifocal VEP recording in normal eye*

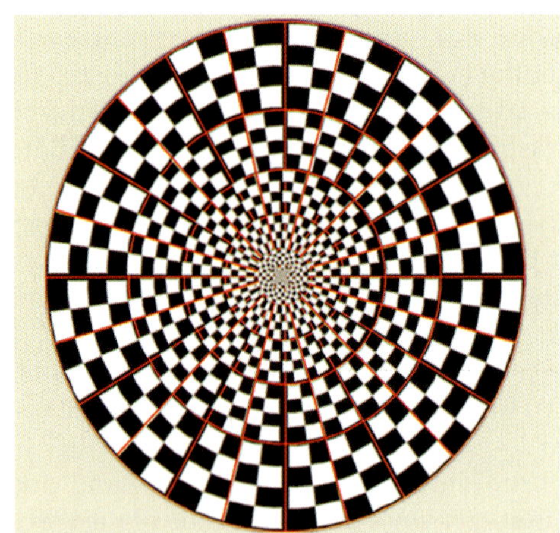

Fig. 11.8 *Dartboard pattern used for recording mfVEP*

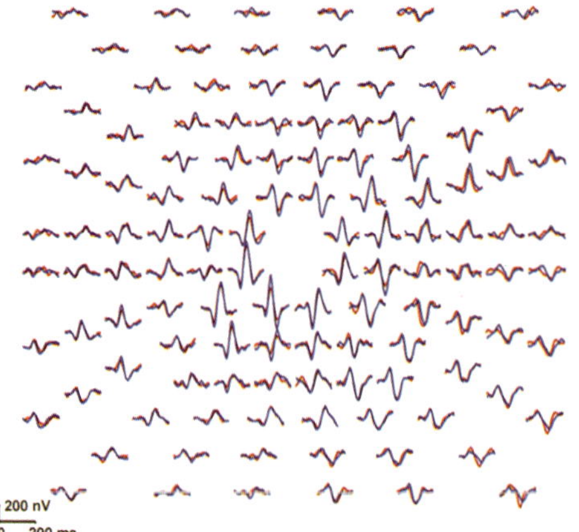

Fig. 11.9 *mfVEP recordings in a normal adult. Waves in red are from right eye and waves in blue are from left eye*

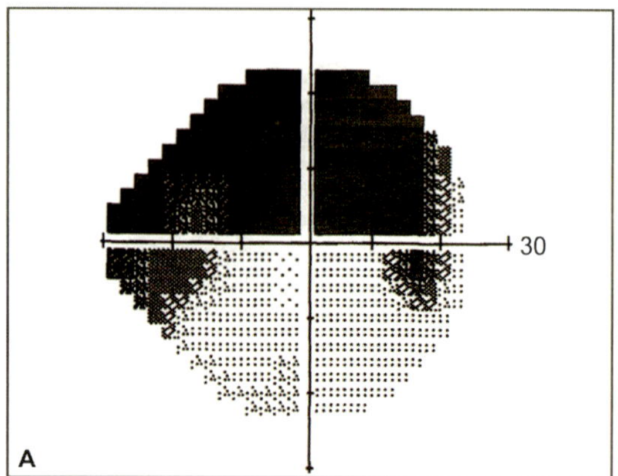

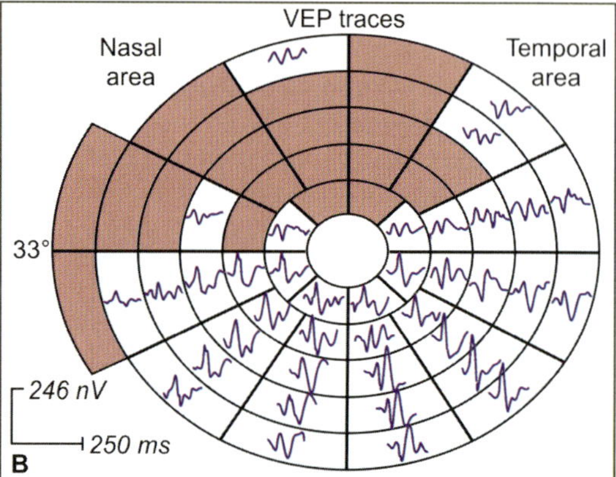

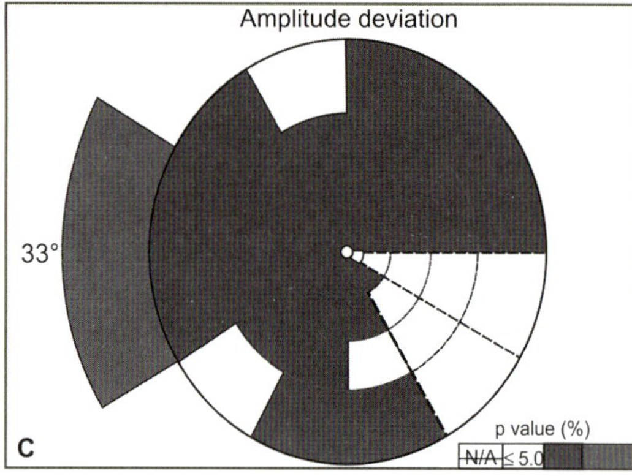

Fig. 11.10 *mfVEP and its corresponding standard automated perimetry (SAP): (A) Superior altitudinal defect on SAP; (B) mfVEP raw data with superimposed grayscale, (C) mfVEP amplitude deviation showing larger superior altitudinal defect*

VEP. A common method is to place two electrodes on the midline one just below the inion and another 3 cm above the inion; and laterally place electrodes 3–4 cm off the midline, several centimeters above the inion. The ground lead can be anywhere on the body.

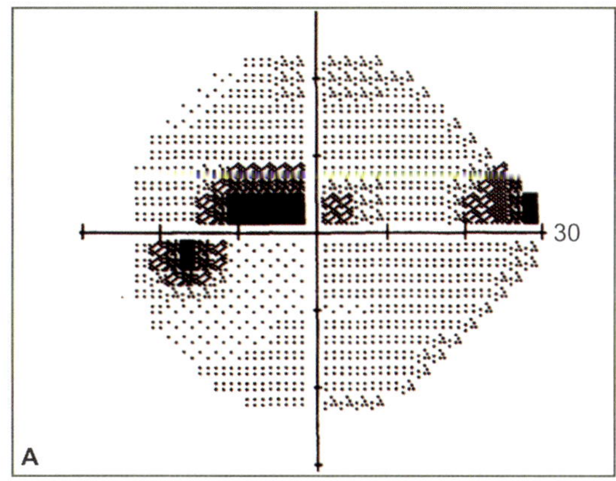

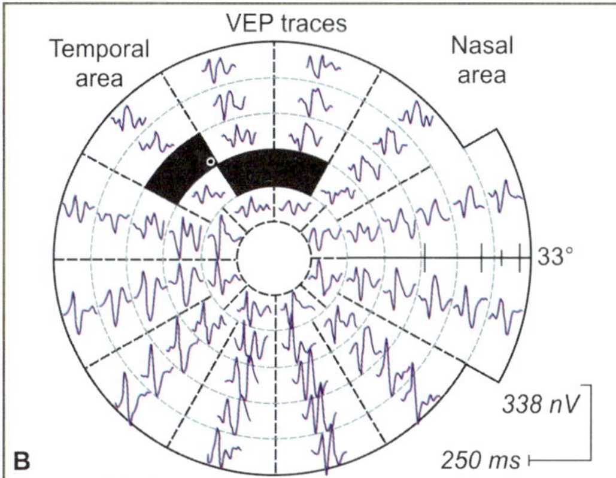

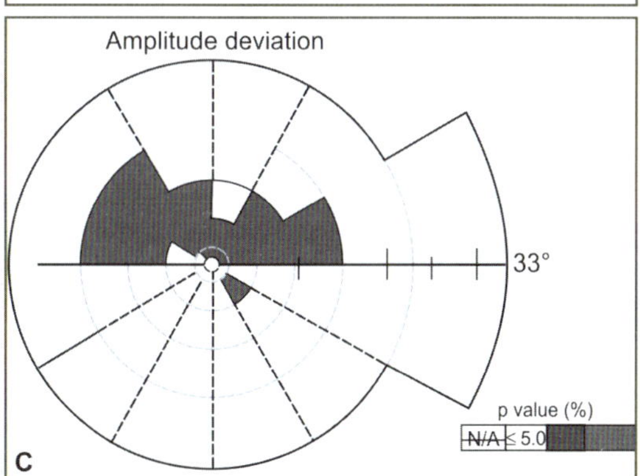

Fig. 11.11 *mfVEP and its corresponding standard automated perimetry (SAP): (A) Superior arcuate defect on SAP; (B) mfVEP raw data with superimposed grayscale; (C) mfVEP amplitude deviation showing larger superior arcuate defect*

Stimulus. The common stimulus for multifocal visually evoked potentials (mfVEPs) is a dartboard pattern with sectors. Each sector contains a contrast reversing check pattern (Fig. 11.8).

Recordings and interpretations. Recordings of multifocal visual evoked potentials from a normal subject are shown in Fig. 11.9. The low amplitude and increased latency of the waveforms may be the first sign of functional damage preceding the structural loss hence can help in early diagnosis of glaucoma. Figures 11.10 and 11.11 depict mfVEPs and its corresponding standard automated perimetry.

Sources of error. Common sources of error during mfVEP recordings can be improper electrode position, poor electrode contact with scalp, refractive error, poor/eccentric fixation, media opacity, miosis or mydriasis.

Role in glaucoma

- Objective evaluation of functional changes of optic nerve in eyes with primary open-angle glaucoma.
- Objective confirmation of findings of standard automated perimetry.
- Clarification of diagnostic dilemma in glaucoma suspects.
- Early diagnosis of functional damage thereby helping early diagnosis and initiation of treatment of glaucoma.
- Objective assessment for follow-up of glaucoma patients.

SUGGESTED READING

1. Bach M. Electrophysiological approaches for early detection of glaucoma. European Journal of Ophthalmology 2001;11(2):541-49
2. Bach M, Ramharter-Sereinig A. Pattern electroretinogram to detect glaucoma: Comparing the PERGLA and the PERG ratio protocols. Doc Ophthalmol 2013 Dec;127(3):227–38.
3. Goyal JL, Sitharam Sudha, Arora Ritu, et al. Electrophysiology in glaucoma, Delhi Journal of Ophthalmology. 2013;23(4):245–49.
4. Thomas Meigan, Michael Bach. Electrophysiology in the diagnosis of glaucoma. In Glaucoma edited by Frenz Ghrehn, Robert Stamper. Essentials of Ophthalmology series editors GK. Krieglstein, RN Wenreb. Springer Science and Business Media, 2006.

CHAPTER 12

OCULAR BLOOD FLOW IN GLAUCOMA

INTRODUCTION

Study of ocular blood flow in relation to glaucomatous optic neuropathy dates back over 100 years when Wagemann and Salzmann first observed vascular sclerosis in glaucoma patients. For more than a century, it has been suspected that disturbed ocular blood flow (OBF) may play a role in the pathogenesis of glaucoma. A century of observation and circumstantial evidence suggesting a vascular component in the pathogenesis of glaucoma is now supported by direct evidence. Reduced OBF has been measured in glaucoma patients by numerous medical centres using a variety of techniques in different tissues of the eye. A decrease in OBF has been proven to be of prognostic value, however, the implementation of this knowledge into clinical practice has been very slow. Vascular problems must be diagnosed and considered when treating known cases of glaucoma.

While we know that OBF is reduced in glaucoma, there is still some discussion as to why this is the case. Some experts focus on perfusion pressure (PP) as the reason. Like the perfusion pressure of any organ, OBF is the result of the relationship between PP and local resistance to blood flow. This explains why not all patients with high IOP or low blood pressure have low OBF.

Some experts believe that mechanical factors (distinguishing between vascular and bio-chemical) are the reasons why OBF is reduced in glaucoma. Another cause for the slow implementation of measuring OBF in clinical practice is the issue of methodology. It is far more challenging to calculate OBF than it is to simply measure IOP.

ASSESSMENT OF OCULAR BLOOD FLOW

Given that OBF outcome measures in different parts of the eye correlate quite well with each other, the selection of the measuring field may not be that relevant. Assessment of OBF can be made by the methods given below.

1. Measuring ocular temperature

Blood flow is an important factor affecting temperature of any organ of the body. Reports indicate that eyes of patients with glaucoma, particularly with normal tension glaucoma (NTG), are cooler than those of patients without glaucoma. Furthermore, reports also show that an increase in ocular blood flow (OBF), induced directly pharmacologically or indirectly by decreasing IOP, increases corneal temperature. Thus, by measuring ocular temperature, the status of OBF can be studied.

2. Fundus fluorescein angiography

Following findings may be observed:

- *Reduction in blood flow velocity* as demonstrated by delayed filling and as prolonged A-V passage time (Fig. 12.1)
- *Increased leakage* indicating impairment of the blood–brain and blood–retinal barriers (Fig. 12.2)
- *Filling defects* in and around, the ONH in peripapillary area (Fig. 12.3).

3. Retinal vessel analysis

Recently retinal vessel analyzer (Fig. 12.4A) has been introduced to quantify the size of retinal arteries and veins along a selected segment over a period of time. Figure 12.4B shows the retinal vessel diameter of a vascular section using the retinal vessel analyzer. This construction resulted after the patient breathed in 100% oxygen. The retinal vessel diameter provides only indirect information about ocular blood flow.

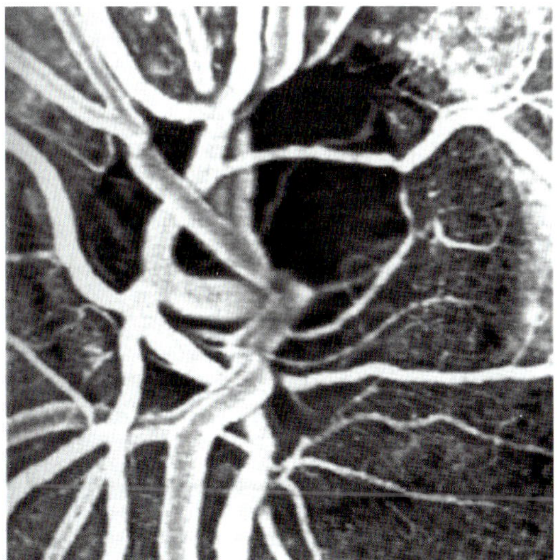

Fig. 12.1 *Fluorescence angiography of a glaucomatous papilla, parts of the optic nerve head are not perfused*

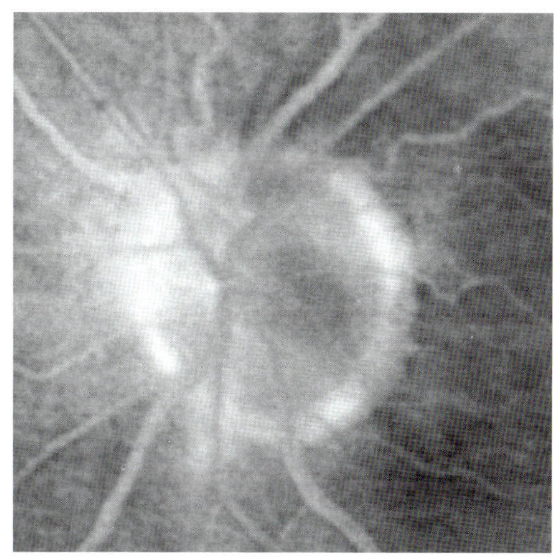

Fig. 12.2 *Fluorescein angiography depicting mild diffuse staining*

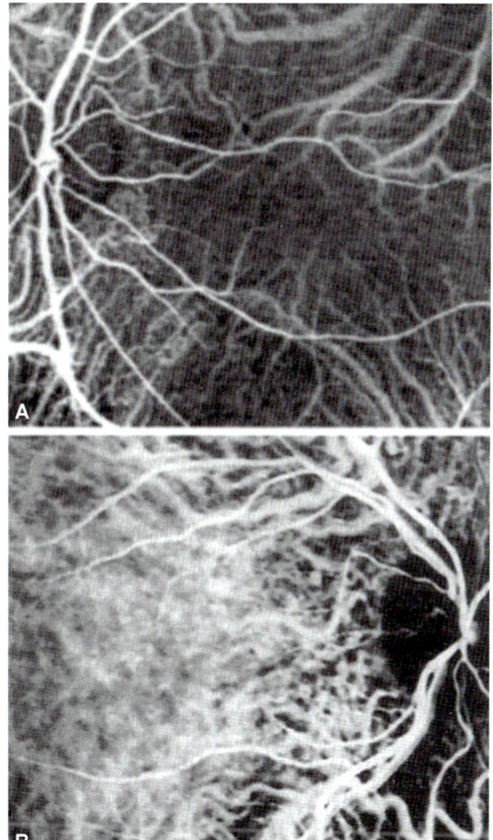

Figs 12.3A and B *Indocyanine angiography in a glaucomatous eye depicting delayed filling of some of the choriocapillaris (From Flammer, 2006)*

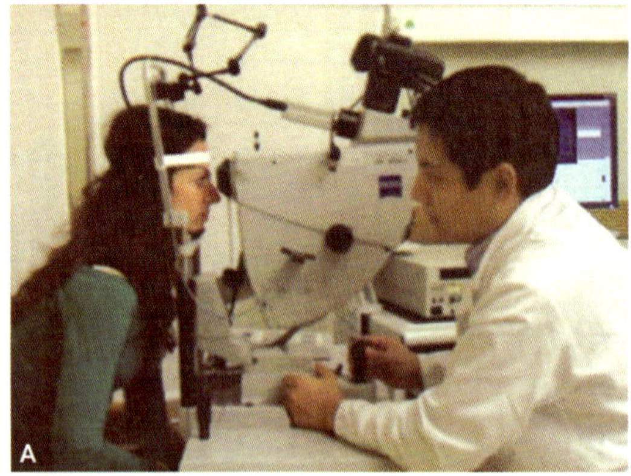

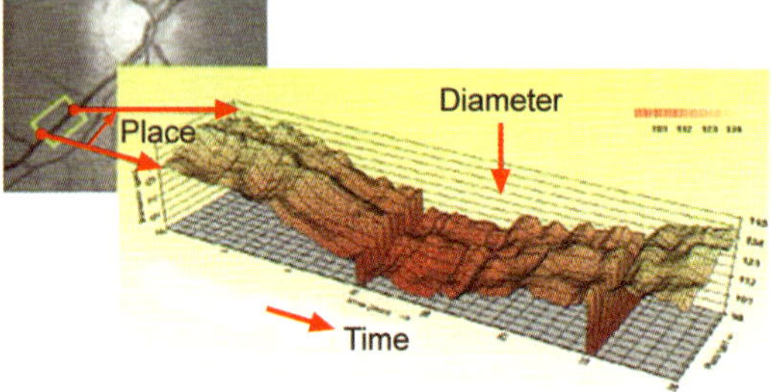

B 100% oxygen breathing healthy subject N35 vts

Fig. 12.4 *Retinal vessel analyzer: (A) Technique of using retinal vessel analyzer in clinical practice; (B) Retinal vessel diameter of a vascular section using the retinal vessel analyzer. Constriction resulted after the patient breathed in 100% oxygen (From Flammer, 2006)*

4. Doppler studies

Principle of Doppler effect

Doppler effect describes a frequency shift of waves of any nature (e.g. light waves, acoustic waves and water waves). Figure 12.5 depicts the principle of Doppler effect. A laser beam reflected by a moving object returns with a frequency change, Δf, known as Doppler shift. The velocity, V, can be determined from Δf.

Methods of Doppler studies

First described by Austrian Scientist Christian Doppler in 1842, the methods of Doppler studies include colour Doppler imaging, laser Doppler velocimetry and laser Doppler flow meter.

i. *Colour Doppler imaging*. Ultrasound is used to measure the blood flow velocity in the retrobulbar vessels, since light cannot reach the tissues behind the eye.

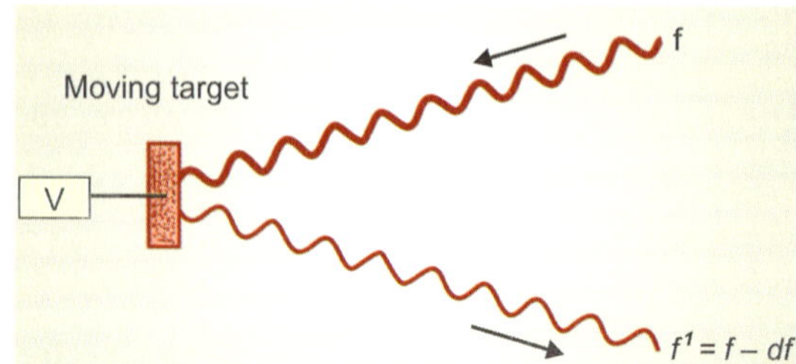

Fig. 12.5 *Principle of the Doppler effect. For explanation see text (From Kaiza and Flammer, 1996)*

Localization of blood flow based on a Doppler principle combined with B-scan imaging forms the colour Doppler device (Fig. 12.6) and is the

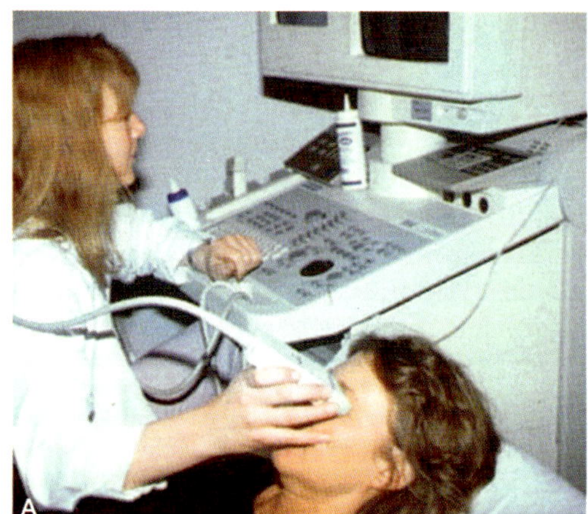

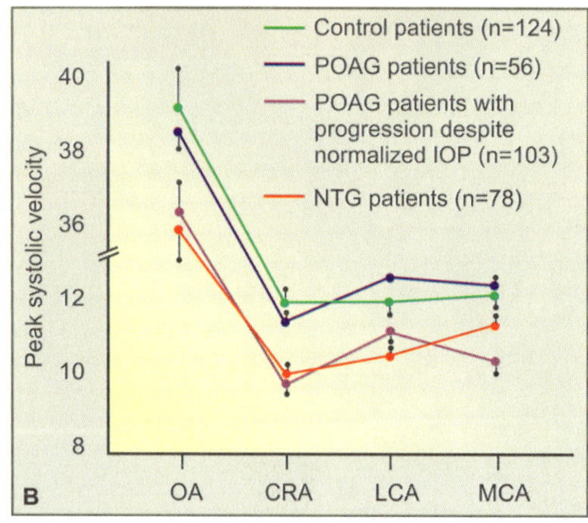

Fig. 12.6 *Colour Doppler imaging: (A) Representation of its clinical use; (B) Peak systolic velocity in the different retro-ocular vessels. The graphs represent the mean with standard deviation (SD) of the different groups. CRA: central retinal artery; LCA: lateral ciliary artery; MCA: medial ciliary artery; OA: ophthalmic artery (From Flammer, 2006)*

most commonly used technique in patients with glaucoma.

ii. ***Laser Doppler velocimetry*** (LDV) measures blood flow velocity by focusing a laser beam at a selected blood vessel. Blood flow can be calculated from the values of blood flow velocity and measured diameter of the vessel wall.

iii. ***Laser Doppler flowmetry*** (Fig. 12.7A) measures the blood flow in capillary beds at a selected point. The laser can be directed to the areas between large vessels, or on the retina or optic nerve head (Fig. 12.7B).

Note. All these tests help to measure blood flow velocity in selected blood vessel. In addition, the capillary bed's colour Doppler also quantifies the blood flow velocity and is used most often today for patients with glaucoma.

5. Pulsatile ocular blood flow

The pulsatile ocular blood flow (POBF) devices, the paradigm systems and others (Fig. 12.8A) utilize a pneumotonometer that measures IOP in real-time. The IOP pulse wave is transformed into an ocular volume wave using the presumed universal relationship. The change in volume over time is reported as the POBF value. The POBF instrument is used in a similar capacity to a Goldmann applanation tonometer (Fig. 12.8B).

The POBF devices utilize a pneumotonometer that measures IOP in real-time. It is based on the principle that blood volume in the eye increases with the systolic pulse and decreases during diastole.

The transient changes in IOP can be used to calculate transient changes in ocular volume. The change in volume over time is reported as POBF value.

6. Detection of visual field changes as a parameter for ocular blood flow

Perimetry is used to measure differential light sensitivity (DLS) in the visual field. The outcome fluctuates in normal eyes and this fluctuation is amplified in patients with glaucoma. In glaucoma, deterioration of the visual field after cold provocation correlates with blood flow deterioration.

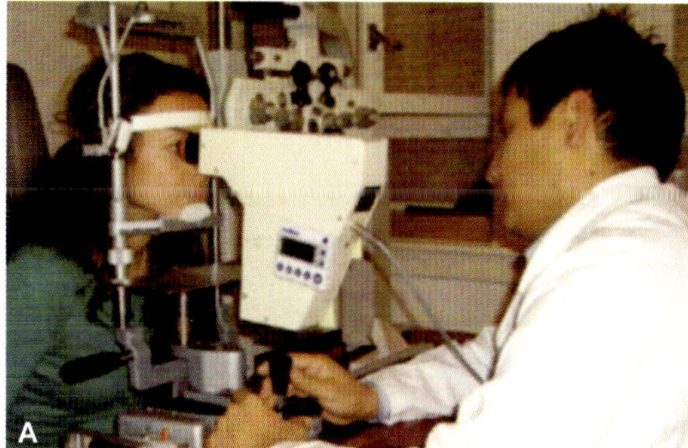

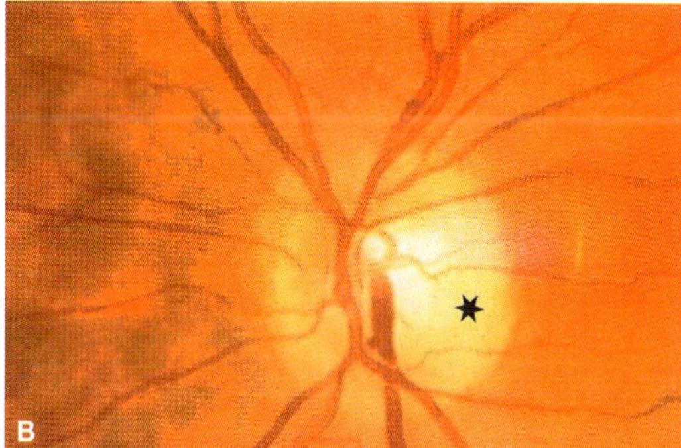

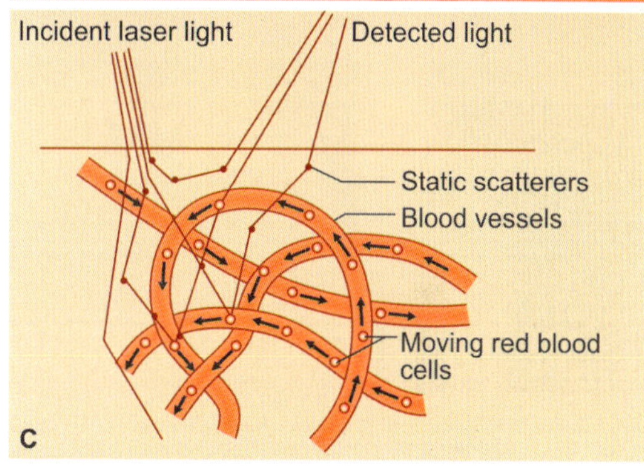

Fig. 12.7 *Laser Doppler flowmetry: (A) Technique in clinical practice; (B) Laser Doppler flowmetry measures flow at a selected point (*); (C) A portion of the scattered light eventually leaves the tissue in the direction of the detector (From Kaiza and Flammer, 1996)*

A relatively quick change in the visual field can, therefore, be an indirect sign of a change in ocular perfusion.

7. Provocative tests

The disturbed blood flow regulation is better tested under challenging stressful conditions. Therefore, provocative tests, which challenge the blood flow may provide more useful information than basal measurements. The

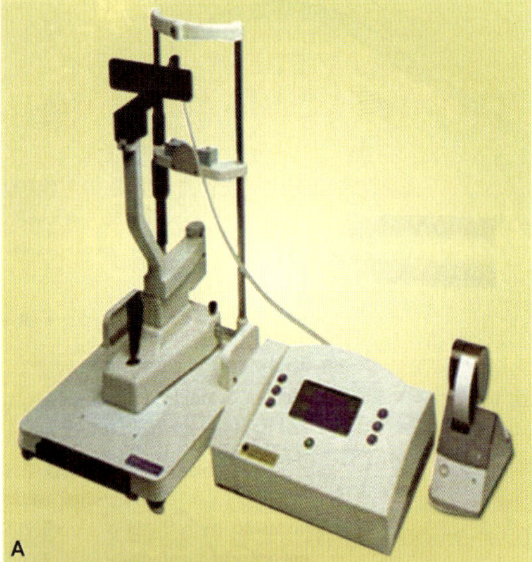

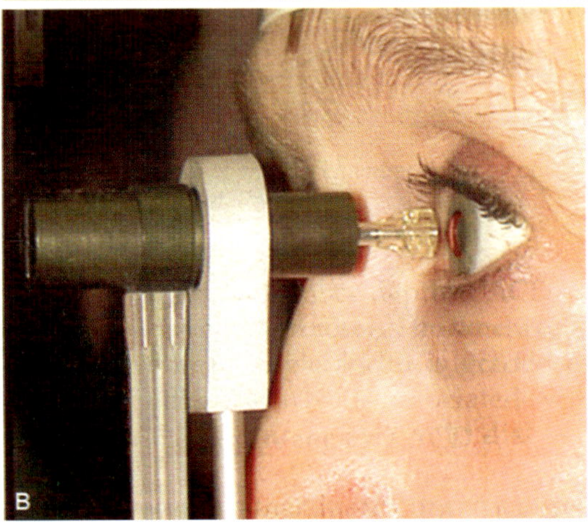

Fig. 12.8 *Pulsatile ocular blood flow device: (A) Profile photograph; (B) Technique of use is similar to applanation tonometer (Courtesy: Harris et al.)*

provocative tests which are used to create stressful challenging conditions include:

- Artificially increasing IOP, e.g. with the help of suction cup.
- Stimulating the automatic nerves with a hand grip, and
- Coldness (e.g. by blowing cold air) which is standard procedure in nail fold capillaro-microscopy.

Note. In patients with vascular dysregulation, blood flow in the fingers correlates very well with ocular blood flow (OBF) and thus can be used as an indirect test.

ROLE OF OCULAR BLOOD FLOW IN GLAUCOMATOUS OPTIC NEUROPATHY

Atherosclerosis

It is well reported that atherosclerosis and its risk factors are also risk factors for an increase in IOP. However, at a given level of IOP, patients with atherosclerosis have only a mildly increased risk for glaucomatous optic neuropathy (GON).

Blood pressure

Many studies have reported arterial hypotension as a risk factor for glaucomatous optic neuropathy (GON). This includes low blood pressure, orthostatic hypotension, and nocturnal dips. On average, patients with NTG or POAG with disease progression tend to have low BP than non-progressive patients, studies indicate that both migraine and low BP are significant risk factors for GON. Interestingly, both migraine and low BP occur more often in patients with vascular dysregulation, i.e. when autoregulation is disturbed.

Vascular dysregulation

Vascular dysregulation is reported in patients with migraine and low blood pressure. Therefore, it has been concluded in the literature that association of GON with migraine and arterial hypotension might be due to vascular dysregulation affecting the ocular blood flow. Vascular dysregulation may be primary or secondary.

1. ***Primary vascular dysregulation*** refers to a genetic predisposition to respond differently to a number of discrete stimuli, such as cold, mechanical or emotional stress. Primary vascular dysregulation (PVD) as a risk factor for GON explains the following facts:

- NTG is more common in women than men as the former are more disposed to PVD.
- GON is more common in patients with migraine a condition frequently associated with PVD.
- NTG is more common in people of Japanese or Korean descent, who are more prone to get PVD.
- Occurrence of splinter haemorrhages on the optic disc more common in NTG than POAG,

and more common in women than men is also explained due to PVD.

- Higher incidence of silent myocardial infarction in patients with NTG may also be due to PVD.

2. ***Secondary vascular dysregulation (SVD)*** refers to vascular dysregulation as a consequence of another disease. SVD is mediated by excessive production of endothelin (vasoactive molecule). Examples of diseases associated with SVD are:

- In patients with arthritis, the synovial cells produce endothelin,
- In multiple sclerosis, the lymphocyte cells produce endothelin, and
- In AIDS, the macrophages produce endothelin.

Effect of endothelin on ocular blood flow is minimal when the blood–retinal barrier is intact. However, in patients with disturbed blood–retinal barrier, endothelin reduces ocular blood flow by causing vasoconstriction of choroidal vessels. Endothelin can also diffuse into the optic nerve head and reduce blood flow to ONH.

CONCLUSION

- There is a need for increased awareness of medication regimens in glaucoma patient population, such as antihypertensive.
- Further advances in tissue oxygenation assessment will improve our understanding of glaucomatous disease pathophysiology.
- Low perfusion pressure and large fluctuation in IOP may be important prognostic factors for glaucomatous progression.
- No current gold standard exists for measuring total ocular blood flow: Therefore, a comprehensive approach is suggested.

SUGGESTED READING

1. Flammer J. The impact of ocular blood flow in glaucoma. Prog Retn Eye Res 2002;21:359–93.
2. Flammer J, Haefliger IO, Resink T. Vascular dysregulation: A principal risk factor for glaucomatous damage. J Glaucoma 1999;8:212–19.
3. Harris A, Kagemann L. Measuring ocular blood flow. J Glaucoma 2009;4:35–39.
4. Resch H, Schmidl D, Hommer A, et al. Correlation of optic disc morphology and ocular perfusion parameters in patients with primary open angle glaucoma. Acta Ophthalmol 2011;89: 544–49.
5. Venkataraman ST, Flanagan JG, Hudson C. vascular reactivity of optic nerve head and retinal blood vessels in glaucoma—a review. Microcirculation 2010;17:568–81.

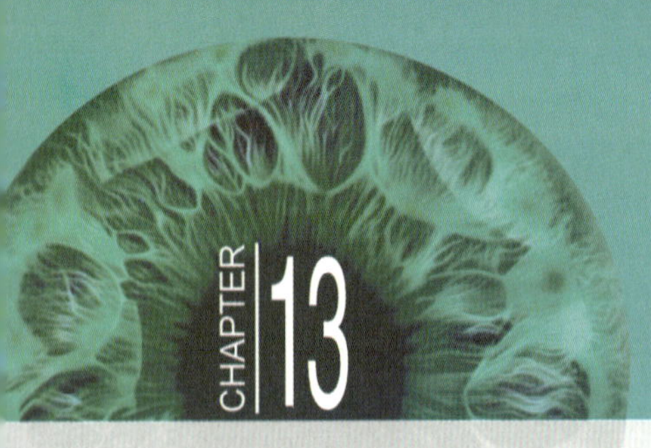

GENETIC TESTING IN GLAUCOMA

INTRODUCTION AND TERMINOLOGY

INTRODUCTION

The etiology of glaucoma is not well understood. The association of primary open-angle glaucoma (POAG) and a positive family history has been known for years. The lifetime risk for first degree relatives of affected individuals to develop POAG is 22% when compared with a 2% risk in controls. It is often felt that people with a family history of blindness go blind with glaucoma.

Primary angle-closure disease (PACD) also has an unusually high incidence among siblings of affected patients. Hence, it has been suggested that genetic factors contribute to the pathology. Previous studies have found that Chinese patients with primary angle-closure glaucoma (PACG) have almost a 50% probability of having narrow angles and the first degree relatives of PACG patients are at 6–9-fold increased risk of developing PACG. However, only 10% of the people with anatomically narrow angles develop PACG suggesting that the pathogenesis of PACG is complex.

Therefore, glaucoma, genetically now has a new definition, a "Complex and multiple gene disease". Genetic testing may, therefore, help to customise the treatment protocol, what is also known as "Personalised Medicine".

Chromosomal location of genes and loci for various forms of open- or closed-angle glaucoma are found throughout the human genome. Only the Y chromosome is believed not to harbour a gene or locus for glaucoma.

TERMINOLOGY

The genetic loci for different types of glaucoma are termed as below:
- GLC1 for POAG
- GLC2 for primary angle-closure glaucomas
- GLC3 for congenital glaucomas

Genetic testing holds the promise to:
- Help assess the risk of an individual developing glaucoma,
- Predict the severity of disease phenotype, and
- Predict the effectiveness of treatment.

APPROACHES TO GENE TESTING

There are various approaches used to identify a single or multiple genes that are involved in inherited disorders. These approaches can also be applied to the discovery of genes underlying treatment outcomes in the field of pharmacogenetics. Pharmacogenetics is the science of how an individual's genes affect the way the individual's body responds to a medication or treatment and pharmacogenomics, the study of drug responses in the context of the entire genome.

SELECTION OF METHOD FOR GENE TESTING

The selection of a particular approach or method depends on the frequency of the disease mutation and the penetrance of the mutation. Two common approaches are:

1. ***Linkage analysis.*** Linkage analysis involves genetic mapping based on contramission of genetic markers and phenotypes from one generation to the next in one or more families.
2. ***Association analysis.*** Association analysis involves comparison of cases to control to assess the relative contribution of genetic variants or environmental effects to the trait being studied. In addition, association studies may also be designed to study a quantitative trait, as IOP, in a single large cohort.

APPLICATIONS

An overview of application of linkage and association approaches to identify genes as markers for complex diseases and quantitative trait is summarized in Fig. 13.1.

TESTS

In 2001, Insite Vision Inc. released OcuGene, the first commercially available genetic testing for glaucoma. Initially it tested for the presence of four mutations of the myocilin gene and featured the Mt-1 single nucleotide polymorphism. The currently available OcuGene kit tests solely for the Mt-1 polymorphism, whose prognostic value for predicting an aggressive phenotype of POAG is controversial.

ENVIRONMENT AND GENES

- Glaucomas are likely the result of a combination of environmental influence and genetic predisposition.
- To date, the studies of numerous families with high rates of glaucoma have revealed 11 unique loci associated with the POAG phenotype (these loci are named GLC 1A through K). In these families, the POAG phenotype is inherited in a simple Mendelian fashion, (autosomal dominant recessive) indicating a single causative gene.
- Recently, genome-wide association studies (GWAS) have identified three susceptibility loci (rs 110224102 in PLEKHA7; rs 3753841 in COL11A1, and rs 1015213 located between PCMTD1 and ST18 on chromosome 8q) for PACG. Association studies also suggest the involvement of several single nucleotide polymorphisms (SNPs) of the matrix metalloproteinase-9 (MMP-9) gene. This gene is involved in the remodelling of the extracellular matrix.
- There is variable penetrance of the phenotype which indicates that there are likely environmental components or effects of modifying genes that contribute to the ultimate development of POAG. Within these 11 loci, three genes have been identified.

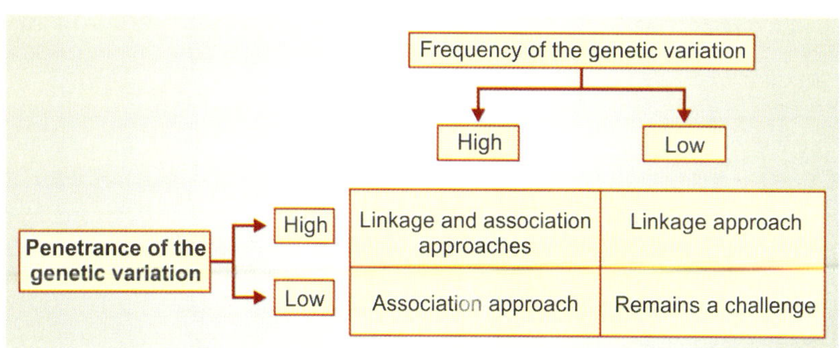

Fig. 13.1 *Summary of applications of linkage and association approach*

TIGR/myocilin (GLC1A), optineurin (GLC1E), and WDR 36 (GLC1G).

- Figure 13.2 depicts that variations in IOP response to glaucoma medical therapy are determined by pharmacokinetic and pharmacodynamic processes (blue arrow) and interaction with the environment, disease, and pathophysiologic process. The sequence variants among pharmacokinetic and pharmacodynamic genes are predicted to have functional consequences that contribute to the genetic component of variance in IOP response (Modified from pharmagkb.org).

GLAUCOMA GENES

Myocilin

In 1997, the first glaucoma gene, myocilin or MYOC, was discovered. It was initially named trabecular meshwork-inducible glucocorticoid response protein gene (TIGR). Genetic linkage was used to localize this gene to chromosome 1q24 and eventually it was cloned. Myocilin is expressed in normal people and is upregulated by corticosteroids, TGF-beta and mechanical stretch of trabecular meshwork cells. There are more than 40 mutations reported in myocilin gene that are associated with a high pressure, POAG phenotype myocilin gene mutation account for approximately 3–5% of POAG.

Recent studies have suggested that the neurotrophin 4 (NTF4) gene located in the 19p13.3 region (GLC1O) may contribute to POAG. Alterations in neurotrophin 4 are predicted to have decreased affinity with its specific receptor, tyrosine kinase receptor B (TrkB), leading to decreased activation of TrkB. Hence, loss of neurotrophic function may be one of the general mechanisms involved in the pathogenesis of glaucoma and that agents activating TrkB may be considered as neuro-protective targets.

CYP1B1

Three chromosomal locations for primary congenital glaucoma are on 2p21 (GLC3A, MIM 231300); 1p36 (GLC3B) and on 14q24.3 (GLC3C). The GLC3A locus colocalises to the CYP1B1 gene (MIM 601771) on chromosome 2p21. CYP1B1 encodes a dioxin inducible member of subfamily I of the cytochrome P450 protein superfamily.

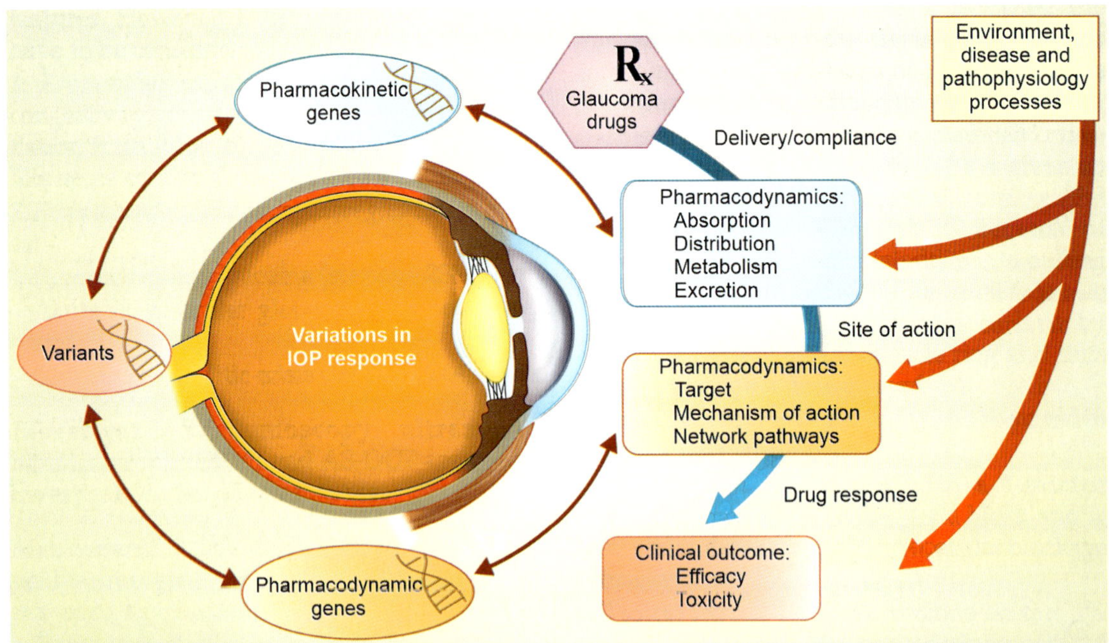

Fig. 13.2 *Factors determining variation in IOP response to glaucoma medical therapy (modified from pharmagkb.org)*

CYP1B1 is thought to be important in the development and regulation of outflow facility of the trabecular meshwork as well as in the secretion of aqueous humour. Mutations may interfere with normal function and could contribute to increased intraocular pressure.

Optineurin

Optineurin may play a role in normal-tension glaucoma, possibly by providing neuroprotection to the retinal ganglion cells. Defects in this gene may mean that retinal ganglion cells are more susceptible to damage or death, leading to glaucoma without pressure necessarily being high. Mutations, including Glu50 → Lys (E50K), Met98 → Lys (M98K), and Arg45 → Gln (R545Q), in OPTN have been found in 16.7% of families with hereditary POAG.

OPTN plays a role in vesicle trafficking and the Golgi organization. The genetic mutation, E50K has been shown to potentiate Golgi fragmentation and cause extensive cell death, a

Table 13.1 *Glaucoma loci defined by linkage studies*

Chromosome location	*Locus*	*Gene*	*Condition*	*Inheritance pattern*
1q24.3–q25.2	GLC1A	MYOC	JOAG and adult-onset POAG	JOAG, AD Adult-onset POAG, complex
1p36.2–p36.1	GLC3B		Congenital glaucoma	AR
2p15–p16	GLC1H		Adult-onset POAG	AD
2p22–p21	GLC3A	CYP1B1	Congenital glaucoma	AR
2cen–q13	GLC1B		Adult-onset POAG	AD
2q11–q14	NN03		Nanophthalmos	AD
3p22–p21	GLC1L		Adult-onset POAG; NTG	AD
3q21–q24	GLC1C		Adult-onset POAG	AD
4q25–q26	RIEG1:IRID2	PITX2	Axenfeld–Rieger syndrome: iridogoniodysgenesis	AD
5q21.3–q22.1	GLC1G	WDR36	Adult-onset POAG	AD: complex
5q22.1–q32	GLC1M		JOAG	AD
6p25	RIEG3: IRID1	FOXC1	Axenfeld–Rieger syndrome: iridogoniodysgenesis	AD
7q35–q36	GLC1F		Adult-onset POAG	AD
7q35–q36	GPDS1		Pigment dispersion syndrome	AD
8q23	GLC1D		Adult-onset POAG	AD
9q22	GLC1J		JOAG	AD
9q34.1	NPS	LMX1B	Nail-patella syndrome	AD
10p15–p14	GLC1E	OPTN	Adult-onset POAG: NTG	AD
11p	NN01		Nanophthalmos	AD
11p13	AN	PAX6	Aniridia	AD
11q23	NN02	MFRP	Nanophthalmos	AR
13q14	RIEG2		Axenfeld–Rieger syndrome	AD
14q24.3	GLC3C		Congenital glaucoma	AR
14q24	GLC3D	LTBP2	Congenital glaucoma	AR
15q11–q13	GLC11		Adult-onset POAG	Complex
15q22	XFS	LOXL1	Exfoliation glaucoma	Complex
15q22–q24	GLC1N		JOAG	AD
19q13.3	GLC10	NTF4	Adult-onset POAG: NTG	Complex
20p12	GLC1K		JOAG	AD

AD: autosomal dominant; AR: autosomal recessive

key occurrence in POAG. These findings may provide an insight into the possible mechanisms why E50K, would exhibit a propensity toward the development of glaucoma.

Other genes have been discovered for systemic diseases where glaucoma is part of the phenotype. Table 13.1 shows glaucoma loci defined by linkage studies.

UTILITY OF GENE TESTING

Knowing the genotype helps in two main ways.

1. ***Realistic prognostic information*** for specific mutation can be obtained, if genotype and resulting phenotype are known, thus helping to focus on surveillance of a patient.
2. ***Guides many decisions,*** e.g. many patients with myocilin mutations particularly those mutations that cause juvenile onset OAG, do better with surgery.

How soon, routine genetic testing can be done for glaucoma remains to be seen. It will be a gradual process, but it is strongly predicted that within a decade, routine genetic testing for glaucoma patients would be possible.

A commercial genetic test for three of the lesser mutations for GLC1A has been available in the USA for sometime. But testing was dramatically altered by Genetic Privacy Act of 2008 (110th Congress, 2008) which prevents insurance from discriminating against applicants on basis of genetic findings alone.

EPIGENETICS

Epigenetics is the study of heritable changes in gene activity that are not caused by changes in the DNA sequence. Stable, long-term alterations in the transcriptional potential of a cell that are not necessarily heritable are studied. Increasing evidence shows that epigenetic alterations influence common pathologic responses including inflammation, ischaemia, neoplasia, aging, and neurodegeneration. Studies have shown that abnormal histone acetylation/ deacetylation may be related to retinal ganglion cell damage in glaucoma. Significant differences in genomic DNA methylation have been found in peripheral mononuclear cells from patients with open-angle glaucoma compared with healthy controls.

SUGGESTED READING

1. Alward WL, Kwon YH, Khanna CL, et al. Variations in the myocilin gene in patients with open-angle glaucoma. Arch Ophthalmol 2002; 120(9):1189–97.
2. Amerasinghe N, Zhang J, Thalamuthu A. The heritability and sibling risk of angle-closure in Asians. Ophthalmology 2011;118(3):480–85.
3. Shastry BS. Genetic susceptibility to primary angle-closure glaucoma (PACG). Discov Med. 2013;15(80):17–22.
4. Wiggs JL. Genetic etiologies of glaucoma. Arch Ophthalmol 2007;125(1):30–37.

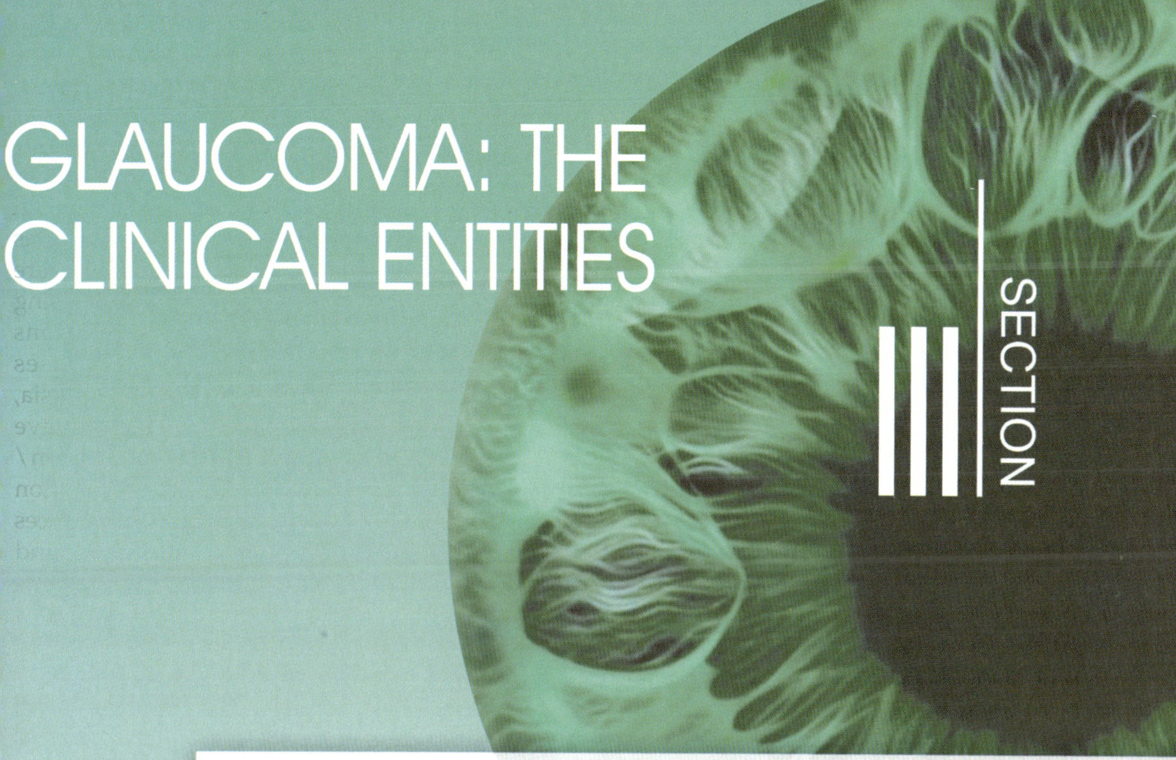

SECTION III

GLAUCOMA: THE CLINICAL ENTITIES

CHILDHOOD GLAUCOMAS

CHAPTER 14

CHILDHOOD GLAUCOMAS

Definition

Classification and terminology

CGRN classification

- Primary childhood glaucoma
- Secondary childhood glaucoma

PATHOGENESIS OF CHILDHOOD GLAUCOMA

PRIMARY CONGENITAL GLAUCOMA

- Terminology
  - Neonatal glaucoma
  - Infantile glaucoma
  - Juvenile glaucoma
- Demography and genetics
- Pathogenesis
- Clinical features
- Differential diagnosis
- Treatment

SECONDARY CHILDHOOD GLAUCOMA

Glaucoma associated with non-acquired ocular anomalies

- Glaucoma associated with iridodysgenesis
- Glaucoma associated with irido-corneal dysgenesis
- Glaucoma associated with other ocular anomalies

Glaucoma associated with non-acquired systemic anomalies

- Glaucoma associated with chromosomal disorders
- Glaucoma associated with ectopia lentis syndromes
- Glaucoma associated with phacomatoses
- Glaucoma associated with metabolic disorders
- Glaucoma associated with connective tissue disorder
- Glaucoma associated with congenital rubella

Glaucoma associated with acquired conditions

Glaucoma following cataract surgery (pseudophakic/aphakic)

CHILDHOOD GLAUCOMAS

DEFINITION

Childhood glaucomas, also referred to as *paediatric glaucomas,* constitute a heterogenous group of disease characterized by symptoms and signs of raised IOP in paediatric age group.

CLASSIFICATION AND TERMINOLOGIES

Childhood glaucomas have been variously classified and as a consequence many confusing terms exist in the literature, especially in relation to the term secondary glaucomas in childhood. Still the terminologies in relation to paediatric glaucoma are inconsistent and confusing.

Presently the Childhood Glaucoma Research Network (CGRN) definition and classification is followed.

Childhood Glaucoma Research Network (CGRN); Definition and Classification

CGRN definition of Glaucoma in children (≥2 of the following)

■ *Intraocular pressure (IOP) >21 mm Hg*, exercise discretion if IOP checked under anesthesia due to variable effects of anesthetic agents.

■ *Optic disc cupping:* Progressive increase in cup-to-disk ratio (CDR)

- Cup disc asymmetry of ≥0.2
- Focal neuroretinal rim (NRR) thinning

■ *Corneal findings*

- Haab's striae
- Diameter ≥11 mm in newborn, >12 mm in child <1 year or >13 mm any age

■ *Progressive myopia*, myopic shift or an increase in ocular dimensions beyond what is expected with normal growth

■ *Reproducible visual field defect* consistent with glaucomatous optic neuropathy with no other observable reason for defects, if the child is old enough to do the field testing.

Glaucoma suspect

No IOP related damage and at least one of the following criteria:
- IOP >21 mm Hg on 2 separate occasions
- Suspicious optic disc appearance for glaucoma
- Suspicious visual field for glaucoma
- Increased corneal diameter and axial length in setting of normal IOP.

CGRN CLASSIFICATION OF CHILDHOOD GLAUCOMA

A. Primary Childhood Glaucoma (without Associated Anomalies)

I. Primary congenital glaucoma (PCG)

1. *Neonatal:* 0–1 month
2. *Infantile:* >1–24 months
3. *Late onset or late recognized:* >2 years
4. Spontaneously arrested cases with normal IOP but typical signs of PCG, can be classified as PCG.

II. Juvenile open angle glaucoma (JOAG)

1. Meets glaucoma definition with open angles
2. No congenital ocular anomalies or syndromes
3. No ocular enlargement.

B. Secondary Childhood Glaucoma (with associated anomalies)

I. Glaucoma associated with non-acquired ocular anomalies

1. *Glaucoma associated with iridodysgenesis*
- Ectropion uveae
- Congenital iris hypoplasia
- Aniridia
- Microphthalmos/microcornea

2. *Glaucoma associated with irido-corneal dysgenesis*
- Posterior embryotoxon
- Axenfeld-Rieger anomaly/syndrome
- Peter's anomaly/syndrome
- Combined Rieger syndrome/Peter anomaly

3. *Glaucoma associated with other ocular anomalies*
- Persistent fetal vasculature (PFV)
- Nevus of Ota
- Ectopia lentis
- Ectopia lentis et pupillae

II. Glaucoma associated with non-acquired systemic anomalies

1. *Glaucoma associated with chromosomal disorders*
- Down syndrome (Trisomy 21)
- Edward syndrome (Trisomy 18)
- Trisomy D syndrome (Trisomy 13–18)
- Turner syndrome (only one X chromosome)

2. *Glaucoma associated with ectopia lentis syndromes*
- Marfan syndrome
- Weill-Marchesani syndrome
- Homocystinuria

3. *Glaucoma associated with phacomatoses*
- Sturge-Weber syndrome (50% cases)
- Von Recklinghausen syndrome (25% cases)

4. *Glaucoma associated with metabolic disorders*
- Lowe syndrome (oculocerebral syndrome)
- Hurler syndrome (mucopolysaccharidosis)
- Zellweger syndrome (Hepato-cerebro-renal syndrome)
- Rubinstein syndrome (disorder of binding protein)

5. *Glaucoma associated with connective tissue disorder*
- Stickler syndrome
- Klippel Trenaunay syndrome

6. *Glaucoma associated with congenital rubella*

III. Glaucoma associated with acquired conditions

1. *Traumatic glaucoma*

i. *Acute onset traumatic glaucoma*
   - Angle concussion glaucoma
   - Hyphaema-induced glaucoma
   - Lens debris or vitreal blockade of trabeculum
   - Ghost cell glaucoma

ii. *Late onset glaucoma with angle recession*

iii. *Arteriovenous fistula*

2. *Glaucoma secondary to intraocular tumours,* such as:
- Retinoblastoma
- Juvenile xanthogranuloma
- Leukaemia
- Iris rhabdomyosarcoma

- Aggressive nevi of the iris

3. ***Inflammatory (uveitis) glaucoma***

i. *Open-angle glaucoma*

ii. *Angle-closure glaucoma*

- Synechial angle-closure
- Iris bombe with pupil block
- Trabecular endothelialization

4. ***Lens-induced glaucoma***

i. *Subluxation–dislocation with pupil block*

- Marfan's syndrome
- Homocystinuria
- Weill-Marchesani syndrome

ii. *Spherophakia with pupil block*

- Weill-Marchesani syndrome
- GEMSS syndrome

iii. *Phacolytic glaucoma*

5. ***Glaucoma after congenital cataract surgery***

- Glaucoma due to lens debris or uveitic blockade of trabeculum
- Pupillary block glaucoma
- Chronic open-angle glaucoma (aphakic or pseudophakic)

6. ***Steroid-induced glaucoma,*** e.g. in patients with vernal keratoconjunctivitis

7. ***Neovascular glaucoma,*** as seen in patients with:

- Retinoblastoma
- Coat's disease
- Medulloepithelioma
- Familial exudative vitreoretinopathy
- Chronic retinal detachment

8. ***Secondary angle-closure glaucoma,*** as associated with:

- Retinopathy of prematurity
- Nanophthalmos
- Microphthalmos
- Persistent fetal vasculature
- Congenital pupillary-iris-lens membrane
- Aniridia
- Iridoschisis
- Cornea plane
- Retinoblastoma
- Iris stromal cysts
- Ciliary body cysts
- Cystinosis
- Topiramate-induced glaucoma

9. ***Glaucoma associated with increased episcleral venous pressure (EVP)***

- Sturge-Weber syndrome
- Cavernous or dural venous fistula
- Orbital space occupying lesions

10. ***Glaucoma secondary to intraocular to infections,*** such as:

- Acute recurrent toxoplasmosis
- Acute herpetic iritis
- Endogenous endophthalmitis
- Opportunistic infections seen in AIDS
- Congenital rubella

11. ***Malignant glaucoma,*** occurring after any intraocular surgery, such as:

- Glaucoma surgery
- Cataract surgery
- Keratoplasty, etc.

IV. Glaucoma following cataract surgery (pseudophakic/aphakic)

- Glaucoma due to lens debris or uveitic blockade of trabeculum
- Pupillary block glaucoma
- Chronic open-angle glaucoma (aphakic of pseudophakic).

PATHOGENESIS OF CHILDHOOD GLAUCOMA

Although the exact pathogenesis of congenital/developmental glaucoma is yet to be elucidated, the disease represents a developmental arrest of the anterior chamber angle tissue derived from the neural crest cells during the late embryonic period. Now it is generally believed that the site of obstruction is the trabecular meshwork itself rather than an imperforate membrane covering it, as proposed earlier (Barkan's membrane theory). Before studying the abnormal development noted in congenital glaucoma, it will be worthwhile to have a brief knowledge of normal development of angle of anterior chamber.

Normal development of anterior chamber angle

Mesenchymal mass of neural crest origin, is now considered to give rise to the cornea, iris and anterior chamber angle rather than that of mesodermal origin (as thought originally).

Three layers of tissue come forward, between the surface ectoderm and developing lens, from the undifferentiated mesenchymal mass of neural crest cell origin and contribute to formation of structures of anterior segments of eyeball as below:

- *First layer* differentiates into primordial corneal endothelium by 8th week and subsequently produces Descemet's membrane as well.
- *Second layer* grows between the corneal epithelium and endothelium and produces corneal stroma.
- *Third layer* insinuates between the developing cornea and lens and gives rise to the pupillary membrane and stroma of iris.

Development of trabecular meshwork occurs by a simple process of growth and differentiation from the mass of the mesenchymal cells of neural crest cell origin forming angle of developing anterior chamber. The concept of anterior chamber angle development proposed by Shields MB (published in Trans Am Ophthalmol Soc. 1983;81:736) is as below (Fig. 14.1A to D):

- *Closed cavity of anterior chamber* is created by a continuous layer of endothelial cells (derived from neural crest cells) at 5th month of gestation (Fig. 14.1A).
- *Anterior surface of iris (i), at* this stage is inserted infront of the primordial trabecular meshwork (TM) (Fig. 14.1A).
- *Endothelial layer progressively disappears,* in the third trimester, from the pupillary membrane (PM) and iris and cavities over the anterior chamber angle (ACA), possibly becoming incorporated in the trabecular meshwork. At the same time, peripheral uveal tissue begins to slide posteriorly in relation to the chamber angle structure (arrow) (Fig. 14.1B).
- *Development of the trabecular lamellar* and intratrabecular spaces begins in the inner posterior aspect of the primordial tissue and progresses towards the developing Schlemm canal (SC), and Schwalbe line (SL) (Fig. 14.1C).
- *Normal anterior chamber angle,* as shown in Fig. 14.1D, is not fully developed until 1 year of age.

Theories of abnormal development of anterior chamber angle in congenital glaucoma

Various theories have been put forward from tissue to tissue to explain the developmental abnormalities in the anterior chamber angle. Most of these have been discarded but are reviewed below for historical academic interest only:

Manon's theory *(1928)* postulated that incomplete atrophy of the anterior chamber mesoderm resulted in retention of abnormal tissue that blocked aqueous outflow.

Barkan's theory *(1955)* postulated that obstruction to aqueous in caused by a transparent membrane representing the undeveloped uveal meshwork; and that the immature angle is functional behind this membrane (Barkan's membrane). It was also postulated that the incision of Barkan's membrane may allow normal aqueous drainage.

Allen and colleagues *(1955)* postulated that incomplete cleavage of mesoderm in the anterior chamber angle resulted in the complete defect.

Maumenee theory *(1959)* postulated that the failure of cleavage of iris from the meridional fibres of the ciliary body closes the trabecular sheets. It was proposed that in goniotomy operation the trabecular ends of these meridional fibres are cut and thus opening the trabecular spaces.

Worst's combined theory *(1966)* included elements of the atrophy and resorption concepts but rejected the cleavage theory.

Smelser and organics *(1971)* postulated that congenital glaucoma occurs as a failure of anterior chamber angle to become properly rearranged into the normal trabecular meshwork.

Note. As mentioned in the beginning, all the above theories have been discarded.

A. PATHOGENESIS OF PRIMARY CHILDHOOD GLAUCOMA (WITHOUT ASSOCIATED ANOMALIES)

Isolated trabeculodysgenesis

Kupffer and colleagues *(1971)* for the first time reported the contribution of the neural crest cells in the development of angle structures, and

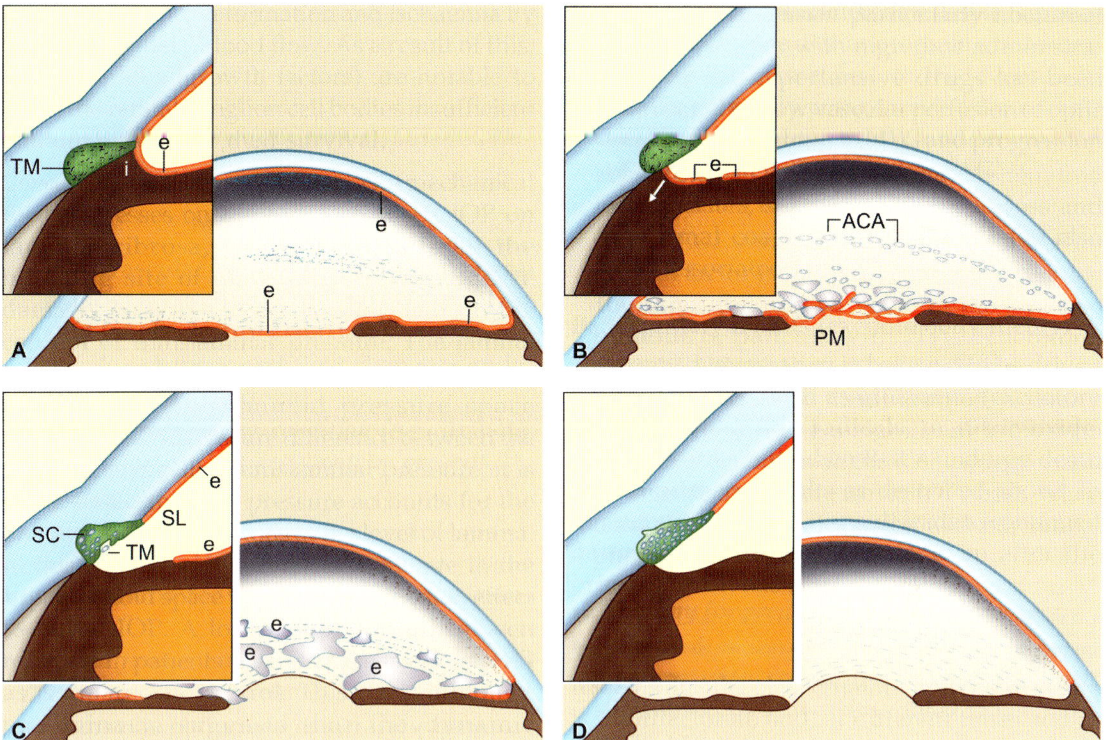

Fig. 14.1 *Development of anterior chamber angle: (A) At 5 months, a continuous layer of endothelium (e) creates a closed cavity of anterior chamber and anterior surface of iris (i) inserts in front of primordial; trabecular meshwork (TM); (B) In third trimester, endothelial layer progressively disappears from pupillary membrane and iris cavitates over the anterior chamber angle (ACA); (C) Development of trabecular lamellae and intertrabecular spaces progressing towards Schlemm's canal (SC) and Schwalbe's line (SL); (D) Normal anterior chamber angle is not developed until 1 year of age. (Source: Redrawn from Shields MB; Published in Trans Am Ophthalmol Soc 1983;81:736.)*

suggested that abnormal development of the angle structures derived from neural crest cells is responsible for various abnormalities in the congenital glaucoma.

Shields *(1983)* has conceptualized the anterior chamber angle development based on various studies and have published a theory of mechanism of Axenfeld–Rieger syndrome and its distinction from the iridocorneal endothelial (ICE) syndrome.

Thus, maldevelopment of trabeculum including the iridotrabecular junction (trabeculodysgenesis) is responsible for impaired aqueous outflow resulting in raised IOP.

In primary congenital glaucoma, the trabeculodysgenesis is not associated with any other major ocular anomalies. Clinically, trabeculodysgenesis is characterized by absence of the angle recess with iris having a flat or concave direct insertion into the surface of trabeculum as follows:

- *Flat iris insertion* is more common than the concave iris insertion. In it, the iris inserts flatly and abruptly into the thickened trabeculum either at or anterior to scleral spur (more often) or posterior to scleral spur. It is often possible to visualize a portion of ciliary body and scleral spur.
- *Concave iris insertion* is less common. In it, the superficial iris tissue sweeps over the iridotrabecular junction and the trabeculum and thus obscures the scleral spur and ciliary body.

B. PATHOGENESIS OF SECONDARY CHILDHOOD GLAUCOMAS

I. Secondary Childhood Glaucoma Associated with Non-acquired Ocular Anomalies

1. Iridotrabeculodysgenesis

Iris anomalies may occur in addition to trabecular malformation. They may involve the anterior stroma, iris vessels, or full thickness of the iris. The trabecular meshwork appearance is similar to that found in isolated trabeculodysgenesis.

- *Anterior stromal defects.* Hypoplasia of the anterior iris stroma is the most common iris defect associated with developmental glaucoma. There is malformation of the collarette with marked reduction of the crypt layer. The pupillary sphincter may appear prominent. Hypoplasia of the anterior iris stroma may be seen in Axenfeld's, Rieger's, and Peters' anomalies. In hyperplasia of the anterior iris stroma, there is a thickened, velvety, pebbled appearance. This condition has only been seen in association with Sturge-Weber syndrome with glaucoma.
- *Anomalous iris vessels.* Vascular anomalies of the iris can present as persistence of the tunica vasculosa lentis or as irregularly wandering superficial anomalous iris vessels. Tunica vasculosa lentis exhibits a regular arrangement of vessels looping into the pupillary axis in front of or behind the lens. Normal radial vessels on the iris surface are also prominent because of associated hypoplasia of the anterior iris stroma.

  Anomalous superficial iris vessels may also wander irregularly over the iris surface with an often distorted pupil. The iris surface has a whorled appearance and the anterior iris stroma is often hypoplastic. Anomalous iris vessels are seen most frequently in eyes that present with glaucoma and cloudy corneas at birth, and are not associated with any particular syndrome.
- *Structural iris defects.* These defects may present as full-thickness holes through the iris with or without sphincter involvement.

2. Corneotrabeculodysgenesis

Congenital corneal defects include peripheral, midperipheral, and central defects, as well as abnormalities in corneal size. There are associated iris abnormalities in the majority of cases. Peripheral corneal lesions extend no more than 2 mm into clear cornea and usually involve the entire corneal circumference. The most common abnormality is Axenfeld's anomaly, which is characterized by posterior embryotoxon and adherent iris tissue.

Midperipheral corneal lesions involve broad areas of iris adhesion. The cornea is frequently opacified in these areas of attachment. Pupillary anomalies and iris holes are often associated. These lesions are generally found in Rieger's anomaly.

Central corneal defects are usually opacified and thinned, with a zone of clear cornea between the defect and limbus. Strands of iris tissue from the collarette may attach to the leukoma. In some cases, there may be lens apposition to the corneal defect. These findings are typically seen in Peters' anomaly.

Microcornea may be seen in microphthalmos, nanophthalmos, Rieger's anomaly, and persistent hyperplastic primary vitreous. Megalocornea may be seen in patients with Axenfeld's syndrome or as an X-linked recessive condition. Megalocornea must be distinguished from corneal enlargement caused by elevated intraocular pressure.

PRIMARY CONGENITAL GLAUCOMA (WITHOUT ASSOCIATED ANOMALIES)

TERMINOLOGY

This group includes those cases which have an isolated maldevelopment of the trabecular meshwork without other developmental ocular or systemic anomalies.

Depending upon the age of onset, following terminologies have been suggested for this entity:

1. ***Neonatal glaucoma*** is labelled when IOP is raised during intrauterine life or within one month of birth. It accounts for about 25% of cases.

2. ***Infantile glaucoma*** is labelled when the disease manifests >1 to 24 months of life. It accounts for about 65% of cases.

- *Late onset or late recognized:* >2 years
- Spontaneously arrested cases with normal IOP but typical signs of PCG, can be classified as PCG.

3. ***Juvenile glaucoma*** is labelled in the rest 10% of cases who develop pressure rise after 3 years and before adulthood. Many glaucoma experts prefer a broad definition of juvenile open-angle glaucoma (JOAG) that includes all forms of primary open-angle glaucoma diagnosed between the age of 10 and 35 years.

Note. When the disease manifests prior to age of 3 years, the eyeball enlarges and so the term ***'buphthalmos'*** (bull-like eyes) is used. As it results due to retention of aqueous humour (watery solution), the term ***'hydrophthalmos'***, has also been suggested.

DEMOGRAPHY AND GENETICS

- Prevalence of primary congenital glaucoma (PCG) is 1 in 10,000 to 20,000 live births in Western countries. The incidence is higher in Middle East due to parental consanguinity. In Indians, incidence as high as 1 in 3300 is reported.
- Accounts for 50 to 70% of all glaucoma.
- Race and geographical predilection is lacking except where consanguinity or small population may play a role.
- *Bilateral occurrence* is seen in 70% cases, though the involvement may be asymmetric.
- *Sex linkage* is not common in inheritance although 65% of patients are males.
- *Sporadic occurrence* is seen in most cases (90%).
- *Autosomal recessive* inheritance with incomplete or variable penetrance and possibly multifactorial inheritance is seen in about 10% cases. Although some pedigrees suggest an autosomal dominant inheritance.
- *Genes.* Three major loci of recessively inherited primary congenital glaucoma genes identified are: GLC3A, GLC3B, and GLC3C on chromosome 14 (14q24.3), respectively. The first gene to be directly implicated in the past pathogenesis of primary congenital glaucoma (Cytochrome P450 1B1, i.e. YP1B1) was mapped to the 2p21 region at the GLC3A locus.
- *Chances of developing congenital glaucoma are.*
  - 5% when one of the parent is affected
  - 5% in a second child when first child is affected
  - 25% per subsequent offsprings, if two siblings are affected.

PATHOGENESIS

As described above (page 175–177) in primary congenital glaucoma there occurs isolated trabeculodysgenesis, i.e. trabeculodysgenesis is not associated with any other major ocular or systemic anomalies.

CLINICAL FEATURES

Congenital glaucoma cases may be referred to the ophthalmologist by the obstetrician, the neonatologist, the paediatrician, or the child's parents.

Symptoms

1. ***Presenting symptoms,*** i.e. *lacrimation, photophobia and blepharospasm* often occur together and form the classic triad of symptoms of congenital glaucoma. Often there is history of rubbing of the eyes. These are thought to be caused by irritation of corneal nerves, which occurs as a result of the elevated IOP. Photophobia is usually the initial sign, but is not enough by itself to arouse suspicion in most cases.

2. ***Other presenting symptoms.*** Depending upon the age of onset and severity of glaucoma, they include:

- *Enlarged globe with diffuse cloudy cornea* in a newborn infant suggests a significantly raised IOP *in utero* (Fig. 14.2).
- *Progressive enlargement of globe with clear cornea* and minimal other symptom may be presentation into older with onset of glaucoma after birth.
- *Progressive defective vision* may be the presenting symptom in older children with late onset of glaucoma, progressive myopia and associated amblyopia.
- *Pain* may be the presenting symptom occasionally, in older children, but this is unusual.
- *Asymptomatic* presentation is not uncommon especially in older children.

Signs

Some signs, e.g. enlarged globe with diffuse corneal haze when present may be obvious, and others may need to be elicited by thorough examination. Older children may allow office

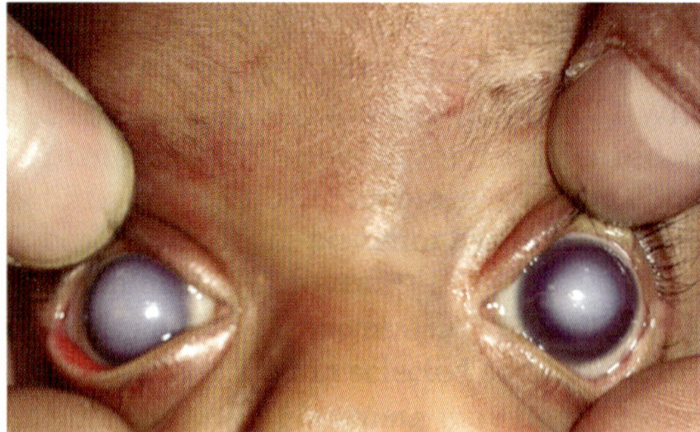

Fig. 14.2 *Bilateral enlarged globe with diffusely cloudy cornea*

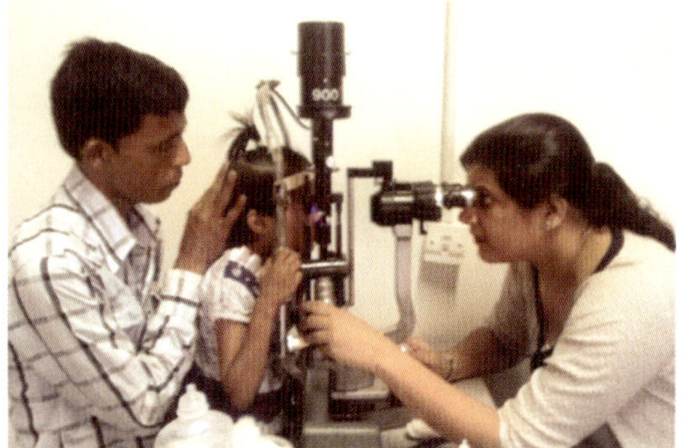

Fig. 14.3 *A 5-year-old PCG child getting Goldmann applanation tonometry done on a slit-lamp*

examination, while smaller may not. Therefore, examination under anaesthesia (EUA) should be carried out in suspected case. Thorough examination under anaesthesia should include:

- *Slit-lamp examination* with a portable slit-lamp or a routine slit-lamp for anterior segment assessment (Fig. 14.3).
- *Measurement of corneal diameter* with caliper
- Gonioscopy,
- Fundus examination, and
- Refraction.

Sequence of evaluation to be carried under general anaesthesia is summarized in Table 14.1.

Table 14.1 *Sequence of EUA*

- External examination
- Anterior segment examination
- Corneal diameter measurement
- Tonometry
- Koeppe gonioscopy (if required)
- Fundus examination

I. Anterior segment sign

Anterior segment signs are best elicited with slit-lamp examination using a portable slit-lamp

1. *Corneal signs.* Corneal signs include its oedema, enlargement and Descemet's breaks.

i. *Corneal oedema.* It is frequently the first sign which arouses suspicion. At first it is subtle and epithelial, but later there is stromal involvement and permanent opacities may occur. Sometimes acute hydrops may occur.

ii. *Corneal enlargement.* It occurs along with enlargement of globe-buphthalmos, especially when the onset is before the age of 3 years. Normal infant cornea measures 10.5 mm. A diameter of more than 13 mm confirms enlargement. Prognosis is usually poor in infants with corneal diameter of more than 16 mm. In children above 2 years of age, corneal enlargement is not a predominant sign of glaucoma.

Vertical corneal diameter measurement is less significant than horizontal corneal diameter, mainly because of the anterior embryotoxon, which makes this measurement inaccurate and difficult to take.

iii. *Tears and breaks in Descemet's membrane (Haab's striae)* (Fig. 14.4). These occur because Descemet's membrane is less elastic than the corneal stroma. The later the development of glaucoma after birth, the less likely tears of the Descemet's membrane will occur; the symptoms are also less severe.

- *Location.* Tears are usually peripheral and concentric with the limbus but may appear in

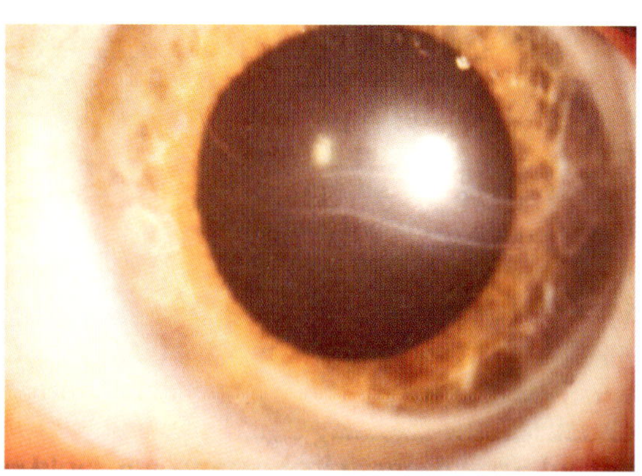

Fig. 14.4 *Parallelepiped Haab's striae*

various orientations near or across the visual axis.

- *Number.* These may be single or multiple.
- *Appearance.* These appear as glassy parallel ridges (*railroad tracks*) on the posterior cornea.
- *Effect.* The Descemet membrane's breaks allow influx of aqueous into the corneal stroma and epithelium resulting in a sudden increase in corneal oedema and haze.
- *Fate.* As the IOP normalizes, the tears are repaired by endothelial overgrowth, the corneal oedema may clear and the linear opacities persist.

iv. *Corneal thickness* is increased due to corneal oedema. Role of pachymetry in congenital glaucoma, though not completely classified, is nevertheless useful in interpretation of IOP as in adults.

v. *Corneal scarring, erosion and ulceration* may from continued enlargement of cornea, when IOP is not controlled appropriately.

2. ***Sclera*** becomes thin and appears blue due to underlying uveal tissue.

3. ***Anterior chamber*** becomes deep. Due to enlargement of the eyeball, posterior segment also deepens and that is why these children are myopic.

4. ***Iris*** is typically normal in primary congenital glaucoma (PCG), although it may have stromal hypoplasia with loss of the crypts. In late stages, it may show iridodonesis and atrophic patches.

5. ***Lens*** becomes flat due to stretching of zonules and may even subluxate.

6. ***Optic disc*** may show variable and rapid cupping, which can be reversed, if IOP is controlled in time but atrophy may happen especially after third year.

7. ***IOP*** is raised which is neither marked nor acute.

8. ***Axial myopia*** may occur because of increase in axial length which may give rise to anisometropic amblyopia.

Measurement of corneal diameter is done with the help of strabismus calliper horizontally from 9 to 3 O'clock position and vertically from 6 to 12 O'clock position. Table 14.2 depicts the normal values and those suggestive of glaucoma at various age groups.

Table 14.2 *Normal values versus those suggestive of glaucoma*

	Corneal diameter in mm	
Age	*Normal values (in mm)*	*Values suggestive of glaucoma (in mm)*
Newborn	9.5–10.5	>11.5
1 year	10–11.5	>12
2 years	11.5–12	>12.5
>3 years	12	>13

II. *Intraocular pressure (IOP)*

Intraocular pressure (IOP) is raised in infants with PCG. Usually such infants present with unanaesthetized IOPs in the range of 30 to 40 mm Hg, although occasionally values may be below or above it.

Normal values of IOP in unanaesthetized children increase with increased mean age. Values reported with increasing age are:

- Up to 1 year 10.6 mm Hg
- 1 to 2 years 12 mm Hg
- 2 to 3 years 12.6 mm Hg
- 3 to 4 years 13.6 mm Hg
- 5 to 12 years 14.2 mm Hg
- 12 to 16 years 14.5 mm Hg

Measurement of IOP should be either with hand-held Perkin's tonometer, Tonopen or I-care tonometer. Non-contact air–puff (e.g. Keeler Pulsair) or Pneumatic tonometer may also be used.

Schiotz tonometer should not be used for IOP measurement in children because:

- The conversion tables for Schiotz tonometry, like those made by Friedenwald, McBain or Prijot, were based on adults' eyes, with normal corneal diameters, and so they are not applicable to children.
- Secondly, the newborn's eye has approximately one-third of the adult's eye volume, the cornea has a more definite curvature, and the ocular walls have a different structure.

IOP measurement under topical anaesthesia may sometimes be possible in older children above 3 years, who may sit for Goldmann applanation tonometry.

IOP measurement under general anaesthesia is part of EUA required in children below 5 years. Most general anaesthetics lower IOP to variable amounts and at variable times (Table 14.3) after administration, except ketamine anaesthesia which raises IOP. IOP is also elevated by endotracheal intubation; therefore, laryngeal mask anaesthesia (LMA) is considered a valuable alternative to tracheal intubation. It is advised that IOP measurement should be done as soon as the airway is secure. Hence, IOP measurements, made under general anaesthesia, do not solely decide diagnosis of glaucoma, or more importantly its management without taking other parameters, such as corneal clarity and diameters, and optic nerve findings into account.

III. *Gonioscopy*

Koeppe direct goniolens is used. Isolated goniodysgenesis is characterized by (Fig. 14.5):

- TM appears as a smooth, homogenous membrane, extending from peripheral iris to Schwalbe's line.
- Peripheral iris is thinner and flatter.
- Open angle with high insertion of iris root.
- Loops of vessels from major arterial circle may be seen over iris root *Loch Ness Monster*.
- Peripheral iris may be covered by a fine fluffy tissue referred to as *Lister's morning mist*.

IV. *Fundus examination*

When measuring IOP, the pupil must never be dilated to see the fundus, because this might modify the IOP. The disc can be easily observed by means of an ophthalmoscope with a small-range diaphragm, with its illumination axis very close to the visual axis. If pupil dilation is necessary, 0.5% tropicamide may be used, not in 1% concentration as it has cycloplegic effect. This examination can be performed on another occasion (at time of cycloplegic retinoscopy).

Table 14.3 *Effect of the anaesthetic agent on IOP*

Anaesthetic agent	*Effect on IOP*
Chloral hydrate	↔
Midazolam	↓
Halothane	↓↓↓
Oxygen	↓
Nitrous-oxygen	↓
Methohexital	↓
Ketamine	↑
Succinylcholine	↑↑↑
Intubation	↑↑↑

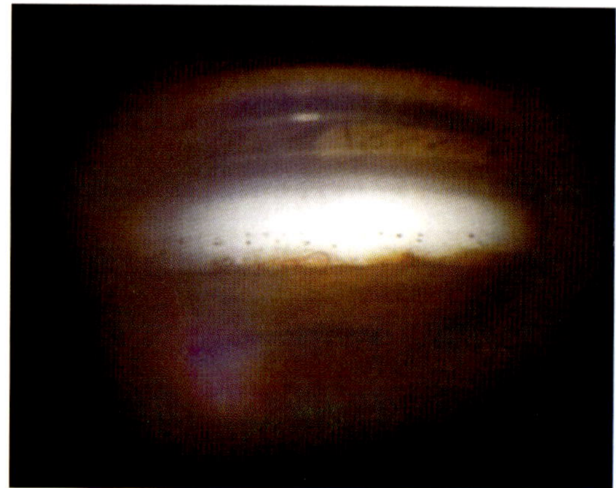

Fig. 14.5 *Goniodysgenesis in a 6-month-old infant with PCG*

DIFFERENTIAL DIAGNOSIS

- A differential diagnosis of epiphora, photophobia, and blepharospasm must be considered before labelling a child as having primary congenital glaucoma.
- Other causes of similar corneal changes include megalocornea, metabolic diseases, corneal dystrophies, trauma, and keratitis.
- Epiphora or photophobia may occur in nasolacrimal duct obstruction, keratitis, iritis, trauma, and corneal dystrophies.
- Optic nerve anomalies simulating a glaucomatous nerve include optic pits, colobomas, and hypoplasia. The diagnosis of primary congenital glaucoma becomes relatively easy when all of the signs and symptoms are considered together.

TREATMENT

The unfortunate combination of delayed presentation and limited management options contribute to the disproportionately high percentage of glaucoma-induced blindness in children: roughly 20% of children in institutions for the blind and 5% of overall paediatric blindness worldwide. The management of an infant or child with glaucoma is challenging. It is a chronic disease affecting children with normal life expectancies. The IOP-reducing benefit of the treatment modality may not persist for lifetime. Surgery is the definitive management.

I. Medical therapy

- *Medical management* plays an adjunctive role:
  - May help clear the cornea
  - Interim period till surgery
  - Postoperative adjunct
- *Oral and topical carbonic anhydrase inhibitors* and β-blockers account for a 25–30% reduction of IOP.
- *Acetazolamide* is effective and can safely be given at a dose of 10–15 mg/day PO. Patients should be monitored for loss of appetite, excessive fatigue, and other signs of metabolic acidosis.
- *Brimonidine* should be avoided.

II. Surgical therapy

1. *Goniotomy*

- Introduced by Barkan in 1938.
- The uveal TM is incised under direct visualization using surgical goniolens and goniotomy knife.
- Basically, in goniotomy, the poorly functioning internal layers of TM are incised; allowing aqueous to exit via Schlemm's canal more easily.
- The abnormal mesodermal tissue has an almost translucent appearance.
- In infants with infantile glaucoma, the iris root has a scalloped, serrated anterior edge, which provides an excellent landmark.
- Incision is placed at the anterior aspect of middle third of TM just posterior to the Schwalbe's line.
- The incision is made clockwise, then the knife is flipped and made anticlockwise, for total of 120° (Fig. 14.6).
- If incision is anterior, goniotomy will not function.
- If placed too posteriorly, results in PI/iridodialysis/intraocular haemorrhage.

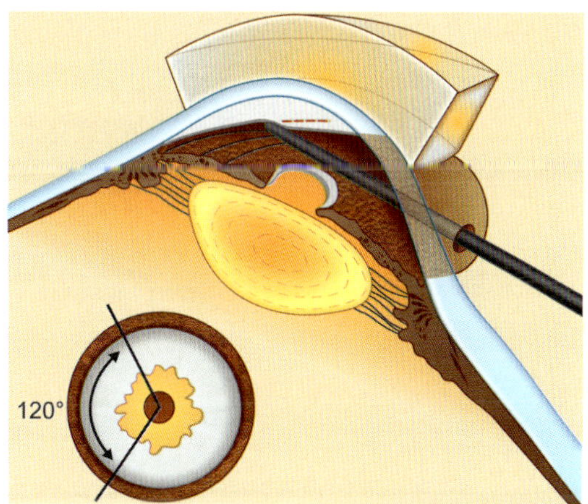

Fig. 14.6 *Goniotomy: Direct incision*

- Small amount of bleeding may be noticed.
- Anti-glaucoma medication may be used to clear the cornea.
- Pilocarpine eyedrops may be used for better visualization.
- Results are evident by 3–6 weeks.
- Goniotomy can be repeated in a different location.
- The success rate is 80–90% after 1–2 procedures.
- Best results seen in primary infantile glaucoma with relatively clear cornea, with onset between 3 months and 1 year of age.

2. *Trabeculotomy*

- It is *ab externo* approach. It creates a direct communication between anterior chamber and Schlemm's canal.
- The Schlemm's canal lies just below the transition from white scleral fibres to blue corneal fibres.
- Radial 2 mm long incision is given. Then careful dissection is carried out layer by layer until the Schlemm's canal is deroofed. The deroofing is confirmed by slow egress of small amount of aqueous humour.
- Two nicks are given circumferentially. Some surgeons use a 10-0 nylon thread and advance it inside the Schlemm's canal.
- Trabeculotomy probes are passed gently in the Schlemm's canal; they should not be forced through.
- Slowly the probe is rotated towards the centre of the cornea, it enters the AC with sudden

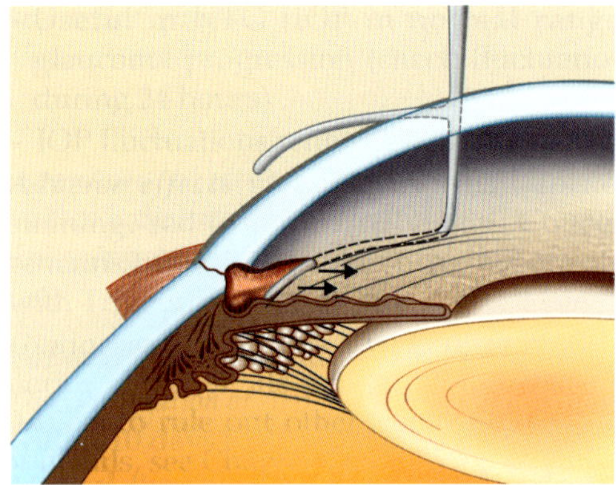

Fig. 14.7 *Trabeculotomy*

gush of aqueous and flattening of AC (Fig. 14.7). This is repeated on the other side.

- Advantages of trabeculotomy: It can be done in cloudy/opaque corneas.
- Disadvantages of trabeculotomy include:
  - Conjunctival scarring
  - Technically difficult
  - Difficult in a buphthalmic eye with a stretched limbus to locate the Schlemm's canal
  - Inadvertent entry into the anterior chamber in the beginning of procedure

3. *Trabeculectomy*

- Usually done when ≥1 angle procedure (goniotomy/trabeculotomy) has failed.
- Success rate varies from 40 to 60%.
- Has low success rate in children due to:
  - Lower scleral rigidity
  - Rapid healing
  - Exuberant scarring processes
  - Enlargement of glaucomatous eyes with thinning and distortion of intraocular anatomy
- Patients must be followed indefinitely for evidence of bleb thinning, and parents need to remain vigilant for signs of infection.

4. *Glaucoma drainage devices*

- Glaucoma implant surgery is an important treatment alternative for children who are poor candidates for goniosurgery and trabeculectomy or who have proven to be refractory to these procedures.
- The superior temporal quadrant is the preferred site to maximize the distance of the drainage plate from the optic nerve and to lessen the risk of postoperative eyelid deformity.
- The drainage plate may be trimmed to accommodate a smaller eye.
- In a subset of refractory glaucoma, one glaucoma drainage device may not adequately control IOP, and either a replacement glaucoma drainage device at the same site or a new glaucoma drainage device at another site may be warranted.

III. Cyclodestruction

Cyclodestructive procedures are selectively used to improve aqueous outflow for childhood glaucoma that has proven refractory to medical therapy and to conventional surgical procedures, and work by decreasing aqueous production.

Conclusion

The care of childhood glaucomas is lifelong. This requires early diagnosis and treatment, repeat examinations (often under anaesthesia), and management of complications, such as amblyopia. Refractive and strabismus amblyopias are important causes of vision loss in children with glaucoma. Early optical and occlusion therapies are important for these children.

SECONDARY CHILDHOOD GLAUCOMA (WITH ASSOCIATED ANOMALIES)

I. GLAUCOMA ASSOCIATED WITH NON-ACQUIRED OCULAR ANOMALIES

1. ***Glaucoma associated with iridodysgenesis***

- Ectropion uveae
- Congenital iris hypoplasia
- Aniridia
- Microphthalmos/microcornea

ANIRIDIA

General features

- Aniridia may be either sporadic or familial.
- Gene for aniridia has been localized to the short arm of chromosome 11; a deletion in this

area results in a syndrome that comprises the ocular findings given above with, in addition, mental retardation, genital anomalies, and a greatly increased risk of Wilms' tumour at a young age.
- Children of parents who have aniridia are at a 50% risk of inheriting the syndrome.

Ocular features

Congenital aniridia is characterized by an obvious iris defect (which varies from an almost complete absence to relatively complete, albeit abnormal, irides), decreased visual acuity with nystagmus, small corneas, small discs, foveal hypoplasia, and cataract.

Glaucoma occurs in 50–75% of patients who have aniridia. Although the majority of children who have aniridia go on to develop glaucoma, most do not do so until late in the first decade of life. This late-onset glaucoma associated with aniridia appears to be the result of a form of angle-closure.

Management

Trabeculectomy or glaucoma drainage devices help control IOP.

2. *Glaucoma associated with irido-corneal dysgenesis*
- Posterior embryotoxon
- Axenfeld-Rieger anomaly/syndrome
- Peter's anomaly/syndrome
- Combined Rieger syndrome/Peter anomaly

Based on the observation that most of the ocular and facial structures involved in these developmental disorders are of neural crest origin, the term ***neurocristopathy*** has been appropriately coined for these disorders.

AXENFELD-RIEGER SYNDROME

Eponyms commonly encountered in scientific literature:
- Limited to peripheral anterior segment defects: Axenfeld's anomaly
- Peripheral abnormalities with additional changes in the iris: Rieger's anomaly
- Ocular anomalies plus systemic developmental defects: Rieger's syndrome

The similarity of anterior chamber angle abnormalities in Axenfeld's anomaly and Rieger's anomaly and syndrome points towards the fact that these three arbitrary categories represent a spectrum of developmental disorders. Hence, nowadays, Axenfeld-Rieger syndrome (A-R syndrome), is used for all clinical variations within this spectrum of developmental disorders.

General features

All patients with the A-R syndrome share the same general features:
- Bilateral, developmental disorder of the eyes
- Frequent family history (autosomal dominant mode of inheritance)
- No sex predilection
- Frequent systemic developmental defects
- High incidence of associated glaucoma.

The age at which the A-R syndrome is diagnosed ranges from birth to adulthood, with most cases becoming recognized during infancy or childhood. The diagnosis is made because of an abnormal iris or other ocular anomaly, signs of congenital glaucoma, reduced vision in older patients, or systemic anomalies.

Ocular features

Ocular defects in the A-R syndrome are typically bilateral. The structures most commonly involved are the peripheral cornea, anterior chamber angle, and iris.

Cornea. The characteristic abnormality is a white line on the posterior cornea near the limbus which corresponds to an anteriorly displaced Schwalbe's line. The cornea is otherwise normal in the typical case of the A-R syndrome, with the exception of occasional patients with variation in the overall size. The corneal endothelium is typically normal.

Anterior chamber angle. Gonioscopic examination reveals a prominent Schwalbe's line, although there is considerable variation among patients in the extent to which Schwalbe's line is enlarged and anteriorly displaced. Tissue strands bridge the anterior chamber angle from the peripheral iris to the prominent ridge

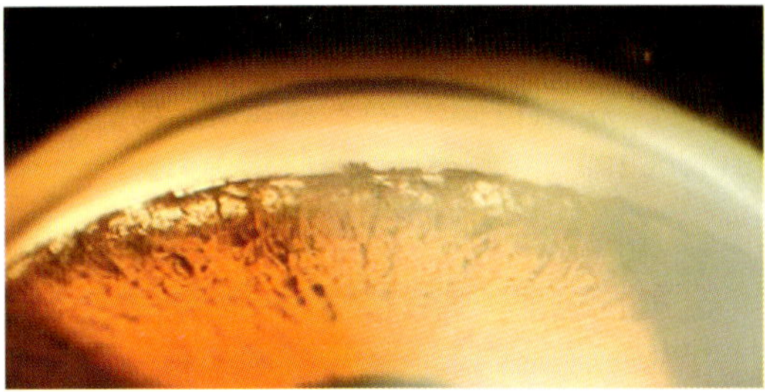

Fig. 14.8 *Gonioscopy shows dense iridocorneal strands*

(Fig. 14.8). These iridocorneal adhesions are typically similar in colour and texture to the adjacent iris. The strands range in size from thread-like structures to broad bands extending for a clock hour or more of the circumference.

Iris abnormalities include peripheral abnormalities, mild stromal thinning (Fig. 14.9) or in some cases, marked atrophy with hole formation, corectopia, and ectropionuveae. In cases with corectopia, the pupil is usually displaced toward a prominent peripheral tissue strand. The atrophy and hole formation occur in the quadrant away from the direction of the corectopia. The progressive changes usually consist of displacement or distortion of the pupil and occasional thinning or hole formation of the iris. In some cases, these progressive iris changes may be confused with those of ICE syndrome.

Other ocular abnormalities include strabismus, limbal dermoids, corneal pannus, cataracts, congenital ectropion uveae, congenital pupillary-iris-lens membrane, peripheral spoke-like transillumination defects of the iris, retinal detachment, macular degeneration, chorio-retinal colobomas, choroidal hypoplasia, and hypoplasia of the optic nerve heads.

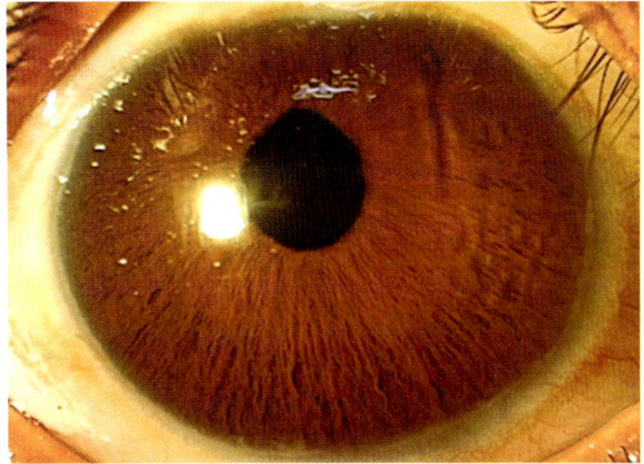

Fig. 14.9 *AR syndrome, note posterior embryotoxon, anterior stromal iris atrophy and up drawn pupil*

Glaucoma. Approximately half of the patients with the A-R syndrome develop glaucoma. The glaucoma may manifest during infancy, although it more commonly appears in childhood or young adulthood. The extent of the iris defects and iridocorneal strands does not correlate precisely with the presence or severity of the glaucoma.

Systemic features

Dental abnormalities. The dental abnormalities include a reduction in crown size (i.e. microdontia), a decreased but evenly spaced number of teeth (i.e. hypodontia), and a focal absence of teeth (i.e. oligodontia or anodontia) The teeth most commonly missing are anterior maxillary and primary and permanent central incisors.

Facial anomalies. These include maxillary hypoplasia with flattening of the midface and a receding upper lip and prominent lower lip, especially in association with dental hypoplasia. Hypertelorism, telecanthus, a broad flat nose, micrognathia, and mandibular prognathism have also been described. Other abnormalities reported in association with the A-R syndrome include redundant periumbilical skin and hypospadias, oculocutaneous albinism, heart defects, middle ear deafness, mental deficiency, and a variety of neurologic, dermatologic, and skeletal disorders.

Genetic linkage

Three chromosomal loci have been linked to A-R syndrome and related phenotypes. These loci are on chromosomes 4q25, 6p25, and 13q14. The genes at chromosomes 4q25 and 6p25 have been identified as PITX2 and FOXC1 (formerly designated FKHL7), respectively.

Differential diagnosis

- ***Iridocorneal endothelial syndrome.*** Clinical features that distinguish the iridocorneal endothelial (ICE) syndrome from A-R syndrome include corneal endothelial abnormalities, unilaterality, absence of family history, and onset in young adulthood. The membrane in the A-R syndrome represents a primordial remnant that of the ICE syndrome results from proliferation of the abnormal corneal endothelium.

- ***Posterior polymorphous dystrophy.*** Differentiation can be made on the basis of the typical corneal endothelial abnormality.
- ***Peters' anomaly.*** The spectrum of disorders that constitutes Peters' anomaly involves the central portion of the cornea, iris, and lens.
- ***Iridogoniodysgenesis.*** Congenital hypoplasia of the iris.
- ***Ectopia lentis et pupillae.*** The corectopia in this disorder may resemble that of the A-R syndrome, but the absence of anterior chamber angle defects is a differential feature.
- Oculodentodigital dysplasia, and
- Aniridia

Management

Intraocular pressure elevation most often develops between childhood and early adulthood, but it may appear in infancy. With the exception of infantile cases, medical therapy should usually be initiated before surgical intervention is recommended. Trabeculectomy is the surgical procedure of choice for most patients with glaucoma associated with the A-R syndrome. These patients must be followed throughout their lives to detect glaucoma. In infants and in cases refractory to medication and trabeculectomy, glaucoma implant surgery and cycloablation remain options for treatment.

PETERS' ANOMALY

General features

The condition is present at birth and is usually bilateral. Most cases are sporadic, although there are reported cases of autosomal recessive inheritance.

Peters' anomaly is considered to be a morphologic finding rather than a distinct entity because of the varied genetic and nongenetic patterns and the spectrum of ocular and systemic abnormalities.

Peters' anomaly can be caused by mutation in the *PAX6* gene, the *PITX2* gene, the *CYP1B1* gene, or the *FOXC1* gene.

Ocular features

Hallmark of Peters' anomaly is a central defect in Descemet's membrane and corneal endothelium with thinning and opacification of the corresponding area of corneal stroma. Bowman's layer may also be absent centrally. Iris adhesions may extend to the borders of this corneal defect.

The disorder has been subdivided into three groups, each of which may have more than one pathogenetic mechanism.

- Peters' anomaly not associated with keratolenticular contact or cataract.

  The defect in Descemet's membrane may represent primary failure of corneal endothelial development.
- Peters' anomaly associated with keratolenticular contact or cataract.

  This variation involves normal development of lens, which gets secondarily pushed forward against the cornea causing the loss of Descemet's membrane. Some cases may result from incomplete separation of the lens vesicle from surface ectoderm.
- Peters' anomaly associated with Axenfeld-Rieger syndrome.

Glaucoma

Approximately one-half of the patients with Peters' anomaly develop glaucoma, which is frequently present at birth. The mechanism of the glaucoma is uncertain, because the anterior chamber angle is usually grossly normal by clinical examination.

Differential diagnosis

- Causes of central corneal opacities: Congenital glaucoma, birth trauma, the mucopolysaccharidoses, and congenital hereditary endothelial dystrophy.
- Posterior keratoconus
- Congenital corneal leukomas and staphylomas

Management

Trabeculotomy or trabeculectomy may be reasonable in milder cases where there is adequate anterior chamber depth, a drainage implant device or cyclodestructive surgery is often needed in refractory or more severely affected cases.

Penetrating keratoplasty is also frequently necessary, although the results are typically poor, which probably is caused in part by the associated glaucoma and its surgical treatment.

II. GLAUCOMA ASSOCIATED WITH NON-ACQUIRED SYSTEMIC ANOMALIES

Developmental glaucoma with some of the important associated systemic anomalies are described briefly.

STURGE-WEBER SYNDROME AND VARIANTS

General features. Classic SWS comprises the triad of port-wine facial telangiectasis (nevus flammeus) in the distribution of the trigeminal nerve that respects the vertical midline, ipsilateral glaucoma, and intracranial angiomata.

Ocular features. Glaucoma occurs in about one-third of patients who have SWS. In patients affected by glaucoma, both the upper and lower lids usually are involved in the facial telangiectasias.

Management. For cases presenting later in life, trabeculectomy, cyclodestruction, and glaucoma drainage devices have been advocated. The presence of choroidal haemangiomas in many of these patients increases the risk of choroidal expansion or haemorrhage intraoperatively.

Less common syndromal associations are described in brief.

MARFAN SYNDROME

General features. Marfan syndrome is characterized by musculoskeletal abnormalities, such as arachnodactyly, hyperextensible joints, and scoliosis, and by cardiovascular disease and ocular abnormalities. Transmission is autosomal dominant with high penetrance, although approximately 15% of cases are sporadic.

Ocular features. These include ectopialentis, microphakia, megalocornea, myopia, keratoconus, hypoplasia of the iris stroma and dilator muscle, retinal detachment, and glaucoma. The zonules are often attenuated and broken, leading to upward subluxation of the lens. The lens may also become dislocated into the pupil or anterior chamber, leading to pupillary-block glaucoma.

In childhood or adolescence, open-angle glaucoma may also develop. It is associated with congenital abnormalities of the anterior chamber angle. Dense iris processes bridge the angle recess, inserting anterior to the scleral spur. This iris tissue sweeping across the recess may have a concave configuration.

Management. If open-angle glaucoma is seen in infancy, it may be treated with goniotomy or trabeculotomy. When the glaucoma occurs in older childhood, medical therapy should be tried first.

HOMOCYSTINURIA

General features. Homocystinuria is an autosomal recessive trait leading to an elevation of homocysteine in the blood and urine. Patients characteristically are lightly pigmented with blond hair and blue eyes and resemble patients with Marfan syndrome in habitus. Systemic manifestations include mental retardation, seizures, skeletal deformities with osteoporosis, and vascular lesions.

Ocular features. Ocular abnormalities include ectopia lentis and retinal detachment. Bilateral lens subluxation usually occurs inferiorly. Anterior lens subluxation or dislocation can lead to pupillary-block glaucoma.

Management. The glaucoma is treated by dilation of the pupil, peripheral iridectomy, and lens extraction, if the lens has dislocated into the anterior chamber. General anaesthesia should be avoided because of the risk of thromboembolism.

NEUROFIBROMATOSIS TYPE 1(NF1)

General features. NF1 has an autosomal-dominant inheritance. It carries a spectrum of findings including café-au-lait spots, freckling of the axial/inguinal area, and sphenoid dysplasia. S-shaped plexiform neurofibromas of the lids, optic nerve gliomas, Lisch nodules and choroidal hamartomas.

Ocular features. Ocular involvement includes S-shaped plexiform neurofibromas of the lids, optic nerve gliomas, Lisch nodules, choroidal hamartomas and glaucoma. Eyes with an associated plexiform neurofibroma have a 50% risk of glaucoma.

Management. Glaucoma can be addressed with trabeculectomy or a drainage device.

OCULOCEREBRORENAL (LOWE) SYNDROME (OCRL)

General features. Lowe syndrome is X-linked recessive. Systemic manifestations include mental retardation, renal tubular dysfunction (Fanconi's syndrome), aminoaciduria and hypotonia.

Ocular features. Ocular manifestations include congenital cataracts and congenital glaucoma. Incidence of glaucoma has been reported to be 47 to 71%.

Management. Glaucoma can be successfully addressed with trabeculotomy or trabeculectomy.

GLAUCOMA ASSOCIATED WITH ACQUIRED SYSTEMIC ANOMALIES

CONGENITAL RUBELLA

General features. Systemic abnormalities associated with congenital Rubella involve the cardiac, auditory, and central nervous systems.

Ocular features. Ocular manifestations may present as glaucoma, cataract, keratitis, uveitis, microcornea, or pigmentary retinopathy.

Management. Glaucoma may occur during infancy with isolated trabeculodysgenesis and responds to goniotomy. The inflammation accompanying active rubella infection may produce elevations in IOP that must be treated with medications rather than surgery.

RUBINSTEIN-TAYBI (BROAD THUMB) SYNDROME

General features. Rubinstein-Taybi syndrome is characterized by large thumbs and large first toes. Patients have mental and motor retardation.

Ocular features. Ocular features include hypertelorism, epicanthus, lid colobomas, and congenital glaucoma.

Management. The glaucoma may be successfully treated by goniotomy or trabeculotomy.

SUGGESTED READING

1. Anderson DR. The development of the trabecular meshwork and its abnormality in primary infantile glaucoma. Tr Am Ophthalmol Soc 1981;79:458–85.
2. Beck AD. Diagnosis and management of pediatric glaucoma. Ophthalmol Clin North Am 2001;14: 501.
3. Khan AO. Conditions that can be mistaken as early childhood glaucoma. Ophthalmic Genet 2011;32(3):129–37.
4. Lister A. Technique of goniotomy. Br J Ophthalmol 1965;49:594–99.
5. Moore DB, Tomkins O, Ben-Zion I. A review of primary congenital glaucoma in the developing world. Surv Ophthalmol 2013;58(3):278–85.
6. Panicker SG, Mandal AK, Reddy ABM, Gothwal VK, Hasnain SE. Correlations of genotype with phenotype in Indian patients with primary congenital glaucoma. Invest Ophthalmol Vis Sci 2004;45:1149–56.
7. Rao KN, Nagireddy S, Chakrabarti S. Complex genetic mechanisms in glaucoma: an overview. Indian J Ophthalmol 2011;59 Suppl:S31–42.
8. Shields MB, Buckley E, Klintworth GK, et al. Axenfeld-Rieger syndrome. A spectrum of developmental disorders. Surv Ophthalmol 1985; 29:387.

CHAPTER 15 PRIMARY ANGLE-CLOSURE DISEASE

TERMINOLOGY AND EPIDEMIOLOGY

TERMINOLOGY

The signs and symptoms of angle-closure disease were first of all described by St. Yves in 1722; but it was in 1923 that the term angle-closure glaucoma was proposed by Raeder.

Primary angle-closure glaucoma, as an entity, is continuously getting enhancement in understanding. Since Curran found that iridectomy relieved pupillary block, Barkan popularized gonioscopy, and Rosengren demonstrated that glaucoma could be divided into cases involving small eyes (later named as angle-closure glaucoma) and large eyes (named as open-angle glaucoma).

Recently, a new nomenclature has been proposed by Foster et al; which has been accepted as new classification of angle-closure by the Association of International Glaucoma Societies (AIGS) in 2006 now termed as International Society of Geographical and Epidemiological Ophthalmology (ISGEO) classifications. Since in the new classification, the word glaucoma is used only when the optic disc and visual field changes are present so the term 'primary angle-closure disease' should preferably replace the term 'primary angle-closure glaucoma'.

Primary angle-closure disease, thus can be considered essentially an anatomical disorder of the anterior segment of the eye characterized by apposition of peripheral iris against the trabecular meshwork (TM) resulting in obstruction of aqueous outflow by closure of an already narrow angle of the anterior chamber. The condition is not associated with any other ocular and systemic abnormalities.

EPIDEMIOLOGY

Salient points regarding epidemiology of primary angle-closure disease as per ISGEO are as below:

1. *Factors affecting incidence and prevalence.* Incidence and prevalence of primary angle-closure disease is affected by a number of risk factors, such as age, sex, race, refractive errors and heredity (For details see etiopathogenesis).

2. *For every 10 occludable angles,* PACS, seen there is only one case of PACG. Thus most occludable eyes do not get glaucoma; and so does not justify prophylactic laser iridotomy in all such cases.

3. *Chronic PACG (asymptomatic)* is more common than acute PAC (symptomatic) (3:1); meaning thereby that most patients do not know they have the disease; justifying need for glaucoma screening.

4. *Ethnic variability* in the prevalence of PACG is marked. The ratio of POAG versus PACG reported for different ethnic groups is as below:

- Europeans, and Africans and Hispanics POAG: PACG = 5:1
- Urban Chinese POAG : PACG = 1:2
- Mongolian POAG : PACG = 1:3
- Asian Indian POAG: PACG = 1:1

5. *Prevalence of PACG* reported in some studies is as below:

- *In Caucasians,* the reported figures are 0.6% in Italy, 0.5% in Wales and 0.1% in Sweden.
- *In Eskimos,* the prevalence is 20 to 40 times higher than whites.
- *In east Asia and southeast Asia,* the reported figure ranges from 1.4 to 4.3% depending upon the age group.

6. *Incidence of acute angle-closure attack* varies widely among different ethnic groups from 4.7/lakh/year in Finland to 11.4 in Japan and 12.2 in Singapore.

7. *Glaucoma blindness* is the second common cause of world blindness. The number of people blinded by PACG is nearly equal to the number blinded by POAG. Presently, there are about 3.9 million bilateral blind people with PACG, and the figure is expected to rise to 5.3 million people in 2020.

ETIOPATHOGENESIS

Etiopathogenesis of primary angle-closure disease can be discussed under the following heads:

A. Predisposing risk factors

B. Pathomechanisms of rise in intraocular pressure (IOP)

PREDISPOSING RISK FACTORS

I. Demographic risk factors

1. *Age.* PACG with pupillary block occurs with greatest frequency in 6th and 7th decades of life. The factors that increase the relative pupillary block with increasing age include increased thickness of lens, more anterior position of lens and senile miosis.

2. *Gender.* Male to female ratio is 1:3. This is believed to be due to higher prevalence of shallow anterior chamber in women.

3. *Race.* In Caucasians, PACG accounts for about 6% of all glaucomas and presents in sixth to seventh decades. It is more common in south-east Asians, Chinese and Eskimos but uncommon in Blacks. In Asians, it presents in the 5th to 6th decades and accounts for 50% of primary adult glaucomas in this ethnic group.

II. Anatomical and ocular risk factors

Eyes anatomically predisposed to develop PACG include:

- Hypermetropic eyes with shallow anterior chamber and short axial length.
- Eyes in which iris–lens diaphragm is placed anteriorly.
- Eyes with narrow-angle of anterior chamber, which may be due to small eyeball, relatively large size of the lens and smaller diameter of the cornea or bigger size of the ciliary body or more anterior insertion of the iris on the ciliary body.
- Plateau iris configuration/thick peripheral iris roll.

To summarize, eyes with following features are considered at risk of developing angle-closure disease:

- Axial length (AL) <22 mm
- Anterior chamber depth (ACD) <2.2 mm

- Lens thickness (LT) > 4.0 mm, and
- LT/AL ratio > 20%

III. Heredity

Most cases of PACG with pupillary block are sporadic in nature. However, predisposing anatomical factors, i.e. shallow anterior chamber and narrow angles have been reported as more common in first degree relatives of the patients.

PATHOMECHANISMS OF RISE IN INTRAOCULAR PRESSURE (IOP)

Three pathomechanisms implicated in the causation of rise in IOP of the eyes at risk of PACG are:

- Pupillary block mechanism
- Plateau iris configuration and syndrome
- Lens-related mechanisms

1. Pupillary block mechanism

Pupillary block mechanism is responsible for causation of rise in IOP in most (70%) of the predisposed patients.

Precipitating factors

In a predisposed patient with occludable angles, the pupillary block causing angle-closure is precipitated by the following factors:

- ***Physiological mydriasis***, e.g. while reading in dim illumination, watching television or cinema in a darkened room, during anxiety and emotional stress (sympathetic overactivity).
- ***Pharmacological mydriasis*** is well documented to precipitate an attack of acute angle-closure. Medications other than topical mydriatics (e.g. phenylephrine, tropicamide, cylopentolate, homatropine and atropine) reported to precipitate the attack include tranquilizers, bronchodilators, antidepressants, vasoconstrictors including common nasal decongestants, antimalarial agents and antispasmodics.
- ***Pharmacological miosis*** induced by drugs, like pilocarpine, is also reported to precipitate an attack of acute PAC.
- ***Induction of Valsalva maneuver*** in day-to-day activities can cause significant narrowing of anterior chamber angle leading to precipitation of angle-closure in predisposed individuals.

Mechanism of rise in IOP after mydriasis

The probable sequence of events resulting in rise of IOP in anatomically predisposed eye is as follows:

- ***Relative pupil block.*** It has been hypothesized that first of all due to the effect of precipitating factors there occurs mid-dilatation of the pupil which increases the amount of apposition between iris and anteriorly placed lens with a considerable pressure due to posterior vector force resulting in relative pupil block (Fig. 15.1A).
- ***Iris bombe formation.*** Consequently, the aqueous collects in the posterior chamber and pushes the peripheral flaccid iris anteriorly resulting in *iris bombe* (Fig. 15.1B).
- ***Appositional angle closure*** due to iridocorneal contact (Fig. 15.1C). Eventually, there occurs rise in IOP which to begin with is transient.
- ***Synaechial angle-closure.*** Slowly the appositional angle-closure is converted into *synaechial angle-closure* (due to formation of peripheral anterior synaechiae) and an attack of rise in IOP may last long.

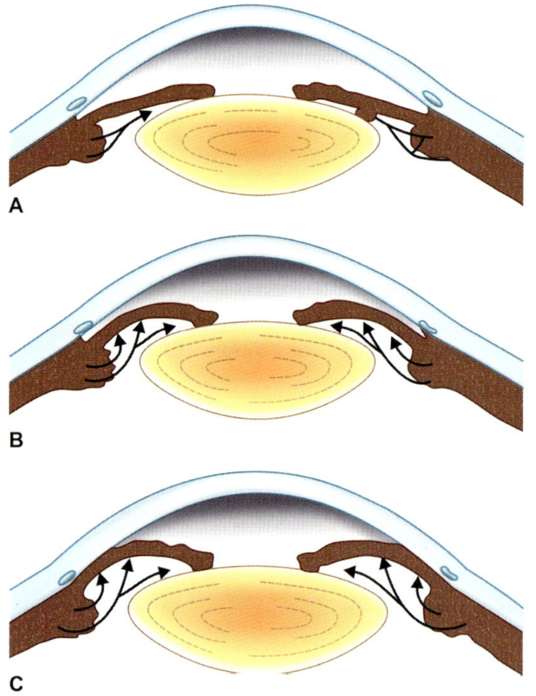

Fig. 15.1 *Mechanism of angle-closure glaucoma: (A) Relative pupil block, (B) Iris bombe formation; (C) Appositional angle-closure*

Note. In some cases, a mechanical occlusion of the angle by the iris is sufficient to block the drainage of aqueous. For this reason, the instillation of atropine in an eye with a narrow angle is dangerous, since it may precipitate an attack of raised IOP.

Mechanism of rise in IOP after miosis

According to another hypothesis, contraction of sphincter muscle is the main factor responsible for increased lens–iris contact. The sphincter muscle contraction exerts a pupil blocking force that is maximum when the size is about 4 mm. Further, the drugs that constrict pupil are also reported to increase pupillary block. Further, these drugs also contract the ciliary muscles allowing the zonules to relax and the lens to move forward. Because of this reason, it is advisable to avoid miotics, such as pilocarpine in the prevention of PACG in predisposed eyes (e.g. fellow eye of patient with acute attack).

2. Plateau iris configuration and syndrome

This mechanism is responsible for a few (10%) of atypical cases of acute angle closure. Acute angle closure associated with plateau iris is atypical in the sense that patients have normal central anterior chamber depth, flat iris plane and minimal pupillary block. It has also been referred in the literature as an angle closure glaucoma without pupillary block (Fig. 15.2 A–D). The anterior chamber angle is closed by a pushing mechanism because of the anterior positioned ciliary processes displacing the peripheral iris anteriorly. Such a situation is called *plateau iris configuration* and iridotomy is sufficient to control IOP in such patients. *Plateau iris syndrome* is labelled when acute angle closure glaucoma occurs either spontaneously or after pharmacological dilation, in spite of patent iridotomy. In such cases, there is high plateau iris configuration on gonioscopy. Studies with ultrasonographic biomicroscopy (UBM) suggest that an anterior position of ciliary process prevents the peripheral iris from falling posteriorly after an iridotomy. Progressive anterior dislocation of the ciliary body with bolstring of the peripheral iris and formation of peripheral anterior synaechial may result in asymptomatic PACG. Such eyes are treated with miotics and laser peripheral iridoplasty to produce thinning of the peripheral iris.

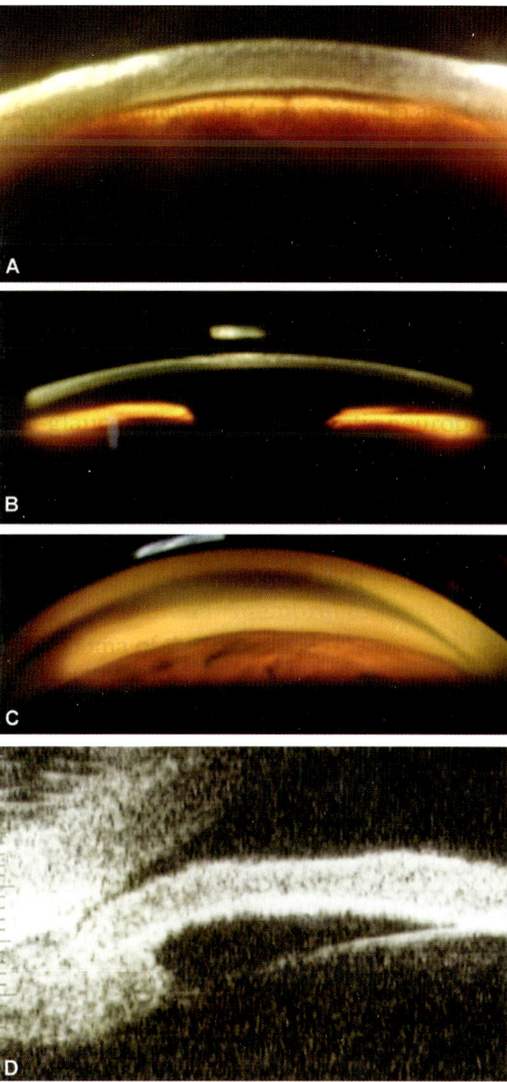

Fig. 15.2 *Plateau iris: (A) Shallow peripheral anterior chamber; (B) Formed central anterior chamber; (C) Flat iris configuration; (D) Anteriorly rotated ciliary process on ultrasound biomicroscopy*

Differential diagnosis of plateau iris

i. *Pseudoplateau iris.* The term pseudoplateau iris is labelled when the peripheral iris is pushed anteriorly by the cysts of the iris or ciliary body epithelium. Clinically, it is difficult to distinguish it from true plateau iris. Such cases are diagnosed on ultrasonographic biomicroscopy (UBM) only (Fig. 15.3).

Treatment is required in the case of significant angle closure and consists of puncture of the cyst with a needle or with Nd:YAG laser. Iridoplasty can also be helpful.

ii. *Swelling of the ciliary body* due to any cause can create a plateau iris configuration and precipitate bilateral angle-closure glaucoma.

Causes. Swelling of the ciliary body with angle-closure glaucoma can be caused by various mechanisms:

- *Dose of sulpha-based oral medication* (e.g. hydrochlorothiazide, oral acetazolamide and topiramate) is reported to cause acute angle closure and the withdrawal of medication is effective in reversing the angle.
- *Scleral buckling* is reported to cause angle closure by causing supraciliary effusion and ciliary body thickening.
- *Other causes of ciliary body swelling* reported are aqueous misdirection, acquired immune-deficiency syndrome (AIDS), and idiopathic uveal effusion syndrome.

3. Lens-related primary angle-closure mechanisms

- Phacomorphic mechanism
- Lens block mechanism

i. *Phacomorphic mechanism.* Phacomorphic mechanism has now been included as one of the three basic PACG mechanisms, along with pupillary block and plateau iris. The abnormal lens may contribute by either causing pupillary block or by pushing the peripheral iris forward into the angle structures. Though the term phacomorphic glaucoma refers to an acute secondary angle-closure glaucoma caused by the intumescent or other lens morphological abnormalities; but now UBM and OCT studies have shown that phacomorphic mechanism may be responsible for initiating acute primary angle- closure glaucoma in predisposed patients (having occludable angle). This also forms the base of lens extraction as a treatment modality for acute primary angle-closure glaucoma.

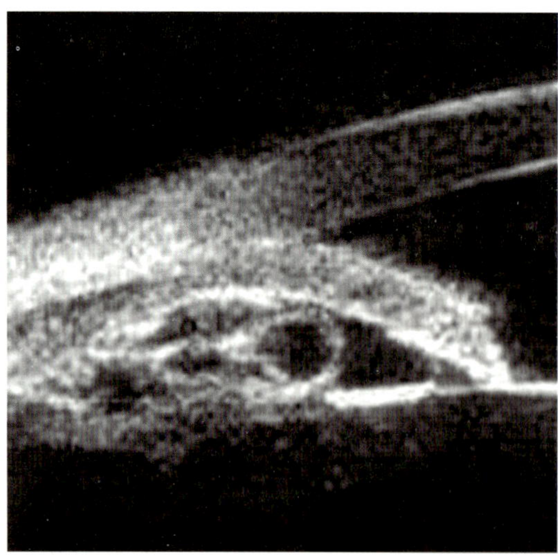

Fig. 15.3 *Ciliary body cyst as seen on UBM*

ii. *Lens block mechanisms.* Lens block describes an underlying mechanism of primary angle closure, in which lens's increased anterior–posterior excursion is due to weakened or lax zonules (*mobile lens syndrome*). This may result in tendency of the lens to rotate forward, especially in the prone position, aggravating the relative pupillary block and the angle closure.

Note. In addition to meticulous gonioscopic examination, the high resolution UBM examination and anterior segment OCT (ASOCT) are very useful in understanding the pathogenesis of the primary angle-closure disease. These investigations are particularly useful in the documentation of plateau iris configuration, plateau iris syndrome, phacomorphic mechanism and post-peripheral iridectomy angle dynamics. Further, these investigations are also helpful in differentiating primary and secondary angle- closure glaucomas.

CLASSIFICATION AND CLINICAL PRESENTATIONS

CLASSIFICATION OF PRIMARY ANGLE-CLOSURE DISEASE

Classifications of primary angle-closure disease in vogue presently are:

A. *Classification based on clinical presentation*

1. Latent primary angle-closure glaucoma (PACG)

2. Subacute (intermittent) PACG
3. Acute PACG
4. Chronic PACG

B. *Classification based on pathomechanism of angle-closure glaucoma*

Apposition of the iris to the trabecular meshwork in ACG may be due to forces acting at three anatomic levels:

1. Pupillary block ACG
2. Plateau iris ACG
3. Phacomorphic ACG
   - Lens-related ACG
   - Lens block ACG

C. *ISGEO classification based on natural history*

1. Primary angle-closure suspect (PACS)
2. Primary angle-closure (PAC)
3. Primary angle-closure glaucoma (PACG)

CLINICAL PRESENTATIONS

World glaucoma experts under the auspices of the "Association of International Glaucoma Societies" (AIGS) in 2006 have proposed the twenty-first century consensus classification which is based on IOP measurements, gonioscopy, disc and visual field evaluation. In this newer classification, the word glaucoma is used only when the optic disc changes and field changes are present. Further, this classification is based only on the signs and has not taken into consideration the presenting symptoms.

The purpose of this new classification is to have a uniform system of case reporting for the purpose of epidemiological and management based studies. Therefore, an effort has been made to integrate the classification based on the clinical presentation into the ISGEO classification (2006) based on natural history. In view of this, it will be worthwhile to denote the entity. 'primary angle-closure glaucoma' as 'primary angle-closure disease' having three stages:

1. ***Primary angle-closure suspect (PACS).*** The term PACS should replace the term 'latent primary angle-closure glaucoma' of clinical presentation based classification.

2. ***Primary angle closure (PAC).*** This stage can be considered to manifest as:
   - *Asymptomatic PAC*
   - *Subacute PAC.* This term should replace the subacute or intermittent primary angle-closure glaucoma of the clinical classification.
   - *Acute PAC.* This term should replace the term acute primary angle-closure glaucoma or acute congestive glaucoma.

3. ***Primary angle-closure glaucoma (PACG).*** This term should replace the term 'chronic angle-closure glaucoma' of clinical presentation based classification.

Note. *The clinical features of these stages of 'primary angle-closure disease', described below are thus the result of integration of old classification based on clinical presentation into the new ISGEO classification based only on the signs.*

I. PRIMARY ANGLE-CLOSURE SUSPECT

Primary angle-closure suspect (PACS), can be considered to replace the term 'latent primary angle-closure glaucoma' of clinical classification.

Clinical features and diagnostic criteria

Symptoms and presenting situations

Symptoms are absent in this stage.

Presenting situations for diagnosis include:

- Suspicious clinical signs on routine ocular examination in patients coming for some other complaints.
- Fellow eye of the patients presenting with acute attack of PAC.
- Glaucoma screening programme.

Suspicious clinical signs

Suspicious clinical signs noted on routine ocular examination include:

1. ***Eclipse sign.*** Eclipse sign, which indicates decreased axial anterior chamber depth, can be elicited by shining a penlight across the anterior chamber from the temporal side and noting a shadow on the nasal side (Fig. 15.4).
2. ***Slit-lamp biomicroscopic signs*** include:
   - Decreased axial anterior chamber depth,
   - Convex-shaped iris lens diaphragm, and
   - Close proximity of the iris to cornea in the periphery.
3. ***Van Herick slit-lamp grading of the angle*** may be used with a fair accuracy. Here, the

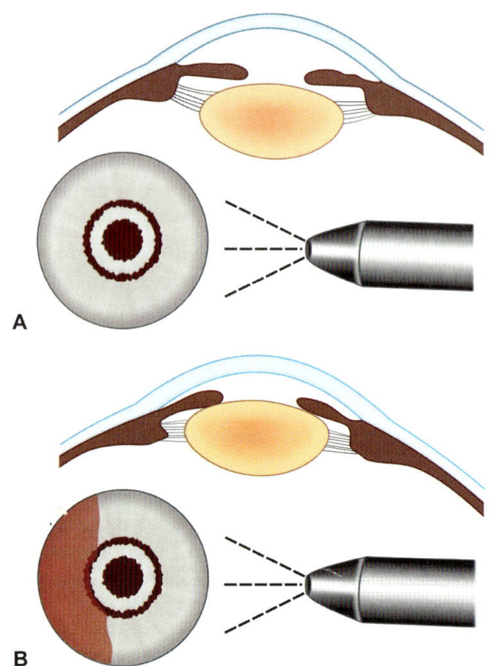

Fig. 15.4 *Estimation of anterior chamber depth by oblique illumination: A; normal, B; shallow*

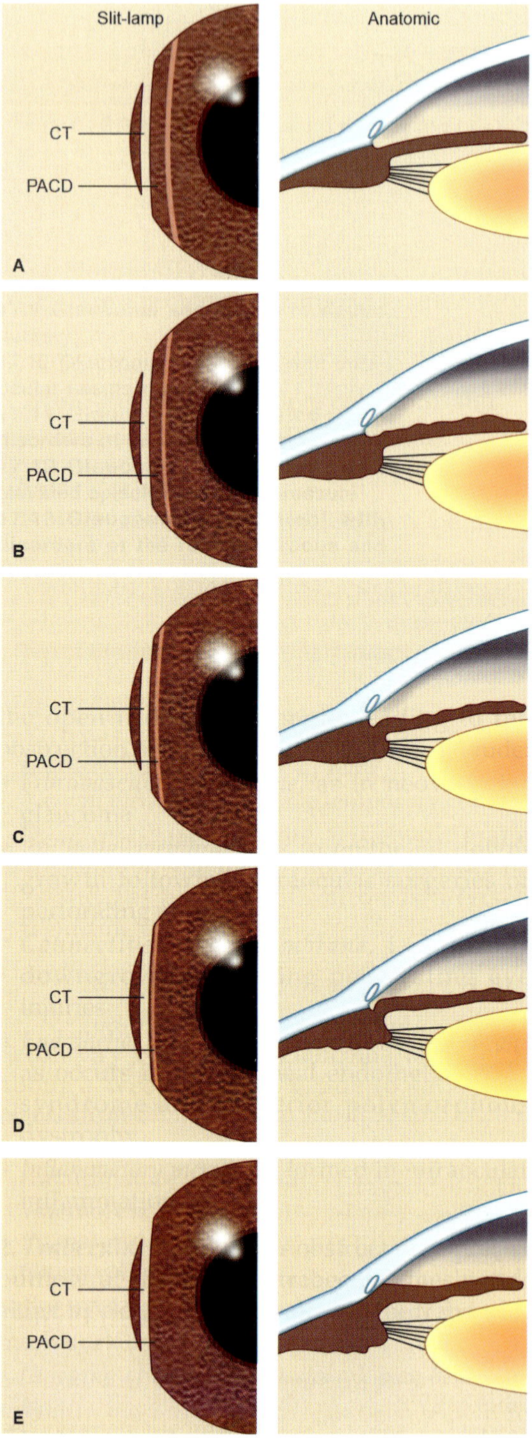

peripheral anterior chamber depth (PACD) is compared to the adjacent corneal thickness (CT) and the presumed angle width is graded as follows (Fig. 15.5):

- Grade 4 (wide open-angle): PACD = ¾ to 1 CT
- Grade 3 (mild narrow-angle): PACD = ¼ to ½ CT
- Grade 2 (moderate narrow-angle): PACD = ¼ CT
- Grade 1 (extremely narrow-angle): PACD <¼ CT
- Grade 0 (closed-angle): PACD = Nil

Diagnostic tests and criteria

Diagnostic tests recommended to confirm the diagnosis include:

- IOP measurement,
- Gonioscopy,
- Ultrasonic biomicroscopy,
- Anterior segment OCT,
- Optic disc evaluation, and
- Visual field analysis.

Fig. 15.5 *Van Herick method of slit-lamp grading of angle width: A, Grade IV; B, Grade III; C, Grade II; and D, Grade I, and E Grade 0. PACD = Peripheral anterior chamber depth; CT = Corneal thickness*

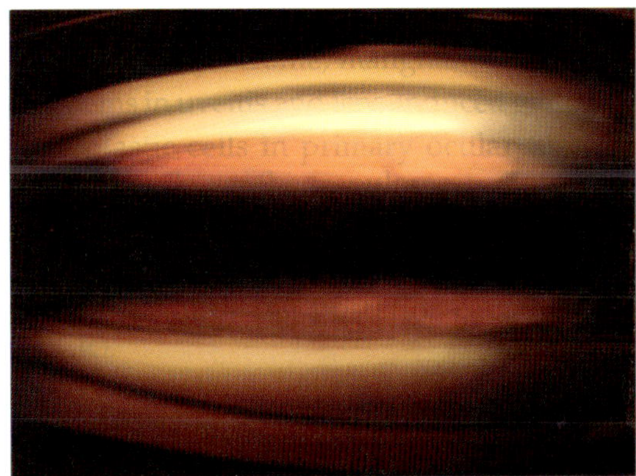

Fig. 15.6 *Occludable angles for 180° on gonioscopy*

Diagnostic criteria for PAC suspect as per ISGEO classification is:

- *Gonioscopy* should reveal iridotrabecular contact in greater than 180° angle and no peripheral anterior synechiae (PAS absent) (Fig. 15.6).
- *IOP* should be normal.
- *Optic disc* should show no glaucomatous change
- *Visual fields* should be normal.

Impression. The angle is at risk of an appositional closure; needs a close watch.

Management

A. Provocative tests

Provocative tests designed to precipitate closure of the angle can be performed in patients with PAC suspect. These tests may be performed in the ophthalmologist's office, where it can be treated promptly.

1. ***Prone-darkroom test*** was the most popular and best physiological provocative test to precipitate the attack of subacute/complete angle closure. In this test, baseline IOP is recorded and patient is made to lie prone in a darkroom for one hour. He must remain awake so that pupils remain dilated. After 1 hour, the IOP is again measured. An increase in IOP of more than 8 mm Hg was considered diagnostic.

2. ***Mydriatic provocative test*** is usually not preferred nowadays because this is not physiological. In this test, either a weak mydriatic (e.g. 0.5% tropicamide) or simultaneously a mydriatic and miotic (10% phenylephrine and 2% pilocarpine) are used to produce a mid-dilated pupil. A pressure rise of more than 8 mm Hg is considered positive.

Inferences from provocative tests include:

- Positive provocative test indicates that angle is capable of spontaneous closure.
- Negative provocative test in the presence of occludable angles on gonioscopy does not rule out a possibility of spontaneous closure. So, patient should be warned of possible symptoms of an acute attack of PAC.

Note. Provocative tests are not considered much reliable and hence sparingly used nowadays.

B. Anterior segment imaging

Anterior segment imaging has become important in the diagnosis of primary angle closure disease spectrum and includes:

1. ***UBM imaging.*** It is especially useful for assessing the glaucoma entities with a structural component to their etiology including acute angle closure. It can demonstrate pupillary block with forward bowing of the iris from the root to the pupillary margin (Fig. 15.7). UBM has become the gold standard to diagnose plateau iris and for imaging ciliary processes.

- *UBM dark room provocative test* enhances sensitivity and specificity, with posterior iris insertion identified as the negative predictor.
- *Valsalva induced angle recess narrowing* with thickening of both ciliary body and iris explains an aspect of PACG in anatomically predisposed eyes.
- *Indentation UBM* by exerting mild pressure on peripheral cornea with skirt of eyecup, can show more details about the angle recess.

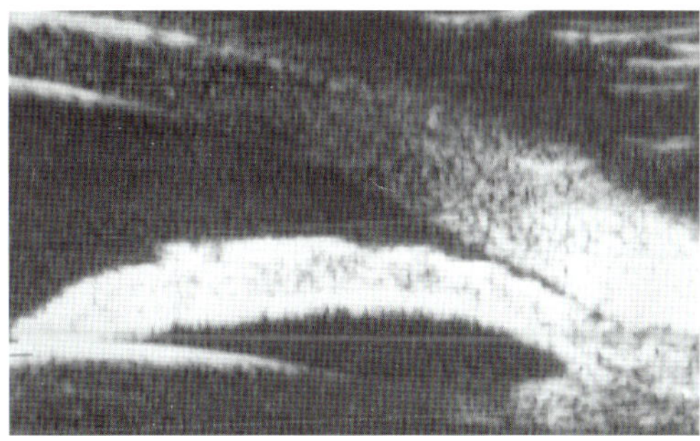

Fig. 15.7 *Pupillary block as seen on UBM*

2. ***Anterior segment OCT.*** Anterior segment OCT also provides useful information in glaucomas with a structural component to their etiology. In addition to the quantification to the angle configuration, the available software also allows recognition of the angles that are potentially at risk of closure. It is also possible to observe and document angle progression over time and patient's crystalline lens thickness.

Treatment

Prophylactic laser iridotomy is warranted, if more than 270° of oppositional iridotrabecular contact is seen on gonioscopy in the fellow eye of all patients presenting with acute PAC or PACG in one eye. If untreated, the risk of conversion to PACG during the next 5 years is about 50%.

Periodic follow-up. Patients with PAC suspect in both eyes need to be followed periodically and educated about the symptoms of the disease.

II. PRIMARY ANGLE-CLOSURE

Defining criteria for primary angle-closure (PAC) are:

- *Iridotrabecular* contact noted on gonioscopy is greater than 180° angle,
- *IOP* elevated and/PAS present,
- *Optic disc:* Normal, and
- *Visual fields:* Normal

Impression. Angle is abnormal either in function (elevated IOP) and/or structure (PAS +ve)

Clinical course. Eyes with PAC may follow any of the following clinical courses:

- May remain as asymptomatic or PAC,
- May manifest as subacute PAC, or
- May manifest as acute PAC, or
- May convert to PACG.

Subacute primary angle-closure

Subacute primary angle-closure may be considered to replace the term subacute (intermittent) angle-closure glaucoma of clinical classification.

In subacute primary angle-closure (subacute PAC), there occurs an attack of transient rise of IOP (40–50 mm Hg) which may last for few minutes to 1–2 hours.

Precipitating factors

Such an attack in a patient with PAC is usually precipitated by:

- *Physiological mydriasis,* e.g. while reading in dim illumination, watching television or cinema in a darkened room, or during anxiety (sympathetic overactivity); or
- *Physiological shallowing of anterior chamber* after lying in prone position.
- *Pharmacological mydriasis* by use of pupil dilating drugs.

Clinical features

Symptoms include:

- *Episode of subacute PAC* is marked by experience of unilateral transient blurring of vision, coloured halos around light, headache, browache and eyeache on the affected side.
- *Self-termination of the attack* occurs possibly due to physiological miosis induced by bright light, sleep or otherwise.
- *Recurrent attacks* of such episodes are not uncommon. Between the recurrent attacks, the eyes are free of symptoms.

Signs. Usually, during examination, the eye is white and not congested. However, all the signs described above in the definition of PAC should be elicited to label PAC.

Diagnosis and treatment

Diagnosis is established as per criteria given for definiting PAC.

Treatment of choice for subacute PAC is laser peripheral iridotomy (LPI).

Differential diagnosis of coloured halos in PAC

Coloured halos during intermittent attacks of raised IOP in PAC occur due to accumulation of fluid in the corneal epithelium and alteration in the refractive condition of the corneal lamellae. Patient typically gives history of seeing colours distributed as in the spectrum of rainbow (red being outside and violet innermost) while watching on a lighted bulb or the moon.

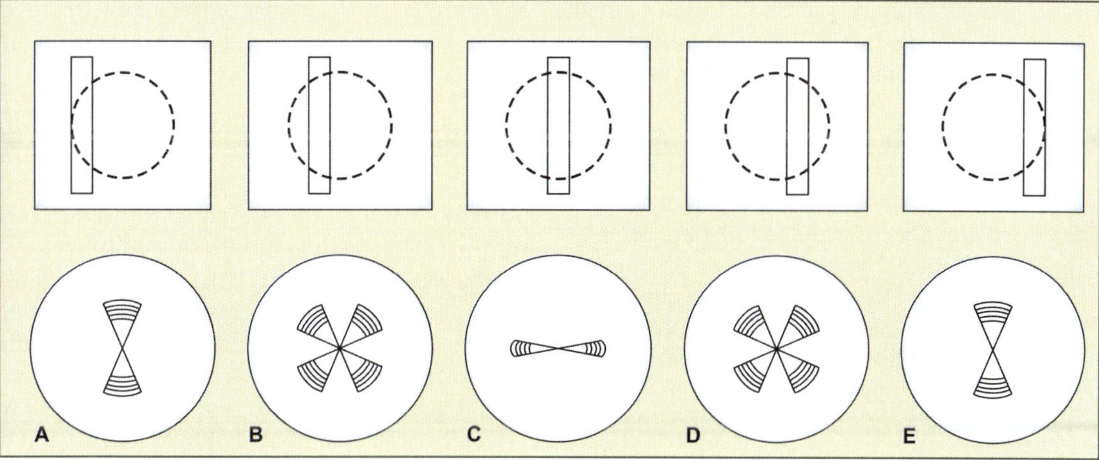

Fig. 15.8 *Emsley-Fincham stenopaic slit test demonstrating breaking up of halos*

The coloured halos in glaucoma must be differentiated from those found in acute purulent conjunctivitis and early cataractous changes. In conjunctivits, the halos can be eliminated by irrigating the discharge. The halos of glaucoma and immature cataract may be differentiated by Fincham's test in which a stenopaic slit is passed across the pupil. During this test, glaucomatous halo remains intact, while a halo due to cataract is broken up into segments (Fig. 15.8).

Acute primary angle-closure

The term acute primary angle-closure may be considered to replace the term acute primary angle closure glaucoma/acute congestive glaucoma of clinical classification. An attack of acute rise in IOP in patients with PAC may occur due to pupillary block causing sudden closure of the angle. It usually does not terminate of its own and thus if not treated lasts for many days. This is a sight-threatening emergency.

Clinical features

Symptoms include:

- *Pain*. Typically acute attack is characterized by sudden onset of very severe pain in the eye and head which radiates along the branches of 5th nerve. The pain is related to the sudden rise in IOP rather than the absolute level of IOP.
- *Nausea, vomiting and prostrations* are frequently associated with pain. These symptoms simulate a migraine attack.
- *Rapidly progressive impairment of vision*, redness, photophobia and lacrimation develop in all cases into different segments.
- *Past history*. About 5% patients give history of typical previous intermittent attacks of subacute angle-closure.

Signs include (Fig. 15.9):

- *Lids* may be oedematous.
- *Conjunctiva* is chemosed, and congested (both conjunctival and ciliary vessels are congested).
- *Cornea* becomes oedematous and insensitive.

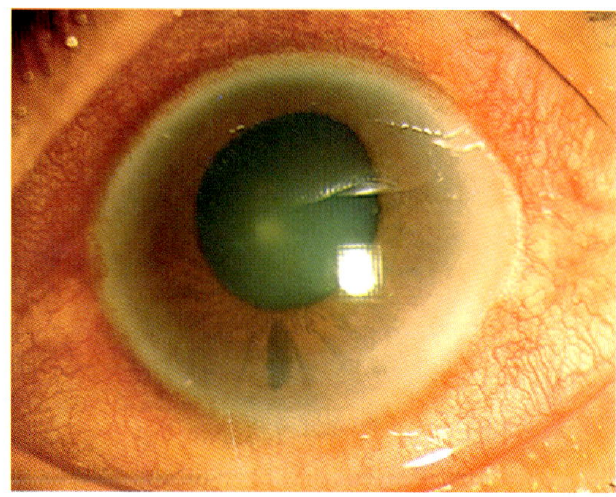

Fig. 15.9 *Clinical photograph of a patient with acute congestive glaucoma. Note ciliary congestion, corneal oedema and mid-dilated pupil*

The oedema may be confined to the corneal epithelium with formation of microcysts; or stromal oedema and thickening may be present.

- *Anterior chamber* is very shallow. Aqueous flare or cells may be seen in anterior chamber.
- *Angle of anterior chamber* is completely closed as seen on gonioscopy (Modified Shaffer grade 0). Topical hyperosmotic agents may be required when the cornea is too cloudy to allow gonioscopic examination. Peripheral anterior synaechiae may also be noted.
- *Iris* may be discoloured.
- *Pupil* is semidilated, vertically oval and fixed. It is non-reactive to both light and accommodation. Pupillary changes result from the ischaemia and paralysis of the sphincter muscle caused by markedly elevated IOP.
- *IOP* is markedly elevated, usually between 40 and 70 mm Hg.
- *Optic disc* is oedematous and hyperaemic.
- *Fellow eye* shows shallow anterior chamber and occludable angle on gonioscopy.

Diagnosis and management

Diagnosis of an attack of acute primary angle closure is usually obvious from the clinical features. However, a *differential diagnosis* may have to be considered:

1. *From other causes of acute red eye.* Acute congestive glaucoma sometimes needs differentiation from other causes of inflamed red eye, like acute conjunctivitis and acute iridocyclitis.
2. *From secondary acute congestive glaucomas,* such as:
   - Phacomorphic glaucoma (*see* page 238),
   - Acute neovascular glaucoma (*see* page 248) and
   - Glaucomatocyclitic crisis (*see* page 244).

Investigations. Gonioscopy, ultrasound biomicroscopy (UBM) and AS-OCT are useful investigations for documentation.

Management. Acute angle closure is a serious ocular emergency condition and needs to be managed aggressively as below:

- Immediate medical therapy to lower IOP
- Definitive treatment
- Prophylactic iridotomy of the fellow eye, and
- Long-term glaucoma surveillance and IOP management of both eyes.

A. *Immediate medical therapy to lower IOP* should include:

1. *Systemic hyperosmotic agents* are required initially, if IOP is more than 40 mm Hg. They reduce IOP by reducing vitreous volume.
   - *Intravenous mannitol* (1 gm/kg body weight) should be preferred in the presence of nausea and vomiting. Caution is needed in patients with cardiovascular and renal disorders.
   - *Oral hyperosmotics,* e.g. glycerol 1 g/kg body weight of 50% solution in lemon juice over ice, may be given, if well tolerated and not contraindicated (as in diabetes mellitus).
2. *Systemic carbonic anhydrase inhibitors,* e.g. acetazolamide 500 mg i.v. stat followed by 250 mg tablet 3 times a day.
3. *Topical anti-glaucoma drugs* to be instilled immediately include:
   - *Beta-blocker,* e.g. 0.5% timolol
   - *Alpha adrenergic agonists,* e.g. brimonidine 0.1–0.2%.
   - *Prostaglandin analogue,* e.g. latanoprost 0.005%.
   - *Role of miotic therapy. Pilocarpine* 2% QID should be started after 1 hour of the commencement of the treatment, i.e. when IOP is lowered, as at higher IOP sphincter is ischaemic and unresponsive to pilocarpine. Intensive miotic therapy is not advised nowadays. Some glaucoma experts have given up the use of pilocarpine entirely in the management of acute PACG because of theoretical concerns that in addition to pulling the iris away from the angle recess, it also increases the axial thickness of lens by constricting the ciliary muscle ring and thus induces anterior lens movement.
4. *Analgesics and anti-emetics* may be required to alleviate the symptoms.
5. *Indentation gonioscopy* with a 4-mirror goniolens may help relieve pupil block and is essential to determine, if the trabecular blockage is reversible.
6. *Topical steroid,* e.g. prednisolone acetate 1% or dexamethasone eyedrops administered 3–4 times a day to reduce the inflammation.

B. ***Definitive therapy*** consists of:

1. *Laser peripheral iridotomy (LPI).* Gonioscopy should be performed as soon as cornea becomes clear. Laser PI should be performed, if PAS are seen in <180° angle. LPI re-establishes communication between posterior and anterior chambers, so it bypasses the pupillary block and immediately relieves the crowding of the angle.

- *LPI* (with Nd:YAG laser or argon laser) should always be preferred over surgical PI. However, if lasers are not available, surgical PI should be done.
- A greater extent of PAS, a high presenting IOP, and a larger cup to disc ratio have been reported as predictors of poor pressure control following LPI in Asian and African eyes.

2. *Laser gonioplasty,* i.e. argon laser peripheral iridoplasty may be useful in PAC especially in eyes with plateau iris. The laser burns are applied on the peripheral iris stroma that contracts and the angle deepens.

3. *Filtration surgery,* i.e. trabeculectomy should be performed in cases where IOP is not controlled with the maximum medical therapy following an attack of acute PAC or when gonioscopy reveals PAS >270° angle and also when peripheral iridotomy is not effective.

Mechanism: Filtration surgery provides an alternative to the angle for drainage of aqueous from anterior chamber into subconjunctival space.

Surgical technique. Trabeculectomy is described in Chapter 20 (see page 311)

4. *Clear lens extraction* by phacoemulsification with intraocular lens implantation has recently been recommended by some workers especially in the presence of phacomorphic etiology of angle-closure (diagnosed on UBM and anterior segment OCT examination). However, these are ethical issues related to clear lens extraction. Beyond doubt in the presence of cataract, lens extraction should be preferred.

C. ***Prophylactic treatment in the normal fellow eye*** should always be advised.

Prophylactic laser iridotomy (preferably) or surgical peripheral iridectomy should be performed on the fellow asymptomatic eye as early as possible.

Note. Chances of acute attack are 50% in such eyes.

D. ***Long-term glaucoma surveillance and IOP management in both eyes*** of a patient with acute PAC is must to ultimately prevent glaucomatous blindness.

- *Eyes treated with LPI* (both affected and fellow eyes) may develop PACG at any time. So it should be treated as and when required.
- *Filtration surgery* may fail any time during the course and hence need to be repeated with antimetabolites.

Sequelae of acute PAC

The clinical status of the eye after an attack of acute PAC with or without treatment is considered a sequela of acute PAC. It may be seen as following clinical settings:

1. ***Postsurgical acute PAC.*** This refers to the clinical status of the eye after laser peripheral iridotomy (LPI) treatment for an attack of acute PAC. It may occur in two clinical settings:

i. *With normalized IOP* after successful laser PI, the eye usually quitens after some time with or without marks of an acute attack (i.e. Vogt's triad, see below).

ii. *With raised IOP* after unsuccessful laser PI, which needs to be treated by trabeculectomy operation.

2. ***Spontaneous angle reopening*** may very rarely occur in some cases and the attack of acute PAC may subside itself without treatment.

- *Treatment* of choice for such cases is laser peripheral iridotomy.

3. ***Ciliary body shut down.*** It refers to temporary cessation of aqueous humour secretion due to ischaemic damage to the ciliary epithelium after an attack of acute PAC.

Clinical features in this stage are similar to acute PAC except that the IOP is low and pain is markedly reduced. Subsequent recovery of ciliary function may lead to chronic elevation of IOP with cupping and visual field defects, i.e. conversion to PACG.

Treatment includes:

- *Topical steroid drops* to reduce inflammation.
- *Laser iridotomy* should be performed when the cornea becomes clear and IOP should be monitored.
- *Trabeculectomy* is required when IOP rises constantly in spite of LPI.

4. *Vogt's triad.* It may be seen in both treated and non-treated cases after an attack of acute PAC. It is characterized by (Fig. 15.10):

- *Glaukomflecken,* i.e. anterior subcapsular lenticular opacity, may appear in the pupillary area following sudden and sustained rise in IOP. These opacities represent areas of lens epithelium necrosis. These are permanent, become dense with time and move deeper in to the anterior cortex.
- *Patches of sectoral iris atrophy.* These result from sector ischaemia of the iris due to closure of iris stromal vessels.
- *Slightly dilated non-reacting pupil* (due to sphincter atrophy).

III. PRIMARY ANGLE-CLOSURE GLAUCOMA

Primary angle-closure glaucoma (PACG) can be considered to replace the term 'chronic primary angle-closure glaucoma' used in clinical classification.

Pathogenesis

Primary angle-closure glaucoma (PACG) results from gradual synaechial closure of the angle of anterior chamber. Untreated patients with PAC may over the period convert to PACG with or without history of subacute or acute attack of PAC.

Clinical features

Clinical features given below are similar to POAG except that angle is narrow:

- *Intraocular pressure (IOP)* remains constantly raised.
- *Eyeball* remains white (no congestion) and painless, except in post-acute angle-closure cases where the eye may be congested and irritable.
- *Optic disc* shows glaucomatous cupping.
- *Visual field defects* similar to POAG occur.
- *Gonioscopy* reveals more than 270° of angle closure along with PAS. The gonioscopic findings provide the only differentiating feature between POAG and chronic PACG.
- *Vogt's triad.* Features of Vogt's triad (Fig. 15.10) may be present in patients having PACG with history of acute PAC in the past.

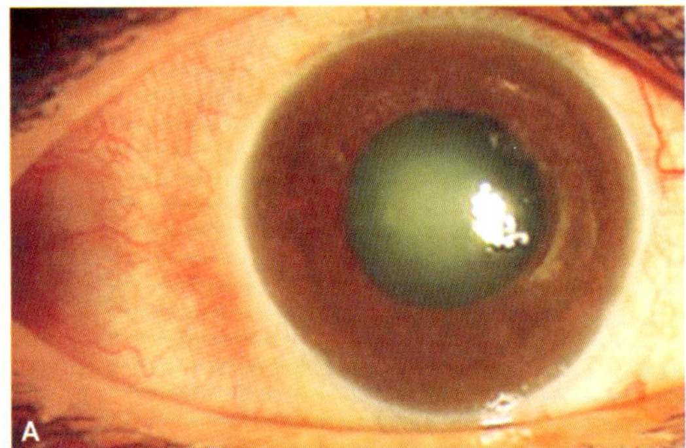

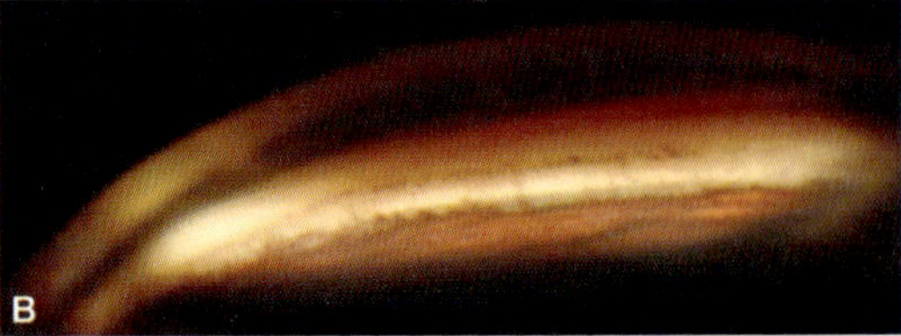

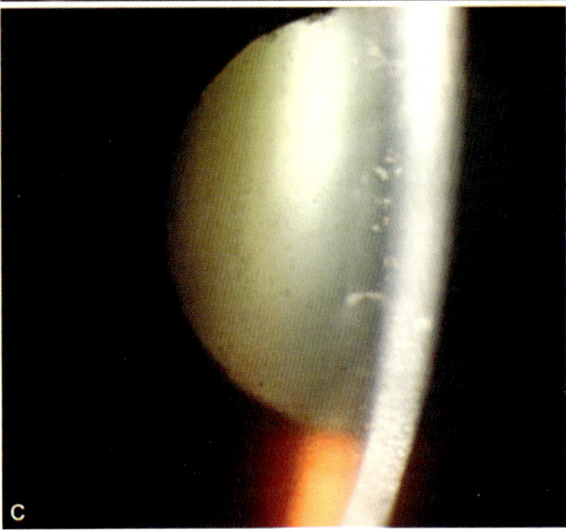

Fig. 15.10 *Primary angle-closure: (A) Patchy iris atrophy and semidilated pupil; (B) Trabecular meshwork pigmentation on gonioscopy suggestive of past attack of angle-closure; (C) Glaucomflecken*

Defining criteria, as per ISGEO classification, for primary angle-closure glaucoma are:

- *Iridotrabecular contact* noted on gonioscopy is greater than 270° of angle
- *PAS* is formed
- *IOP* is elevated
- *Optic disc* shows glaucomatous damage, and
- *Visual fields* show typical glaucomatous defects.

Impression: Angle is abnormal in function (elevated IOP) and structure (PAS +ve) with optic neuropathy.

Note. In circumstances where advanced PACG disease with compromised media prohibits disc and visual field testing, e.g. cataract or corneal disease, a coarser definition holds for PACG whereby an IOP >24 mm Hg and visual acuity of <3/60 or a history of prior glaucoma surgery, will suffice.

Investigations and treatment

Investigations include:

- Gonioscopy
- Anterior segment imaging with UBM and ASOCT

Treatment consists of:

- *Laser iridotomy* alone or along with medical therapy similar to POAG should be tried first.
- *Trabeculectomy* (filtration surgery) is needed when the above treatment fails to control IOP.
- *Prophylactic laser iridotomy* in fellow eye must also be performed.

Sequelae of Primary Angle-closure Glaucoma

Primary angle-closure glaucoma, when untreated, gradually passes into the final phase of absolute primary angle closure glaucoma.

Clinical features

- *Painful blind eye.* The eye is painful, irritable and completely blind (no light perception).
- *Perilimbal reddish blue zone,* i.e. a slight ciliary flush around the cornea due to dilated anterior ciliary veins.
- *Caput medusae,* i.e., a few prominent and enlarged vessels are seen in long-standing cases.
- *Cornea* in early cases is clear but insensitive. Slowly it becomes hazy and may develop epithelial bullae (bullous keratopathy) or filaments (filamentary keratitis).
- *Anterior chamber* is very shallow.
- *Iris* becomes atrophic.
- *Pupil* becomes fixed and dilated and gives a greenish hue.
- *Optic disc* shows glaucomatous optic atrophy.
- *Intraocular pressure* is high; eyeball becomes stony hard.

Management of absolute glaucoma

1. *Retrobulbar alcohol injection:* It may be given to relieve pain. First, 1 ml of 2% xylocaine is injected followed after about 5–10 minutes by 1 ml of 80% alcohol. It destroys the ciliary ganglion.
2. *Destruction of secretory ciliary epithelium* to lower the IOP may be carried out by *cyclocryotherapy* or *cyclodiathermy* or *cyclophotocoagulation.*

Complications

When not treated, due to prolonged high IOP, following complications may occur:

1. *Corneal ulceration.* It results from prolonged epithelial oedema and insensitivity. Sometimes, corneal ulcer may even perforate.
2. *Staphyloma formation.* As a result of continued high IOP, sclera becomes very thin and atrophic and ultimately bulges out either in the ciliary region (ciliary staphyloma) or equatorial region (equatorial staphyloma).
3. *Atrophic bulbi.* Ultimately, the ciliary body degenerates, IOP falls, and the eyeball shrinks.

SUGGESTED READING

1. American Academy of Ophthalmology, Preferred Practice Pattern. San Francisco, Primary Angle Closure, 2005.
2. Bonomi L, Marchini G, Marrafa M, et al. Epidemiology of angle-closure glaucoma. Prevalence, clinical types, and association with peripheral anterior chamber depth in the Egna-Neumarkt Glaucoma Study. Ophthalmology 2000;107:998–1003.
3. Cheng JW, Zong Y, Zeng YY, Wei RL. The prevalence of primary angle closure glaucoma in adult asians: a systematic review and meta-analysis. PLoS One 2014 Jul 24;9(7):e103222.
4. Dandona L, Dandona R, Mandal P, et al. Angle-closure glaucoma in an urban population in southern India. The Andhra Pradesh Eye Disease Study. Ophthalmology 2000;107:1710–16.
5. Foster PJ, Buhrmann R, Quigley HA, Johnson GJ. The definition and classification of glaucoma in prevalence surveys. Br J Ophthalmol 2002;86:238–42.
6. Quigley HA, Silver DM, Friedman DS, et al. Iris volume decreases with pupil dilation and its dynamic behavior is a potential risk factor in angle closure. J Glaucoma 2009;18:173–179.

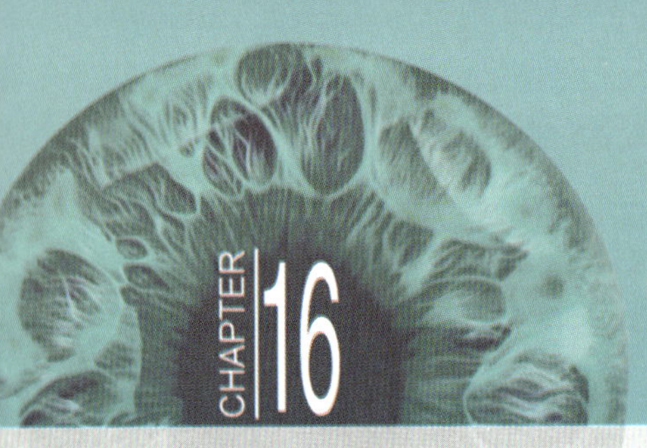

PRIMARY OPEN-ANGLE GLAUCOMA AND RELATED CONDITIONS

PRIMARY OPEN-ANGLE GLAUCOMA

DEFINITION AND EPIDEMIOLOGY

DEFINITION OF POAG

American Academy of Ophthalmology (2005)-POAG-Preferred Practice Pattern defines primary open-angle glaucoma (POAG) as a multifactorial, progressive chronic optic neuropathy of adult onset typically characterized by:

- Characteristic acquired optic disc changes
- Specific visual field defects
- Slowly progressive raised IOP (>21 mm Hg recorded at least a few occasion) as the main risk factor.
- Open, normal appearing anterior chamber angle on gonioscopy, and
- Absence of identifiable contributing systemic or ocular factors of the secondary open-angle glaucomas (e.g. pigment dispersion, pseudo-exfoliation, etc.).

EPIDEMIOLOGY

Salient points regarding epidemiology of POAG are:

- Glaucoma is the second most frequent cause of blindness, after cataract.
- Most common single form of glaucoma world-wide is POAG. More than 2 million people develop the disease each year.

- Worldwide, more than 3 million people are bilaterally blind because of POAG.
- Prevalence ratio of POAG versus PACG reported for different ethnic groups is as below:

Ethnic groups	*POAG: PACG*
Europian, African and Hispanics	5:1
Indian	1:1
Urban Chinese	1:2
Mongolian	1:3

- Prevalence in general population older than 40 years worldwide is between 1 and 2% in the most studies. However, reports vary considerably according to the population studied and the diagnostic criteria and screening techniques used.
- Prevalence increases with increasing age, i.e. from 1–2% in above 40 years to up to 11% in those above 80 years.
- Prevalence of POAG reported in major Indian studies is shown in Table 16.1.
- Prevalence of POAG in blacks is three times the prevalence in whites.

ETIOPATHOGENESIS

Etiopathogenesis of POAG is not known exactly. Some of the facts which need to be considered are:

- Risk factors
- Pathogenesis of rise in IOP, and
- Pathogenesis of optic neuropathy

A. RISK FACTORS

I. **Major risk factors** identified for POAG in various studies are: Elevated IOP, older age, family history of glaucoma, race (African or Latino ancestry) and thinner central corneal thickness.

1. ***IOP.*** Elevated IOP is the most important and only modifiable risk factor for development of POAG. Population surveys also support the increase in prevalence of POAG with increasing IOP with following conclusions:

- Prevalence of POAG rises with increasing IOP.
- A person with IOP of 28 mm Hg is about 15 times more likely to develop visual field defects than a person with IOP of 22 mm Hg.
- IOP is the only risk factor amenable to intervention.
- Lowering of IOP, by whatever means, slows down the visual field loss.

2. ***Age.*** Advancing age is reported as an independent risk factor in overall population-based studies.

- People older than 40 years are at a greater risk to develop this disease.
- Subjects aged over 60 years are seven times more likely to develop POAG than those aged less than 40 years.
- Prevalence of POAG is reported to increase with advancing age, i.e. from 1 to 2% in above 40 years to even 11% above 80 years.
- Even in Japanese people in whom IOP does not increase with advancing age, POAG does increase in prevalence with age.
- The ocular hypertension treatment study (OHTS) revealed that age is also a risk factor for the conversion from ocular hypertension to POAG.

Table 16.1 *Prevalence of POAG in India reported in some popular studies*

	APEDS	*ACES*	*CGS (rural)*	*ACGS (urban)*	*WBGS*
40–49	1.27	0.34	0.63	2.26	-
50–59	2.31	1.57	1.62	3.57	2.55
60–69	4.89	1.83	2.58	4.08	2.69
> 70	6.32	2.88	3.25	6.42	4.76
Prevalence %	2.56	1.7	1.62	3.51	2.99

Possible reasons for higher prevalence with increasing age may be:

- Older people had elevated IOP for a larger period than younger people.
- Optic nerve may become more susceptible to damage due to microvascular perfusion defects.
- Altered connective tissue integrity of the lamina cribrosa with increasing age.

3. ***Race.*** Black race (African and Latino ancestry) is another important risk factor. POAG is significantly more common (4 to 8 times), develops earlier and is more severe in blacks than whites (accounting for 4 times more blindness in blacks than whites). Average prevalence of POAG reported in some races is as below:

- Blacks: 4.74%
- Whites: 1.29%
- South Indians: 1.6%
- Japanese: 0.58%
- Mongolian: 0.5%

Possible reasons for higher prevalence and aggressive nature of POAG among black races may include:

- Higher level of IOP in black population
- Large size of optic nerve head and higher incidence of vascular abnormalities of the optic nerve
- Increased central corneal thickness in blacks (OHTS).

4. ***Family history (hereditary)*** is also an important risk factor for POAG. The approximate risk of getting disease is 10 times in the siblings, and 4 times in the offsprings of the patients with POAG than the general population.

However, unlike juvenile open-angle glaucoma (JOAG), which is typically inherited as autosomal dominant, the genetics of POAG is complex. POAG has a polygenic inheritance. Approximately two dozen loci have been, identified for POAG. Among those, only three genes, myocilin (MYOC), optineurin (OPTN), and WD repeat domain 36 (WDR 36) have been cloned presently.

5. ***Corneal thickness.*** Thinner central corneal thickness (CCT) apart from causing IOP underestimation by Goldmann tonometry is being considered an independent and a significant risk factor for POAG. A person with a CCT of less than 555 µm has a three times greater risk of developing POAG as compared to a person with CCT of greater than 588 µm. OHTS found CCT to be a powerful predictor for the development of POAG from ocular hypertension (the relative risk of POAG increased 81% for every 40 microns thinner cornea). Whether a thin cornea per se makes an eye more susceptible to glaucoma is unclear.

II. Other risk factors which are not so strongly associated with POAG, such as IOP, age, race, family history and thinner cornea, but have been considered as important risk factors include the following:

1. ***Characteristics of optic nerve head*** have been implicated as a risk factor for glaucoma in several epidemiological studies. Large discs with high cup:disc ratios have been found to be a risk factor for field defects in Collaborative Initial Glaucoma Treatment Study (CIGTS). Both horizontal and vertical ratios correlate positively with subsequent field defects.

2. ***Myopia.*** It has been reported to be associated with POAG in many studies. A survey reported two- to three-fold increased prevalence of myopia in individuals with POAG. However, an association between myopia and development of POAG was not observed in OHTS. An association of POAG with myopia may complicate both diagnosis and management as below:

- Assessment of cupping becomes difficult of broad shallow cups, tilting of disc and posterior staphyloma in myopia. In addition, the magnification factor in myopia also interferes with optic disc evaluation.
- Unreliable tonometry, especially Schiotz, because of low ocular rigidity in myopia. Goldmann applanation tonometry gives false low reading because of thinner cornea in myopes.
- Visual field changes may become difficult to interpret due to defects caused by myopic retinal changes. Further, accurate perimetry evaluation and its interpretation becomes difficult due to high refractive error (refractive scotoma).

- It has been postulated that higher IOPs and alterations in the optic nerve collagen and extracellular matrix may be the possible contributory factors for the higher prevalence of glaucoma in myopia.

3. ***Diabetes mellitus.*** Higher prevalence of POAG as well as OHTN is reported among the diabetics in various studies, e.g. Blue Mountain Eye Study in Australia, the Rotterdam study and Bever Dam Eye study in Wisconsin. Though the explanation of relationship is not documented, some authorities believe that small vessel involvement in diabetes may render the optic disc more susceptible to glaucomatous damage. However, diabetes was not associated with an increased risk of progression to glaucoma in OHTS, though patients with retinopathy were not enrolled in the trial.

4. ***Cardiovascular disease.*** It has been reported that high blood pressure lowers the incidence of POAG and low blood pressure (to be more precise low perfusion pressure) increases the risk of POAG.

5. ***Thyroid diseases.*** An association between thyroid diseases and POAG, NTG and OHTN has been reported, possibly secondary to orbital changes and raised episcleral venous pressure.

6. ***Migraine.*** Some studies, such as The Blue Mountain Eye study, have reported association between migraine and NTG.

7. ***Sleep apnoea*** has been linked with POAG in some studies. It has been proposed that transient episodes of nocturnal hypoxia in patients with sleep apnoea may predispose the optic nerve to damage. However, many studies have not confirmed association between sleep apnoea and POAG.

B. PATHOGENESIS OF RISE IN IOP

Decreased aqueous outflow facility beyond doubt increases the resistance to aqueous outflow leading to a rise in the IOP.

Sites of the increased resistance to the aqueous outflow in POAG are trabecular meshwork and endothelium of Schlemm's canal. It has been hypothesized that the main site of resistance to the aqueous outflow is probably in juxtacanalicular meshwork.

Possible causes of increased resistance to aqueous outflow

- *Accumulation of foreign material* in the trabecular meshwork and juxtacanalicular tissue is being considered an important cause of increased resistance to aqueous out flow. The accumulated foreign materials include glycosaminoglycan, amorphous material, pigment and extracellular lysosomes.
- *Loss of trabecular endothelial cells* is reported in glaucomatous eyes as compared to normal eyes leading to depression in the normal functioning.
- *Loss of giant vacuoles in the inner wall endothelium* of Schlemm's canal reported by some workers accounts for increased outflow.
- *Reduction in pore density and size* in the inner wall of Schlemm's canal has been reported by some workers as cause of increased resistance to aqueous outflow.

Changes in the trabecular meshwork and other components of the conventional aqueous drainage reported on histopathological studies on the tissue obtained during surgeries in patients with POAG include:

- Thickening and sclerosis of trabecular meshwork with faulty collagen tissue
- Narrowing of intratrabecular spaces
- Accumulation of amorphous material in the juxtacanalicular tissue
- Collapse of Schlemm's canal and absence of gain vacuole in the endothelium cells limiting it
- Narrowing of collector channels.

Mechanism of changes in aqueous outflow system

Mechanisms suggested for changes in the aqueous outflow system are:

1. ***Theory of acceleration of normal aging process.*** The aforementioned histopathological changes reported to corroborate the hypothesis regarding possible causes of increased resistance to aqueous outflow. Probably all the factors contribute to increased resistance. Further,

similar changes are also reported in older, nonglaucomatous eye. Consequently, workers have proposed that the changes reported in the aqueous outflow system of patients with POAG could be an acceleration of the normal aging process.

2. ***Theory of immunogenic mechanism.*** Detection of increased gammaglobulin and plasma cells in trabecular meshwork on immunohistochemistry and positive antinuclear antibody reaction in some cases support an immunogenic mechanism in POAG.

3. ***Theory of altered corticosteroid metabolism*** has also been reported to contribute to the changes in the trabecular meshwork. Researchers postulated that endogenous corticosteroids affected trabecular meshwork function by altering prostaglandin metabolism, glycosaminoglycan catabolism, release of lysosomal enzymes, synthesis of cyclic adenosine monophosphate or inhibition of phagocytosis.

4. ***Theory of dysfunctional adrenergic control*** in the form of increased sensitivity to adrenergic agonists has been suggested as a cause of diminished outflow facility in patients with POAG. While other workers have failed to confirm an increased sensitivity to adrenergic agonists.

5. ***Theory of oxidative damage.*** It has been reported that the trabecular meshwork contains glutathione. Which may be protective to the endothelial cells from the effect of oxidants including hydrogen peroxide (H_2O_2). It is being postulated that the oxidative insults secondary to inactivation of protective mechanism may be responsible for the changes trabecular meshwork leading to increased resistance to aqueous outflow.

6. ***Theory of toxic influence of transforming growth factor (TGF)*** has also been postulated in the pathogenesis of trabecular meshwork changes in POAG. It has been shown that there occurs a three-fold increase in the aqueous plasminogen activator inhibitor in the aqueous humour of patients with POAG as compared to normal patients; indicating thereby that perhaps this protein may play some role in the pathogenesis of POAG.

Summary of pathogenesis of rise in IOP

- Rise in IOP occurs due to increased resistance to aqueous outflow.
- Juxtacanalicular trabecular meshwork is probably the main site of increased resistance.
- The exact cause of trabecular dysfunction is still not clear.
- No single theory can explain the pathogenesis of rise in IOP.

C. PATHOGENESIS OF OPTIC NEUROPATHY

It has now been recognized that progressive optic neuropathy results from the death of retinal ganglion cells (RGCs) in a typical pattern which results in characteristic optic disc appearance and corresponding visual field defects.

Pathogenesis of retinal ganglion cell death

Retinal ganglion cell death is initiated when some pathologic event blocks the transport of growth factors (neurotrophins) from the brain to the RGCs.

The blockage of these neurotrophins initiates a damaging cascade, and the cell is unable to maintain its normal function. The RGCs losing their ability to maintain normal function undergo apoptosis and also trigger apoptosis of adjacent cells. Apoptosis is a genetically controlled cell suicide programme whereby irreversibly damaged cells die, and are subsequently engulfed by neighbouring cells, without eliciting any inflammatory response.

Retinal ganglion cell death is, of course, associated with loss of retinal nerve fibres. As the loss of nerve fibres extends beyond the normal physiological overlap of functional zones, the characteristic optic disc changes and specific visual field defects become apparent over the time.

Etiological factors

Factors involved in the etiology of retinal ganglion cell death and thus in the etiology of glaucomatous optic neuropathy can be grouped as below.

A. Primary insults

1. ***Mechanical theory.*** Raised IOP causes mechanical stretch on the lamina cribrosa leading to axonal deformation and ischaemia by altering capillary blood flow. As a result of this, neurotrophins (growth factors) are notable to reach the retinal ganglion cell bodies insufficient amount needed for their survival.

Concept of translaminar pressure. The mechanical theory stresses on the effect of raised IOP on lamina cribrosa, which is considered the initiating site of glaucomatous optic nerve damage. Now the stress is being laid on the concept of translaminar pressure. The lamina separates the higher IOP space anteriorly from the lower subarachanoid pressure space posteriorly. The pressure difference between the two spaces is called translaminar pressure, it is being stated that this pressure accounts for the damage to the RGC axons at the level of lamina. In this context, a reduced CSF pressure in the subarachnoid space would exert the same effect as raised IOP. A low CSF pressure has been reported in patients with POAG as well as NTG as compared to control. This data, although preliminary, suggests that the dynamic interplay between these fluid spaces may explain why some individuals with normal IOP may develop glaucoma and others with elevated IOP may not.

2. *Vascular insufficiency theory*. Factors affecting vascular perfusion of optic nerve head in the absence of raised IOP have been implicated in the glaucomatous optic neuropathy in patients with NTG. However, these may be the additional factors in cases of raised IOP as well. These factors include:

i. *Failure of autoregulatory mechanism of blood flow*. The retina and optic nerve share a peculiar mechanism of autoregulation of blood flow with rest of the central nervous system. Once the autoregulatory mechanisms are compromised, blood flow may not be adequate beyond some critical range of IOP (which may be raised or in normal range).

ii. *Vasospasm* is another mechanism affecting vascular perfusion of optic nerve head. This hypothesis gets credence from the convincing association between NTG and vasospastic disorders (migranous headache and Raynaud's phenomenon).

iii. *Systemic hypotension* particularly nocturnal dips in patients with nigh-time administration of antihypertensive drugs has been implicated for low vascular perfusion of optic nerve head resulting in NTG and progression of damage in patients with POAG.

iv. *Other factors,* such as acute blood loss and abnormal coagulability profile have also been associated with NTG.

B. Secondary insults (excitotoxicity theory)

Neuronal degeneration is believed to be driven by toxic factors, such as glutamate (excitatory toxin), oxygen free radicals, or nitric oxide, which are released when RGCs undergo death due to primary insults as described above. In this way, the secondary insult leads to continued damage mediated apoptosis, even after the primary insult has been controlled.

Summary of pathogenesis of optic neuropathy

It seems that the glaucomatous optic neuropathy is multifactorial, and, at different times and in different eyes, may involve:

- Genetic susceptibility factors
- Mechanical factors including concept of translaminar pressure
- Loss of neuropathic factors and neurotoxicity
- Inability of the astroglial cells to prevent or repair injury to the ganglion cells or its extracellular matrix regardless of the source of initial insult.

CLINICAL FEATURES

SYMPTOMS

1. *Asymptomatic*. The disease is rightly called the "Sneak thief of sight" as it is insidious and usually asymptomatic, until it has caused a significant loss of visual field. Therefore, periodic eye examination is required after middle age. The few exceptions to this rule include the occasional patients who may notice some of the symptoms described below.

2. *Headache and eyeache* of mild intensity may be experienced in the course of the disease.

3. *Scotoma* (defect in the visual field) may be noticed occasionally by some observant patients.

4. ***Difficulty in reading and close work,*** often persistently increasing, is experienced by most patients. This occurs due to increasing accommodative failure as a result of constant pressure on the ciliary muscle and its nerve supply. Therefore, patients usually complain of frequent changes in presbyopic glasses.

5. ***Halo vision and discomfort*** may occasionally be reported by young patients who develop sudden and severe rise in IOP with corneal oedema.

6. ***Delayed dark adaptation*** may develop, a disability which becomes increasingly disturbing in the late stages.

7. ***Significant loss of vision and blindness*** is the end result of undiagnosed and/or untreated cases of POAG.

SIGNS

I. Anterior segment signs

Ocular examination including slit-lamp biomicroscopy may reveal normal anterior segment.

Pupillary signs. Relative afferent pupillary defect (RAPD) may be seen in patients with asymmetric or unilateral glaucoma. In late stages, pupil reflex becomes sluggish.

Corneal signs. Cornea may show slight haze. A thin (<555 μm) central corneal thickness (CCT) is a significant risk factor for POAG.

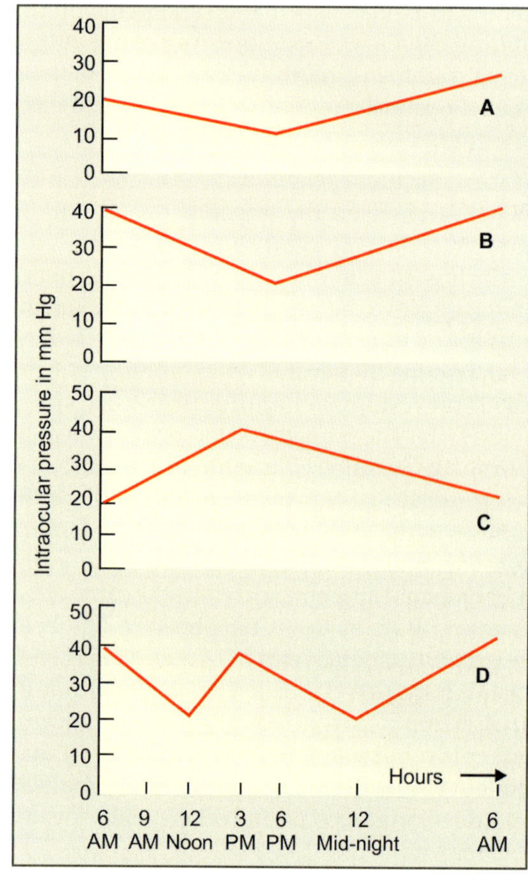

Fig. 16.1 *Patterns of diurnal variations of IOP: A, normal slight morning rise; B, morning rise seen in 20% cases of POAG; C, afternoon rise seen in 25% cases of POAG; D, biphasic variation seen in 55% cases of POAG*

II. Intraocular pressure changes

In the initial stages, the IOP may not be raised permanently, but there is an exaggeration of the normal diurnal variation. Therefore, repeated observations of IOP (every 3–4 hour), for 24 hours, is required during this stage (Diurnal variation test; DVT). In most patients, IOP falls during the evening, contrary to what happens in closed-angle glaucoma. Different patterns of diurnal variation of IOP shown in Fig. 16.1 are:

- Morning rise in IOP—20% of cases
- Afternoon rise in IOP—25% of cases
- Biphasic rise in IOP—55% of cases

A variation in IOP of over 6 mm Hg is suspicious and over 8 mm Hg is suggestive of glaucoma. In later stages, IOP is permanently raised above 21 mm Hg and ranges between 30 and 45 mm Hg. Most patients have fairly symmetric IOP readings, but asymmetric POAG does occur.

III. Glaucomatous Optic disc changes

Optic disc changes, usually observed on routine fundus examination, provide an important clue for suspecting POAG. These are typically progressive, asymmetric and present a variety of characteristic clinical patterns. It is essential, therefore, to record the appearance of the nerve head in such a way that will accurately reveal subtle glaucomatous changes over the course of follow-up evaluation.

Examination and recording techniques

Examination techniques. Careful assessment of disc changes can be made by direct ophthalmoscopy, slit-lamp biomicroscopy using a +90D lens or a +78D (best method) or +60D lens.

Recording and documentation techniques include:

- Serial drawings, photography and photogrammetry.
- *Confocal scanning laser topography (CSLT)*, i.e. Heidelberg retinal tomograph (HRT) is an accurate and sensitive method for this purpose.
- *Other advanced imaging techniques* include optical coherence tomography (OCT) and scanning laser polarimetry, i.e. Nerve Fibre Analyser (NFA; GDx).

Note. These techniques are described in detail in Chapters 8 and 9.

Description of glaucomatous disc changes

Glaucomatous changes in the optic disc can be described as early changes, advanced changes and glaucomatous optic atrophy. Figure 16.2 shows normal disc configuration.

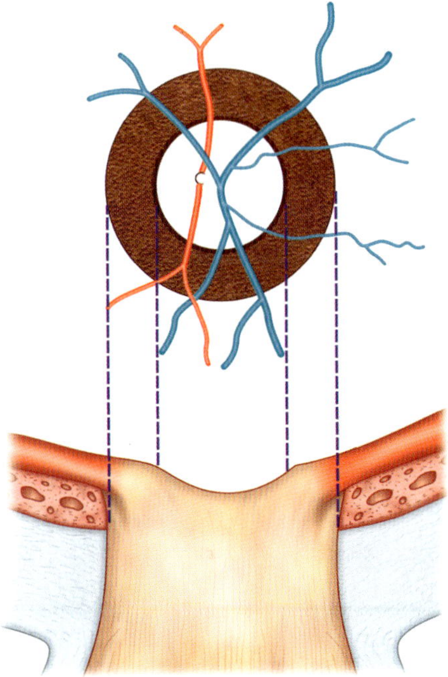

Fig. 16.2 *Normal disc configuration*

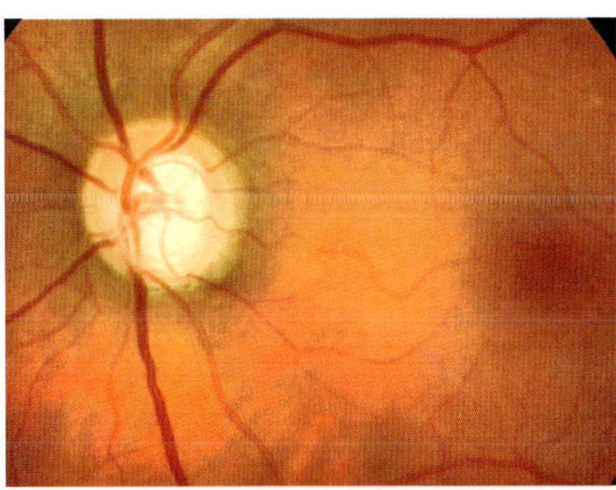

Fig. 16.3 *Inferior notching of the disc*

A. *Early glaucomatous changes* should be suspected to exist, if fundus examination reveals one or more of the following signs:

- *Vertically oval cup* due to selective loss of neural rim tissue in the inferior and superior poles (Fig. 16.3).
- *Asymmetry of the cups.* A difference of more than 0.2 between two eyes is significant.
- *Large cup*, i.e. 0.6 or more (normal cup size is 0.3 to 0.4) may occur due to concentric expansion.
- *Splinter haemorrhages* present on or near the optic disc margin (Fig. 16.4).
- *Pallor areas* on the disc.
- *Atrophy of retinal nerve fibre layer* which may be seen with red free light.

B. *Advanced glaucomatous changes in the optic disc* include:

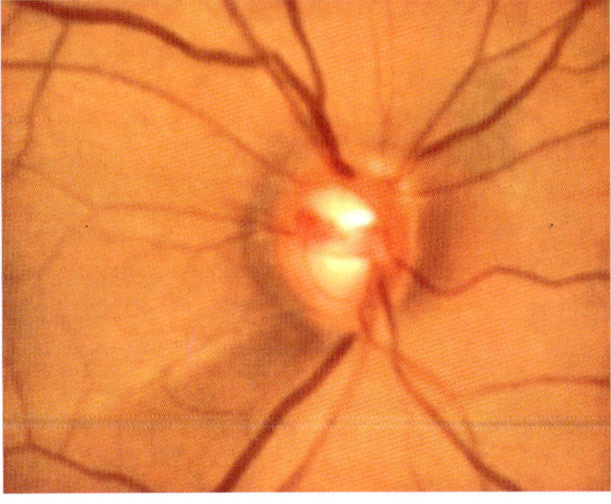

Fig. 16.4 *Splinter haemorrhage*

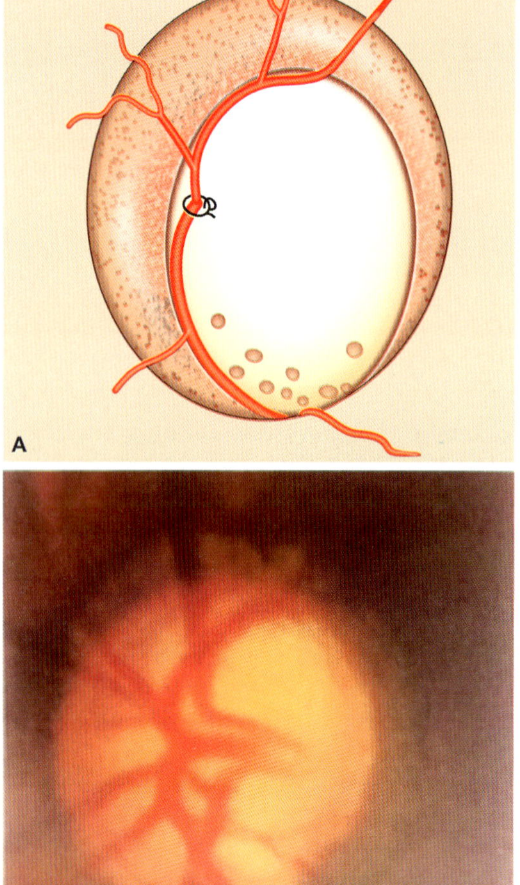

Fig. 16.5 *Excavation of the cup involving the disc margin: (A) Diagrammatic depiction; (B) Disc photograph*

- *Marked cupping* (cup size 0.7 to 0.9), excavation may even reach the disc margin, the sides are steep and not shelving (c.f. deep physiological cup) (Fig. 16.5).
- *Thinning of neuroretinal rim* which occurs in advanced cases is seen as a crescentic shadow adjacent to the disc margin. Normally, the thickest to thinnest parts of the neuroretinal rim of the optic disc are inferior, superior, nasal and temporal (ISNT rule). Any variation from this helps to detect glaucoma. Notching of the rim specially the disc margin is pathognomonic.
- *Nasal shifting of retinal vessels* which have the appearance of being broken off at the margin is an important sign (Bayonetting sign). When the edges overhang, the course of the vessels as they climb the sides of the cup is hidden.
- *Pulsations of the retinal arterioles* may be seen at the disc margin (a pathognomonic sign of glaucoma), when IOP is very high.
- *Lamellar dot sign*. The pores in the lamina cribrosa are slit-shaped and are visible up to the margin of the disc.

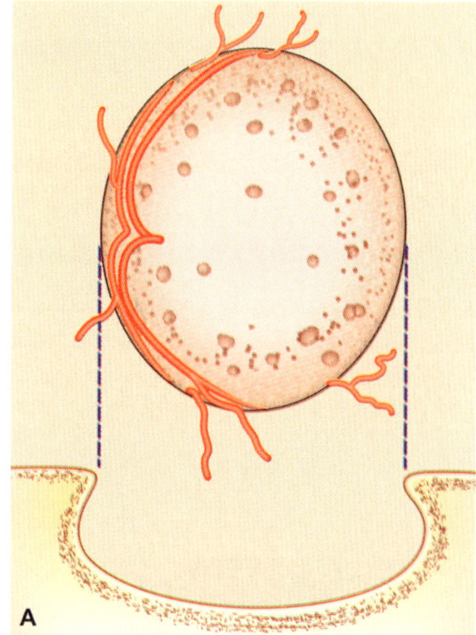

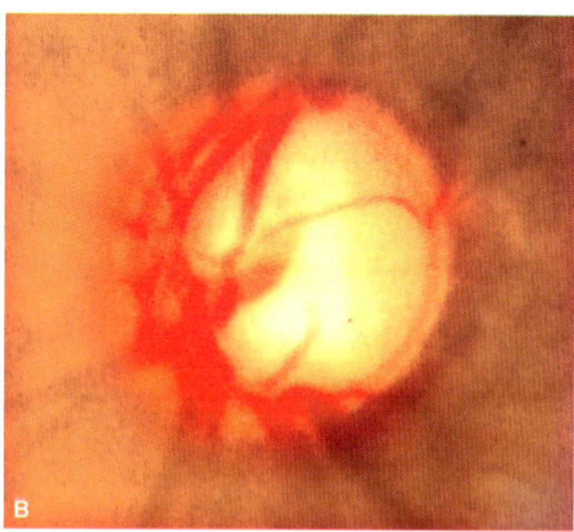

Fig. 16.6 *Bean pot cupping (glaucomatous optic atrophy) (A) Diagrammatic depiction; (B) Disc photograph*

C. ***Glaucomatous optic atrophy.*** As the damage progresses, all the neural tissues of the disc are destroyed and the optic nerve head appears white and deeply excavated (Fig. 16.6).

IV. Glaucomatous visual field defects

Visual field defects appear only after about 40% of axons have been damaged and subsequently the field defects usually run parallel to the changes at the optic nerve head and continue to progress, if IOP is not controlled. These can be described as early and late field defects.

Anatomical basis of field defects

For better understanding of the actual field defects, it is mandatory to have a knowledge of their anatomical basis.

A. ***Distribution of retinal nerve fibres*** (Fig. 16.7).

- Fibres from nasal half of the retina come directly to the optic disc as superior and inferior *radiating fibres* (srf and irf).
- Fibres from the macular area come horizontally as *papillomacular* bundle (pmb).
- Fibres from the temporal retina arch above and below the macula and papillomacular bundle as superior and inferior *arcuate fibres* with a horizontal raphe in between (saf and iaf).

B. ***Arrangement of nerve fibres within optic nerve head*** (Fig. 16.8). Those from the peripheral part of the retina lie deep in the retina but occupy the most peripheral (superficial) part of the optic disc. While fibres originating closer to the nerve head lie superficially in the retina and occupy a more central (deep) portion of the disc. The arcuate nerve fibres occupy the superior and inferior temporal portions of optic nerve head and are most sensitive to glaucomatous damage; accounting for the early loss in the corresponding regions of the visual field. Macular fibres are most resistant to the glaucomatous damage and explain the retention of the central vision till end.

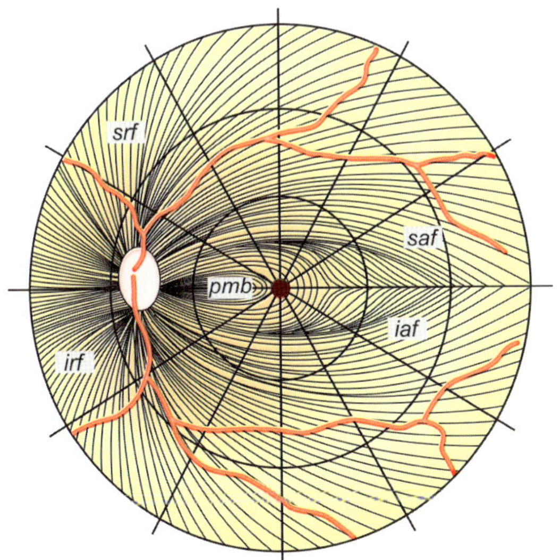

Fig. 16.7 *Distribution of retinal nerve fibre layers*

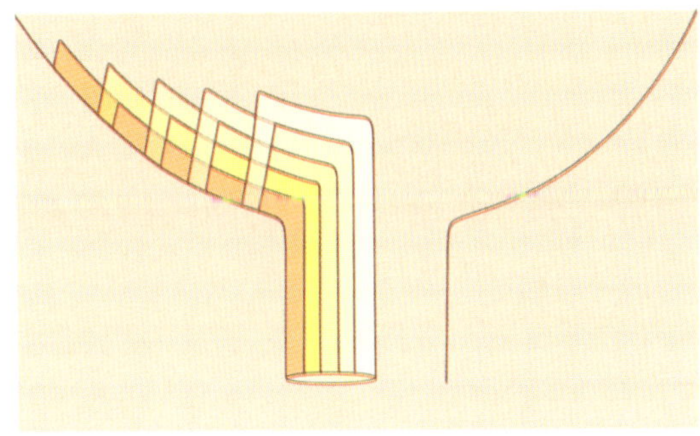
Fig. 16.8 *Arrangement of nerve fibres within the optic nerve head*

Progression of field defects

Visual field defects in glaucoma are initially observed in Bjerrum's area (10–25° from fixation) and correlate with optic disc changes. The natural history of the progressive glaucomatous field loss, more or less, takes the following sequence:

1. ***Isopter contraction.*** It refers to mild generalized constriction of central as well as peripheral field. It is the earliest visual field defect occurring in glaucoma. However, it is of limited diagnostic value, as it may also occur in many other conditions.

2. ***Baring of blind spot.*** It is also considered to be an early glaucomatous change, but is very non-specific and thus of limited diagnostic value. Baring of the blind spot means exclusion of the blind spot from the central field due to inward curve of the outer boundary of 30° central field (Fig. 16.9A).

3. ***Small wing-shaped paracentral scotoma*** (Fig.16.9B). It is the earliest clinically significant

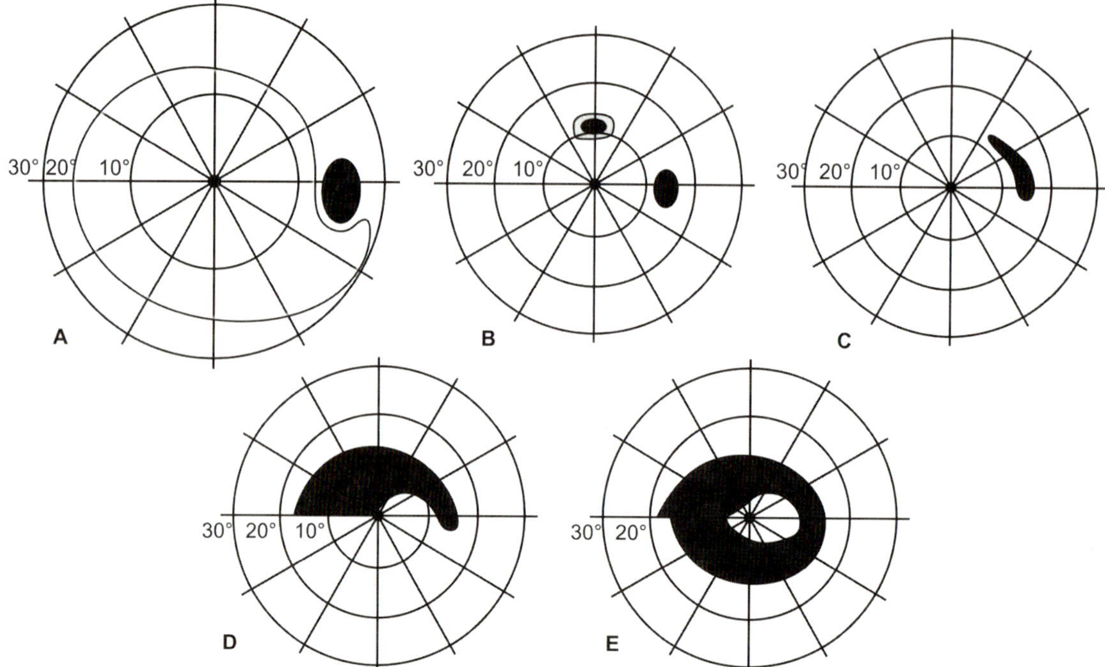

Fig. 16.9. *Field defects in glaucoma: (A) Baring of blind spot; (B) Superior paracentral scotoma; (C) Seidel's scotoma; (D) Bjerrum's scotoma; (E) Double arcuate scotoma and Roenne's central nasal step*

field defect. It may appear either below or above the blind spot in Bjerrum's area (an arcuate area extending above and below the blind spot to between 10° and 20° of fixation point).

4. ***Seidel's scotoma.*** With the passage of time, paracentral scotoma joins the blind spot to form a sickle-shaped scotoma known as Seidel's scotoma (Fig. 16.9C).

5. ***Arcuate or Bjerrum's scotoma.*** It is formed at a later stage by the extension of Seidel's scotoma in an area either above or below the fixation point to reach the horizontal line (Fig. 16.9D). Damage to the adjacent fibres causes a peripheral breakthrough.

6. ***Ring or double arcuate scotoma.*** It develops when the two arcuate scotomas join together (Fig. 16.9E).

7. ***Roenne's central nasal step.*** It is created when the two arcuate scotomas run in different arcs and meet to form a sharp right-angled defect at the horizontal meridian (Fig. 16.9E).

8. ***Peripheral field defects.*** These appear some times at an early stage and sometimes only late in the disease. The peripheral nasal step of Roenne's results from unequal contraction of the peripheral isopter.

9. ***Advanced glaucomatous field defects.*** The visual field loss gradually spreads centrally as well as peripherally, and eventually only a small island of central vision (tubular vision) and an accompanying temporal island are left. With the continued damage, these islands of vision also progressively diminish in size until the tiny central island is totally extinguished. The temporal island of the vision is more resistant and is lost in the end leaving the patient with no light perception.

Diagnosis of glaucoma field defects on HFA single field printout

Glaucomatous field defects should always be interpreted in conjunction with clinical features (IOP and optic disc changes). Further, before final interpretation, the fields must be tested twice, as there is often a significant improvement in the field when plotted second time (because patients become more familiar with the machine and test process).

Table 16.2 *Hodapp-Anderson-Parrish criteria for glaucomatous field defects*

Parameter	*Criteria for glaucomatous field defects*		
	Early defects	*Moderate defects*	*Severe defects*
Mean deviation (MD)	< – 6 dB	– 6 dB – 12 dB	> – 12 dB
Corrected pattern standard deviation (CPSD)	Depressed to p < 5%	Depressed to p <5%	Depressed to the p <5%
Pattern deviation plot			
• Points depressed below the p <5% or	<18 (25%)	<37 (50%)	>37 (>50%)
• Points depressed below the p <1%	<10	<20	>20
Glaucoma hemifield test (GHT)	Outside normal limits	Outside normal limits	Outside normal limits
Sensitivity in central 5 degrees	No point <15 dB	One hemifield may have point with sensitivity <15 dB No point has 0 dB	Both hemifields have points with sensiti-vity <15 dB Any point has 0 dB

Criteria to grade glaucomatous field defects. The criteria to label early, moderate and severe glaucomatous field defects from the HFA central 30-2 test, single printout is depicted in Table 16.2.

Note. For proper understanding of Table 16.2, evaluation of the Humphrey single field printout described on page 147–154. Chapter 10, should be revised. For details of visual field defects and perimetry, see Chapter 10.

OCULAR ASSOCIATIONS

POAG may sometimes be associated with:

- High myopia
- Fuchs' endothelial dystrophy
- Retinitis pigmentosa
- Central retinal vein occlusion, and
- Primary retinal detachment.

INVESTIGATIONS AND DIAGNOSIS

1. *Tonometry.* Goldmann applanation tonometry is the gold standard for measurement of IOP. (for details see Chapter 6).

2. *Central corneal thickness* (CCT) measurement is essential in the work-up for glaucoma since a thinner cornea underestimates and a thicker cornea overestimates the IOP on applanation tonometry. A low CCT (<545 microns) is an independent risk factor for conversion of OHTN to POAG.

3. *Diurnal variation test* is especially useful in detection of early cases.

- ***SENSIMED Triggerfish Contact lens sensor (CLS)*** (Lausanne, Switzerland), is a silicone soft contact lens, designed from the 1967 model. It monitors 24 hours ocular volume changes and IOP. It is a FDA approved device and consists of a silicone lens incorporating 2 platinum-titanium sensing-resistive strain micro-gauges which record circumferential changes in the corneoscleral junction, microprocessor and an antenna. With dimensions of 14.1 mm diameter, 585 μm cen-tral and 260 μm peripheral thickness, it is available in steep (8.4 mm), regular (8.7 mm) and flat (9 mm) base curves.
- Power is derived from and information transmitted to antenna adhered to the patient's orbit. Information of 300 readings over a 30-second period every 5 minutes with aggregate 288 points over a 24-hour period, is transferred to a portable recorder, worn by the patient.
- Uses include:
  - Measurement of diurnal IOP without waking patient

- Useful in NTG (IOP in normal range), glaucoma progression (check fluctuations during 24 hours)
- IOP fluctuations with sleep and posture.

- ***Adverse effects*** include: Transient corneal staining, red eye, blurred vision. Concern remains of anti-glaucoma drug absorption, with Triggerfish CLS in situ.

4. ***Gonioscopy.*** It reveals a wide open angle of anterior chamber. Its primary importance in POAG is to rule out other forms of glaucoma (for details, see Chapter 7).

5. ***Documentation of optic disc changes*** is of utmost importance (for details see Chapters 8 and 9).

6. ***Slit-lamp examination*** of anterior segment to rule out causes of secondary open angle glaucoma.

7. ***Perimetry*** to detect the visual field defects (for details, see Chapter 10).

8. ***Nerve fibre layer analyzer*** (NFLA) is a recently introduced device which helps in detecting the glaucomatous damage to the retinal nerve fibre before the appearance of actual visual field changes and/or optic disc changes (for details, see Chapter 9).

9. ***Provocative tests*** are required in borderline cases. The test commonly performed is water drinking test. Other provocative tests not frequently performed include combined water drinking and tonography, bulbar pressure test, prescoline test and caffeine test.

Water drinking test. It is based on the theory that glaucomatous eyes have a greater response to water drinking. In it, after an 8-hour fast, baseline IOP is noted and the patient is asked to drink one litre of water, following which IOP is noted every 15 min for 1 hour. The maximum rise in IOP occurs in 15–30 min and returns to baseline level after 60 min in both normal and the glaucomatous eyes. A rise of 8 mm Hg or more is said to be diagnostic of POAG.

DIAGNOSIS

Depending upon the level of IOP, glaucomatous cupping of the optic disc and the visual field changes the patients are assigned to one of the following diagnostic entities (Fig. 16.10):

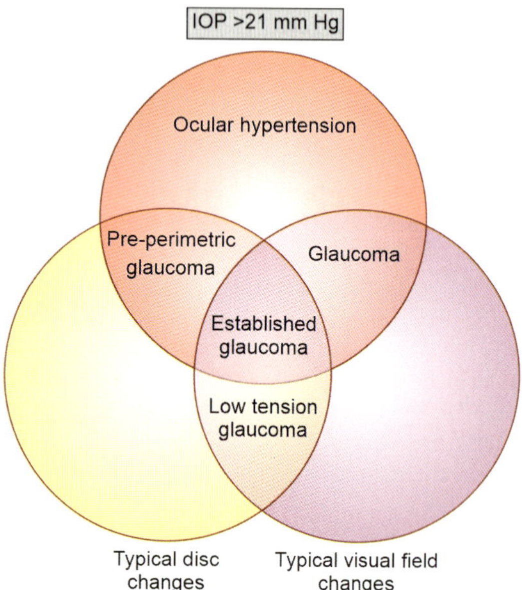

Fig. 16.10 *Triad of abnormalities in optic disc, visual fields and intraocular pressure for diagnosis of glaucoma*

1. ***Primary open-angle glaucoma; POAG.*** Characteristically, POAG is labelled when raised IOP (>21 mm Hg) is associated with definite glaucomatous optic disc cupping and visual field changes. Patients with raised IOP and typical disc changes but no field defects are also labelled as having ***pre-perimetric POAG***.

2. ***Ocular hypertension; OHTN.*** This term is used when a patient has an IOP constantly more than 21 mm Hg but no optic disc and visual field changes (for details, see page 227).

3. ***Normal tension glaucoma; NTG or low tension glaucoma; LTG.*** It is diagnosed when typical glaucomatous disc cupping with or without visual field changes is associated with an IOP consistantly below 21 mm Hg (for details, see page 230).

MANAGEMENT

BASELINE EVALUATION AND THERAPEUTIC OPTIONS

Baseline evaluation and grading of severity of glaucoma

The aim of treatment is to lower intraocular pressure to a level where (further) visual loss does not occur. The management thus requires careful and regular periodic supervision by an ophthalmologist. Therefore, it is important to perform a good baseline examination with which future progress can be compared. The initial data should include: visual acuity, slit-lamp examination of anterior segment, tonometry (preferably with an applanation tonometer); measurement of central corneal thickness, optic disc evaluation (preferably with fundus photography), gonioscopy and visual field charting.

American Academy of Ophthalmology (AAO) grades severity of glaucoma damage into mild, moderate and severe (Table 16.3).

Table 16.3 *Severity of glaucoma damage*

Degree	*Description*
Mild	Characteristic optic-nerve abnormalities are consistent with glaucoma but with normal visual field.
Moderate	Visual field abnormalities in one hemifield and not within 5° of fixation.
Severe	Visual-field abnormalities in both hemifields and within 5° of fixation

Source: AAO 2000

Therapeutic options

Therapeutic options include:

- Medical therapy,
- Selective laser trabeculoplasty or argon laser trabeculoplasty, and
- Surgical therapy.

A. MEDICAL THERAPY OF POAG

Initial therapy of POAG is still medical, with surgery as the last resort.

Basic principles of medical therapy of POAG

1. ***Identification of target pressure.*** From the baseline evaluation data, a 'target pressure' (below which glaucomatous damage is not likely to progress) should be identified for each patient. The target pressure is identified taking into account the severity of existing damage, the level of IOP, age and general health of the patient. Although it is not possible to predict the safe level of IOP, however, progression is uncommon if IOP is maintained at less than 16 to 18 mm Hg in patients having mild to moderate damage. Lower target pressures (12–14 mm Hg) are required in patients with severe damage.

2. ***Single drug therapy.*** One topically instilled antiglaucoma drug should be chosen after due consideration to the patient's personal and medical factors. If the initial drug chosen is ineffective or intolerable, it should be replaced by the drug of second choice.

3. ***Combination therapy.*** If one drug is not sufficient to control IOP, then a combination therapy with two or more drugs should be tried.

4. ***Monitoring of therapy*** by disc changes and field changes and tonometry is most essential on regular follow-up. In the event of progress of glaucomatous damage, the target pressure is reset at a lower level.

Treatment regimes

There are no clear-cut prescribed treatment regimens for medical therapy of POAG. However, at present, considerations are as follows:

Single drug therapy

1. ***Topical beta-blockers*** are being recommended as the first drug of choice for medical therapy of POAG in poor and average income patients. These lower IOP by reducing the aqueous secretion due to their effect on beta-2 receptors in the ciliary processes.

Preparations. In terms of effectiveness, there is little difference between various beta-blockers. However, each offers a slight advantage over the other, which may help in choosing the particular medication as follows:

- *Timolol maleate*, a non-selective beta blocker (0.25, 0.5%: 1–2 times/day), is most popular as initial therapy in patients who cannot afford prostaglandin therapy. However, it should not be used in patients having associated bronchial asthma and/or heart blocks.
- *Betaxolol* (0.25%: 2 times/day). Being a selective beta-1 blocker, it is preferred as initial

therapy in patients with asthma and other pulmonary problems.

- *Levobunolol* (0.25, 0.5%: 1–2 times/day). Its action lasts the longest and so is more reliable for once a day use than timolol.
- *Carteolol* (1%: 1–2 times/day). It raises triglycerides and lowers high density lipoproteins the least. Therefore, it is the best choice in patients with POAG having associated hyperlipidemias or atherosclerotic cardiovascular disease.

2. *Prostaglandin analogues.* These decrease the IOP by increasing the uveoscleral outflow of aqueous. Presently, prostaglandin analogues are the drug of first choice for the treatment of POAG (provided patient can afford to buy it). Further, these form a very good adjunctive drug to beta-blockers, dorzolamide and even pilocarpine when additional therapy is indicated. The available preparations include:

- Latanoprost (0.005%) to be used HS
- Travoprost (0.004%) to be used HS
- Bimatoprost (0.03%, a prostamide) to be used HS
- Unoprostone (0.15%) to be used BID
- Tafluoprost HS (0.0015%) to be used HS

3. *Adrenergic drugs.* Role in POAG is as follows:

i. *Epinephrine hydrochloride* (0.5, 1, 2%: 1–2 times/day) and dipivefrine hydrochloride (0.1%: 1–2 times/day). These drugs lower the IOP by increasing aqueous outflow by stimulating alpha receptors in the aqueous outflow system. These are characterized by a high allergic reaction rate. Their long-term use has also been recognized as a risk factor for failure of filtration glaucoma surgery. For these reasons, epinephrine compounds are no longer being used as first-line or second line drug. However, dipivefrine may be combined with beta-blockers in patients where other drugs are contraindicated.

ii. *Brimonidine* (0.2%; 0.15%; 0.1%: 3 times/day). It is a selective alpha-2-adrenergic agonist and lowers IOP by decreasing aqueous production and also by increasing uveoscleral outflow. Because of increased allergic reactions and tachyphylaxis rates, it is not considered the drug of first choice in POAG. It is used as second drug of choice and also for combination therapy with other drugs.

4. *Topical carbonic anhydrase inhibitors*

- *Dorzolamide* (2%: 3 times/day). It is a topical carbonic anhydrase inhibitor which lowers IOP by decreasing aqueous production by altering ion transport along the ciliary process epithelium.
- *Brinzolamide* (1%: 3 times/day). This is a recently introduced topical carbonic anhydrase inhibitor with better adverse effect profile than dorzolamide.

5. *Pilocarpine* (1, 2, 4%: 3–4 times/day). It is a very effective drug and had remained as the sheet anchor in the medical management of POAG for a long time. However, presently it is not preferred as it causes problems due to spasm of accommodation and miosis. Most, but not all, older patients tolerate pilocarpine very well; however, axial lenticular opacities when present preclude its use in many such patients. Therefore, presently pilocarpine is considered only as an adjunctive therapy where other combinations fail.

Mechanism of action. Pilocarpine contracts longitudinal muscle of ciliary body and opens spaces in trabecular meshwork, thereby mechanically increasing aqueous outflow.

Combination topical therapy

If one drug is not effective, then a combination of two drugs—one drug which decreases aqueous production (timolol or other beta-blocker, or brimonidine or dorzolamide) and other drug which increases aqueous outflow (latanoprost or brimonidine or pilocarpine) may be used.

Oral carbonic anhydrase inhibitors

Acetazolamide and methazolamide are not recommended for long-term use because of their side effects. However, acetazolamide 250 mg TDS may be added to control IOP for short term.

Neuroprotective agents

Neuroprotection is an IOP independent method of treating the retinal ganglion cells (RGCs) that are damaged in glaucoma. Some currently available neuroprotective agents have shown effects in vitro and in animal models, however, results in human clinical trials are either lacking or inconclusive.

Note. For details of anti-glaucoma drugs and medical therapy of glaucoma, *see* Chapter 18.

B. LASER TRABECULOPLASTY

Laser trabeculoplasty can be done using argon laser (ALT), or diode laser (DLT) and selective laser trabeculoplasty (SLT). It should be considered in patients where IOP is uncontrolled despite maximal tolerated medical therapy. It can also be considered as primary therapy where there is non-compliance to medical therapy.

Note. For details of laser therapy of glaucoma, see Chapter 19.

Technique and role of argon (ALT) or diode laser trabeculoplasty (DLT) in POAG

It has an additive effect to medical therapy. Its hypotensive effect is caused by increasing outflow facility, possibly by producing collagen shrinkage on the inner aspect of the trabecular meshwork and opening the intratrabecular spaces. It has been shown to lower IOP by 8–10 mm Hg in patients on medical therapy and by 12–16 mm Hg in patients who are not receiving medical treatment.

Treatment regime usually employed consists of 50 spots on the anterior half of the trabecular meshwork over 180°.

Complications. These include transient acute rise of IOP, which can be prevented by pretreatment with apraclonidine or brimonidine (an alpha agonist) and/or acetazolamide; and inflammation which can be lessened by use of topical steroids for 3–4 days. Less commonly haemorrhage, uveitis, peripheral anterior synaechiae and reduced accommodation may occur.

Selective laser trabeculoplasty (SLT)

Selective laser trabeculoplasty (SLT), based on the principle of selective photothermolysis, targets selectively pigmented trabecular meshwork (TM) cells without causing thermal or collateral damage to non-pigmented cells or structures unlike ALT or DLT. SLT is performed using Q-switched frequency doubled, 532 nm ND:YAG laser with a pulse duration of 3 nsec, a spot size of 400 microns and energy setting of 0.8 ms. Pressure lowering effect of SLT is similar to ALT with the advantage of not causing scarring and damage to TM. Further, SLT can be used in patients treated with ALT.

C. SURGICAL THERAPY

Indications

1. *Uncontrolled glaucoma* despite maximal medical therapy and laser trabeculoplasty.
2. *Non-compliance* of medical therapy and non-availability of ALT/SLT.
3. *Failure of medical therapy and unsuitable for ALT* either due to lack of cooperation or inability to visualize the trabeculum.
4. *Eyes with advanced disease,* i.e. having very high IOP, advanced cupping and advanced fieldloss should be treated with filtration surgery as primary line of management.

Types of surgery

Surgical treatment of POAG primarily consists of a fistulizing (filtration) surgery which provides a new channel for aqueous outflow and successfully controls the IOP (below 21 mm Hg). Trabeculectomy is the most frequently performed filtration surgery nowadays. The details of filtration operations are described in Chapter 20.

Note. For details of surgical procedures of glaucoma, see Chapter 20.

OCULAR HYPERTENSION

DEFINITION

Ocular hypertension versus glaucoma suspect

Ocular hypertension (OHTN) term is used when a patient has an IOP constantly more than 21 mm Hg but no optic disc and visual field changes. These patients should be carefully monitored by an ophthalmologist and should be treated as cases of POAG in the presence of high-risk factors.

Glaucoma suspect. Shaffer (1977) introduced the term 'glaucoma suspect' for the patients likely to develop either POAG or NTG over the period. A glaucoma suspect is defined as an adult having normal open angle on gonioscopy and anyone of the following findings in at least one eye:

1. *Elevated IOP,* consistently more than 21 mm Hg by applanation tonometry.
2. *Glaucomatous disc changes,* in any of the follows forms enlarged (0 >0.3) cup–disc ratio, asymmetric cup–disc ratio (difference >0.2), notching or narrowing of the neuroretinal rim, a disc haemorrhage, or suspicious alteration in the nerve fibre layer.
3. *Visual fields* consistent with glaucomatous damage.

Terminology

Based on the above signs, the clinical diagnosis is made as below (Fig. 16.10)

- *Ocular hypertension.* Only no. 1 positive
- *Glaucoma suspect.* Any one of 1, 2, or 3 positive
- *Pre-perimetric glaucoma.* 1 and 2 positive
- *Primary open-angle glaucoma.* 1 and 2 or 1 and 3 or 1, 2 and 3 positive
- *Normal tension glaucoma.* Only 2 and 3 positive

Note. The term glaucoma suspect should not be confused with 'primary angle-closure suspect' (PACS) which is a term used for suspicion of developing primary angle-closure glaucoma. For definition, see page 195.

EPIDEMIOLOGY

As mentioned above, the term OHTN is used when IOP is constantly more than 21 mm Hg but the visual fields, optic disc are normal along with a normal and open angle of the anterior chamber and absence of any ocular or systemic disorder contributing to elevated IOP. Epidemiological aspects of OHTN include:

- *Prevalence.* In general, 4 to 10% of the population over 40 years is reported to have ocular hypertension.
- *Race.* The reported figures of prevalence in the patients above 40 years, of different race are: Black African—18.4%, mixed race—13.6% and 4.6%.
- *Conversion to glaucoma.* About 0.5–1% of the OHTN patients per year develop visual field loss.
- *Ocular hypertension treatment study (OHTS)* concluded that over 5 years conversion to POAG occurred in 1% per years of treated patients (topical ocular hypertensive drugs) and 2% per year of not treated (observed) patients and in 3 to 5% per year of patients having high-risk factors.

RISK FACTORS FOR DEVELOPMENT OF POAG

High-risk factors for development of POAG reported by OHTS and European Glaucoma Prevention Study (EGPS) are;

- IOP consistently >30 mm Hg
- Corneal thickness <550 μm
- Vertical cup disc ratio of more than 0.7
- Increased age
- Increased pattern standard deviation (PSD) on Humphrey visual field test
- Disc haemorrhage, i.e. splinter haemorrhages over or near the disc.

Other reported risk factors are:

- Family history of glaucoma or know genetic predisposition
- Fellow eye of the unilateral POAG
- Other ocular conditions include suspicious disc appearance, myopia, positive diurnal variation, steroid responder, and low optic nerve perfusion pressure
- Systemic risk factors include diabetes mellitus, sleep apnoea, hypertension, cardiovascular disease, hypothyroidism, migranous headache and vasospasm.

Note. The risk of developing POAG cannot be predicted from a single risk factor. The multivariate analysis of the risk factors is more useful in predicting the development of POAG in glaucoma suspect.

Risk calculators

Risk calculators have been developed to calculate the risk of developing POAG in ocular hypertensive patients. The risk calculators have been developed by incorporating the data from OHTS, EGPS, longitudinal population studies, such as Barbados Incidence Study of Eye Disease (BISED) and the Diagnostic Innovation in Glaucoma Study (DIGS); and are based on multivariate analysis of the risk factors.

Examples of risk calculators

1. ***STAR II risk calculator:*** Screening Tool for Assessing Risk (STAR) by Pfizer Corporation (Fig. 16.11). It is based on the model of risk calculator developed by Medeiros and Colleagues (2005). They have valide this model in prospective study implemented of the OHTS group of patients.
2. ***Dever's OHTN to glaucoma risk calculator*** (Fig. 16.12) is available of the Dever's Eye Institute Website (www.devereye.org/gre_web/gre.(fm)

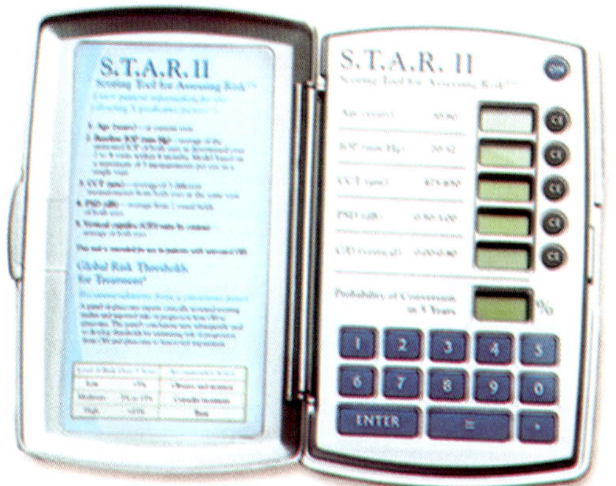

Fig. 16.11 *STAR risk calculator*

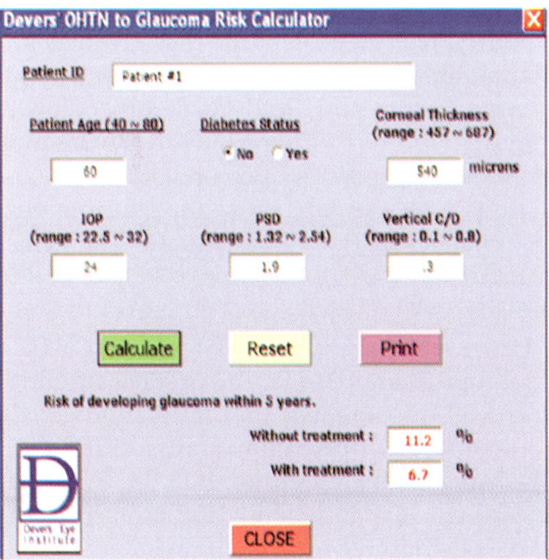

Fig. 16.12 *Devers' OHTN to glaucoma risk calculator*

Facts about utility and limitations of risk calculators

- *Availability* of the risk calculators on internet (website of the provider).
- *Underlying basis* of most current risk calculator is the result of an OHTS multivariate regression model. Five variables predictive for conversion of OHTN to POAG are age, CCT, IOP, PSD and vertical cup disc ratio. The number of combination between these five variables is enormous and the risk calculator helps to simplify the decision tree.
- *Applicability*. Since most risk calculators are based on risk factor uncovered with the OHTS population, and thus their results are most applicable to the patients who resemble the OHTS population in term of age, IOP level, having an open-angle and normal visual field, etc. without risk calculator, the ocular hypertension is frequently over and under treated.

  Since the present risk calculators are designed for patients with ocular hypertension, these cannot be used as glaucoma screening devices.
- *Utility*. Risk calculator helps in deciding whether or not to treat patient with OHTN. In general, a 15% or greater risk of developing glaucoma from OHTN over 5 years is considered a high-risk and treatment is recommended.
- *Limitation* of risk calculators are:
  - Calculation may not apply to the patients who are younger than 40 years, non-white or of African descent, and do not have an IOP of 22 mm Hg or higher.
  - Do not provide critical information that may guide therapy, such as life expectancy and psychological and social factors.
  - Factors not included in the risk calculators are also important and should be taken into account when deciding whether to initiate treatment in an ocular hypertensive.

TREATMENT

Indications of treatment

To decide when to treat a glaucoma suspect in complex process. Following guidelines may be

Table 16.4 *American Academy of Ophthalmology (2005) guidelines for follow-up of a glaucoma suspect*

Treatment examination	*Target IOP ONH/RNFL evaluation*	*High-risk*	*Follow-up interval (in months)*	
No	NA	No	6–24	6–24
No	NA	Yes	3–12	6–18
Yes	Yes	Yes	3–12	6–18
Yes	Yes	Yes	<4	3–12

(IOP, intraocular pressure; NA, not applicable; ONH, optic nerve head; VF, visual fields)
(*Source:* American Academy of Ophthalmology (2005), available at http://www.aao.org/ppp))

useful in glaucoma suspects with elevated IOP (ocular hypertensive).

Stratify patients as those with low, moderate and high-risk of progression to glaucoma and process as below:

- Patients with high-risk of progression must be treated on the lines of POAG (see page 216–219).
- Patients with moderate risk of progression need to analyzed critically and treatment can be initiated, if appropriate or patient should be monitored closely.
- Patients with high-risk of progression need to be monitored for IOP as well as optic nerve structure and function, and treated on evidence of progression.

Goals of treatment

Goal of treatment of glaucoma suspects is to prevent conversion to glaucoma. OHTS reported that on reducing IOP by at least 20% (and to 24 mm Hg), 4.45% of the treatment group advanced to POAG as compared to 9.5% in the not treated (observation) group. The results indicate that the number needed to treat (NNT) in OHTS was 16 ocular hypertensives to prevent one case of conversion to glaucoma

Treatment modalities

1. ***Medical therapy*** remains the mainstay of treatment. Based on social, economic and systemic health of the patient, the antiglaucoma drug may be chosen out of prostaglandins, beta-blockers, carbonic anhydrase inhibitors or alpha agonists. As a therapeutic trial, the medication should be started in one eye. Monotherapy is desirable with maximum of two drugs most of the times.

2. ***Laser trabeculoplasty.*** Selective laser trabeculoplasty (SLT) can be considered as an adjuvant, if medical therapy fails or is not tolerated.

3. ***Glaucoma surgery*** is rarely required in a glaucoma suspect.

Guidelines for follow-up

The follow-up guidelines recommended by American Academy of Ophthalmology (AAO) in its 2005 Preferred Practice Pattern for treated and non-treated (observed) cases of glaucoma suspect are depicted in Table 16.4.

NORMAL TENSION GLAUCOMA

DEFINITION

The term normal tension glaucoma (NTG), also referred to as low tension glaucoma, is labelled when typical glaucomatous disc changes and visual field defects are associated with an intraocular pressure (IOP) constantly below 21 mm Hg (Fig. 16.10). Characteristically, the angle of anterior chamber is open on gonioscopy and there is no secondary cause for glaucomatous disc changes. NTG is a variant of POAG which accounts for 16% of all cases of POAG and its prevalence above the age of 40 years is 0.2%.

However, it is still not clear whether NTG is a subtype (variant) of POAG or separate entity. It is well documented that mechanism of the glaucomatous optic neuropathy shifts from predominantly elevated IOP in POAG to additional IOP independent factors in NTG, with considerable overlap of causative factors. Further, it is also being considered that probably NTG is not one entity but several different conditions with similar clinical features.

EPIDEMIOLOGY

- NTG in reported to account for 16% of all cases of POAG.
- Prevalence of NTG above the age of 40 years reported is 0.2%.
- *Age*. As a rule, NTG in seen in older individuals usually above 60 years, although rarely, it may be seen below 50 years. Average age for NTG is 10 years more than that for POAG.
- *Sex*. Females are more commonly affected than males.
- *Race*. Japanese have very high incidence of NTG to that extent that about 75% cases of POAG have IOP <21 mm Hg.
- *Heredity*. Most cases are sporadic. However, a family history of some forms of glaucoma is reasonably common in patients with NTG.
- *Laterality*. Left eye is 2.5% times more affected than right.

PATHOGENESIS

Exact pathogenesis of NTG is still not clear. Following views have been put forward.

1. *Variant of POAG.* Many workers believe that NTG is variant of POAG, except that the optic disc demonstrate greater vulnerability to the effects of IOP with considerable overlap of causative factors.

2. *Chronic low vascular perfusion of optic disc* which makes it susceptible to normal IOP is being considered by many workers as the basic pathogenesis. This view is supported by following association with NTG:

- Raynaud phenomenon, i.e. peripheral vascular spasm on cooling.
- Migraine
- Nocturnal systemic hypotension and over-treated systemic hypertension.
- Reduced blood flow velocity in the ophthalmic artery (as revealed on transcranial Doppler ultrasonography).
- Hemodynamic crisis, prevalence is higher in patients with NTG.
- Hypercoagulability, increased blood viscosity and elevated blood cholesterol and lipids are also reported with NTG.
- Carotid artery diseases, slowed parapapillary, choroidal and retinal circulations have also been reported as association.

Note. Some studies have found no difference in the prevalence of vascular diseases in NTG and POAG. Other workers have commented that even if vascular disease occurs somewhat more frequently in NTG, it does not imply different pathogenesis of NTG and POAG.

3. *Autoimmune mechanism* has also been suggested by few workers. They have reported association of NTG with abnormal immuno-proteins such as anti-Ro/SS-A positivity and heat shock protein antibodies.

4. *Genetic mutation.* Mutations in the optineurin gene located on chromosome 10 have also been reported in about 15% of Japanese patients with NTG compared to 5% in normal population. Further, it has been reported the patients of NTG with mutation in optineurin gene seemed to have a more severe disease and progressive course than those without this mutation.

CLINICAL FEATURES

Clinical features of NTG are similar to POAG, except that IOP is consistently below 21 mm Hg.

A. Peculiarities of clinical features in NTG

1. *Intraocular pressure*

- *Higher side of normal range.* IOP, though consistently lower than 21 mm Hg, in most patients tends to be on higher side of normal range as compared to normal healthy population.
- *Influence of IOP on progression of visual field* and damage to neuroretinal rim is reported in many studies.
- *IOP reduction by 30% is associated with* protection of visual field and optic nerve head status, validating the concept that IOP is a contributing factor in the optic neuropathy of NTG.
- *Wider fluctuation of IOP* is reported in NTG by many workers, while others have floated this observation.

2. Optic disc changes

Characteristics of optic disc changes in NTG are reported with following differences than POAG:

- *Thinning of neuroretinal rim* is more significant specially inferiorly and inferotemporally.
- *Splinter haemorrhages at disc* are more frequent in patients with NTG than those with POAG, suggesting the possibility of vascular disease as a contributing factor.
- *Retinal nerve fibre layer (RNFL)* defects are more localized and close to macula in NTG as compared to more diffuse defects in POAG.

Sclerotic versus ischaemic optic neuropathy. Some authorities have divided NTG into 2 groups based on disc appearance:

- *Senile sclerotic group* with shallow, pale slopping of neuroretinal rim (primarily in older patients with vascular diseases).
- *Focal ischaemic group* with deep focal notching in neuroretinal rim.

3. Visual field changes

- *Visual field defects* tend to be deeper, steeper, more localized and closer to fixation point (Fig. 16.13).
- *Initial field defects* are more often in superior hemifield especially in the superonasal quadrant.

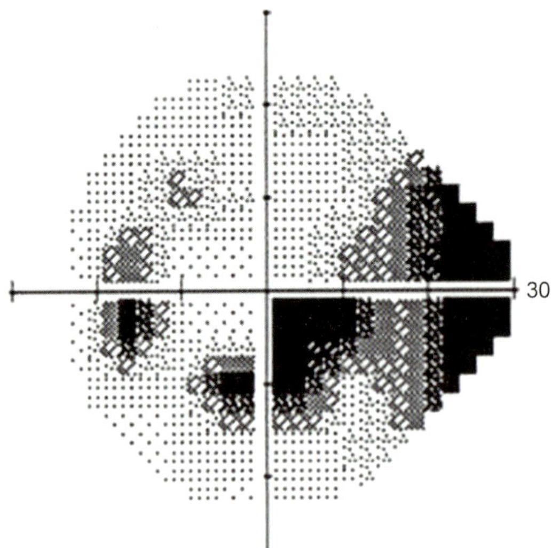

Fig. 16.13 *Deep and steep visual field defects close to fixation in an NTG patient*

- *Progression rate of field defects* is greater in NTG vis-a-vis POAG.
- *Pattern of progression* in field defects is initially in area and later in depth in POAG while in NTG progression is equal in area and depth.

4. Ocular vascular abnormalities

Ocular vascular abnormalities reported in patients with NTG are:

- *Increased resistance of ophthalmic artery* is reported in NTG and not in POAG, as measured by a variety of indirect methods, including Doppler velocity.
- *Reduced diastolic ophthalmodynamometry* levels and ocular pulse amplitude.
- *Focal arteriolar narrowing* around the disc, diffuse and focal hypofluorescence of the disc and abnormal transit time are reported on fluorescein angiography.

5. Systemic vascular and haematological abnormalities

One or more of the systemic vascular abnormalities mentioned in pathogenesis (page 231) may be detected as clinical features on critical analysis of the case. Therefore, the clinician should inquire about any history of haemodynamic crisis including episodes of blood loss, hypotension, anaemia, syncope, blood transfusions and falls.

Neurological symptoms, such as weakness in extremities, dizziness, headache, loss of consciousness and diplopia must also be noted. If elicited, the presence of neurological symptoms may indicate the need for neuro-ophthalmological evaluation to rule out neurological diseases that may masquerade as NTG.

Those of younger age at initial observation (<50 years), with decreased visual acuity (VA poorer than 20/40), specific visual field defects respecting the vertical midline or pallor greater than cupping are the ideal candidates for such investigations.

B. Progressive versus non-progressive NTG

Drance and co-workers (1973) have described two types of NTG—progressive and non-progressive.

1. ***Progressive NTG.*** It is a comparatively more common form and is believed to result from chronic vascular insufficiency of the optic nerve head due to one or more of the factors mentioned in the pathogenesis of NTG (page 231).

2. ***Non-progressive*** or stable form of NTG is comparatively rare and is usually associated with previous haemodynamic crisis, such as episodes of acute blood loss, arrhythmia, and acute hypotension. Drance and co-workers have also labelled them as cases of shock-induced optic neuropathy. Such patients are not likely to develop progressive visual field loss.

DIFFERENTIAL DIAGNOSIS

Differential diagnosis of NTG needs to be made from other conditions which produce visual field loss and an abnormal appearance of the disc without an elevated IOP. Such condition can be broadly described into two groups: undetected high tension glaucoma and non-glaucomatous optic neuropathy.

I. Undetected high tension glaucoma

Undetected high tension glaucomas which can be mistaken for NTG are:

1. POAG ***with misleading IOP.*** In some cases of POAG, IOP can be misleading because of:

- Wide diurnal variation
- Decreased CCT
- Low sclera rigidity
- Systemic medications that may decreases IOP

All these factors should be investigated to rule out POAG.

2. ***Glaucomas with intermittent rise in IOP,*** which may be mistaken for NTG include:

- Intermittent angle-closure glaucoma
- Glaucomatocyclitic crisis

3. ***Previous episodes of glaucoma*** which might have caused visual field changes and abnormal disc appearance with normal IOP on presentation include:

- *Past secondary glaucoma,* e.g. corticosteroid-induced glaucoma, uveitic glaucoma, pigmentary glaucoma, traumatic glaucoma, post-intraocular surgery glaucoma.
- *Previous elevated IOP,* which may have caused damage in the past and now may be in remission because of hyposecretion of aqueous humour that may occur in aged and in diseased eye.

4. ***Tonometric errors*** either iatrogenic or due to thinner CCT or low scleral rigidity in other high tension glaucoma.

5. ***Misleading compliance to medications*** only on the day when the patient is seen by ophthalmologist.

II. Non-glaucomatous optic neuropathy

Non-glaucomatous causes of optic neuropathy which can mimic NTG can be further divided into two groups: congenital and acquired conditions.

1. ***Congenital disorders of optic disc,*** which need to be considered in differential diagnosis include:

- Coloboma of the optic disc
- Optic disc pit
- Oblique insertion of the optic disc

2. ***Acquired causes of the non-glaucomatogenous optic neuropathy,*** which need to be differential are:

- Compressive lesions of the optic nerve include tumours, aneurysms and cysts.
- Shock optic neuropathy, associated with previous hemodynamic crisis, arrhythmias and hypotension. Some workers label these cases as non-progressive cases of NTG.
- Anterior ischaemic optic neuropathy (AION), which may be arteritic or non-arteritic.
- Retinal disorders, such as retinitis pigmentosa, vascular occlusion and chorioretinitis
- Methyl alcohol poisoning
- Traumatic optic neuropathy, and
- Optic nerve drusens.

TREATMENT

The Collaborative Normal Tension Glaucoma Study Group (CNTGSG) evaluated whether IOP should be reduced in patients with NTG. After the five-year trial, CNTGSG results found that 12% (7/61) of medically or surgically treated patients versus 35% (31/79 controls) of untreated patients exhibited visual field or optic disc progression. Their results showed a positive benefit from a 30% reduction of IOP with disease progression.

I. Medical treatment

1. ***Medical treatment to lower IOP.*** The aim of the treatment is to lower IOP by 30%, i.e. to achieve IOP levels of about 12–14 mm Hg. Some important facts about medical treatment of NTG are:

- *Dorzolamide* may be considered the drug of choice because in addition to lowering IOP it also increases optic nerve blood flow.
- *Beta blockers* should better be avoided (as these cause nocturnal systemic hypotension and are likely to affect adversely the optic nerve-perfusion).
- *Brimonidine.* The collaborative normal tension glaucoma study (CNTGS) looked at visual field progression with monotherapy of brimonidine tartrate 0.2% vs. timolol maleate 0.5% (both dosed BID). Despite similar average IOP-lowering effects from both the drugs, the brimonidine treatment group had a much lower rate (9.1%) of visual field progression as compared to the timolol group (39.2%).
- *Prostaglandin analogues* tend to have a greater ocular hypotensive effect in eyes with normal IOP.

2. ***Systemic calcium channel blockers*** (e.g. nifedipine) may be useful because of the possible beneficial effects of increasing capillary perfusion of the optic disc head. Studies involving patients with NTG receiving concurrent calcium channel blockers have demonstrated a significant reduction in the rate of disc and field progression, compared with similar NTG groups who were not receiving concomitant therapy.

3. ***Monitoring of systemic blood pressure*** should be done for 24 hours. If nocturnal dip is detected, it may be necessary to avoid night dose of antihypertensive medication.

4. ***Nutritional supplements and phytochemicals.*** These have been used as adjunctive therapies for NTG. One of the more commonly used phytochemicals is ginkgo biloba. Ginkgo biloba has vasorelaxant and anti-oxidative properties. Another phytochemical currently under investigation is resveratrol—a naturally-occurring polyphenol commonly found in berries, nuts and the skin of red grapes with reported anti-oxidative and anti-inflammatory properties. Resveratrol has also been shown to be helpful in preventing damage of trabecular meshwork cells in the setting of chronic oxidative stress.

II. Surgical treatment

Trabeculectomy may be considered when progressive field loss occurs despite IOP in lower teens.

SUGGESTED READING

1. Cheng JW, Cai JP, Wei RL. Meta-analysis of medical intervention for normal tension glaucoma. Ophthalmology 2009;116(7):1243–49.
2. Dielemans I, Vingerling JR, Wolfs RCW, et al. The prevalence of primary open-angle glaucoma in a population-based study in the Netherlands: The Rotterdam study. Ophthalmology 1994;101: 1851.
3. Hayreh SS. Effect of nocturnal blood pressure reduction on retrobulbar hemodynamics in glaucoma. Graefes Arch Clin Exp Ophthalmol 2002;240:867–68.
4. Jonas JB, Wang N. Intracranial pressure and glaucoma. J Glaucoma 2013;22 Suppl 5:S13–14. 16.
5. Klein BEK, Klein R, Sponsel WE, et al. Prevalence of glaucoma: The Beaver Dam eye study. Ophthalmology 1992;99:1499.
6. Leske MC, Heijl A, Hyman L, et al. Predictors of long-term progression in the Early Manifest Glaucoma Trial. Ophthalmology 2007;114:1965–72.
7. Lichter PR, Musch DC, Gillespie BW, et al., and the CIGTS Study Group. Interim clinical outcomes in the Collaborative Initial Glaucoma Treatment Study comparing initial treatment randomized to medications or surgery. Ophthalmology 2001;108:1943–53.
8. Mansberger S, Cioffi GA. The probability of glaucoma from ocular hypertension determined by ophthalmologists in comparison to a risk calculator. J Glaucoma 2006;15:426–31.
9. Mansouri K, Liu JH, Weinreb RN, Tafreshi A, Medeiros FA. Analysis of continuous 24-hour intraocular pressure patterns in glaucoma. Invest Ophthalmol Vis Sci 2012;53:8050–56.

10. Medeiros FA, Weinreb RN, Sample PA, et al. Validation of a predictive model to estimate the risk of conversion from ocular hypertension to glaucoma. Arch Ophthalmol 2005;123:1351–60.
11. Sommer A, Tielsch JM, Katz J, et al. Relationship between intraocular pressure and primary open angle glaucoma among white and black Americans. The Baltimore Eye Survey. Arch Ophthalmol 1991;109:1090–95.
12. Takako Nakagami, Yoshio Yamazaki, Fukuko Hayamizu. Prognostic Factors for Progression of visual field damage in patients with normal-tension glaucoma. Japanese Journal of Ophthalmology 2006;50(1):38–42.

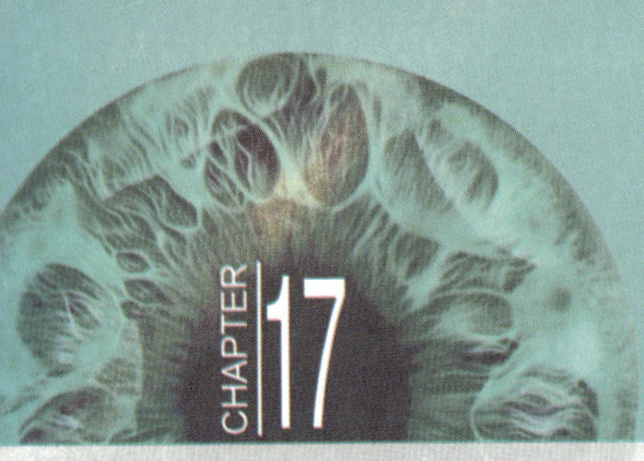

SECONDARY GLAUCOMAS

TERMINOLOGY AND CLASSIFICATION

TERMINOLOGY

Secondary glaucoma per se is not a disease entity, but a group of disorders in which rise of intraocular pressure (IOP) is associated with some primary ocular or systemic disease. Therefore, clinical features comprise that of primary disease and that due to effects of raised IOP.

CLASSIFICATION

A. Depending upon the mechanism of rise in IOP

I. *Secondary open-angle glaucomas*

Secondary open-angle glaucomas (SOAG) are characterized by an open-angle on gonioscopy. Depending upon the anatomical position in relation to the trabecular meshwork, the elements obstructing aqueous outflow leading to raised IOP can be grouped as:

- Pretrabecular mechanisms,
- Trabecular mechanisms, and
- Post-trabecular mechanisms.

1. ***Pretrabecular mechanisms*** are characterized by formation of a membrane that extends across the open iridocorneal angle, leading to the obstruction of aqueous outflow. These include:

- *Fibrovascular membrane*, as in neovascular glaucoma
- *Epithelial membrane*, as in epithelial downgrowth following intraocular surgeries or perforating injuries
- *Connective tissue membrane*, i.e. fibrous downgrowth following penetrating eye injuries
- *Endothelial layer with Descemet's like membrane* as occurs in iridocorneal endothelial (ICE) syndrome and posterior polymorphous dystrophy
- *Inflammatory membrane* formed in intraocular inflammation.

2. ***Trabecular mechanisms*** obstruct the aqueous outflow at the level of trabecular meshwork either by clogging it or by altering the trabecular meshwork tissue.

a. *Clogging of trabecular meshwork may be caused by:*

- Red blood cells (RBCs) in haemorrhagic, ghost cell and sickle cell glaucoma
- Macrophages in haemolytic, phacolytic and melanoma lytic glaucoma

- Pigment particles in pigmentary glaucoma, exfoliation syndrome, malignant melanoma
- Proteins in uveitis and lens-induced glaucoma
- Neoplastic cells in primary ocular tumours and juvenile xanthogranuloma
- Viscoelastic agents following cataract or other intraocular surgeries
- Vitreous following posterior capsular rent (PCR).

b. *Alteration of the trabecular meshwork tissue may occur in following conditions:*

- Steroid-induced glaucoma
- Uveitis
- Scleritis
- Alkali burns
- Trauma with subsequent scarring
- Toxic reactions associated with intraocular foreign bodies

3. *Post-trabecular mechanisms* are characterized by obstruction to aqueous flow distal to the meshwork as below:

a. *Increased resistance in Schlemm canal*, due to:

- Collapse of Schlemm canal, or
- Absence of Schlemm canal, or
- Obstruction of the canal with sickled red blood cells in the patients with sickle cell anaemia.

b. *Elevated episcleral venous pressure* in the conditions, like:

- Carotid cavernous fistula
- Cavernous sinus thrombosis
- Retrobulbar tumours
- Thyroid ophthalmopathy
- Superior vena cava obstruction
- Mediastinal tumours, and
- Sturge-Weber syndrome

II. *Secondary angle-closure glaucomas*

Secondary angle-closure glaucoma mechanisms include situations in which the peripheral iris is in apposition for the trabecular meshwork or peripheral cornea. These situations can be grouped as below:

1. *Anterior (pulling) mechanism.* These cause narrowing of the angle by pulling the peripheral iris due to:

i. *Contracture of the membranes* as in:

- Neovascular glaucoma,
- ICE syndrome
- Posterior polymorphous dystrophy
- Penetrating and non-penetrating trauma

ii. *Contracture of inflammatory precipitates*, as in anterior uveitis.

2. *Posterior (pushing) mechanism.* With the posterior mechanism, pressure behind the iris, lens, or vitreous causes the peripheral iris to be pushed into the anterior chamber angle. The causes of posterior mechanism can be grouped as below:

a. *With pupillary block*

- Lens-induced mechanism
- Phacomorphic glaucoma due to intumescent lens
- Subluxation of the lens
- Mobile lens syndrome
- Posterior synaechiae
- Uveitis with posterior synaechiae
- Intraocular lens block in pseudophakia
- Iris–vitreous block in aphakia

b. *Without pupillary block*

i. Ciliary block (malignant) glaucoma

ii. Lens-induced mechanism

- Intumescent lens
- Subluxation of lens
- Mobile lens syndrome

iii. Pseudoplateau iris

iv. After lens extraction (forward vitreous thrust)

v. Anterior rotation of the ciliary body following

- Sclera buckling, or
- Panretinal photocoagulation

vi. Intraocular tumours pushing lens–iris diaphragm:

- Malignant melanoma
- Retinoblastoma

vii. Retrolenticular tissue contracture

- Retinopathy of prematurity
- Persistent hyperplastic primary vitreous

B. Depending upon the causative primary disease

Secondary glaucomas are named as below:

1. Lens-induced (phacogenic) glaucomas

2. Inflammatory glaucoma (glaucoma due to intraocular inflammation)
3. Pigmentary glaucoma
4. Neovascular glaucoma
5. Glaucoma associated with intraocular tumours
6. Pseudoexfoliative glaucoma
7. Steroid-induced glaucoma
8. Traumatic glaucoma
9. Glaucoma secondary to ocular surgery
10. Glaucomas associated with intraocular haemorrhage
11. Glaucomas associated with disorders of corneal endothelium
12. Glaucoma associated with episcleral venous pressure
13. Glaucoma associated with disorders of retina, vitreous and choroid

17.1 LENS-INDUCED (PHACOGENIC) GLAUCOMAS

In lens-induced glaucomas (LIGs), the IOP is raised secondary to some disorders of the crystalline lens. Lens-induced glaucoma can be classified as below:

I. ***Lens-induced secondary angle-closure glaucoma***

- Phacomorphic glaucoma (due to swollen lens)
- Phacotopic glaucoma (due to anterior lens displacement)

II. ***Lens-induced secondary open-angle glaucoma***

- Phacolytic glaucoma
- Lens particle glaucoma
- Phacoantigenic glaucoma

LENS-INDUCED SECONDARY ANGLE-CLOSURE GLAUCOMA

PHACOMORPHIC GLAUCOMA

Phacomorphic glaucoma is an acute secondary angle-closure glaucoma caused by intumescent lens, i.e. swollen cataractous lens due to rapid maturation of cataract or sometimes following traumatic rupture of the lens capsule.

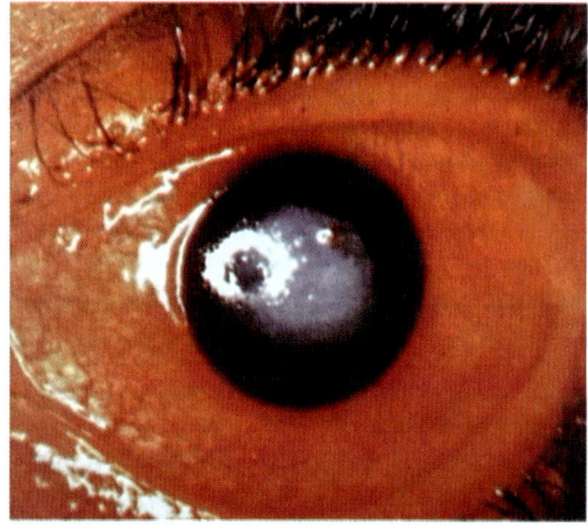

Fig. 17.1 *Phacomorphic glaucoma. Note ciliary congestion, fixed dilated pupil and intumescent senile cataractous lens*

Pathogenesis. The swollen lens pushes the iris forward and obliterates the angle resulting in secondary acute angle-closure glaucoma. Further, the increased iridolenticular contact also causes potential pupillary block and iris bombe formation.

Clinical presentation. Phacomorphic glaucoma presents as an acute congestive glaucoma with features almost similar to acute primary angle-closure (see page 207) except that the lens is always cataractous and swollen (Fig. 17.1). Demonstration of deep anterior chamber and open-angle in the fellow eye helps in differentiating it from the acute primary angle-closure glaucoma.

Treatment should be immediate and consists of:

- *Medical treatment* to:
  - Control IOP by i.v. mannitol, systemic acetazolamide and beta blockers, and
  - Control inflammation by topical steroids.
- *Laser iridotomy* may be effective in breaking the angle-closure attack.
- *Cataract extraction* with implantation of PCIOL (which is the main treatment of phacomorphic glaucoma) should be performed once the eye becomes quiet.

GLAUCOMA DUE TO SUBLUXATED LENS

Subluxation (partial zonular dehiscence) of the lens may cause lens-induced angle-closure glaucoma.

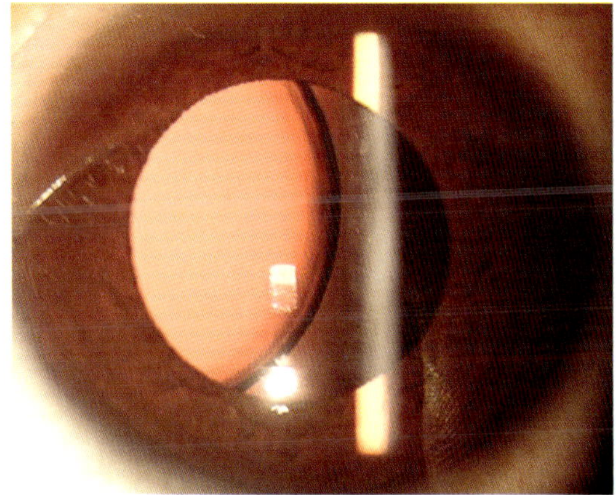

Fig. 17.2 *Ectopia lentis*

Causes of subluxation of lens

Causes of the subluxation may be grouped as:

1. *Congenital subluxations* which include:
   - Simple ectopia lentis,
   - Ectopia lentis et pupillae,
   - Ectopia lentis (Fig. 17.2) with systemic anomalies, such as Marfan's syndrome, Weill-Marchesani syndrome, Ehler-Danlos syndrome, homocystinuria, hyperlysinaemia, etc.
2. *Traumatic subluxations* are common with closed globe trauma
3. *Spontaneous or consecutive subluxations* occur secondary to some intraocular diseases giving rise to mechanical stretching, inflammatory disintegration or degeneration of the zonules. A few common conditions associated with spontaneous subluxation are: hypermature cataract, buphthalmos, high myopia, staphyloma, intraocular tumours, uveitis and exfoliative syndrome.

Mechanism of glaucoma

- *Pupil block* may be caused by a lens dislocated into the pupil or anterior chamber or subluxated or tilted forward against the iris without entering the anterior chamber. Pupillary block may also be caused by the vitreous herniation.
- *Peripheral anterior synaechiae* may develop from a long-standing pupillary block and produce chronic IOP elevation.

Management

- *Antiglaucoma medical treatment* with hyperosmotic agents, carbonic anhydrase inhibitors and β-blockers may be helpful in breaking the attack.
- *Cycloplegics* may relieve the attack by dilating the pupil, when the lens has subluxated into the pupil.
- *Laser PI* helps by providing bypass to aqueous in the presence of pupillary block.
- *Laser peripheral iridoplasty* may also be helpful in some cases of angle-closure glaucoma.
- *Surgical removal of the lens* may be required when the lens is in anterior chamber or lens extraction is needed to relieve the glaucoma or improve vision. Patient must be informed about the surgical risks with guarded prognosis.

PUPILLARY BLOCK GLAUCOMA DUE TO MICROSPHEROPHAKIA

Pupillary block glaucoma due to microspherophakia needs special mention. Microspherophakia is often familial and may occur as an isolated condition or as part of either Weill-Marchesani or Marfan's syndrome.

Mechanism of glaucoma. As the name indicates in microspherophakia, the lens has a spherical or globular shape which may cause pupillary block and angle-closure glaucoma.

Management. Cycloplegics dilate the pupil, tighten the zonules, flatten the lens and pull it posteriorly, breaking the pupillary block.

Note. Miotics are contraindicated, as these may make the condition worse by increasing the pupillary block and by rotating the ciliary body forward, loosening the zonules and allowing the lens to become more globular. Since the glaucoma caused by microspherophakia is relieved by cycloplegics and worsens by miotics, it is also called inverse glaucoma or paradoxical glaucoma.

LENS-INDUCED SECONDARY OPEN-ANGLE GLAUCOMAS

Lens-induced secondary open-angle glaucomas include three clinical entities:

- Phacolytic glaucoma,
- Lens particle glaucoma, and
- Phacoantigenic glaucoma.

1. PHACOLYTIC GLAUCOMA (LENS PROTEIN GLAUCOMA)

Phacolytic glaucoma in hypermature cataract

Pathogenesis. It is a type of secondary open-angle glaucoma, in which trabecular meshwork is clogged by the lens proteins and macrophages which have phagocytosed the lens proteins and inflammatory debris. Leakage of the lens proteins occurs through the microscopic openings of an intact capsule in the hypermature (Morgagnian) cataractous lens (Fig. 17.3A, B).

Clinical features. The condition is characterized by (Fig. 17.3A):

- *Features of acute congestive glaucoma* due to an acute rise of IOP in an eye having hypermature cataract.
- *Anterior chamber* may become deep and aqueous may contain fine white protein particles, which settle down as pseudo-hypopyon.
- *Anterior chamber angle* is open on gonioscopy.

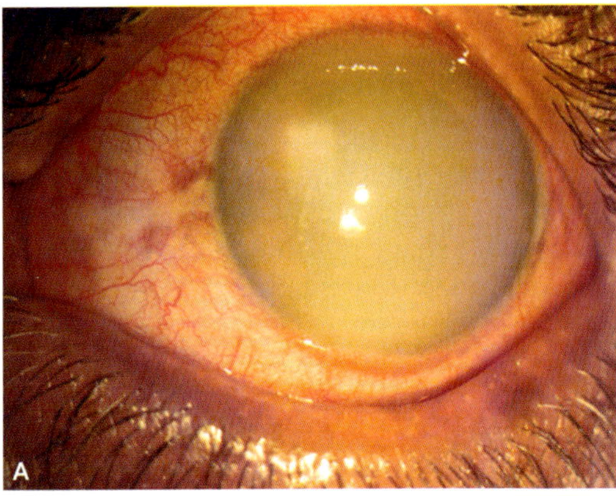

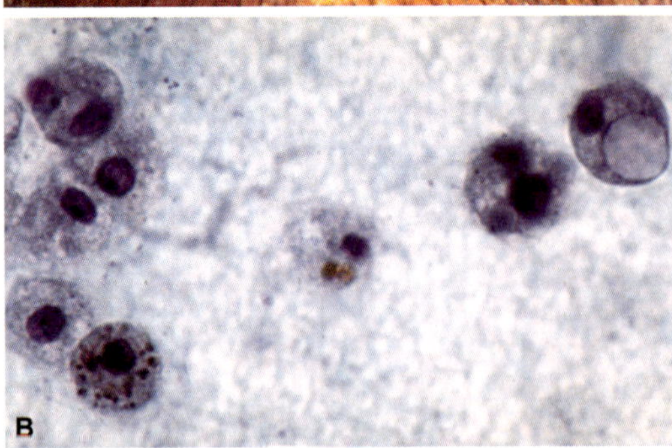

Fig. 17.3 *Phacolytic glaucoma: (A) Clinical photograph; (B) Microscopic appearance of macrophages which have phagocytosed the lens proteins and inflammatory debris*

Management. It consists of;

- *Medical therapy* to lower the IOP followed by,
- *Surgical extraction* of the mature, hypermature cataractous lens with PCIOL implantation.
- *Topical and oral steroids* must be started preoperatively to reduce the inflammation.

Phacolytic glaucoma due to posteriorly dislocated lens

Sometimes the lens dislocated into the vitreous cavity undergoes degenerative changes with release of material that obstructs the aqueous outflow.

Management

- *Medical therapy* to control the IOP.
- *Surgical removal of the posteriorly dislocated lens* by pars plana lensectomy with vitrectomy, is the only definitive treatment.

2. LENS PARTICLE GLAUCOMA

Pathogenesis. It is a type of secondary open-angle glaucoma, in which trabecular meshwork is blocked by the lens particles floating in the aqueous humour. It may occur due to lens particles left after accidental or planned extracapsular cataract extraction or following traumatic rupture of the lens. However, the associated inflammation, whether in response to the surgery, trauma or retained lens material may contribute to glaucoma in this condition.

Clinical features. Symptoms of acute rise in IOP associated with lens particles in the anterior chamber (Fig. 17.4).

Management includes:

- *Medical therapy* to lower IOP,
- *Irrigation–aspiration* of the lens particles from the anterior chamber may be required
- *Cycloplegics and topical steroids* to control inflammation.

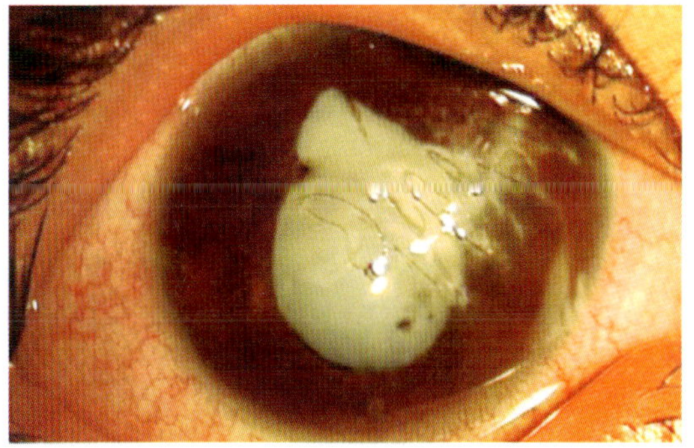

Fig. 17.4 *Lens particle glaucoma secondary to post-traumatic rupture of anterior lens capsule*

3. PHACOANTIGENIC GLAUCOMA

Pathogenesis. As in the case of lens particle glaucoma, there is usually a preceding disruption of lens capsule by extracapsular cataract extraction, penetrating injury, or leak of proteins from the capsule. Distinguishing feature is a latent period during which sensitization to the lens proteins occurs. IOP is then raised due to inflammatory reaction of the uveal tissue excited by the lens matter. Basically, it is also a type of secondary open-angle glaucoma where trabecular meshwork is clogged by both inflammatory cells and the lens particles.

Clinical features. Phacoantigenic glaucoma (previously known as phacoanaphylaxis) is a rare entity. In this condition, there occurs:

- Fulminating acute inflammatory reaction due to antigen (lens protein)–antibody reaction.
- Typical finding is a granulomatous inflammation in the involved eye after it goes surgical trauma.
- KPs are present on the corneal endothelium. In addition, a low grade vitritis, synaechial formation and residual lens material in the anterior chamber may be found.

Management consists of:

- *Medical therapy* to lower IOP.
- *Treatment of iridocyclitis* with steroids and cycloplegics.
- *Irrigation–aspiration* of the lens matter from anterior chamber (if required) should always be done after proper control of inflammation.

17.2 GLAUCOMAS DUE TO UVEITIS

Intraocular pressure can be raised by varied mechanisms in inflammations of the uveal tissue (iridocyclitis). Even in other ocular inflammations, such as keratitis and scleritis, the rise in IOP is usually due to secondary involvement of the anterior uveal tract.

Types of inflammatory glaucoma

Inflammatory glaucoma can be classified as below:

I. *Non-specific inflammatory glaucomas*
   1. Open-angle inflammatory glaucoma
   2. Angle-closure inflammatory glaucomas

II. *Specific hypertensive uveitis syndromes*
   1. Fuch's uveitis syndrome
   2. Glaucomatocyclitic crisis

NON-SPECIFIC INFLAMMATORY GLAUCOMAS

These include all cases of inflammation of the uveal tract associated with raised IOP, other than the specific hypertensive uveitis syndromes, but inclusive of postoperative inflammation.

Based on the mechanism of rise in IOP, the inflammatory glaucoma can be:

- Open-angle inflammatory glaucoma
- Angle-closure inflammatory glaucomas

1. OPEN-ANGLE INFLAMMATORY GLAUCOMA

Clinically, the open-angle inflammatory glaucoma may manifest as:

- Acute, or
- Chronic entity.

Acute open-angle inflammatory glaucoma

Mechanisms of rise in IOP include:

- *Trabecular clogging* by inflammatory cells, exudates and turbid aqueous humour,
- *Trabecular oedema* due to associated trabeculitis, and
- *Prostaglandin*-induced rise in IOP.

Most cases of anterior uveitis are idiopathic, but uveitis commonly associated with open-angle inflammatory glaucoma include herpes zoster iridocyclitis, herpes simplex, kerato-uveitis, toxoplasmosis, rheumatoid arthritis, and pars planitis.

Clinical features. It is characterized by features of acute iridocyclitis associated with raised IOP with open-angle of anterior chamber IOP, usually returns to normal after acute episode of inflammation.

Management includes:
- Treatment of iridocyclitis by topical steroids and cycloplegics
- Medical therapy to lower IOP by use of hyperosmotic agents, oral acetazolamide and topical antiglaucoma medications (pilocarpine and prostaglandin agonists are contra-indicated).

Chronic open-angle inflammatory glaucoma

Mechanisms of rise in IOP include:
- Chronic trabeculitis, and
- Trabecular scarring

Clinical features include:
- Raised IOP
- Open-angle on gonioscopy
- No active inflammation but signs of previous episode of uveitis are often present.
- Some chronic cases may also have signs of glaucomatous disc changes and field defects.

Treatment consists of:
- Medical therapy with topical beta blockers, and/or carbonic anhydrase inhibitors and alpha agonist may be useful. Preferably avoid pilocarpine and prostaglandin agonists.
- Trabeculectomy under cover of steroids may be tried, if medical treatment fails. The results are usually poorer than POAG, but can be improved by augmented trabeculectomy or tube procedures.
- Cyclodestructive procedures may need to be considered, if surgical treatment fails.

Note. Steroid-induced glaucoma may occur in some patients during treatment of uveitis and it needs to be considered as a differential diagnosis of open-angle inflammatory glaucoma. It is important to note that raised IOP due to steroids requires a reduction in the potency and frequency of topical steroids or even use of steroid sparing agents; whereas if raised IOP is due to uncontrolled inflammation, the dose of steroid needs to be increased.

Grant's syndrome

Grant's syndrome is a type of chronic secondary open-angle glaucoma (SOAG) with following key features.

Etiology. The condition is either idiopathic or could be associated with systemic conditions, such as sarcoidosis, ankylosing spondylitis, and rheumatic arthritis.

Mechanism of glaucoma is blockage of trabecular meshwork due to inflammatory trabecular oedema and blockage by inflammatory debris.

Clinical features include:
- *Clinical presentation* is similar to POAG with bilateral rise in IOP, with no complaints.
- *Eyes appear white and quite* with minimal inflammatory signs in the anterior segment.
- *Gonioscopy* reveals open-angle with grey to yellowish inflammatory precipitates present over the trabecular meshwork, which is crucial in differentiating it from POAG.

Treatment consists of:
- *Topical antiglaucoma drugs* alone are not effective in lowering IOP.
- *Topical steroids.* IOP shows excellent response with disappearance of inflammatory precipitates and IOP returning to normal level within 1 to 2 weeks of therapy.

2. ANGLE-CLOSURE INFLAMMATORY GLAUCOMAS

i. Secondary angle-closure inflammatory glaucoma with pupil block

Mechanism. Pupillary block due to 360° synaechiae or seclusio-pupillae leads to iris bombe formation followed by appositional angle-closure (Fig. 17.5). If not treated, over the period PAS are formed causing synaechial angle closure.

Clinical features include:
- Raised IOP,

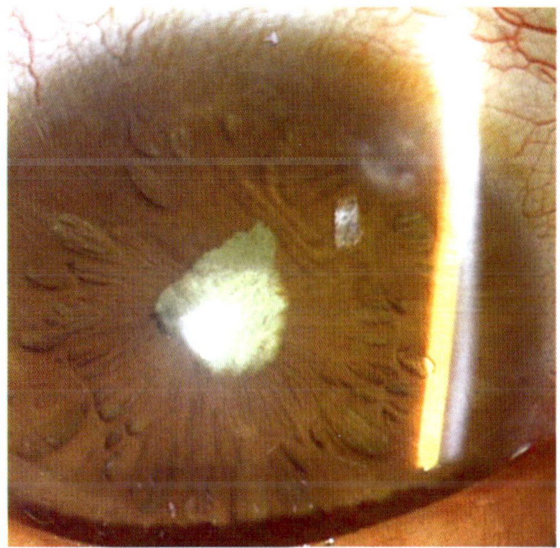

Fig. 17.5 *Secondary angle-closure with pupil block*

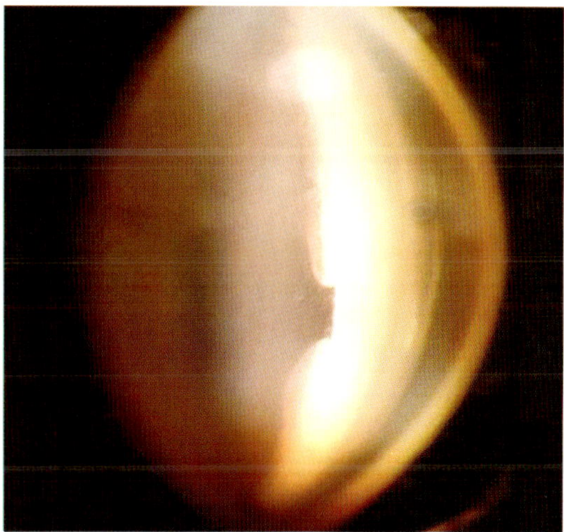

Fig. 17.6 *Broad based goniosynaechiae*

- Seclusio-pupillae,
- Iris bombe, and
- Shallow anterior chamber.

Management. It includes prophylaxis and curative treatment.

1. *Prophylaxis*. Acute iridocyclitis should be treated energetically with topical steroids and atropine to prevent formation of synaechiae.
2. *Curative treatment*. It consists of:

- *Medical therapy* to lower IOP (miotics are contraindicated).
- *Laser iridotomy* may be useful in pupil block without synaechial angle-closure. Laser PI should be large (or multiple) than is necessary for primary acute angle-closure.
- *Surgical PI* may need to be considered when laser PI closes.

ii. Secondary angle-closure inflammatory glaucoma without pupil block

Mechanism. It occurs due to organization of the inflammatory debris in the angle, which on contraction pulls the iris over the trabeculum. It is followed by gradual and progressive synaechial angle-closure with eventual elevation of IOP. Risk of synaechial angle-closure increases in the presence of granulomatous inflammation and also in patients with pre-existing narrow angle. Also in cases of chronic uveitis with rubeosis iridis, there may occur fibrovascular growth at the angles leading to a decrease in the aqueous outflow.

Clinical features include:

- Raised IOP
- Shallow anterior chamber
- PAS with angle-closure (Fig. 17.6), and
- Signs of previous inflammatory episodes.

Treatment options are:

- *Medical therapy* with topical beta blockers, carbonic anhydrase inhibitors and alpha agonists may reduce IOP.
- *Surgical treatment* is required when medical therapy fails. Trabeculectomy with metabolites or drainage implants (tube shunts) may be required.

SPECIFIC HYPERTENSIVE UVEITIS SYNDROME

FUCH'S HETEROCHROMIC UVEITIS SYNDROME

Clinical features

Presenting symptoms include:

- *Gradual blurring of vision* due to posterior subcapsular cataract (PSC) is the most common presenting symptoms.
- *Floaters* and difference in the colour of the two eyes are other presenting symptoms.

Signs include:

1. ***Keratic precipitates (KPs)*** are typically fine stellate present all over the endothelium with

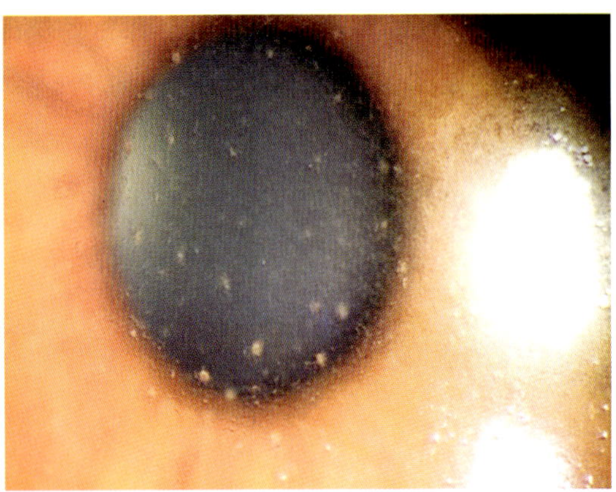

Fig. 17.7 Keratic precipitates in Fuchs' heterochromic uveitis syndrome

filaments in between them, and possibly are pathognomonic of FUS (Fig. 17.7).

2. ***Anterior chamber signs***
   - *Aqueous flare* is usually faint.
   - *Aqueous cells* are never more than +2

3. ***Iris signs*** include:
   - *Heterochromia iridis* is an important and common sign.
   - *Diffuse stromal atrophy* gives rise to washed-out appearance (moth-eaten appearance). Radial iris vessel becomes more visible as stroma is atrophied.
   - *Posterior pigment layer iris atrophy* is patchy and best detected by retroillumination as transillumination defects.
   - *Iris nodules* may be present along the pupillary border.
   - *Iris crystals.* Small, refractile iris crystals called Russell bodies can be seen on the surface of the iris. Russell bodies are aggregations of spherical immunoglobulin.
   - *Rubeosis iridis* may be seen in the form of fine irregular fragile vessels on the iris surface. Recurrent hyphaema may occur as a result of bleeding from the fragile vessels (Amsler's sign).
   - *Posterior synaechiae* are conspicuously absent.

4. ***Cataract*** (posterior subcapsular cataract) is a common complication of Fuch's uveitis syndrome having a chronic long-lasting course. Most of the time, blurring of vision due to posterior subcapsular cataract is the presenting symptom.

5. ***Glaucoma in FUS*** occurs in about 30% of the cases, with following key features:
   - *Mechanism.* Secondary open-angle glaucoma, occurring probably due to trabecular sclerosis. Prolonged steroid use may also contribute in causation of glaucoma as well as cataract.
   - *Raised IOP*, initially intermittent, later becomes constant. Occasionally, the IOP rise may be precipitated by cataract surgery.
   - *Gonioscopy* reveals open-angle with ± twig-like neovascularization of the angle.

Treatment

Uveitis in FUS is typically resistant to steroids, though steroids are still used to provide comfort.

- *Mydriatics* are not required since posterior synaechiae are seldom formed.
- *Posterior subtenon injection of long-acting steroids* (triamcinolone) may be useful for the annoying floaters.

Glaucoma is treated similar to POAG. However, pilocarpine and prostaglandin analogous are avoided.

- *Medical therapy.* Glaucoma is resistant to hypotensive agents in many cases (with 73% failing to respond to maximal medical therapy).
- *Surgery* (trabeculectomy with antimetabolites or a drainage device) is the main line of treatment.

POSNER-SCHLOSSMAN SYNDROME

Posner-Schlossman syndrome (glaucomatico-cyclitic crisis) is characterized by recurrent attacks of unilateral acute rise of IOP. Both eyes may be involved at different times but very rarely contemporaneously.

Etiology

- Cause of acute rise in IOP is presumed to be acute trabeculitis, possibly secondary to HSV, CMV or *Heliocobacter pylorii.*
- A direct correlation between elevated levels of prostaglandins (prostaglandin E) in the aqueous humour and the level of IOP has been found during acute attacks of glaucomato-cyclitic crisis.

- Condition typically affects young adult males much more than females, 40% of whom are positive for HLA-BW 54.

Clinical features

Presenting symptoms include mild discomfort, haloes around light and slight blurring of vision without any redness and pain.

Signs seen on examination:

- *No congestion*, i.e. the eye is typically white.
- *IOP is markedly raised* (40–50 mm Hg) during the attacks, but becomes normal in between the attacks. The rise of IOP is out of proportion to the severity of the uveitis, and this rise in IOP precedes the identifiable inflammatory reaction, often by several days.
- *Cornea* shows epithelial oedema due to a high IOP, and fine KPs on the back. Fine keratic precipitates appear after 2–3 days of elevated IOP and resolve rapidly. Fresh precipitates may appear with each episode of increased IOP.
- *Anterior chamber* shows few aqueous cells with minimal flare, no posterior synaechiae.
- *Gonioscopy* reveals open-angle with no PAS (a differentiating point from other inflammatory glaucomas).

Course. The recurrent attacks are unilateral, however, about 50% patients do give history of bilateral attacks at times. The interval between the attacks becomes longer with time. Many patients develop chronic open-angle glaucoma as a result of damage to the trabecular meshwork caused by recurrent attacks.

Investigations

- *PCR analysis of aqueous humor* to rule out CMV/HSV/VZV. OCTA.
- *Laser Doppler flowmeter* to rule out ONH decreased perfusion.

Treatment

Uveitis is treated by:

- *Typical steroids* mainly.
- *Oral NSAIDs* may also be helpful.
- *For CMV DNA positive cases:* Ganciclovir eye drops 0.15%/2% or Oral Valganciclovir 900 mg BD × 2 weeks, followed by additional 450 mg BD maintenance. Intravitreal injection-ganciclovir 2.0 mg in 0.05 cc or valganciclovir can be tried.

Glaucoma may be treated by:

- *Topical antiglaucoma drugs,* such as beta blockers, alpha-2 agonists, and carbonic anhydrase inhibitors.
- *Oral acetazolamide* may be added according to IOP level.

17.3 PIGMENTARY GLAUCOMA

DEFINITIONS

- ***Pigment dispersion syndrome (PDS):*** Dispersion of iris pigments on the corneal endothelium, midperipheral transillumination defects in the iris and heightened pigmentation of the trabecular meshwork.
- ***Pigmentary ocular hypertension (POH):*** PDS with elevated IOP but no glaucomatous optic neuropathy.
- ***Pigmentary glaucoma (PG):*** PDS with glaucomatous optic neuropathy, with or without elevated IOP. It is a secondary open angle glaucoma.

ETIOPATHOGENESIS

It is a type of secondary open-angle glaucoma wherein clogging up of the trabecular meshwork occurs by the pigment particles. About 50% of patients with the pigment dispersion syndrome (PDS) develop glaucoma (pigmentary glaucoma).

Genetics. PDS is inherited as an autosomal dominant trait (Ch 7q36) with a possible second locus on Ch18q; the exact gene(s) have not yet been identified.

Race. PDS is more common among Caucasians. Africans and Asians are less affected as they have thicker iris stroma which is less predisposed to shedding pigment, but once affected they develop more severe form of glaucoma.

- Family history of glaucoma
- Young male; 20–40 years
- Myopia (80% of cases)
- Presenting IOP >21 mm Hg
- Exercise
- Accommodation
- Frequent blinking

Pathogenesis. Exact mechanism of pigment shedding is not known. It is believed that, perhaps, pigment release is caused by mechanical rubbing of the posterior pigment layer of iris with the zonular fibrils. Part of iris in contact with the lens acts as a simple flap-valve allowing aqueous to pass from the posterior chamber (PC) to the anterior chamber (AC), but not in the opposite direction. Probably, a physiological event causes aqueous to be pumped through the flap valve of the iris from the PC to the AC leading to a higher pressure within the AC (relative to the PC) that causes the flap valve of the iris to close leading to "*reverse pupillary block*". The aqueous trapped at a higher pressure in the AC results in posterior bowing of the peripheral iris leading to irido-zonular contact and subsequent pigment dispersion.

Due to bowing of the mid-periphery, this unusual iris configuration may be due to 'reverse pupil block' (Fig. 17.8) causing an increase in anterior chamber pressure (relative to the posterior chamber). This assumption is supported by an observation that neutralization of reverse pupil block with peripheral iridotomy flattens the iris and decreases iridozonular contact.

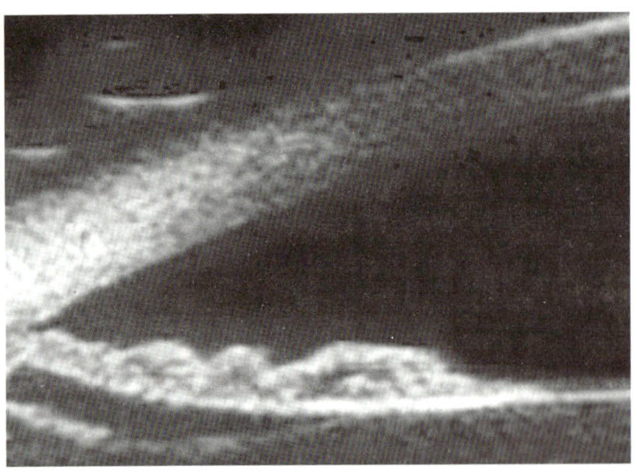

Fig. 17.8 *Reverse pupil block due to posterior bowing of iris*

CLINICAL FEATURES

The condition typically occurs in young myopic males.

Stages of pigment dispersion include:

- Inactive pigment dispersion with stable IOP
- Active pigment dispersion with stable IOP
- Active pigment dispersion with progressive glaucoma and elevated IOP
- Inactive pigment dispersion with progressive glaucoma and normal/elevated IOP.

Characteristic glaucomatous features are similar to POAG, associated with deposition of pigment granules in the anterior segment structures, such as:

1. ***Posterior surface of cornea*** shows pigment dispersal in the form of vertical spindle known as Krukenberg spindle (Fig. 17.9). The Krukenberg spindle, although common, is neither universal nor pathognomonic of PDS.

Endotheliopathy: Endothelial cells in PDS show pleomorphism and polymegathism. However, the endothelial cell count is normal with normal corneal thickness.

2. ***Anterior chamber*** shows pigments floating in the aqueous humour.

3. ***Iris*** shows fine pigments deposited preferentially within its furrows. The iris becomes

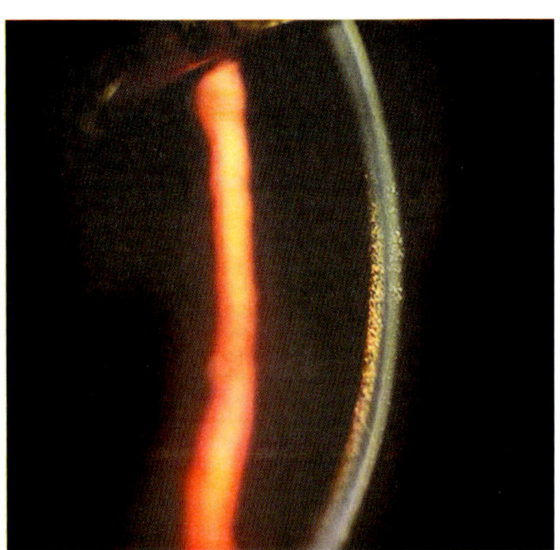

Fig. 17.9 *Krukenberg's spindle*

progressively darker resecting in the heterochromia iridis. Atrophy of the pigment epithelium of the iris occurs due to shedding of the pigment from the mid-periphery. Due to this atrophy, the iris transillumination shows radial slit-like transillumination defects in the mid-periphery (pathognomonic features of PDS). In asymmetric cases, the eye with the greater iris transillumination may have a larger pupil (Anisocoria) due to hyperplastic dilator muscle that is associated with the loss of iris pigment epithelium in eyes with PDS.

4. ***Lens*** shows fine pigment granules scattered on the anterior surface and accumulated in the form of a line at the site of vitreolenticular adhesion on the posterior surface. Pigmentation of lens equator or posterior lens capsule, classically occurs in the shape of a line known as Scheie's line or Zentmayer's line (Fig. 17.10).

5. ***Gonioscopy*** reveals:

- Wide open-angle with characteristic mid-peripheral iris concavity
- Pigment deposition along the Schwalbe's line especially inferiorly (Sampolesi's line)
- Pigment deposition is seen on and within the trabecular meshwork (most marked over the posterior trabeculum) along the entire circumference of the angle uniformly (Fig. 17.11). The pigment is fine and homogeneous in PDS in contrast to the coarse pigments seen in pseudoexfoliation (PEX).

6. ***Fundus examination*** may show:

- *Pigment deposition* in the peripheral retina
- *Lattice degeneration* areas, which may be responsible for an increased risk of retinal detachment.

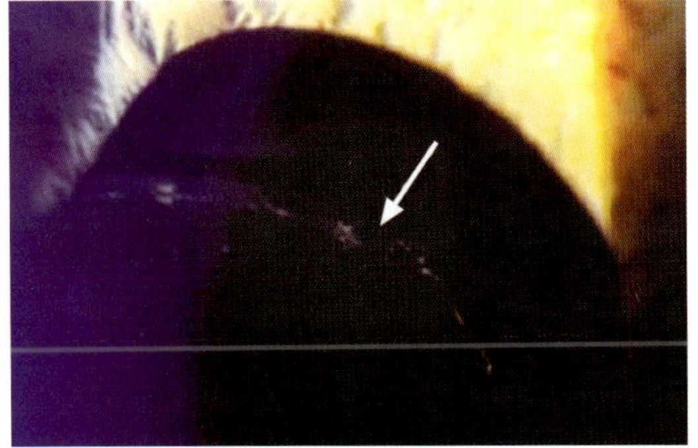

Fig. 17.10 *Zentmayer's line*

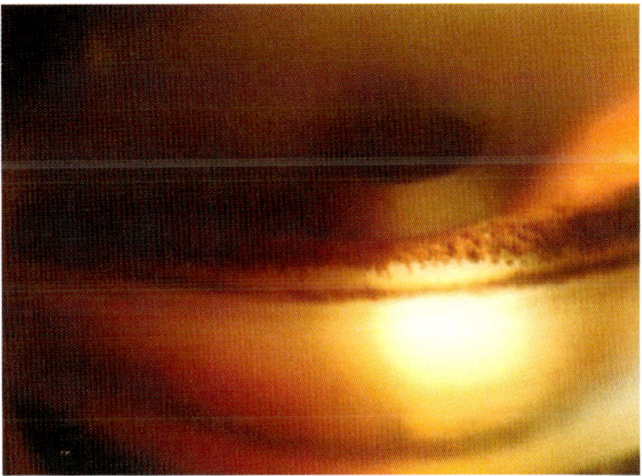

Fig. 17.11 *Heavily pigmented angle on gonioscopy*

- Retinal breaks occur more frequently than in normal eyes (12–15%).
- Incidence of retinal detachments is also higher in PDS for the degree of myopia.

Differential diagnosis

Pseudoexfoliation syndrome (PEXS), uveitis, iris/ciliary body cyst and iris/ciliary body melanoma must be differentiated from PDS. PDS is usually bilateral while PEXS is unilateral.

Investigations

- *Ultrasound biomicroscopy (UBM)* is very helpful in confirming the peripheral posterior bowing of the iris and showing iridozonular contact.
- *Anterior segment OCT* both, pre and post laser iridotomy, is useful.

Treatment

1. ***Medical therapy*** is similar to POAG. Miotics in addition to controlling IOP (by facilitating aqueous outflow) may also decrease the iridozonular contact (or theoretical benefit), but tend to be poorly tolerated in this age group and carry a small risk of inducing retinal detachment (myopic patients with lattice degeneration). Therefore, beta-blockers and PG analogues are still the commonest drugs used for this condition.

2. ***Laser trabeculoplasty*** is especially good in young patients and is effective easily on with a more than 50% failure rate by 5 years.

3. ***Laser peripheral iridotomy (LPI)*** can be used as a prophylactic measure in young myopic caucasian males with heavily pigmented eyes with type A personality. It decreases the iris-lens touch and thus prevents the 'reverse pupil block'. However, still there is no trial data to support its use.

4. ***Trabeculectomy.*** Results are good with a success rate similar to POAG. However, there is risk of hypotensive maculopathy (especially if augmented).

17.4 NEOVASCULAR GLAUCOMA (NVG)

It is an intractable glaucoma which results due to formation of neovascular membrane involving the angle of anterior chamber. In the past, a variety of other terms have been used to describe this condition, including thrombotic glaucoma, haemorrhagic glaucoma, diabetic haemorrhagic glaucoma, congestive glaucoma and rubeotic glaucoma, but since 'neovascular glaucoma' fits most appropriately with the pathophysiology of the entity, it is the most accepted term these days.

ETIOLOGY

It is usually associated with neovascularization of iris (rubeosis iridis). Neovascularization develops following retinal ischaemia, which is a common feature of:

- Diabetic retinopathy
- Central retinal vein occlusion
- Sickle-cell retinopathy, and
- Eales' disease.
- Other rare causes are chronic intraocular inflammations, intraocular tumours, long-standing retinal detachment and central retinal artery occlusion.

CLINICAL PROFILE

Clinical stages

NVG occurs in three stages:

1. *Pre-glaucomatous stage*, i.e. stage of rubeosis iridis; is characterized by formation of new vessels which leak leading to formation of membrane over the angle.
2. *Open-angle glaucoma stage* occurs due to formation of a pretrabecular neovascular membrane.
3. *Secondary angle-closure glaucoma* occurs due to goniosynaechiae resulting from contracture of the neovascular membrane (zipper-angle closure).

Clinical features

Symptoms include:

- *Pain* is often a feature and may be severe. It can be associated with watering, if there is an acute rise of IOP.
- *Symptoms of underlying predisposing condition* may be present, or may be suggested by the history (e.g. history of sudden loss of vision a couple of months ago may be given by a patient with CRVO).

Signs include:

- *Conjunctiva* may be congested.
- *Corneal oedema* may be present.
- *Neovascularization of iris (NVI) or rubeosis iridis*, i.e. presence of abnormal/non-radial vessels on the iris, initiating near the pupil. Florid NVI may be associated with ectropion uvea (Fig. 17.12).
- *IOP* is often raised.
- *Anterior chamber* may show flare and/or cells. Hyphaema may be associated.
- *Gonioscopy*. Depending upon the stage, gonioscopy may reveal:
  - Neovascularization of angle NVA (Fig. 17.13), (preglaucomatous stage), or
  - Fibrovascular membrane overlying the trabeculum (open-angle glaucoma stage), or

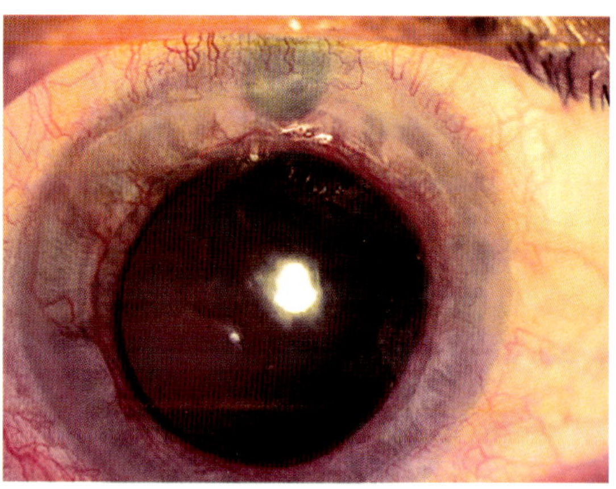

Fig. 17.12 *Florid neovascularization of iris (NVI) with ectropion uvea*

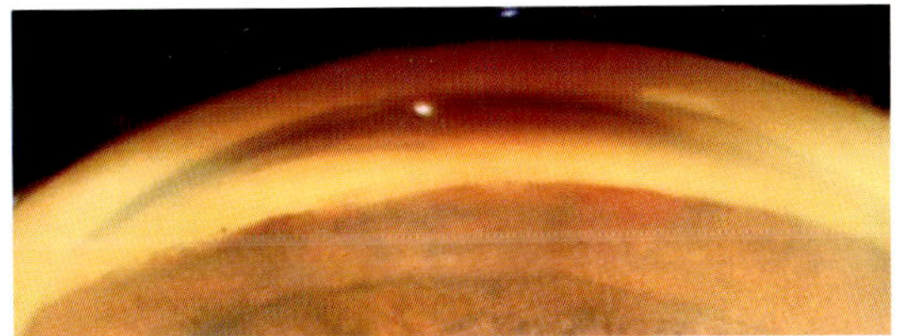

Fig. 17.13 *Neovascularization of angle*

- Fibrovascular membrane with peripheral anterior synaechiae (PAS) and zipping angle shut (angle-closure glaucoma).

- *Optic disc* changes and field changes similar to POAG may be present.
- *Signs of predisposing condition* (e.g. diabetic retinopathy, CRVO, etc.) may be present.

INVESTIGATIONS AND TREATMENT

Investigation

Investigations for predisposing conditions include:

- *Detailed fundus examination including indirect ophthalmoscopy* is essential.
- *FFA* may be performed as per indication.
- *Carotid Doppler* in suspected cases of carotid artery disease, especially when there is no underlying rational pathology or there is asymmetric diabetic retinopathy.
- *B-scan ultrasonography* is indicated to rule out intraocular tumour, retinal detachment, inflammation and other pathologies in patients with marked hazy media due to associated cataract or otherwise.
- *Optical coherence tomography angiography (OCTA):* Now-a-days, OCTA is being used for monitoring of ischaemic retinal disorders and the neovessels regression as well as detecting NVI. OCTA has approximately 79% sensitivity and 97% specificity against FFA, for diagnosing NVG.

Treatment

Treatment of NVG is often frustrating, but is undergoing a positive transformation with the advent of anti-VEGF therapies.

I. ***Medical therapies to control IOP and inflammation*** include:

- *Antiglaucoma drugs* topical as well as systemic similar to POAG. Pilocarpine should be avoided as it will exacerbate the inflammation. Prostaglandin analogs are also less effective because access to the uveoscleral route is generally compromised from angle closure.
- *Topical steroids and atropine* may be required for associated inflammation.
- *Anti-VEGF therapy.* Vascular endothelial growth factor is found in concentrations 40–100 times the normal value in the aqueous humour of patients with NVG. Therefore, anti-VEGF therapy with intravitreal bevacizumab and ranibizumab is being considered to have a significant impact on neovascularization in the form of regression of vessels and decrease in IOP, both when used alone or in combination with pan retinal photocoagulation (PRP).

II. ***Therapy for predisposing conditions,*** e.g.

- *Panretinal photocoagulation (PRP)* is required aggressively to abolish the angiogenic stimulus in patients with retinal ischaemia.
- *Retinal reattachment surgery* is required for patients with retinal detachment.
- *Carotid end artereotomy* may be required for suitable carotid artery stenosis.

III. ***Surgical therapy for intractable glaucomas*** includes:

- *Trabeculectomy with mitomycin (MMC)* may be effective in some cases.
- *Glaucoma drainage device* (Valve implant) surgery is a preferable option in inflamed eyes since conventional trabeculectomy with antimetabolites has a high chance of failure. Glaucoma implants can be inserted either in the anterior chamber or in pars plana if combined with vitrectomy.
- *Glaucoma drainage devices* may control the IOP.
- *Vitrectomy* might be required for associated vitreous haemorrhage and other proliferative disorders of vitreous and retina.
- *For painful blind eye,* consider diode cyclophotocoagulation.

Presently, trans-scleral diode laser (810 nm wavelength) or endoscopic cyclophotocoagulation (ECP) is preferred.

Prognosis

Even when circumstances are favourable, the diagnosis of NVG has a guarded prognosis, and success depends on prevention and early treatment. Hence, all patients with diabetes mellitus or CRVO must be counselled for the need for regular ophthalmological follow-up with patient education regarding the risks and dangers of NVG.

17.5 GLAUCOMA ASSOCIATED WITH INTRAOCULAR TUMOURS

Undoubtedly, glaucoma may sometimes be the presenting sign in a patient with intraocular tumour, but in general, the number of patients of glaucoma associated with intraocular tumours are small. Further, once diagnosed, the management of glaucoma becomes of secondary importance to the treatment of tumour itself.

MECHANISMS OF GLAUCOMA

An intraocular tumour may produce glaucoma by one or more of the following mechanisms:

A. *Secondary open-angle glaucoma,* may be caused by:

- *Pigment dispersion glaucoma* occurring due to the blockage of the trabecular meshwork by the pigment granules.
- *Melanocytic glaucoma* occurring due to blockage of trabecular meshwork by the pigment laden macrophages.
- *Inflammatory glaucoma* occurring as a result of blockage of outflow system by the inflammatory cells due to necrotic tumour-induced inflammation.
- *Tumour cell glaucoma* caused by the blockage of trabecular meshwork by the tumour cell seeding.
- *Haemorrhagic glaucoma* occurring secondary to recurrent intracameral haemorrhage from a tumour.
- *Direct invasion* of the angle by the invading tumour.
- *Elevated episcleral venous pressure (EVP)* may occur due to orbital extension of tumours and lead to a rise in IOP.

B. *Secondary angle-closure glaucoma* may be caused by the following mechanisms:

- *Mechanical angle-closure* caused by anterior displacement of the iris–lens diaphragm by:
  - Posterior tumour mass effect, or
  - As a result of associated suprachoroidal haemorrhage
- *Neovascular angle-closure glaucoma* occurring as a result of tumour associated neovascularization of the angle.
- *Synaechial angle-closure* may occur due to tumour cell-induced peripheral anterior synaechiae formation.
- *Angle-closure by pseudoplateau iris mechanism,* as in primary cysts of the ciliary body or iris.

CLASSIFICATION OF INTRAOCULAR TUMOURS CAUSING GLAUCOMA

A. Primary ocular tumours

I. *Tumours of uvea*

1. *Tumours of choroid*

a. *Benign.* Naevus, haemangioma, melanocytoma, choroidal osteoma

b. *Malignant:* Melanoma

2. *Tumours of ciliary body*

a. *Benign.* Hyperplasia, benign cyst, medulloepithelioma

b. *Malignant.* Melanoma

3. *Tumours of iris*

a. *Benign.* Naevus, benign cyst, naevoxanthoendothelioma

b. *Malignant.* Melanoma

II. *Tumours of retina*

1. *Neuroblastic tumours.* These arise from sensory retina (retinoblastoma and astrocytoma) and pigment epithelium (benign epithelioma and melanotic malignant tumours).
2. *Mesodermal angiomata,* e.g. cavernous haemangioma.
3. *Phakomatoses.* These include: angiomatosis retinae (von Hippel-Lindau disease), tuberous sclerosis (Bourneville's disease), neurofibromatosis (von Recklinghausen's disease and encephalotrigeminal angiomatosis (Sturge-Weber syndrome).

III. Intraocular tumours of optic nerve

Melanocytoma

B. Secondary ocular tumours

Choroid and/or retina can be involved in the following metastatic tumours:

1. *Metastatic carcinomas* from the GIT, lungs, breast, pancreas and genitourinary tract,
2. *Metastatic sarcomas,*
3. *Metastatic melanomas* from the skin, and
4. Leukaemic infiltration.

Note. Details of intraocular tumours are not described here and can be seen in the relevant books/chapters.

GENERAL PRINCIPLES OF DIAGNOSIS AND MANAGEMENT

Glaucoma secondary to intraocular tumours should be considered in all cases of unilateral or markedly asymmetric glaucoma, especially when certain features, such as iris heterochromia, lack of response to antiglaucoma agents, or lack of response to steroids in inflammatory glaucoma (may indicate pseudouveitis) are present.

Ocular examination

Thorough ocular examination including indirect ophthalmoscopy is a must to diagnose intraocular tumours. Indirect ophthalmoscopy allows three-dimensional stereoscopic view of the lesion. It also depicts the presence of shifting fluid which is pathognomonic of exudative retinal detachment seen with intraocular tumours.

Examination under anaesthesia (EUA) should always be taken up in children with suspected intraocular tumour. The examination should include fundus examination of both eyes with full mydriasis (direct as well as indirect ophthalmoscopy), measurement of IOP and corneal diameter.

Investigations

Certain investigations mentioned below are essential to demonstrate the presence of an intraocular tumour, especially when it is masked by a cataract, vitreous haemorrhage, retinal detachment or other opacity in the ocular media.

1. ***Transillumination test.*** It indicates a tumour mass and thus helps to differentiate from choroidal detachment and simple retinal detachment.
2. ***Ultrasonography.*** Both A and B scans help to outline the tumour mass in the presence of hazy media.
3. ***Fluorescein angiography*** is of limited diagnostic value because there is no pathognomonic pattern.
4. ***Radioactive tracer.*** It is based on the fact that the neoplastic tissue has an increased rate of phosphate (^{32}P) uptake.
5. ***MRI.*** Choroidal melanomas are hyperintense in T1-weighted and hypointense in T2-weighted images.

Management

Once diagnosed that the case with secondary glaucoma under investigation is due to an intraocular tumour, immediately the emphasis shifts from the prevention of blindness to the preservation of life. However, care needs to be taken in eyes with benign lesions to avoid loss of vision from unnecessary treatment. Outlines of treatment options are given below:

1. ***Enucleation of the eyeball*** is indicated to limit the morbidity and mortality in many cases. In such patients, the management of glaucoma is not an issue.
2. ***Conservative treatment,*** for example, in case of melanoma of choroid to salvage the eyeball, should be instituted when there is no doubt of diagnosis and the tumour is not very large. However, when the diagnosis is doubtful, observation is indicated especially for small asymptomatic lesions with absence of suspicious features (i.e. associated subretinal fluid/detachment, lipofuscin on the surface, thickness >2 mm). Methods used for conservative treatment and their indications are:
   i. *Brachytherapy* using cobalt-60 or iodine-125 plaques surgically placed externally on the sclera is usually the treatment of choice in tumours less than 10 mm in elevation and less than 16 mm in basal diameter. Supple-

mental transpupillary thermotherapy may be required to enhance the results.

ii. *External beam radiotherapy (EBRT)* with protons or helium ions is indicated in tumours unsuitable for brachytherapy either because of size or posterior location to within 4 mm of disc or fovea.

iii. *Transpupillary thermotherapy (TTT)* with diode laser is indicated in selected small tumours.

3. ***Management of glaucoma*** may be necessary in eyes that are likely to retain good vision with conservative management and will not/do not require enucleation.

i. *Medical management of glaucoma* with anti-glaucoma agents may be effective in many eyes with ocular tumours.

ii. *Laser therapy* is controversial, due to possibility of intraocular spread of tumour cells and the low success of achieving intraocular pressure control.

iii. *Surgical therapy* may be needed to control IOP in some conservatively treated cases of intraocular tumours:

- *Filtration surgery* may be appropriate for eyes with benign tumours, but should be better avoided in eyes with malignant tumours, because of the potential risk of extraocular spread.
- *Tube shunt surgery* may induce a lower risk of intraocular spread.

17.6 PSEUDOEXFOLIATIVE GLAUCOMA (GLAUCOMA CAPSULARE)

Pseudoexfoliation syndrome (PXF) is a systemic condition characterized by deposition of whitish amorphous dandruff-like material over the anterior segment structures of eye and other organs, such as skin, heart, lungs, kidneys and meninges. PXF is associated with secondary open-angle glaucoma in about 25% of the cases.

DEMOGRAPHY AND GENETICS

Age. PXF occurs after about 40 years of age and secondary glaucoma mostly presents after 60 years of age.

Sex. PXF is more common in females, but the glaucoma occurs more commonly in males.

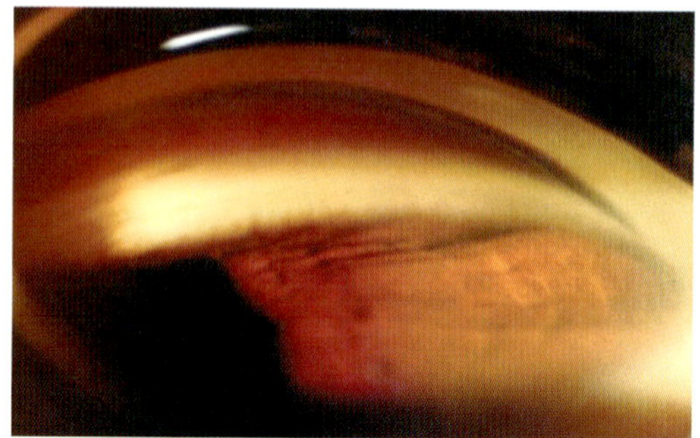

Fig. 17.14 *Benign iris cyst*

Race. More common in Scandinavians Caucasians (up to 20% in general population and up to 90% of glaucoma patients). However, it occurs in all races.

Genetics. A significant association between common single nucleotide polymorphisms (SNPs) 1 intronic (rs2165241) and 2 nonsynonymous (SNPs) (rs1048661, R141L; rs3825942, G153D) in exon 1 of the lysyl oxidase-like protein 1 gene (LOXL1) have been found. They represent a major susceptibility variant for PXF and support the idea that the variant confers risk of glaucoma by causing pseudoexfoliation syndrome.

Laterality. Involvement is asymmetric, i.e. one eye shows full blown picture while other eye quite often shows subclinical changes.

PATHOGENESIS AND RISK FACTORS FOR GLAUCOMA

Pathogenesis

Although exact nature of the white dandruff-like material is not known, it appears to include abnormal elastic microfibrills, basement membrane material and glycosaminoglycan. The fibrillogranular material is homogenous, PAS positive, eosinophilic and rich in polysaccharides. It is supposed to be secreted by pre-equatorial lens epithelium, traverses the lens capsule and reaches the anterior surface. It is deposited over the ciliary body, zonules, anterior face of the vitreous, anterior lens capsule and trabeculum.

Mechanisms of glaucoma postulated are:

- *Secondary open-angle glaucoma* results due to blockage of trabecular meshwork by the exfoliative material

- *Secondary chronic angle-closure glaucoma* may (very rarely) be superadded over the open-angle. Weak zonules with anterior movement of the lens–iris diaphragm may be followed by PAS formation.

Risks of developing glaucoma in patients with PXF

- 5% risk at the end of 5 years of PXF.
- 15% risk at the end of 10 years of having PXF
- 50% risk at the end of 5 years in the fellow eye with PXF of a patient with pseudo-exfoliative glaucoma in one eye
- Very small risk in the normal eye of a patient with exfoliative glaucoma in one eye.

CLINICAL FEATURES

A. Features of pseudoexfoliation

1. *Cornea* shows:

- *Deposition of dandruff-like material* at the back of cornea which may mimic keratic precipitates.
- *With polymegathism of endothelial cells* along with predisposing the cornea for decompensation with moderate rise of IOP.
- *Pigment deposition* on endothelium is usually diffuse, but occasionally Krukenberg spindle may be present.

2. *Anterior chamber angle* on gonioscopy reveals deposition of PXF material on the angle. Pigmentation may be seen ahead of the Schwalbe's line and also over the trabeculum (more marked inferiorly).

3. *Anterior chamber.* Slit-lamp examination may reveal mild flare due to breakdown of blood–aqueous barrier (pseudouveitis).

4. *Iris* shows:

- *Dandruff-like material* distributed on the pupillary border (Fig. 17.15).
- *Peripupillary transillumination* defects and moth-eaten appearance due to sphincter atrophy. It is associated with poor prognosis.
- *Pigment dispersion* may be present in a whorl-like configuration on the sphincter diffusely scattered on the periphery. Mydriasis during surgery usually precipitates the pigment dispersion.

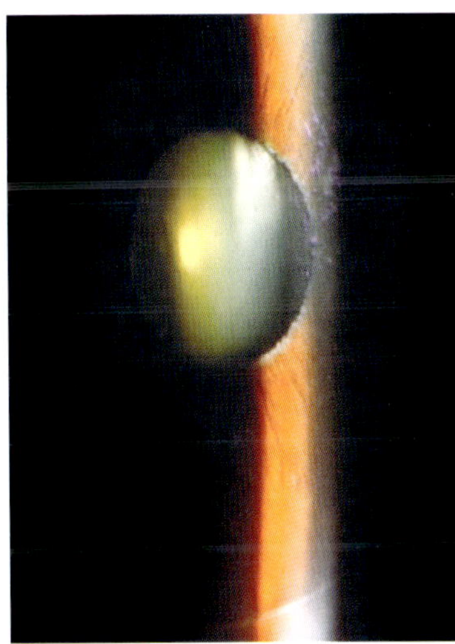

Fig. 17.15 *Pseudoexfoliative deposits at pupillary border*

- Intrastromal haemorrhages may occur in the iris, especially on pharmacological mydriasis.
- Posterior synaechiae may also be develop and contribute to poor mydriasis

5. *Lens* may show:

I. *Deposition of dandruff-like material* on the anterior lens capsule (Fig. 17.16) may occur centrally and peripherally with a clear intermediate zone, thus deviding the anterior lens surface into these zones:

- *Central disc-like area* of exfoliative material deposit is translucent and well demarcated.

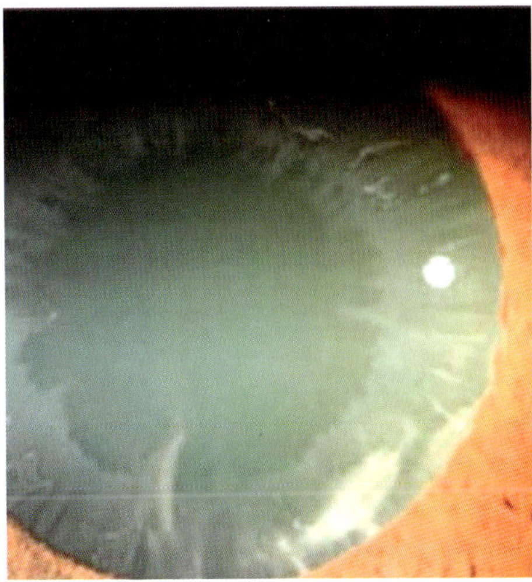

Fig. 17.16 *Pseudoexfoliation seen on anterior lens surface*

It may be absent in 20% cases of PXF.

- *Intermediate clear zone* is formed due to constant rubbing of the pupil which scrapes the dandruff-like material off the mid-zone of the lens.
- *Peripheral band,* outside the intermediate zone, clear shows granular deposits and has a well-delineated inner border with multiple radial striations. The peripheral band is seen on mydriasis.

II. *Zonular instability* is a common feature of PXF and gives rise to phacodonesis and even subluxation. Risk of zonulodialysis during cataract surgery is a matter of concern while operating such cases.

III. *Nuclear cataract* is a common association of pseudoexfoliation syndrome.

B. Features of glaucoma

I. *Secondary open-angle glaucoma* with features almost similar to POAG characterizes the pseudoexfoliative glaucoma (glaucoma capsulare). The only difference being that the disease is often unilateral, the course is more severe with poorer response to medication and more frequent need for surgery.

II. *Secondry narrow-angle glaucoma* is reported to occur occasionally. Even in eyes with open-angle, the IOP may become elevated with pharmacological mydriasis.

MANAGEMENT

1. *Medical therapy*, similar to POAG, is the first choice. However:

- Chances of failure with medical therapy are more than POAG.
- Theoretically, the use of miotics (pilocarpine) may decrease the pseudoexfoliation as it constricts the pupil and iris excursion in the lens.

2. *Laser trabeculoplasty* is very effective initially but after 5 years, failure rate is more than 50%.

3. *Trabeculectomy* is as effective as in POAG.

17.7 STEROID-INDUCED GLAUCOMA

It is a type of secondary open-angle glaucoma which develops following topical, periocular, intraocular and systemic steroid therapy. Even excess endogenous production of glucocortico-steroids (Cushing's syndrome) can also cause an increase in IOP. In 1954, Francois for the first time reported increase in IOP after long-term therapy with corticosteroids. Becker and Mills (1963) reported that steroids not only produce a glaucoma-like state in otherwise healthy eyes but also exacerbate the pre-existing glaucoma.

ETIOPATHOGENESIS

Genetics and steroid responsiveness

Genetics. It has been postulated that the response of IOP to steroids is genetically determined and that based on the response to 6 weeks use of steroids the population can be divided into three groups:

- *High steroid responders,* (5% of normal population), i.e. those who develop an increase in IOP of >15 mm Hg.
- *Moderate steroid responders* (35% of normal population), i.e. those who develop an increase in IOP of 6–15 mm Hg.
- *Low or nonsteroid responders* (60% of normal population), i.e. those in which IOP does not rise ≥6 mm Hg.

Incidence of steroid responsiveness is summarized in Table 17.1.

Theories of pathogenesis

Following theories have been put forward:

Table 17.1 *Incidence of steroid responsiveness (in percentage %)*

Steroid responsiveness	*Normal population*	*POAG patients*	*POAGA's siblings*	*POAGM's offspringes*
High (IOP 73 mm Hg)	05	90	30	25
Moderate (IOP 22–30 mm Hg)	35	10	50	70
Low (IOP <21 mm Hg)	60	20	20	05

1. *Glycosaminoglycans (GAG) theory.* Corticosteroids inhibit the release of hydrolases (by stabilizing lysosomal membrane). Consequently, the GAGs present in the trabecular meshwork cannot depolymerize and they retain water in the extracellular space. This leads to narrowing of trabecular spaces and decrease in aqueous outflow.

2. *Endothelial cell theory.* Under normal circumstances, the endothelial cells lining the trabecular meshwork act as phagocytes and phagocytose the debris from the aqueous humour. Corticosteroids are known to suppress the phagocytic activity of endothelial cells leading to collection of debris in the trabecular meshwork and decreasing the aqueous outflow.

3. *Prostaglandin theory.* Prostaglandin E and F (PGE and PGF) are known to increase the aqueous outflow facility. Corticosteroids can inhibit the synthesis of PGE and PGF leading to decrease in aqueous outflow facility and increase in IOP.

Trabecular Meshwork (TM) Cell Function: Inhibition of phagocytosis resulting in increased cellular debris and elevation of intraocular pressure (IOP).

TM cell morphology changes include:
- Activation of TM cells
- Increased TM cell and nucleus size
- Altered gap junction morphology
- Increased resistance to cytoskeleton disruption

TM extracellular matrix (ECM) changes include:
- Increased deposition of ECM in TM cells
- Increased expression of select ECM molecules
- Increased expression of fibronectin, collagen and elastin
- Altered expression of glycosaminoglycans (GAGs)
- Thickening of the trabecular beams, resulting in increased resistance

TM cell gene expression include:
- Increased glaucoma gene expression MYOC [Trabecular meshwork-induced glucocorticoid response (TIGR)] at locus GLC1A.
- Decreased expression of matrix metalloproteins (MMP's).

Risk factors

Risk factors for steroid-induced glaucoma reported are:
- Primary open-angle glaucoma (exacerbation)
- Family history of glaucoma
- High myopia
- Diabetes mellitus
- Connective tissue disease
- Traumatic angle recession
- Adrenal hyperplasia or neoplasia

CLINICAL FEATURES

Steroid-induced glaucoma usually develops following weeks of topical therapy with strong steroids and months of therapy with weak steroids. Steroid-induced glaucoma typically resembles POAG, i.e.
- Patients are usually asymptomatic,
- IOP is elevated,
- White and painless eyes,
- Open and normal appearing angle on gonioscopy,
- Optic disc cupping, and
- Visual field defects occur in long-standing cases.

Acute presentation, though rare, is reported after intensive steroid therapy, especially with systemic steroids. With acute presentation patient may experience corneal oedema.

IOP elevating potency of steroids. Table 17.2 shows comparison of anti-inflammatory and

Table 17.2 *Anti-inflammatory and intraocular pressure elevating potencies of various steroids*

Potency	*Steroid*	*Glaucoma risk*
	Betamethasone	
High	Dexamethasone	
	Fluocinonide	
Moderate	Triamcinolone	
	Fluorometholone	
	Loteprednol etobonate	
	Dexamethasone sodium phosphate	
	Hydrocortisone	
Low	Rimexolone	
	Medrisone	

intraocular pressure elevating potencies of various steroids.

MANAGEMENT

Prevention of steroid-induced glaucoma involves judicious use of steroids and a regular monitoring of IOP when steroid therapy is a must.

Treatment consists of:
- *Discontinuation of steroids.* IOP may normalise within 10 days to 4 weeks in 98% of cases.
- *Medical therapy with 0.5% timolol maleate* is effective during the normalization period.
- *Anecortave acetate injection* into the anterior subtenon space in eye with uncontrolled steroid-related ocular hypertension following intravitreal or subtenon injections of triamcinolone acetonides a possible new treatment under investigation. It is actually a cortisone, free of glucocorticoid and mineralo-corticoid activity.
- *Filtration surgery* is required occasionally in intractable cases. Tube shunt, excision of the subtenon steroid depot, explantation of steroid implant and pars plana vitrectomy for removal of intravitreal depot may be required.

17.8 TRAUMATIC GLAUCOMA

Glaucoma can occur in almost all types of injuries which include:
- Mechanical injuries
- Chemical injuries
- Electrical injuries
- Radiational injuries

A. GLAUCOMA IN MECHANICAL INJURIES

American Ocular Trauma Society has classified the mechanical ocular injuries as below:

1. ***Closed globe injury*** is one in which the eyewall (sclera and cornea) does not have a full thickness wound but there is intraocular damage. It includes contusion and lamellar laceration.
- *Contusion* refers to the closed-globe injury resulting from blunt trauma. Damage may occur at the site of impact or at a distant site.
- *Lamellar laceration* is a closed globe injury characterized by a partial thickness wound of the eyewall caused by a sharp object or blunt trauma.

2. ***Open-globe injury*** is associated with a full thickness wound of the sclera or cornea or both. It includes rupture and laceration of eye wall.

i. *Rupture* refers to a full-thickness wound of eyewall caused by the impact of blunt trauma. The wound occurs due to markedly raised intraocular pressure by an inside-out injury mechanism.

ii. *Laceration* refers to a full-thickness wound of eyewall caused by a sharp object. The wound occurs at the impact site by an outside-in mechanism. It includes penetrating and perforating injuries.

- *Penetrating injury* refers to a single laceration of eyewall caused by a sharp object.
- *Perforating injury* refers to two full thickness lacerations (one entry and one exit) of the eyewall caused by a sharp object or missile. The two wounds must have been caused by the same agent.
- *Intraocular foreign body injury* is technically a penetrating injury associated with retained intraocular foreign body. However, it is grouped separately because of different clinical implications.

Mechanisms of traumatic glaucoma

Mechanisms producing traumatic glaucoma are as below:

Open-angle traumatic glaucoma

I. Acute open-angle traumatic glaucomas

Causes of acute open-angle traumatic glaucoma include:

1. *Hyphaema, e.g.*
   - Red blood cell glaucoma, or
   - Haemorrhagic glaucoma
2. *Inflammatory glaucoma*
3. *Lens particle glaucoma*
4. *Pigment disposition in trabecular meshwork*

II. Chronic open-angle traumatic glaucomas

Causes of chronic open-angle traumatic glaucoma include:

1. ***Ghost cell glaucoma*** (see page 271)

2. ***Angle recession glaucoma.*** Angle recession refers to rupture in the ciliary body face (between scleral spur and iris root). Unilateral open-angle glaucoma usually occurs after years (may be 10 years) of blunt trauma. Angle recession is not the cause of glaucoma but just indicator of old trauma. Glaucoma occurs due to slowly induced fibrosis of trabecular meshwork.

Angle recession may be:

- *Shallow.* Characterized by increased visibility of the ciliary body and the scleral spur.
- *Moderate.* Tear extends between the longitudinal and circular fibres of the ciliary bodies.
- *Deep.* Gonioscopically angle recession is characterized by an irregular widening of the ciliary body band (Fig. 17.17).

Lifetime risk of developing glaucoma in patients with angle recession is as below:

- Angle recession <180° : 4%
- Angle recession >180% : 22%
- Fellow eye has a 50% greater risk of developing glaucoma

III. Glaucoma due to effect of retained IOFB

The retained iron and copper foreign bodies may produce siderosis and chalcosis, respectively and cause glaucoma by producing structural changes in trabecular meshwork.

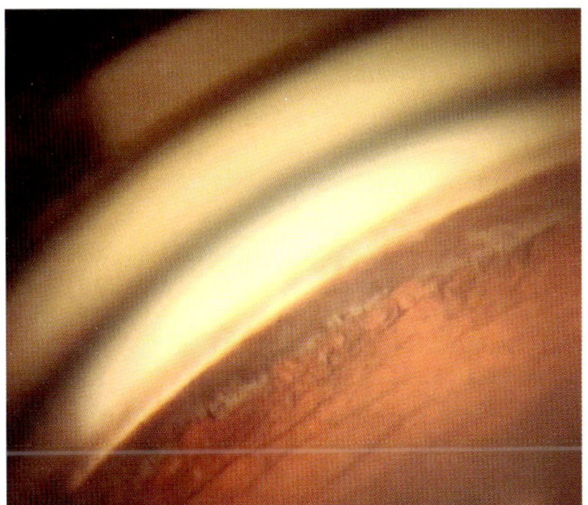

Fig. 17.17 *Angle recession*

Angle-closure traumatic glaucoma

1. ***Acute angle-closure traumatic glaucoma*** may occur due to:
   - Peripheral anterior synaechiae
   - Lens subluxation
   - Lens intumescence
   - Uveal effusion
2. ***Chronic angle-closure glaucoma*** may occur due to:
   - Peripheral anterior synaechie
   - Posterior synaechiae
   - Epithelial ingrowth, and
   - Fibrovascular downgrowth

Note. All mechanisms that can elevate IOP after closed globe trauma (blunt trauma) can also lead to increased IOP in eyes with open globe trauma (rupture or penetrating or perforating injuries). The mechanisms of raised IOP pertinent to open globe trauma include fibrous ingrowth, epithelial downgrowth and intraocular foreign bodies (IOFB).

Investigations

- *B scan ultrasound:* To rule out intraocular foreign body, vitreous haemorrhage, retinal detachment.
- *Ultrasound biomicroscopy:* Can be useful in the identification of a ciliary body cleft.
- Anterior segment optical coherence tomography (OCT), computed tomography (CT) and magnetic resonance imaging (MRI) (if a magnetic foreign body is ruled out).

Management of glaucoma in mechanical trauma

1. ***Medical antiglaucoma therapy.*** Medical therapy, depending upon the level of IOP, may include topical and systemic aqueous suppressants and systemic hyperosmotic agents.
2. ***Treatment of causative mechanism,*** i.e.
   - Hyphaema
   - Uveal inflammation
   - Subluxated lens
   - Lens particles due to ruptured lens in the anterior chamber
3. ***Filtration surgery*** may be required in glaucomas non-response to above measures.

i. *Trabeculectomy:* Trabeculectomy with anterior chamber washout and peripheral iridectomy may be a beneficial primary surgical treatment for traumatic hyphema unresponsive to medical management with antiglaucomatous agents.

ii. *Glaucoma drainage devices:* In cases such as refractory angle recession glaucoma, after a failed trabeculectomy, the insertion of a glaucoma drainage device may be considered. In cases with insufficient conjunctiva, a conjunctival autograft from other eye or amniotic membrane graft can be planned.

iii. *Microinvasive glaucoma surgery:* iStent Trabecular Micro-Bypass Stent, ab interno trabeculotomy using the Trabectome, and gonioscopy-assisted transluminal trabeculotomy (GATT) have shown good results in patients with traumatic glaucoma, so in some cases these can also be tried.

B. GLAUCOMA IN CHEMICAL INJURIES

Glaucoma is more common after alkali burns but is also seen after severe acid burns.

Mechanisms of glaucoma

1. *Early rise of IOP* is caused by:
   - Shrinkage of collagen tissue, cornea and sclera, and
   - Increase in uveal blood flow.
2. *Intermediate rise of IOP* is caused by intraocular inflammatory changes. Hypopyon may also develop and contribute to rise of IOP.
3. *Late rise of IOP* is caused by intraocular damage and formation of PAS or other intraocular scarring. Delayed pressure rise is also caused by prostaglandin release.

Management

I. *Medical therapy*

1. *Antiglaucoma agents*, especially topical and systemic aqueous suppressants, are quite useful. Miotics and prostaglandin should usually be avoided.
2. *Antiprostaglandins*. The presence of prostaglandins during the delayed pressure rise suggests that the early use of drugs, such as indomethacin and imidazoles, which inhibit prostaglandin synthesis, may be beneficial.

II. *Surgical therapy*

1. *Filtration surgery* may be required, but may be difficult due to scarring of conjunctiva and episcleral tissue.
2. *Glaucoma drainage device procedure*, such as Ahmed or Molteno valve should be considered when external scarring is present.
3. *Cyclodestructive procedures* may be considered as a last resort.

C. GLAUCOMA IN ELECTRICAL INJURIES

Transient rise of IOP is reported after electrical injury, cardioversion, and electroshock therapy.

Mechanisms of glaucoma in electric shock include;

- *Venous dilatation*
- *Contraction of the extraocular muscle*, and
- *Pigment dispersion*.

Treatment. Usually no treatment is required as the rise in IOP is transient. If required, topical and systemic aqueous suppressants may be given; miotics and prostaglandins are usually avoided.

D. GLAUCOMA IN RADIATIONAL INJURIES

Rise in IOP has been reported radiation injury to the eyeball following radiation therapy to the structures near the eye.

Mechanisms of rise in IOP following radiation injury to the eyeball include:

- *Neovascularization of the angle*
- *Structural damage to trabecular meshwork* causing secondary open-angle glaucoma associated with diffuse conjunctival telangiectasia
- *Ghost cell glaucoma* following radiation retinopathy and intraocular haemorrhage.

Management includes:

- *Medical therapy* with topical and systemic aqueous suppressants may be useful.
- *Surgical therapy needed* includes:
  - *Filtration surgery*, chances of success are less
  - *Cyclodestructive procedures* are often required to control IOP.

17.9 GLAUCOMA SECONDARY TO OCULAR SURGERY

Secondary glaucoma after ocular surgery is not uncommon and may occur after operative procedures for cataract, glaucoma, corneal transplantation and vitreoretinal surgery. The common entities described are:

- Glaucoma in aphakia/pseudophakia
- Malignant glaucoma
- Glaucoma associated with epithelial downgrowth and fibrous ingrowth
- Glaucomas associated with corneal surgery
  - Glaucoma after penetrating keratoplasty
  - Glaucoma after lamellar keratoplasty
  - Glaucoma after keratoprosthesis
- Glaucoma associated with procedures for vitreous and retinal diseases:
  - Glaucoma after pars plana vitrectomy,
  - Glaucoma after scleral buckling procedure, and
  - Glaucoma after retinal photocoagulation

GLAUCOMA IN APHAKIA/PSEUDOPHAKIA

IMPORTANT FACTS

- *Terms aphakic and pseudophakic* glaucomas have been discarded as the causative conditions differ in their pathogenesis, clinical features and treatment.
- Ideally, even the *term glaucoma-in-aphakia/pseudophakia* should also not be considered as a clinical entity for the same reasons. However, the glaucomas considered in this section are related by the fact that they develop after cataract extraction.
- Incidence of glaucoma after cataract surgery has dropped significantly in recent years as microsurgical techniques have improved and the vitreous disturbance when occurs is being efficiently managed by vitrectomy.
- *Uncomplicated phacoemulsification* with IOL implantation usually produces a late sustained reduction in IOP.

TYPES/CAUSES OF GLAUCOMA IN APHAKIA/PSEUDOPHAKIA

A. Open-angle glaucoma

i. ***Early onset (within first postoperative week),*** usually self-limiting may be caused by:

- Viscoelastic material
- Hyphaema debris
- Inflammation
- Idiopathic (may be trabecular meshwork oedema, or distortion of outflow channels by suture)
- Pre-existing (undiagnosed) POAG

ii. ***Intermediate onset (after first postoperative week).*** It includes:

- Steroid-induced glaucoma
- Lens-particle glaucoma
- Ghost cell glaucoma
- Pigmentary glaucoma
- Hyphaema
- Vitreous in anterior chamber
- Pre-existing (undiagnosed POAG)

iii. ***Late onset glaucoma (occurring after 2 months postoperatively)***

- Chronic inflammation
- Pigmentary glaucoma
- Ghost cell glaucoma
- Late occurring haemorrhage
- Post-Nd:YAG laser capsulotomy
- Pre-existing (undiagnosed POAG)

B. Angle-closure glaucoma

i. ***With pupillary block***

Pupil block is caused by adhesions of the pupil with structure lying posterior to it, which depending upon the circumstances (aphakia, pseudophakia with ACIOL, pseudophakia with PCIOL (with zonular dehiscence or posterior capsular rent or post-Nd:YAG capsulotomy), may be:

- Vitreous
- Posterior capsule
- Anterior chamber or iris supported IOL
- Posterior chamber IOL

ii. ***Without pupillary block***

Angle closure with peripheral anterior synaechiae (PAS) are formation may occur without pupillary block in the following conditions:

- Ciliary block glaucoma
- Prolonged anterior chamber shallowing
- Inflammatory angle-closure glaucoma
- Neovascular angle-closure glaucoma
- Epithelial downgrowth
- Fibrous downgrowth
- Endothelial proliferation
- Proliferation of iris melanocytes across the trabecular meshwork
- Pre-existing angle-closure glaucoma

CLINICAL FEATURES AND MANAGEMENT

Clinical features

Clinical features of glaucoma in aphakia/pseudophakia depend upon the type and cause of glaucoma and are the same as described for different types, e.g. lens particle glaucoma, inflammatory glaucoma, steroid-induced glaucoma, etc.

Management

1. *Prevention of IOP rise after cataract surgery*

The risk of postoperative glaucoma can be significantly reduced by:

i. *Meticulously performed surgery as below:*

- *Gentle handling of the tissues* reduces the risk of inflammation, pigment dispersion and haemorrhage
- *Judicious use and thorough removal of viscoelastic material* decrease the risk of postoperative rise of IOP.

ii. *Prophylactic use of IOP lowering drugs,* such as oral acetazolamide and topical timolol maleate in immediate postoperative period, is quite useful.

2. *Treatment of the cause of IOP elevation*

Efforts should be made to find out the cause and treat it (as described in different types of secondary glaucoma, e.g.:

- *Pars plana vitrectomy and removal of lens fragments* will solve the problem when uveitis and glaucoma are due to retained lens fragments in the vitreous.
- *Laser PI* is useful in pupil block glaucoma
- *Withdrawal of steroids* is useful in controlling the steroid-induced glaucoma.

3. *Medical therapy*

Medical therapy similar to POAG may be needed in cases of glaucoma in aphakia/pseudophakia due to:

- Pre-existing (undiagnosed) POAG,
- Pigmentary glaucoma,
- Glaucoma capsulare, and
- Idiopathic open-angle glaucoma.

4. *Surgical therapy*

Indications. Surgical therapy needs to be undertaken when the medical therapy fails.

Caution. Surgical therapy in these eyes is less successful and has a higher complication rate than in phakic eyes.

Surgical procedures include:

- *Trabeculectomy with mitomycin* C can result in long-term IOP control, but the use of an antimetabolite increases the risk of post-operative complications.
- Glaucoma drainage implants may be useful in cases where trabeculectomy fails or in cases with excessive conjunctival scarring.

MALIGNANT GLAUCOMA

TERMINOLOGY

Malignant glaucoma. This term was coined by Von-Grafe in 1869, to denote a condition characterized by marked rise in IOP associated with shallow anterior chamber, occurring after surgery (peripheral iridectomy or filtration surgery) in patients with angle-closure glaucoma. The condition has nothing to do with any neoplastic diseases. Over the years, many alternative terms have been suggested and many other causative conditions have been added.

Alternative terms suggested by different workers based on the postulated mechanism of rise in IOP are:

- Ciliary block glaucoma
- Aqueous misdirection syndrome, and
- Direct lens block glaucoma

Conclusion. Till date there is no universal consensus for any term. However, over the period, many workers prefer the term *'aqueous* *misdirection syndrome*'. In this text, the original term malignant glaucoma is used for the purpose of description. In the international literature, a common term used to describe a flat anterior chamber is "athalamia."

PATHOMECHANISM OF MALIGNANT GLAUCOMA

Exact pathogenesis is still not clear. The postulated mechanisms with supportive mechanisms are described below.

1. Posterior pooling of aqueous

Shaffer (1954) postulated that an accumulation of aqueous behind a posterior vitreous detachment (PVD) causes a forward movement of the iris–lens or iris–vitreous diaphragm leading to shallowing of anterior chamber and angle-closure. This concept was later expanded to include the collection of aqueous as pockets in the vitreous body (Fig. 17.18). Since aqueous misdirection was considered the causative factor, so the condition was also termed as 'aqueous misdirection syndrome'.

Mechanisms of posterior misdirection of aqueous

i. *Ciliary block mechanism.* Many clinicians believe the anterior rotation of the ciliary body with ciliary processes pressed against the lens along with anterior displacement of the vitreous is responsible for the aqueous misdirection (Fig. 17.18A). The anterior displacement of the vitreous puts it in apposition to the ciliary processes contributing to the misdirection. Because of this concept, the term 'ciliary block glaucoma' has been suggested as alternative to malignant glaucoma.

ii. *Anterior hyaloid face block mechanism.* Some workers have suggested that the block to anterior aqueous flow is caused by the intact anterior vitreous face which is compressed against the ciliary process and breaks in the hyaloid near the vitreous base allow the aqueous to be diverted posteriorly in the vitreous body.

iii. *Choroidal expansion mechanism.* It has been suggested that the precipitating event is an increase in the choroidal volume which pushes the vitreous body and thus the iris–lens and iris–vitreous diaphragm forward causing flattening of the anterior chamber and angle-closure.

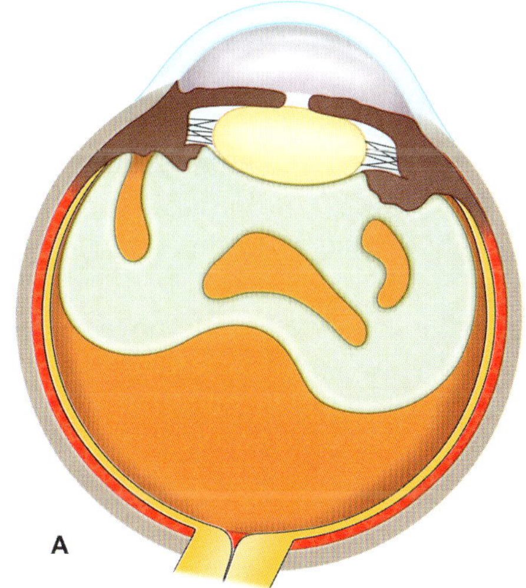

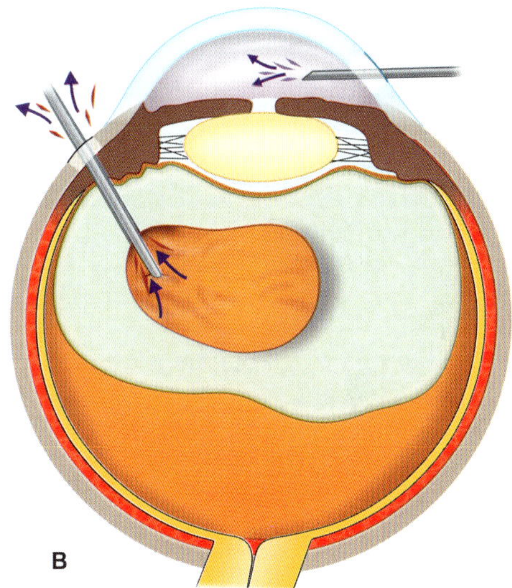

Fig. 17.18 *Malignant glaucoma: (A) Mechanism of ciliolenticular block with collection of aqueous as pockets in the vitreous and behind the posterior hyaloid face; (B) Management by vitreous aspiration and air injection in the anterior chamber*

Consequently, the aqueous which cannot move forward collects behind the vitreous which further moves forward, carrying the lens and iris further with it.

2. Direct lens block angle-closure mechanisms

Chandler and Grant (1962) postulated that the forward movement of iris lens diaphragm occurs as a result of laxity of lens granules. Many other workers have also corroborated this theory and suggested the laxity of lens zonules might be caused by any of the following situations:

- Severe and prolonged angle-closure
- Ciliary muscle spasm induced by surgery, miotics, inflammation, trauma or other known factors.

Since in this concept, the lens moves forward directly due to the laxity, so the term 'Direct lens block angle-closure glaucoma' has also been suggested as an alternative to malignant glaucoma.

CLINICAL PROFILE

Symptoms and signs

Symptoms. Typically, following an intraocular operation (usually after surgical peripheral iridectomy, filteration surgery, i.e. trabeculotomy in patients with primary angle-closure glaucoma), patients develop following symptoms:

- *Sever pain* in the eye with associated headache, nausia and sometimes vomiting.
- *Blurring of vision* and sometimes marked loss of vision.

Signs of ciliary block glaucoma noted are:

- *Flat anterior chamber*, usually persistent after the intraocular surgery.
- *Markedly raised IOP*, in early postoperative period.
- *Negative Seidel's test* indicating absence of any leak in the section.
- *Absence of papillary block*, confirmed by a patent iridectomy.
- *Absence of suprachoroidal haemorrhage.*
- *Miotics* are unresponsive or even aggravate the condition.
- *Cycloplegics and mydriatics* may relieve the condition.

Clinical forms

Different clinical forms of malignant glaucoma described are:

1. ***Classic malignant glaucoma*** refers to the typical clinical features described above after an incisional surgery (filtration surgery or surgical peripheral iridectomy) in patients with primary angle-closure glaucoma (Fig. 17.19).

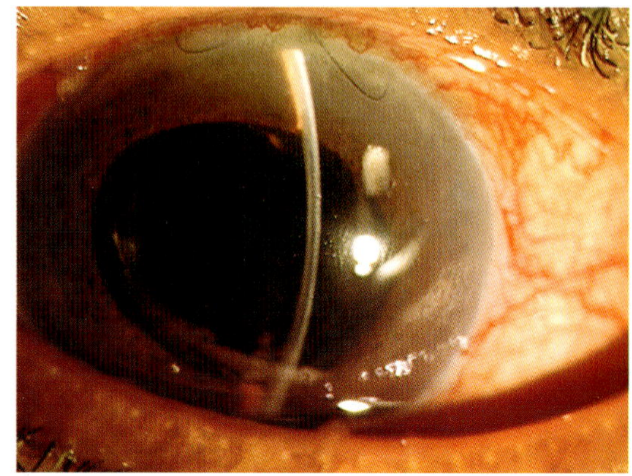

Fig. 17.19 *Classic malignant glaucoma: Shallow central anterior chamber in a post-trabeculectomy patient*

2. ***Aphakic/pseudophakic malignant glaucoma*** refers to the disease occurring after cataract surgery as a result of ciliovitreal block or cilio-IOL block. It occurs in eyes with or without pre-existing angle-closure glaucoma.
3. ***Other clinical forms of malignant glaucoma*** reported are:
   - i. *Miotic-induced malignant glaucoma* has been reported to occur in patients with prior surgery (iridectomy or filtration) or without any prior surgery.
   - ii. *Malignant glaucoma following laser treatment*
     - After laser iridotomy
     - After laser suture lysis following trabeculectomy
     - After Nd:YAG cyclophotocoagulation
   - iii. *Malignant glaucoma associated with retinal diseases*, such as:
     - Retinopathy of prematurity
     - After retinal detachment surgery
     - After central retinal vein occlusion
   - iv. *Malignant glaucoma associated with inflammation and infection*, e.g. in association with:
     - Traumatic or non-traumatic uveitis
     - Endophthalmitis caused by fungal keratomycosis
     - Endophthalmitis caused by *Nocardia asteroides*
   - v. *Spontaneous malignant glaucoma* may rarely occur without any known cause (previous

surgery, miotic therapy, or other apparent cause).

MANAGEMENT

Differential diagnosis of malignant glaucoma

Classic malignant glaucoma needs to be differentiated from other causes of post-filtration surgery, shallow anterior chamber which include:

- Pupillary block glaucoma,
- Serous choroidal detachment, and
- Suprachoroidal haemorrhage.

Treatment

1. ***Medical therapy*** forms the first-line of treatment and consists of:
   i. *Topical cycloplegics* preferably 1% atropine instilled four times a day help by moving the lens–iris diaphragm back and breaking the ciliary block.
   ii. *Hyperosmotic agents* especially mannitol 2 g/kg intravenously over 45 minutes help by reducing the pressure exerted by the vitreous.
   iii. *Aqueous suppressants,* such as topical β blockers or α2 agonists (or both) and oral or topical anhydrase inhibition, help by decreasing aqueous production.

Note.

- *Prolonged maintenance on atropine* with a very slow taper is required after the attack is broken because of high-risk of recurrence.
- *Miotics are contraindicated,* as the y may cause or contribute to aqueous misdirection.

2. ***Laser therapy*** constitutes the second line of treatment and includes:
   i. *Argon laser photocoagulation of the ciliary processes* that can be visualized through an iridectomy.
   ii. *Trans-scleral diode laser cyclophotocoagulation* has been reported to relieve malignant glaucoma presumably by breaking the ciliolenticular block.
   iii. *Nd:YAG laser iridotomies and anterior hyaloidotomy* are helpful in aphakic/ pseudophakic malignant glaucoma by releasing the trapped aqueous from the vitreous and re-establishing normal aqueous flow. Several openings should be made peripherally, i.e. not directly behind the optic. The placement of iridotomies should be peripheral since the underlying etiology is an abnormal relationship between the hyaloid and the ciliary processes.

3. ***Surgical measures*** are needed when medical and laser therapy fails. These include:
   i. *Surgical disruption of the anterior hyaloid face* with the help of a sharp needle through a transcorneal approach with reformation of anterior chamber may be tried in aphakic/ pseudophakic patients especially when Nd:YAG laser is not available.
   ii. *Vitreous aspiration and air injection in anterior chamber* (Fig. 17.18B) was described by Chandler (1964) using 18-gauge needle via posterior sclerotomy (3 mm behind the limbus) with reasonably good results in many patients.
   iii. *Pars plana vitrectomy with or without lensectomy* (as the case may be) is presently being considered the treatment of choice due to improved microsurgical equipment and techniques.

Management of the fellow eye

It is important to note that the fellow eye is also prone to meet the same fate. So a laser PI should be performed as prophylaxis.

GLAUCOMA ASSOCIATED WITH EPITHELIAL DOWNGROWTH AND FIBROUS INGROWTH

Epithelial downgrowth or fibrous ingrowth or both together may occur following any anterior segment incisional surgery (e.g. cataract surgery, glaucoma surgery, penetrating keratoplasty, etc.) or penetrating trauma. Ofcourse, their incidence has decreased markedly in recent years owing to improved microincisional surgery and suturing techniques.

GLAUCOMA IN EPITHELIAL DOWNGROWTH

Pathogenesis

Conjunctival and corneal epithelial cells may downgrowth into the anterior chamber following either surgical or traumatic wound under following conditions:

- *Penetration of epithelium* into the anterior chamber usually occurs through a fistula which may be associated with incarceration of iris, lens material or vitreous strands in the wound (surgical or traumatic).
- *Implantation of epithelial cells* into the anterior chamber from surgical instruments or sutures.

Clinical features

Epithelial downgrowth into the anterior chamber may proliferate in three forms: pearl tumour, epithelial cyst and epithelial downgrowth.

- ***Pearl tumours*** usually occur after penetrating trauma associated with implantation of a cilium along with epithelial elements. The epithelial walls of the pearl tumour are keratinized and so give a pearly appearance. The pearl tumours may remain stationary for a long time or may enlarge, till the anterior chamber and cause secondary angle-closure glaucoma.
- ***Epithelial cysts***, also known as epithelial inclusion cysts, are formed when the surface epithelial cells are implanted in the anterior chamber following surgical or accidental trauma. It is believed that iris tissue provides nutritional support for the epithelial cells to grow as a cyst in months or even years. These cysts appear as translucent, non-vascular anterior chamber cysts. The cyst wall shows varying degrees of pigmentation. The cysts may remain stationary or may enlarge to fill the pupil and anterior chamber.
- ***Epithelial downgrowth*** presents as greyish sheet with rolled edges, growing from the wound margin along the posterior surface of the cornea, trabecular meshwork, iris surface and ciliary body. This sheet is formed when the surface epithelium gets opportunity to grow into the anterior chamber through the wound which is not properly closed, e.g. when iris tissue or vitreous strands are incarcerated. It is usually associated with persistent inflammation that does not respond to steroid therapy. It was common occurrence after cataract surgery when the wound size used to be large and non-valvular closed with 3 to 7 sutures. The suspected epithelization can be confirmed by applying a shot of argon laser photocoagulation to the iris which turns white.

Note. Specular microscopy and confocal microscopy allow direct visualization of epithelial cells.

Mechanism of glaucoma

Epithelial downgrowth may cause glaucoma by following mechanisms:

- *Secondary open-angle glaucoma,* due to epithelial membrane covering the trabecular meshwork.
- *Secondary angle-closure glaucoma* following contraction of the membrane with PAS formation.
- *Pupillary block glaucoma* may occur when the epithelial membrane advances across the pupil to the anterior vitreous face.

Management

I. *Treatment of epithelial downgrowth* is often frustrating. An early diagnosis is essential to avoid later enucleation. It is advisable to determine the extent of epithelization by applying argon-laser shots before taking up any of the following surgical measures to treat the epithelial downgrowth:

- *Surgical excision* of the membrane through a limbal incision along with fistulectomy (when present).
- *Cryotherapy* of the involved posterior corneal surface using a double freeze-thaw technique.
- *Swabing with absolute alcohol* of the involved corneal surface.
- *Scrapping the membrane* off the corneal surface.
- *Pars plana vitrectomy approach* to remove the iris membrane off the ciliary body combined with unipolar diathermy and end photocoagulation. Alternatively, after removal of membrane and involved iris, intraocular air may be inserted and cryotherapy applied in the transcorneal and trans-scleral fashion.

II. *Postoperative treatment to control inflammation and IOP* should include topical:

- Steroid eyedrops
- Cycloplegic eyedrops
- Aqueous suppressants

III. *Treatment of pearl tumours and epithelial cysts* is as below.

- *Pearl tumours* rarely need treatment, as they remain stationary for a long period.

- *En bloc surgical excision of an anterior chamber cyst and involved iris* is indicated when enlargement threatens other intraocular structures. Post-traumatic epithelial cysts usually require surgical excision for progressive enlargement.

IV. ***Surgical treatment of glaucoma*** is often required, is mostly difficult and consists of:

- *Filtration surgery* with intraoperative use of Mitomycin C or postoperative 5-fluorouracil may be tried.
- *Glaucoma drainage device* may be the treatment of choice in many cases with glaucoma secondary to epithelial downgrowth.
- *Enucleation* was required in the past, in many eyes with painful blind eye due to intractable glaucoma associated with epithelial downgrowth. However, with improved diagnosis and early treatment, the need for enucleation is decreasing.

GLAUCOMA IN FIBROUS INGROWTH

Fibrous ingrowth, also known as stromal ingrowth or stromal outgrowth, occurs under similar circumstances as epithelial downgrowth and may occur alone or in association with epithelial downgrowth. Unlike epithelial downgrowth, the fibrous ingrowth is slow to progress and may be self-limited. Because of this relatively indolent nature of fibrous ingrowth, vis-à-vis epithelial downgrowth, comparatively a smaller number of eyes require enucleation.

Pathogenesis

Two forms of this condition have been described: fibrous ingrowth and retrocorneal membrane.

1. ***Pathogenesis of fibrous ingrowth.*** Like epithelial downgrowth, the fibrous ingrowth also occurs when there is inadequate wound closure after intraocular surgery or penetrating trauma. It follows a break in the corneal endothelium and Descemet's membrane, which allows fibroblasts to enter the anterior chamber from subepithelial connective tissue or from corneal or limbal stroma. The ingrowth of connective tissue is inhibited when the inner wound margins are bridged by the endothelium by the second postoperative break. Thus, one can say that damaged corneal endothelium is also a risk factor for stromal ingrowth even after well- opposed wound.

2. ***Pathogenesis of retrocorneal membrane.*** Inflammatory and traumatic insults to the cornea are reported to result in the formation of retrocorneal membrane. Descemet's membrane is typically intact and the metaplastic corneal endothelium and blood mononuclear cells are believed to contribute the fibrous tissue.

Clinical features

I. ***Fibrous ingrowth*** presents as a thick greyish white, translucent, vascular, retrocorneal membrane. The edges of this membrane have tongue-like projections rather than scalloped edges of epithelial membrane. Overall the appearance of fibrous membrane resembles a woven cloth.

II. ***Glaucoma.*** Initially, *secondary open-angle glaucoma* develops from associated inflammation and haemorrhage. But the frequent complication is *secondary angle-closure glaucoma* which occurs when the fibrous ingrowth involves the angle and, on contraction leads to formation of PAS and the destruction of trabecular meshwork.

III. ***Posterior segment involvement*** may occur due to tractional forces produced by the fibrous membrane and induce retinal tears or detachments and cystoid macular oedema.

Management

I. ***Fibrous ingrowth*** has no specific treatment per se. Therefore, attention needs to be given to the complicating sequelae without efforts to eradicate the membrane.

II. ***Glaucoma*** should be managed medically or surgically as necessary.

III. ***Release of vitreous traction*** by vitrectomy or Nd:YAG laser lysis may be required to prevent further posterior segment complications.

IV. ***Penetrating keratoplasty*** may be required for visual rehabilitation.

GLAUCOMA ASSOCIATED WITH CORNEAL SURGERY

Glaucoma associated with corneal surgery includes:

- Glaucoma after penetrating keratoplasty
- Glaucoma after lamellar keratoplasty
- Glaucoma after keratoprosthesis

GLAUCOMA AFTER PENETRATING KERATOPLASTY

Glaucoma associated with penetrating keratoplasty (PK) is a common and growing problem. Its incidence varies widely depending upon the pre-existing status of the eye and indication of PK; in general being more common in aphakic eyes, combined cataract and keratoplasty, and repeat PK. Glaucoma after PK is of concern not only because of difficulty in management but also because of associated graft failure.

Pathogenesis and mechanisms of post-PK glaucoma

Risk factors

Risk factors for developing post-PK glaucoma can be divided into preoperative, intraoperative and postoperative factors.

I. *Preoperative factors* are as below:

1. *Preoperative glaucoma*, even if controlled, is a major risk factor for developing postoperative raised level of IOP.
2. *Other preoperative factors* associated with increased incidence of post-PK glaucoma are:
   - *Phakic vs aphakic/pseudophakic status*. Though secondary glaucoma is reported to occur in all circumstances but the chances are more in aphakics (60–70%) than pseudophakics (20–50%), which is more than phakic eyes.
   - *Indications of PK associated with an increased incidence of post-PK raised IOP* reported in a decreasing chronological order are: Peter's anomaly (60%), scarr in an aniridia (56%), ulcerative disease (50%), corneal regraft (50%), trauma (45%), viral keratitis (45%), Fuch's dystrophy (37%), acanthamoeba keratitis (36%), keratoconus (0–12%) and congenital hereditary endothelial dystrophy (0–3%).

II. *Intraoperative factors* that influence the risk of post-PK glaucoma are:

- *Technical skill* of performing the surgery is a critical factor as it affects the PAS formation and wound distortion. However, this factor has not been studied much.
- *Choice of viscoelastic* at the time of surgery may have a role in minimizing the formation of PAS.
- *Size of corneal graft.* The literature reports a protective effect of the oversize graft to some extent.

III. *Postoperative factors*, which increase the risk of post-PK rise in IOP are:

- *Corticosteroids-induced glaucoma* may occur in steroid responders, as these are to be used for a very long time.
- *PAS formation* and progressive angle-closure in the postoperative period has been reported to increase the incidence of rise in IOP. This is particularly important among the patients without any preoperative glaucoma.

Clinical spectrum and mechanisms of post-PK glaucoma

I. *Glaucoma in early postoperative period* may occur due to the following mechanisms:

1. *Pressure elevating mechanisms similar to other intraocular procedures* (e.g. cataract surgery) which can raise IOP in early post-PK period are:
   - Uveal inflammation,
   - Intraocular haemorrhage,
   - Pupillary block mechanism, and
   - Steroid responsiveness.
2. *Pressure elevating mechanisms peculiar* to penetrating keratoplasty are:
   - *Collapse of trabecular meshwork* which may occur due to loss of anterior support as a result of incision in the Descemet's membrane. The trabecular collapse occurs more in aphakic patients where posterior support is also reduced due to loss of zonular tension.
   - *Compression of the anterior chamber angle* may occur with conventional techniques of PK.

II. *Glaucoma in late postoperative period* may occur due to the following mechanisms:

- Gradual flattening of the anterior chamber and angle-closure is reported in the late post-operative period especially in aphakic eyes with intact anterior hyaloid face. Prophylactic vitrectomy should be performed to avoid this complication.
- Graft rejection may be associated with glaucoma due to inflammatory reaction.
- Pigment dispersion glaucoma may occur especially in pseudophakic eyes. An inferior pigmented linear line may be seen on the endothelium and should not be confused with an allograft rejection.
- Epithelial ingrowth and fibrous downgrowth may also cause late onset glaucoma.
- Other factors which cause late onset glaucoma include PAS formation and long-term steroid use.
- Idiopathic late onset glaucoma is also known to occur after PK.

Management

Glaucoma assessment

Essential points to be considered in glaucoma assessment in patients with keratoplasty are:

- *Monitoring* the status of keratoplasty associated glaucoma can be challenging due to the presence of corneal disease.
- *Measurement of IOP* by Goldmann Applanation Tonometry (GAT) may not be reliable in post-keratoplasty glaucoma and other devices, such as Tono-Pen and Pneumotonometer may provide more accurate pressure measurements.
- *Useful information about glaucoma* generated from visual field testing and neuroretinal examinations may not be available due to corneal disease.
- *Gonioscopy*, though essential for glaucoma assessment in general, is a very important component of the evaluation of postkeratoplasty glaucoma patient to assess the status and structure of the filtering angle.

Medical treatment

Medical treatment is being considered the first choice. Surgery should be the option when maximal medical therapy fails or in the presence of specific conditions, like pupillary block. Medical treatment is on the general lines with the following comments;

- *β-blockers and α-agonists* are useful drugs particularly in the early postoperative period.
- *Miotics* may occasionally be of value. However, their effectiveness is markedly reduced in the presence of significant synaechial angle-closure.
- *Prostaglandin analogs* are effective drugs, but their role in the presence of inflammation and their influence on graft survival and graft clarity remains unclear.
- *Dorzolamide* has been shown to decrease corneal endothelial dysfunction and to increase the corneal thickness.

Laser therapy

- *Laser PI* is quite useful in pupillary block glaucoma and also to confirm the presence of malignant glaucoma.
- *Laser hyaloidotomy* may be useful in aphakic and pseudophakic malignant glaucomas. The presence of a patent PI is necessary to rule out pupillary block mechanism before treatment of malignant glaucoma can be initiated.
- *Laser iridoplasty/gonioplasty* may be useful to prevent progressive synaechial angle-closure after keratoplasty.
- *Laser trabeculoplasty* may be helpful in selective cases.

Surgical therapy

- *Trabeculectomy* is reported to be successful in 27–80% cases. Graft failure at 3 years post-trabeculectomy is reported in 11–20% cases.
- *Glaucoma drainage devices* may be required in patients where trabeculectomy appears to be of little use.
- *Cyclodestructive procedures* may be required in refractory cases of glaucoma. Laser cyclophotocoagulation is preferred over cyclocryotherapy because of reduced side effects.

GLAUCOMA AFTER LAMELLAR KERATOPLASTY

Lamellar keratoplasty, such as deep lamellar endothelial keratoplasty (DLEK) and Descemet stripping endothelial keratoplasty (DSEK) may be associated with glaucoma in 0–15% of cases.

Mechanisms of glaucoma

- *Pupillary block by air bubble* may occur in immediate postoperative period.
- *Steroid-induced glaucoma* may occur due to their long-term use.

Management

- *Medical therapy* to lower the IOP.
- *Paracentesis* may be required for release of air in cases with pupillary block.

GLAUCOMA AFTER KERATOPROSTHESIS

Keratoprosthesis is required in patients with severe corneal opacification and vascularization, e.g. after chemical burns, with the intention to provide some vision in these cases. Presently, the Boston keratoprosthesis and osteo-odonto-keratoprosthesis are being preferred.

- *Pre-existing glaucoma* is quite common in such cases.
- Measuring IOP in such cases remains problematic.

Management

- *Glaucoma drainage devices* need to be implanted along with keratoprosthesis surgery in most cases having pre-existing glaucoma.
- *Medical therapy* is required to control the IOP rise in early postoperative period.
- *Trans-scleral diode laser photocoagulation* may be useful, if IOP is not controlled with medical therapy.

GLAUCOMA ASSOCIATED WITH SURGICAL PROCEDURES FOR VITREOUS AND RETINAL DISEASES

Commonly seen glaucoma associated with surgical procedure for vitreous and retinal diseases include:

- Glaucoma after pars-plana vitrectomy,
- Glaucoma after scleral buckling procedure, and
- Glaucoma after retinal photocoagulation.

GLAUCOMA AFTER PARS PLANA VITRECTOMY

Secondary glaucomas which may be seen after pars plana vitrectomy (PPV) are described below briefly.

1. Glaucoma associated with intravitreal air or gas tamponade

Mechanism. Long-acting gases, such as sulphur hexachloride (SF_6) and octofluorocyclopropane (C_3F_8) are injected for tamponade after PPV. These gases expand and may cause glaucoma by following mechanisms:

- Acute angle-closure (more common), and
- Acute pupillary block (less common).

Clinical features

- Sudden post-PPV rise in IOP may be up to 80 mm Hg.
- Usually occurs on very first postoperative day.
- Glaucoma is usually secondary angle-closure types rarely may be pupillary block glaucoma.

Management

- *Vitreous tap* to reduce pressure may be required for abrupt rise in IOP.
- *Medical therapy* can achieve temporary control.
- *Daily pressure checking* with Goldmann applanation tonometry should be performed as the gas expands. Caution is advised regarding travel by air.

2. Secondary open-angle glaucoma associated with pars plana vitrectomy

Secondary open-angle glaucoma may occur about a week after PPV due to following mechanisms:

- Red cell glaucoma (associated with hyphaema)
- Inflammatory glaucoma
- Haemolytic glaucoma
- Phacolytic glaucoma
- Ghost cell glaucoma
- Pre-existing POAG

3. Glaucoma associated with silicon oil

Silicon oil injected after PPV may cause secondary glaucoma in 50–60% cases, 2–4 weeks postoperatively.

Mechanisms of glaucoma include:

- Pupillary block, and

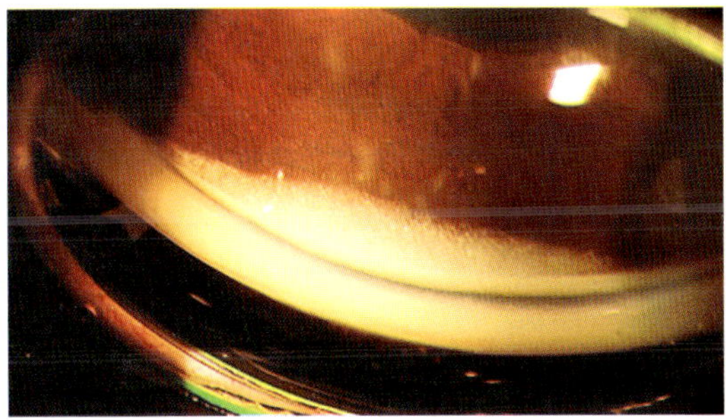

Fig. 17.20 *Emulsified silicon oil in the angle*

- Blockage of trabecular meshwork by silicon oil in the anterior chamber seen as inverse hypopyon (Fig. 17.20).

Management includes:

- *Inferior peripheral iridectomy* to relieve pupillary block.
- *Medical therapy* is usually effective.
- *Surgical therapy* indicated in non-responsive cases includes:
  - Removal of silicon oil,
  - Glaucoma drainage device (if indicated) should be placed inferiorly with intra-operative viscoelastic to prevent loss of silicon oil.

4. Neovascular glaucoma

Neovascular glaucoma is also reported to occur 2–4 weeks after pars plana vitrectomy.

GLAUCOMA AFTER SCLERAL BUCKLING PROCEDURES

Scleral buckling procedure performed in retinal detachment cases is reported to produce raised IOP and narrowing of the anterior chamber in about 15–50% cases.

Mechanisms

1. ***Anterior movement of the lens–iris diaphragm caused*** by the raised intravitreal pressure following scleral buckle and encirclage bands.

2. ***Anterior movement of the lens–iris diaphragm caused by anterior rotation of the ciliary body*** at the scleral spur as a result of ciliochoroidal effusion and detachment. Fluid accumulation in the suprachoroidal space may result from occlusion of vortex veins, inflammation and relative ischaemia.

3. ***Peripheral anterior synaechiae (PAS)*** may be formed following prolonged narrowing of the angle.

Treatment

1. ***Cycloplegics and steroids*** given topically reduce inflammation, ciliary spasm and prevent synaechiae formation.
2. ***Antiglaucoma drops***, such as β-blockers, α_2-agonists and carbonic anhydrase inhibitors, may be used to control IOP.
3. ***Surgical measures*** are indicated as below:
   - *Drainage of ciliochoroidal fluid* and air injection in anterior chamber may be required in persistent shallow anterior chamber.
   - *Loosening of the buckle* may be required when the above measures fail.

17.10 GLAUCOMA ASSOCIATED WITH INTRAOCULAR HAEMORRHAGES

Intraocular haemorrhage includes hyphaema and/or vitreous haemorrhage.

Types of glaucoma associated with intraocular haemorrhage

I. Glaucoma associated with hyphaema

II. Glaucoma associated with degenerated blood, which includes:
   - Ghost cell glaucoma,
   - Haemolytic glaucoma, and
   - Haemosiderotic glaucoma.

I. GLAUCOMA ASSOCIATED WITH HYPHAEMA

Causes of hyphaema

- ***Traumatic hyphaema*** is of common occurrence in blunt trauma and may also occur following penetrating injuries.
- ***Hyphaema associated with intraocular surgery*** may occur during operation in the early or late postoperative period.
- ***Spontaneous hyphaema*** may be associated with intraocular neovascularization in diseases,

like diabetic retinopathy, CRVO, sickle cell retinopathy, chronic uveitis and intraocular tumours, etc.

Mechanism of glaucoma

- ***Obstruction of trabecular meshwork*** in hyphaema results in secondary open-angle glaucoma. Although fresh red cells are known to pass through the conventional aqueous outflow system with relative ease, it appears to be overwhelming number of cells, combined with plasma, fibrin and debris, that may lead to a transient obstruction of aqueous outflow. This is why glaucoma associated with fresh blood in the anterior chamber has also been referred to as 'Red cell glaucoma' by some workers. Glaucoma is more frequent with total hyphaema.
- ***Pupil block glaucoma*** may also occur, though rarely in hyphaema. Formation of clot (eight-ball hyphaema) may be associated with pupil block.
- ***Other factors*** may also contribute to glaucoma in hyphaema. Release of melanin into the anterior chamber with trauma may prolong the course of hyphaema and affect the rate of rebleeding. Other factors associated with traumatic glaucoma may also contribute to the glaucoma associated with traumatic hyphaema.

Clinical features

- ***IOP*** is also reported to be raised in about 50% cases with total hyphaema, in 25% cases with hyphaema filling more than half of AC and in about 13% of cases with hyphaema filling less than half of the AC. Although IOP may be raised after the initial bleed, but is more common in cases of recurrent haemorrhages. Acutely elevated IOP may pose as a threat for vision as a result of corneal staining or optic nerve damage.
- ***Blood staining of the cornea*** may develop, if raised IOP associated with hyphaema is not lowered within a few days. Cornea becomes reddish brown (Fig. 17.21) or greenish in colour and in later stages simulates dislocation of the clear lens in the anterior chamber. Once corneal staining occurs, it clears very slowly from the periphery towards the centre, and the whole, process may take even more than 2 years.

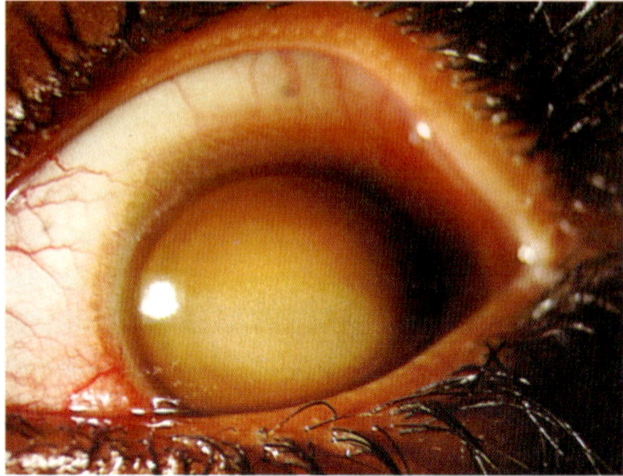

Fig. 17.21 *Full chamber hyphaema with corneal staining*

- ***Optic nerve damage*** may occur with acute rise of IOP associated with hyphaema. Optic atrophy at only slightly elevated IOP has been reported in patients with hyphaema associated with sickle cell haemoglobinopathies. Suboptimal blood flow to the optic nerve on the basis of sickling has been proposed as a mechanism for this sensitivity.

Management

1. ***Conservative management of hyphaema and medical control of IOP*** include:
   - *Rest* and limiting patients ambulation
   - *Topical steroids and cycloplegics* to control inflammation
   - *Aqueous suppressants*, topical and systemic to control IOP.
2. ***Measures to accelerate hyphaema clearance*** include:
   - *Hyperosmotic agents*, e.g. i.v. mannitol may accelerate resorption of clotted hyphaema.
   - *Tissue plasminogen activator* (clot specific fibrinolytic agent) when given intracamerally has been reported to accelerate the clearance of experimental hyphaema in rabbits, although it may increase the risk of rebleed.
3. ***Prevention of rebleeding*** can be done by:
   - *Antifibrinolytic agents* (tranexamic acid and aminocaproic acid) have been reported to decrease the incidence of rebleed by delaying the natural lysis of the clot.

- *Lowering of systemic blood pressure and elevation of head end of bed* is also reported to decrease rebleed and accelerate clearance of hyphaema.
- *Avoidance* of aspirin and NSAIDs for the first week after hyphaema or till hyphaema clears is useful.

4. ***Surgical removal of hyphaema.*** When conservative measures fail to prevent vision loss from damage to optic nerve and corneal staining, surgical measures are required to remove hyphaema and control the IOP.

Proposed guideline for surgical removal of hyphaema is that an IOP threatening the optic nerve, like 60 mm Hg for 2 days or 50 mm Hg for 5 days or 35 mm Hg for 7 days, requires intervention.

Timing for surgical intervention. It is advisable (if possible), to delay the evacuation of hyphaema until the 4th day, because at this time, the clot is somewhat retracted and less adherent to the surrounding structures.

Surgical techniques used in the literature include anterior chamber washout, clot expression, delivery of the clot with a cryoprobe, automated hyphaemectomy and ultrasonic emulsification and aspiration.

- *Paracentesis and manual irrigation–aspiration* using two-way Simcoe's canula is a simple and safe procedure.
- *Viscodissection of the clot* from the iris and expression of the anterior chamber may be used for a clot.
- *Removal of the clot with vitrectomy instruments* is also considered a safe and effective procedure.

5. ***Adjunctive surgical procedures along with hyphaema removal*** have included:

- *Peripheral iridotomy* in the setting of pupillary block resulting from the clot.
- *Trabeculectomy* has also been used for control of IOP.
- *Cyclodiathermy* to control recurrent bleeding has also been described.

II. GLAUCOMAS ASSOCIATED WITH DEGENERATED OCULAR BLOOD

Glaucomas associated with degenerated ocular blood include:

- Ghost cell glaucoma,
- Haemolytic glaucoma, and
- Haemosiderotic glaucoma

1. GHOST CELL GLAUCOMA

Ghost cell glaucoma, initially described by Campbell et al (1976), is a type of secondary open-angle glaucoma in which the trabecular meshwork is blocked by the ghost cells (described below) and is associated with vitreous haemorrhage.

Mechanism of glaucoma

One to three weeks after vitreous haemorrhage (from any cause, trauma, surgery, retinal disease) the RBCs degenerate, loose their pliability and become khaki-coloured cells called the ghost cells. Histopathologically, ghost cells have thin walls and appear hollow except for clumps of denatured haemoglobin called 'Heinz bodies' (Fig. 17.22). Once developed, the ghost cells remain in the vitreous cavity for months. Whenever there occurs disruption of the anterior hyaloid face (situations as mentioned below), the ghost cells pass from the vitreous into the anterior chamber unlike fresh RBCs, the ghost cells are not able to pass through the trabecular meshwork causing its blockage, leading to rise in IOP.

Specific situations for disruption of anterior hyaloid face include:

- Pre-existing pseudophakia or aphakia (before vitreous haemorrhage)
- Cataract surgery performed after vitreous haemorrhage

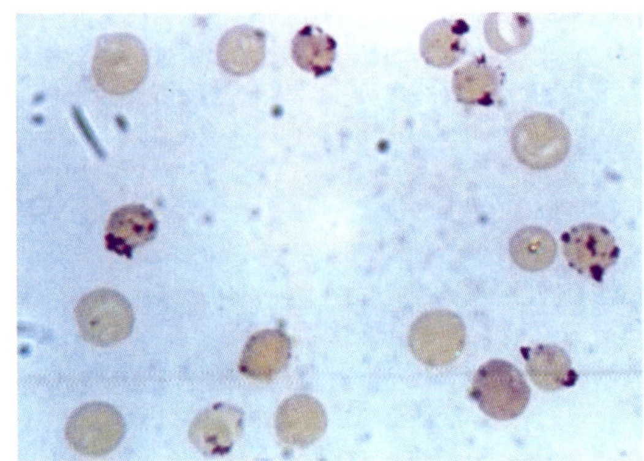

Fig. 17.22 *Heinz bodies*

- Vitrectomy operation
- Traumatic with presumed disruption of anterior hyaloid face

Clinical features

- *IOP*, depending upon the number of ghost cells in the anterior chamber, may vary from normal to marked elevation associated with pain and corneal oedema.
- *Cornea* may show oedema and/or characteristic khaki-coloured cells on the endothelium.
- *Anterior chamber*, on slit-lamp examination, may reveal:
  - *Ghost cells* in the aqueous humour
  - *Pseudohypopyon* due to settling down of ghost cells when present in abundance. Occasionally, pseudohypopyon may be associated with a layer of fresh RBCs (known as 'candy-stripe sign').
- *Angle of anterior chamber*, on gonioscopy, is open and may appear normal or may show a layer of deposited khaki-coloured cells.

Differential diagnosis

Differential diagnosis needs to be made from phacolytic glaucoma, haemosiderotic glaucoma, secondary open-angle neovascular glaucoma and inflammatory glaucoma.

Clinical diagnosis of ghost cell glaucoma is made from the typical history and signs on examination as described above.

Laboratory confirmation of ghost cell glaucoma is made on examination of ghost cells in the aqueous aspirate. This examination may be performed with:

- Phase contrast microscopy, or
- Routine light microscopy of a paraffin embedded specimen stained with H & E.

Management

1. ***Medical therapy***, similar to POAG, may be effective in more than half of the cases.
2. ***Surgical therapy,*** required when medical therapy fails, includes:
   i. *Anterior chamber wash*, using two-way irrigation–aspiration canula, is the surgery of choice and is most effective. It may be repeated when required.
   ii. *Pars plana* vitrectomy may be required in unresponsive patients to ensure complete removal of blood components trapped in the vitreous body.
   iii. *Trabeculectomy* is sparingly required.

2. HAEMOLYTIC GLAUCOMA

Haemolytic glaucoma, described first of all by Fenton and Zimmerman (1963), is a type of glaucoma associated with intraocular haemorrhage.

Pathogenesis

It is an acute secondary open-angle glaucoma due to the obstruction (clogging) of the trabecular meshwork caused by macrophages laden with lysed RBC debris.

Pathology

Microscopic study of the enucleated eyes with haemolytic glaucoma revealed the trabecular meshwork to be occluded by RBCs, debris and macrophages laden with blood pigments. The endothelial cells of trabecular meshwork were degenerated and had phagocytosed the blood.

Clinical features

- ***IOP*** is acutely raised causing pain, nausea and even vomiting.
- ***Cornea*** may show oedema.
- ***Anterior chamber*** is normal in depth and on slit-lamp examination shows numerous reddish cells in the aqueous humour.
- ***Angle of anterior chamber*** on gonioscopy is open, with reddish-brown pigment covering the trabecular meshwork.

Diagnosis

- ***Clinical diagnosis*** is made from the history suggestive of intraocular haemorrhage associated with the above signs.
- ***Confirmation of diagnosis*** is made by anterior chamber paracentesis, which reveals pigment-containing macrophages laden with rather than khaki-coloured ghost cells.

Management

1. ***Medical therapy*** in the form of topical and systemic aqueous suppressants may be needed

for some time to control IOP, otherwise, the condition is self-limiting and does not need prolonged therapy.

2. ***Surgical therapy*** is rarely needed:

i. *Anterior chamber washout* may be required in occasional cases, where IOP is not controlled by medical therapy.

ii. *Filtration surgery* may be considered in non-responsive cases.

iii. *Cyclodestructive procedures* may be required in painful blind eyes.

3. HAEMOSIDEROTIC GLAUCOMA

Haemosiderotic glaucoma is a rare secondary open-angle glaucoma associated with intra-ocular haemorrhage.

Pathogenesis

It is a rare variety of secondary glaucoma occurring due to sclerotic changes in trabecular meshwork caused by the iron from the phagocytosed haemoglobin by the endothelial cells of trabeculum. Thus, we can say that haemosiderosis is similar to siderosis bulbi, except that the source of iron in haemosiderosis is degenerating RBCs rather than a retained intraocular foreign body.

Clinical features

Clinical features of this rare secondary open-angle glaucoma are similar to POAG, except that it is associated with a history of intraocular haemorrhage.

Management

1. ***Medical therapy*** with aqueous suppressants to control the IOP.

2. ***Trabeculectomy*** may be required in non-responsive cases.

17.11 GLAUCOMA ASSOCIATED WITH THE DISORDERS OF THE CORNEAL ENDOTHELIUM

Primary disorders of corneal endothelium associated with glaucoma include:

- Iridocorneal endothelial syndrome
- Posterior polymorphous corneal dystrophy
- Fuchs' endothelial dystrophy

IRIDOCORNEAL ENDOTHELIAL SYNDROME

Iridocorneal endothelial syndrome (ICE) is characterized by an abnormal corneal endothelium associated with iris atrophy, corneal oedema and secondary angle-closure glaucoma. Originally, it was described that ICE includes three clinical entities, viz. progressive iris atrophy, Chandler's syndrome and Cogan-Reese (iris naevus) syndrome, which were distinguished on the basis of changes in the iris. However, presently it is considered that the three clinical variants represent a spectrum of ICE syndrome rather than distinct clinical entities.

Pathogenesis

Formation of endothelial membrane. The characteristic features of ICE syndrome is the presence of corneal endothelial cells which proliferate to form a membrane which covers the angle of the anterior chamber and to some extent the anterior surface of the iris. Contraction of this membrane leads to the following changes:

- *Secondary angle-closure glaucoma*, due to the formation of PAS
- *Iris defects*, such as corectopia, stretch holes and iris nodules
- *Ischaemia of iris* may occur secondary to contraction, which may lead to the 'melt holes'

What causes the abnormal corneal endothelium is still not clear. Absence of positive family history and the presence of postnatal layer of Descemet's membrane suggest that it is an acquired disorder. Following views were put forward:

- *Abnormal proliferation of neural crest cells* has been held responsible for abnormal endothelial cells by some workers.
- *Viral theory*, blaming HSV has been put forward based on the electron micrographic, immunohistochemical and serological studies while in some studies Epstein-Barr virus has been blamed. The viral theory is attractive and might explain the unilaterality of the syndrome in majority of the patients.

Clinical features

General features

Age and sex. ICE syndrome typically affects middle-aged females (20–40 yrs) more often.

Laterality. The condition is almost always unilateral. However, subclinical abnormalities of corneal endothelium are reported in the fellow eye.

Clinical presentation

Presenting features include reduced visual acuity, pain, corneal oedema, abnormalities of iris and raised IOP.

Glaucoma occurs in about 50% cases.

Signs

1. ***Corneal signs*** include:
   - *Fine hammered silver appearance* of the posterior cornea, similar to Fuchs' endothelial dystrophy is seen on slit-lamp examination.
   - *Abnormal endothelial cells* on specular microscopy appear dark with a light central spot and light peripheral zone with varying degree of pleomorphism in shape and size and less of clear hexagonal margins.
   - *Corneal oedema* occurs when IOP is raised.
2. ***Iris signs*** are pathognomonic of various clinical variants of ICE syndrome as described below.
3. ***Lens signs.*** The retrocorneal membrane may grow over the anterior surface of the lens. It simulates anterior lens capsule and may create confusion while creating a capsulorrhexis during cataract surgery.
4. ***Peripheral anterior synaechiae*** (PAS), usually extending to or beyond the Schwalbe's line seen on gonioscopy, are characteristic feature of ICE syndrome.
5. ***IOP*** rises when PAS becomes extensive. On occasion, IOP may be raised despite open-angle due to pretrabecular membrane before contraction.

Clinical spectrum of ICE syndrome

Depending upon the characteristic features, the three clinical variants (now considered to be the spectrum of ICE syndrome) are as below:

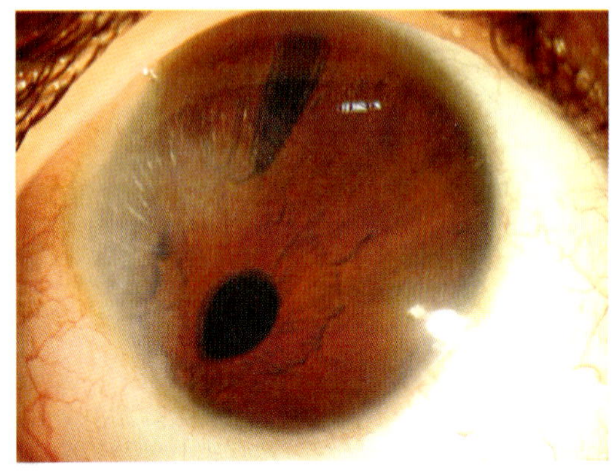

Fig. 17.23 *Essential iris atrophy*

1. ***Progressive essential iris atrophy*** (Fig. 17.23). The iris features predominate with:
   - Marked *correctopia, iris atrophy* and ectropion uveae that usually occurs toward the quadrant with most prominent PAS.
   - *Iris holes* which are of two types:
     - *Stretch holes*, caused by traction, occur in the quadrant away from the direction of pupillary displacement.
     - *Meet holes*, ischaemic in nature, occur without correctopia.
2. ***Chandler's syndrome*** is characterized by:
   - *Iris changes* are minimal to absent.
   - *Corneal changes* are marked and oedema may occur even at normal IOP.
3. ***Cogan-Reese syndrome*** is characterized by nodular or diffuse pigmented lesions of the iris. Therefore, it is called iris naevus syndrome. Ultrastructure of the iris nodules is similar to that of the underlying iris stroma and is always surrounded by the continuation of the retrocorneal membrane. Corneal oedema may or may not be associated.

Management

A. Treatment of glaucoma

1. ***Medical therapy*** with aqueous suppressants may be effective in early cases. However, failure with medical therapy is common.
2. ***Surgical therapy*** is often required.
   i. *Trabeculectomy with mitomycin C use* may be useful. Failure of trabeculectomy with endothelialization of the filtering bleb is not uncommon. Repeat trabeculectomy may be

considered. The success rates for repeated trabeculectomies are comparable to those of the initial procedure and similar to repeat procedures in patients with POAG.

ii. *Glaucoma drainage devices* may be tried in cases with failure of repeat trabeculectomy.

iii. *Cyclodestructive procedures* are last resort considerations.

B. Treatment of corneal oedema

1. *Lowering of IOP*, as described above, clears the corneal oedema in most of the cases.
2. *Hypertonic saline* solution may be used for early clearance of corneal oedema.
3. *Penetrating keratoplasty* is required in non-responsive cases.

C. Treatment of underlying mechanism

1. *Role of antiviral drugs* needs to be evaluated, if the viral theory of etiology is proved.
2. *Role of immunotoxin drugs* is being evaluated to inhibit the proliferation of human corneal endothelium in tissue culture.

Prognosis. Overall prognosis of ICE syndrome is not good inspite of the best efforts.

GLAUCOMA IN POSTERIOR POLYMORPHOUS CORNEAL DYSTROPHY

Clinical features

Posterior polymorphous dystrophy is a congenital condition, usually with an autosomal dominant inheritance pattern. The cornea, iris, and anterior chamber angle are involved, but there is a wide variation in expression of this dystrophy both within and between affected families.

- It can be stationary or slowly progressive.
- Although the condition is bilateral, involvement may be so asymmetric as to be clinically evident in only one eye.
- *Corneal oedema* may be associated.
- *Iris involvement* may occur including mild correctopia and iridocorneal adhesions.
- *Glaucoma* occurs in 10–15% of cases of PPCD and is thought to be caused by PAS formation and iridocorneal adhesions as a result of retrocorneal membrane formation similar to ICE syndrome. Glaucoma is also reported in eyes with open-angle associated with a high insertion of the iris into the posterior aspect of the trabecular meshwork.

Differential diagnosis

Corneal lesions of PPCD need to be differentiated from that seen in:

- Fuch's corneal dystrophy
- Congenital hereditary corneal dystrophy (CHCD)
- Posterior amorphous corneal dystrophy (PACD)

Iridocorneal adhesions when present in PACD, the differential diagnosis should be considered from:

- Axenfeld-Rieger syndrome, and
- ICE syndrome.

Management

A. *No treatment* is required as majority of patients with PPMD are asymptomatic.

B. *Treatment of corneal oedema,* when present includes:
- *Conservative treatment* with hypertonic saline and bandage soft contact lenses may be effective.
- *Penetrating keratoplasty (PK)* may be required in non-responsive cases with guarded visual prognosis. The presence of iridocorneal adhesions is a risk factor for failure of keratoplasty. Recurrence of PPMD has been reported after PK.

C. *Treatment of glaucoma* includes:
- *Medical therapy* with aqueous suppressants
- *Laser trabeculoplasty* is not effective in such patients
- *Surgical therapy* is required when medical therapy fails and includes:
  - Filtration surgery
  - Glaucoma drainage devices (when trabeculectomy fails)
  - Laser cyclodestruction may be tried as a last resort.

GLAUCOMA IN FUCHS' ENDOTHELIAL DYSTROPHY

Clinical types

- POAG is rarely associated with Fuchs' dystrophy.

- Secondary angle-closure glaucoma, though rare, but is more frequently associated with Fuchs' dystrophy than the POAG.

Management

Lowering of IOP with aqueous suppressants is useful in reducing corneal oedema even in the absence of glaucoma. Topical carbonic anhydrase inhibitors (CAIs) should better be avoided, as they are reported to cause further decompensation of cornea.

POAG when associated, may need peripheral iridotomy or filtration surgery.

17.12 GLAUCOMA ASSOCIATED WITH ELEVATED EPISCLERAL VENOUS PRESSURE

The normal episcleral venous pressure (EVP) is approximately 8 to 10 mm Hg, and plays a significant role in aqueous humour dynamics. The aqueous outflow through a trabecular meshwork depends upon the difference between the IOP and EVP and the resistance (R) at the canalicular meshwork. Thus aqueous flow = [IOP–EVP] R. Though the relationship between IOP and EVP is complex, but to simplify, it may be concluded that with increase in IOP, the aqueous flow decreases which leads to an increase in IOP. Thus, any condition which raises episcleral venous pressure (EVP) also raises IOP by obstructing the post-trabecular flow of aqueous humour. It is generally thought that for every 1 mm Hg increase in EVP, IOP increases by 0.8–1 mm Hg.

Causes of elevated EVP

Causes of raised EVP can be grouped as below:

I. *Conditions causing venous obstruction*

1. *Episcleral venous obstruction* may occur in:
   - Vasculitis involving episcleral veins in scleritis and episcleritis
   - Chemical burns, and
   - Radiation
2. *Orbital causes of venous obstruction* are:
   - Retrobulbar tumours,
   - Thyroid associated ophthalmopathy,
   - Pseudotumour of the orbit
   - Orbital phlebitis, and
   - Orbital amyloidosis
3. *Cavernous sinus thrombosis*
4. *Superior vena cava syndrome*. Malignancy is reported to be the underlying cause in 97% cases of this syndrome. Other associated causes include aortic aneurysm, enlarged hilar nodes and thyroid disease.
5. *Irregular vein obstruction* as occurs in inflammatory jugular phlebostenosis
6. *Pulmonary venous obstruction*

II. *Arteriovenous fistulas*

1. *Carotid-cavernous sinus fistula*, which can be:
   - Traumatic fistula, or
   - Spontaneous fistula
2. *Orbital varices*
3. *Sturge-Weber syndrome*
4. *Dural fistula*

III. *Idiopathic episcleral venous pressure elevation*

Pathomechanisms of raised IOP with elevated EVP

Following mechanisms causing glaucoma have been associated with different causes of raised EVP.

1. *Direct effect.* As explained in the introduction, the raised EVP per se causes an almost equal rise in IOP.

2. *Increase in outflow resistance* due to extracellular deposits and hyalinization of the trabecular meshwork is reported to occur following prolonged elevation of EVP.

3. *Acute angle-closure* due to forward shift of lens–iris diaphragm following serous choroidal detachment or suprachoroidal haemorrhage is reported to occur in patients with raised EVP associated with AV fistulas.

4. *Neovascular glaucoma* is also reported in some cases of elevated EVP. This occurs following ocular ischaemia associated with reduced arterial flow in such cases.

Salient features of causative conditions

Salient features of common conditions associated with elevated EVP are described in the relevant sections.

Management

1. *Treatment of the underlying cause of elevated EVP* is the definitive treatment.

2. *Management of glaucoma* in idiopathic cases and as conservative measures in cases with treatable cause is on general lines with antiglaucoma agents and surgery as and when indicated.

17.13 GLAUCOMAS ASSOCIATED WITH DISORDERS OF THE RETINA, VITREOUS AND CHOROID

- Neovascular glaucoma (see page 248)
- Glaucoma associated with retinal detachment
- Glaucoma with haemorrhagic retinal or choroidal detachment
- Glaucoma with ciliochoroidal effusion
- Glaucoma with retinopathy of prematurity
- Glaucoma with persistent hyperplastic vitreous (PHPV)
- Glaucoma with retinal dysplasia
- Glaucoma with retinitis pigmentosa

GLAUCOMA ASSOCIATED WITH RETINAL DETACHMENT

In a patient with retinal detachment, the IOP is typically low, but may be normal or even high;

Hypotony is reported in about 65% of cases and is caused by posterior flow of aqueous through the retinal hole.

Normal IOP in patients with rhegmatogenous RD is reported in about 25% of cases.

Elevated IOP (glaucoma) is reported in only about 10% of cases with RD.

Causes of raised IOP in retinal detachment

Causes of elevated IOP at presentation with RD can be grouped as below:

1. *Elevated IOP preceding RD*
   - Ocular hypertension
   - Primary open-angle glaucoma (POAG) (genetic linkage)
   - Other secondary glaucoma (a chance occurrence), e.g. pigmentary glaucoma

2. *Elevated IOP and RD due to common underlying mechanisms*
   - Traumatic glaucoma and RD
   - Glaucoma and RD in aphakia/pseudophakia
   - Glaucoma and RD due to proliferative retinopathies, e.g. in diabetic retinopathy
   - Glaucoma and RD occurring in retinopathy of prematurity (ROP)
   - Stickler's syndrome
   - Angle-closure glaucoma and RD occurring in nanophthalmos and uveal effusion

3. *Elevated IOP caused by retinal detachment*
   - Schwartz's syndrome
   - Ghost cell glaucoma due to retinal tear and vitreous haemorrhage in RD
   - Chronic retinal detachment may be complicated by:
     - Neovascular glaucoma
     - Secondary angle-closure due to iritis, posterior synaechiae and pupillary block

Note. Only few of the above entities are described briefly.

Primary open-angle glaucoma and retinal detachment

A much high incidence of POAG (4%) is reported in patients with rhegmatogenous retinal detachment as compared to general population (1%). It has been suggested that the two diseases might be related genetically by multifactorial inheritance.

Important considerations regarding co-existence of POAG and RD are:

- *Reduction in IOP due to RD* may mark the pre-existing POAG. A careful optic disc evaluation is important in patients with RD.
- *Miotics.* Although their role in the pathogenesis of rhegmatogenous RD has not been clearly established; it is better to avoid these drugs in

patients with POAG, predisposed to develop RD.

- *Steroids* should be used cautiously post-operatively in such patients operated for RD.
- *Success of retinal detachment surgery* in such patients is not affected by the presence of POAG, but visual outcome may be worse.

Pigmentary glaucoma and retinal detachment

Incidence of pigment dispersion syndrome reported in patients with RD is higher than the general population.

Considerations regarding co-existence of pigmentary glaucoma and RD are same as described above for POAG and RD.

Schwartz's syndrome

Characteristic features of Schwartz's syndrome are:

- Rhegmatogenous retinal detachment
- Unilateral secondary open-angle glaucoma in the affected eye with IOP varying between 30–55 mm Hg
- Presence of aqueous cells and flare
- Normal contralateral eye
- Raised IOP with iritis, both poorly respond to medical therapy consisting of anti-glaucoma drugs and steroids.
- IOP is controlled within days to weeks of the repair of RD.

Theories of mechanism. Exact mechanism of elevated IOP is not clear. Following theories have been put forward:

- *Schwartz's hypothesis.* Iridocyclitis complicating long-standing RD reduces the aqueous outflow facility resulting in glaucoma.
- *Davidorf hypothesis.* Retinal pigment cells released from the break migrate anteriorly and block the trabecular meshwork.
- *Matsuo et al (1986),* based on microscopic evidence, have proposed that the predominant mechanism in obstruction of the trabecular meshwork by photoreceptor outer segments, which pass through the retinal break and migrate anteriorly.

Management includes:

- *Anti-glaucoma* drugs may be used to lower IOP temporarily.
- *Surgical repair of RD* resolves glaucoma within few days.

GLAUCOMA WITH HAEMORRHAGIC RETINAL OR CHOROIDAL DETACHMENT

Causes

Sudden haemorrhagic retinal or choroidal detachment is reported to occur under following circumstances:

I. *Spontaneously* in patients with;

- Systemic hypertension
- Primary clotting disorders
- Systemic use of anticoagulants and thrombolytic agents

II. *During or after intraocular surgery,* especially filtering surgery, with associated IOP elevation and flattening of the anterior chamber.

Mechanism of glaucoma

Sudden forward displacement of lens–iris diaphragm by the massive haemorrhagic retinal or choroidal detachment leads to acute angle-closure glaucoma.

Management

- *Medical therapy* to lower IOP
- *Cyclodestructive* procedures may be required in non-responsive cases.

GLAUCOMA WITH CILIOCHOROIDAL EFFUSION

Mechanism

Secondary angle-closure glaucoma occurs with ciliochoroidal effusion due to forward rotation of the lens–iris diaphragm.

Causes

Causes of ciliochoroidal effusion can be grouped as below:

- Nanophthalmos
- Uveal effusion syndrome, and
- Other causes of ciliochoroidal effusion

Nanophthalmos

Characteristic features

Nanophthalmos refers to an otherwise normal but small-sized eyeball (approximately two-thirds of normal), with normal sized crystalline lens. Thus, its characteristic features are:

- *Axial length* is usually less than 20.5 mm. Vertical and horizontal diameters are also small.
- *Volume* is reduced to about two-thirds of the normal eyeball.
- *High hyperopia* with corrected visual acuity is most common presentation. Rarely lesser ranges of hypermetropia and even emmetropia may be there.
- *Cornea* is small, but may be normal.
- *Crystalline lens* is normal in size with a high lens-to-eye volume ratio.
- *Anterior chamber* is shallow with normal angle.
- *Sclera* is thickened and its permeability to proteins is reduced.
- *Uveal tissue* is thickened with choroidal effusion occurring posteriorly.

Mechanism of glaucoma

In nanophthalmos, glaucoma may occur by the following mechanisms:

- *Angle-closure glaucoma either phacomorphic and/or pupillary block type* may occur due to progressive shallowing of the chamber and narrowing of the angle width (usually between 4th to 6th decades of life).
- *Angle-closure glaucoma due to spontaneous ciliochoroidal effusion* is also common with nanophthalmos. Uveal effusion is caused by reduced scleral permeability to proteins by the thickened sclera or compression of the venous drainage channels by the dense collagen around vortex veins.

Ciliochoroidal effusion with retinal detachment in nanophthalmos may occur under the following situations:

- *Spontaneously* in asymptomatic nanophthalmos during 4th to 6th decades of life causing acute angle-closure glaucoma.
- *Intraoperatively*, during glaucoma or cataract surgery, manifesting an operative hard eye.
- *Postoperatively*, the ciliochoroidal effusion causes flat anterior chamber with raised IOP, similar to malignant glaucoma.

Management of glaucoma due to ciliochoroidal effusion

- *Medical therapy* to lower IOP. Pilocarpine 2% may cause pupillary block.
- *Laser iridotomy and laser gonioplasty* have the highest success rate and are the procedures of choice.
- *Prophylactic scleral resection* with or without vortex vein decompression is recommended 2 months before the planned anterior segment surgery (elective cataract and/or filtration surgery).

Uveal effusion syndrome

Characteristic features. Uveal effusion syndrome is characterized by features of ciliochoroidal effusion occurring in nanophthalmos except that the eyeball is normal in size and otherwise also.

Management is also similar to that of ciliochoroidal effusion in nanophthalmos.

Other conditions associated with ciliochoroidal effusion

Other conditions associated with ciliochoroidal effusion as causes of secondary angle closure are:

- Arteriovenous malformation,
- Inflammatory conditions,
- Trauma,
- Ocular surgery
- Intraocular tumours, and
- Certain drugs (sulphonamides), such as acetazolamide and topiramate (as anticonvulsant drug).

GLAUCOMA IN RETINOPATHY OF PREMATURITY

Retinopathy of prematurity (ROP) is a bilateral proliferative retinopathy, occurring in premature infants with low birth weight who often have been exposed to high concentration of oxygen.

Mechanism of glaucoma. Glaucoma in ROP can occur by multiple mechanisms:

- *Angle-closure glaucoma* typically occurs following contracture of the retrolental mass in ROP at 3 to 6 months of age. However, angle closure may occur later in childhood or even in young adulthood.
- *Developmental glaucoma* may occur in some cases as evidenced by associated developmental angle anomalies reported, such as hypopigmentation of the iris root (73%), a translucent or Barkan's type membrane (69%), detectable posterior synaechiae (62%), prominent iris convexity (58%), visible iris or angle vessels (46%), pigment clumping in the angle recess (40%), prominent Schwalbe's line (15%) and greater than 180° of angle-closure (in 12%).
- *Other reported mechanisms of glaucoma in ROP* are ciliary block, neovascularization and inflammatory changes.

Management of glaucoma in ROP is difficult:

- *Medical therapy* with antiglaucoma drugs alone is usually not effective. However, when used with cycloplegic agents and topical steroids some success may occur.
- *Iridectomy or trabeculectomy* may be effective in some cases.
- *Lens aspiration with vitrectomy* may be useful in controlling IOP, relieving pain and thus avoiding enucleation. There is little hope for useful vision up to this stage of ROP.

GLAUCOMA IN PRIMARY HYPERPLASTIC PERSISTENT VITREOUS

Primary hyperplastic persistent vitreous (PHPV) results from failure of the primary vitreous structure to regress combined with the hypoplasia of the posterior portion of the vascular meshwork. It is often associated with microphthalmos and elongated ciliary processes.

Mechanisms of glaucoma in PHPV

1. ***Secondary angle-closure glaucoma*** may occur due to forward displacement of lens–iris diaphragm due to the following mechanisms:

- Contracture of the fibrous retrolenticular mass
- Swollen cataractous lens
- Swelling of the lens due to intralenticular haemorrhage

2. ***Secondary angle-closure glaucoma*** may occur due to:

- Intraocular haemorrhage (ghost cell glaucoma)
- Chronic uveal inflammation (inflammatory glaucoma)
- Associated developmental angle anomalies

Management

- *Aspiration of lens and removal of fibrovascular mass* with vitrector or scissors is the recommended surgical measure to prevent or eliminate the angle-closure glaucoma.
- *Visual rehabilitation* is not easy and treatment to avoid amblyopia is generally required.
- *Monitoring of fellow eye* is also important, since occurrence of POAG is reported in the normal fellow eye.

SUGGESTED READING

17.1 Lens-induced (phacogenic) glaucomas

1. Ellant JP, Obstbaum SA. Lens-induced glaucoma. Doc Ophthalmol 1992;81(3):317–38.
2. Gadia R, Sihota R, Dada T, Gupta V. Current profile of secondary glaucomas. Indian J Ophthalmol Jul-Aug 2008;56(4):285–89.
3. Moisseiev E, Kinori M, Glovinsky Y, Loewenstein A, Moisseiev J, Barak A. Retained lens fragments: nucleus fragments are associated with worse prognosis than cortex or epinucleus fragments. Eur J Ophthalmol. Nov-Dec 2011;21(6):741–47.
4. Rosenbaum JT, Samples JR, Seymour B, Langlois L, David L. Chemotactic activity of lens proteins and the pathogenesis of phacolytic glaucoma. Arch Ophthalmol Nov 1987;105(11):1582–84.
5. Schaal S, Barr CC. Management of retained lens fragments after cataract surgery with and without pars plana vitrectomy. J Cataract Refract Surg May 2009;35(5):863–67.

17.2 Glaucomas due to uveitis

1. Asrani S, Moore DB, Jaffe GJ. Paradoxical changes of retinal nerve fiber layer thickness in uveiticglaucoma. JAMA Ophthalmol. 2014; 132(7):877–80.

2. Horsley MB, Chen TC. The use of prostaglandin analogs in the uveitic patient. Semin Ophthalmol 2011;26(4-5):285–89.
3. Rachmiel R, Trope GE, Buys YM, Flanagan JG, Chipman ML. Ahmed glaucoma valve implantation in uveitic glaucoma versus open-angle glaucoma patients. Can J Ophthalmol. 2008;43(4):462–67.
4. Siddique SS, Suelves AM, Baheti U, Foster CS. Glaucoma and uveitis. Surv Ophthalmol. 2013; 58(1):1–10.

17.3 Pigmentary glaucoma

1. Lichter PR, Shaffer RN. Diagnostic and prognostic signs in pigmentary glaucoma. Trans Am Acad Ophthalmol Otolaryngol 1970;74(5): 984–98.
2. Roberts DK, Lukic A, Yang Y, Wilensky JT, Wernick MN. Multispectral diagnostic imaging of the iris in pigment dispersion syndrome. J Glaucoma 2012;21(6):351–57.
3. Reistad CE, Shields MB, Campbell DG, Ritch R, Wang JC, Wand M. The influence of peripheral iridotomy on the intraocular pressure course in patients with pigmentary glaucoma. J Glaucoma 2005;14(4):255–59.
4. Siddiqui Y, Ten Hulzen RD, Cameron JD, Hodge DO, Johnson DH. What is the risk of developing pigmentary glaucoma from pigment dispersion syndrome? Am J Ophthalmol 2003;135(6):794–99.

17.4 Neovascular glaucoma

1. Hayreh SS. Neovascular Glaucoma. Progress in Retinal and Eye Research, 2007;26(5):470–85.
2. Ichhpujani P, Ramasubramanian A, Kaushik S, Pandav SS. Bevacizumab in glaucoma: a review. Can J Ophthalmol 2007;42(6):812–15.
3. Shazly TA, Latina MA. Neovascular glaucoma: etiology, diagnosis and prognosis. Semin Ophthalmol 2009;24(2):113–21.
4. Shen CC, Salim S, Du H, Netland PA. Trabeculectomy versus Ahmed GlaucomaValve implantation in neovascular glaucoma. Clin Ophthalmol 2011;5:281–86.

17.5 Glaucoma associated with intraocular tumours

1. Bianciotto C, Shields CL, Kang B, Shields JA. Treatment of iris melanoma and secondary neovascular glaucoma using bevacizumab and plaque radiotherapy. Arch Ophthalmol 2008; 126(4):578–79.
2. Jakobiec FA. Intraocular tumors and glaucoma. In: Principles and Practice of Ophthalmology, 1999.
3. Johnson DL, Altaweel MM, Neekhra A, Chandra SR, Albert DM. Uveal melanoma masquerading as pigment dispersion glaucoma. Arch Ophthalmol 2008;126(6):868–69.
4. Radcliffe NM, Finger PT. Eye cancer related glaucoma: current concepts. Surv Ophthalmol 2009;54(1):47–73.
5. Shields CL, Shields JA, Shields MB, Augsburger JJ. Prevalence and mechanisms of secondary intraocular pressure elevation in eyes with intraocular tumors. Ophthalmology 1987;94(7):839–46.

17.6 Pseudoexfoliative glaucoma

1. Fingert JH, Alward WL, Kwon YH, Wang K, Streb LM, Sheffield VC, et al. LOXL1 mutations are associated with exfoliation syndrome in patients from the midwestern United States. Am J Ophthalmol 2007;144(6):974–75.
2. Jeng SM, Karger RA, Hodge DO, Burke JP, Johnson DH, Good MS. The risk of glaucoma in pseudoexfoliation syndrome. J Glaucoma 2007; 16(1):117–21.
3. Ritch R. Exfoliation syndrome: the most common identifiable cause of open angle glaucoma. J Glaucoma 1994;3:176–78.

17.7 Steroid-induced glaucoma

1. Bartlett JD, Woolley TW, Adams CM. Identification of high intraocular pressure responders to topical ophthalmic corticosteroids. J Ocul Pharmacol 1993;9:35–45.
2. Becker B, Chevrette L. Topical corticosteroid testing in glaucoma siblings. Arch Ophthalmol 1966;76:484–87.
3. Haller JA et al. for the OZURDEX GENEVA Study Group. Randomized, sham controlled trial of dexamethasone intravitreal implant in patients with macular edema due to retinal vein occlusion. Ophthalmology 2010;117:1134–46.
4. Robin AL, Suan EP, Sjaarda RN, Callanan DG, Defaller J; Alcon Anecortave Acetate for IOP Research Team. Reduction of intraocular pressure with anecortave acetate in eyes with ocular steroid injection-related glaucoma. Arch Ophthalmol 2009;127(2):173–78.

17.8 Glaucoma in ocular trauma

1. Bai HQ, Yao L, Wang DB, Jin R, Wang YX. Causes and treatments of traumatic secondary glaucoma. Eur J Ophthalmol 2009;19(2):201–06.
2. Campbell DG, Simmons RJ, Grant WM: Ghost cells as a cause of glaucoma. Am J Ophthalmol 1976:81:441.
3. Manners T, Salmon JF, Barron A, Willies C, Murray AD. Trabeculectomy with mitomycin C in the treatment of post-traumatic angle recession glaucoma. Br J Ophthalmol 2001;85(2): 159–63.

17.9 Glaucoma secondary to ocular surgery

1. Ayyala RS. Penetrating keratoplasty and glaucoma. Surv Ophthalmol 2000;45(2):91–105.
2. Costarides AP, Alabata P, Bergstrom C. Elevated intraocular pressure following vitreoretinal surgery. Ophthalmol Clin N Am 2004; 17(4): 507–12.
3. Gedde SJ. Management of glaucoma after retinal detachment surgery. Curr Opin Ophthalmol. 2002;13(2):103–09.
4. Han DP, Lewis H, Lambrou FH Jr, et al. Mechanisms of intraocular pressure elevation after pars plana vitrectomy. Ophthalmology 1989;96:1357.
5. Ichhpujani P, Jindal A, Katz JL. Silicone oil-induced glaucoma: a review. Graefes Arch Clin Exp Ophthalmol 2009;247(12):1585–93.
6. Panda A, Prakash VJ, Dada T, Gupta AK, Khokhar S, Vanathi M. Ahmed glaucoma valve in post-penetrating-keratoplasty glaucoma: a critically evaluated prospective clinical study. Indian J Ophthalmol 2011;59(3):185–89.

17.10 Glaucoma associated with intraocular haemorrhages

1. Campbell D, Shields MB, Liebmann JM. Ghost cell glaucoma. In: Ritch R, Shields B, Krupin T, (eds). The Glaucomas Vol 2. 1989:1239–47.
2. Shields MB. Glaucomas associated with intraocular hemorrhage and glaucomas associated with ocular trauma. In: Textbook of Glaucoma 1992:381–99.
3. Shingleton BJ, Hersh PS. Traumatic hyphema. In: Eye Trauma 1991:104–16.
4. Walton W, Von Hagen S, Grigorian R, Zarbin M. Management of traumatic hyphema. Surv Ophthalmol 2002;47(4):297–334.

17.11 Glaucoma associated with disorders of the corneal endothelium

1. Bourgeois J, Shields MB, Thresher R: Open-angle glaucoma associated with posterior polymorphous dystrophy: A clinicopathologic study. Ophthalmology 1984:91;420.
2. Rodrigues MM, Phelps CD, Krachmer JH, Weingeist TA. Glaucoma due to endothelialization of the anterior chamber angle: A comparison of posterior polymorphous dystrophy of the cornea and Chandler's syndrome. Arch Ophthalmol 1980;98:688.
3. Shields MB. Progressive essential iris atrophy, Chandler's syndrome, and the iris nevus (Cogan-Reese) syndrome: A spectrum of disease. Surv Ophthalmol 1979;24:3.

17.12 Glaucoma associated with elevated episcleral venous pressure

1. Audren F, Abitbol O, Dureau P, Hakiki S, Orssaud C, Bourgeois M, et al. Non-penetrating deep sclerectomy for glaucoma associated with Sturge-Weber syndrome. Acta Ophthalmol Scand Oct 2006;84(5):656–60.
2. Bellows AR, Chylack LT Jr, Epstein DL, Hutchinson BT. Choroidal effusion during glaucoma surgery in patients with prominent episcleral vessels. Arch Ophthalmol 1979;97:493–97.
3. Bloom PA, Tsai TC, Sharma K, et al. "Cyclodiode". Trans-scleral cyclodiode laser cyclophotocoagulation in the treatment of advanced refractory glaucoma. Ophthalmology. 1997;104:1508–19.
4. Eibschitz-Tsimhoni M, Lichter PR, Del Monte MA, et al. Assessing the need for posterior sclerotomy at the time of filtering surgery in patients with Sturge-Weber syndrome. Ophthalmology 2003;110:1361–63.
5. Higginbotham E, Parrish RK. Uveal effusion syndrome. J Glaucoma 1996;5(1):63–67.

17.13 Glaucomas associated with disorders of the retina, vitreous and choroid

1. Blinder KJ, Friedman SM, Mames RN. Diabetic iris neovascularization. Am J Ophthalmol 1995; 120:393–95.
2. Hayreh S, March W, Phelps CD. Ocular hypotony following retinal vein occlusion. Arch Ophthalmol 1978;96:827–33.
3. Tasman W, Magargal LE, Augsburger II. Effects of argon laser photocoagulation on rubeosis

iridis and angle neovascularization. Ophthlmology 1980;87:400–02.

4. Priluck IA, Robertson DM, Hollenhorst RW. Long-term follow-up of occlusion of the central retinal vein in young adults. Am J ophthalmol 1980;90:190–202.
5. Zegarra H, Gutman FA, conforto J. The natural course of central retinal vein occlusion. Ophthalmology 19779;86:1931–42.
6. Laatikainen L, Blach RK. Behavior of the iris vasclature in central retinal vein occlusion: a fluorescein angiographic study of the vascular response of the retina and iris. Br J Ophthlmol 1977;61:272–77.
7. Nguyen NX, Kuchle M. Aqueous flare and cells in eyes with retinal vein occlusion—correlation with retinal fluorescein angiographic findings. Br J Ophthlmol 1993;77:280–83.
8. Servais GE, Thompson HS, Hayreh SS. Relative afferent pupillary defect in central retinal vein occlusion. Ophthalmology 1986;93:301–03.
9. Bloom PA, Papakostopoulos D, Gogolitsyn Y, et al. Clinical and infrared pupillometry in central retinal occlusion. Br J Ophthalmol 1993; 77:75–80.
10. Sabates R, Hirose T, McMeel JW. Electroretinography in the prognosis and classification of cenral retinal vein occlusion. Arch Ophthalmol 19883;101:232–35.

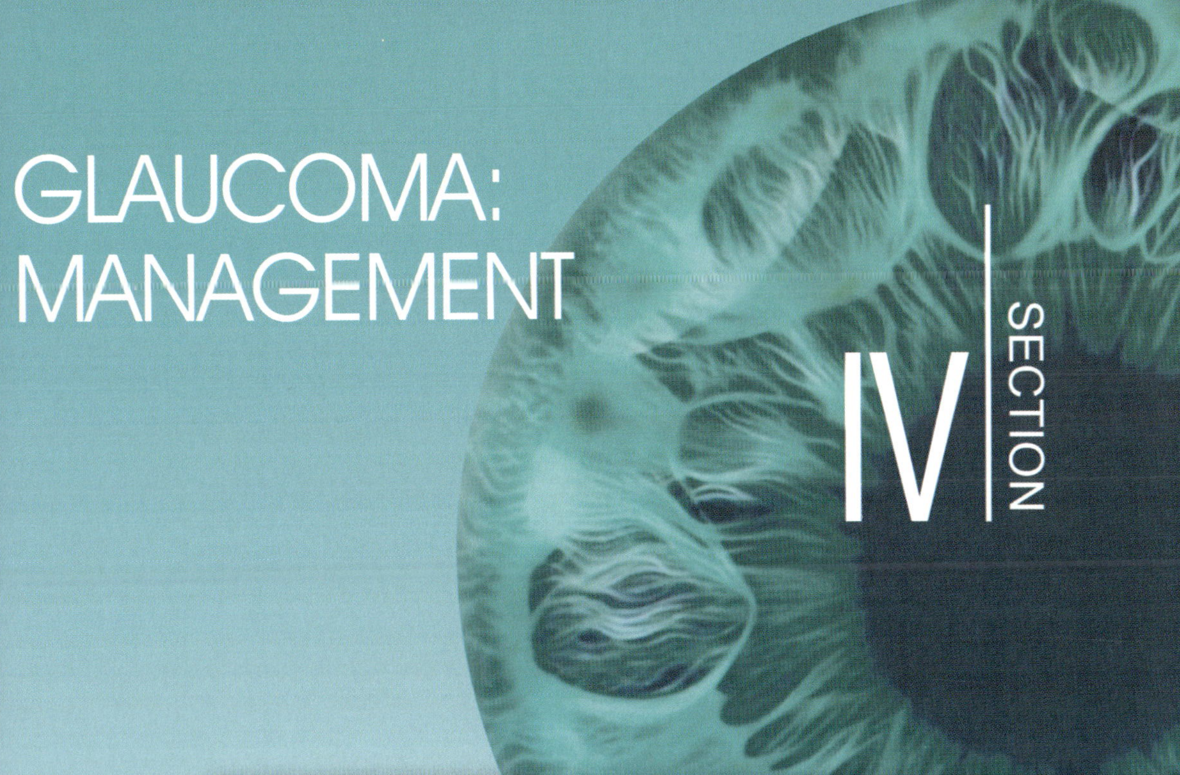

GLAUCOMA: MANAGEMENT

SECTION IV

MEDICAL MANAGEMENT OF GLAUCOMA

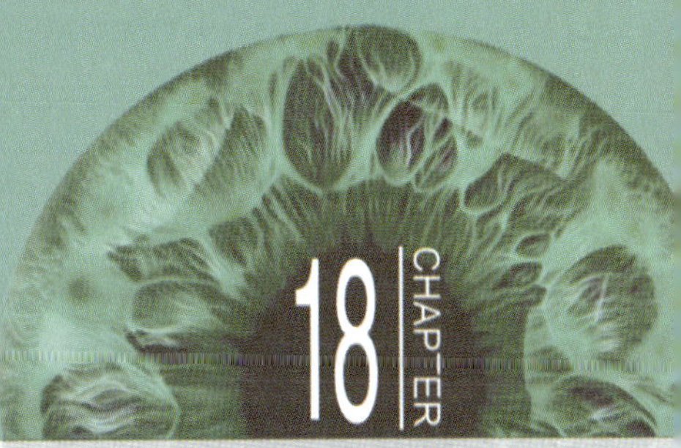

INTRODUCTION

Primary open-angle glaucoma is a pressure sensitive, progressive, chronic optic neuropathy characterized by acquired atrophy of the optic nerve and loss of retinal ganglion cells and their axons.

Three major theories regarding the pathogenesis of glaucoma are:

1. *Mechanical* (intraocular pressure-related damage)
2. *Vascular* (decrease in blood supply to optic nerve head), and
3. *Biochemical* (decrease in neurotrophic factors/ increased levels of neurotoxins).

Three possible therapeutic options would, therefore, be to:

- Decrease intraocular pressure (IOP)
- Increase perfusion to the optic nerve head, and
- Provide neuroprotection to retinal ganglion cells.

Note. As of today, the only feasible option is to reduce IOP by medical, laser or surgical therapy. In addition, one needs to address non-IOP dependent systemic factors, such as blood pressure, diabetes, sleep apnoea, lipids and vasospasm which can contribute to a worsening of glaucomatous optic neuropathy.

MEDICAL MANAGEMENT: GENERAL CONSIDERATIONS

INDICATIONS AND RISK FACTORS FOR TREATMENT

When to treat Glaucoma?

Decision to initiate therapy to lower intraocular pressure is a serious issue that has far-reaching consequences. Once started, therapy generally is continued for the rest of the patient's life. Patients may be subjected to untoward side effects, significant costs, and altered quality of life from the use of glaucoma medications. In addition, the public health impact of treatment is enormous; therapy is expensive and requires regular medical attention.

Determining when to start treatment is a complex decision-making process, which must be individualized for each patient. Any decision to initiate therapy must weigh the patient's risk factors for the development or progression of glaucoma against the risk of side effects, and inconveniences of treatment.

Main goals of glaucoma therapy are to preserve functional vision and quality of life.

As a general rule, treatment should be started, if there is documented progressive structural change in the optic nerve head or retinal nerve fibre layer with or without visual field defects on automated perimetry.

Concept of "Glaucoma continuum"

There are three fluid phases of the continuum, characterized by accelerated retinal ganglion cell death, subsequent axonal loss and optic nerve damage, and visual field loss. These are:

- Undetectable disease
- Asymptomatic disease
- Functional impairment

The earliest stages of glaucoma are generally undetectable. At diagnosis, many patients will present with intermediate-stage glaucoma.

By diagnosing glaucoma in its earliest stages, one can only improve patient awareness of the disease process. In addition, early diagnosis gives the clinician more time to sufficiently monitor the patient such that one can assess the rate of disease progression. Insufficient treatment is likely less problematic in the early stage as compared with the late stage of the disease; early diagnosis provides the practitioner with the luxury of time when it comes to adjusting therapy.

While conclusive evidence of an association between early diagnosis and the prevention of glaucoma-associated vision loss is lacking, the prevailing opinion in the glaucoma community remains that identifying patients earlier along the glaucoma continuum reduces the likelihood of vision loss and blindness.

Risk factors to be considered for treatment

Extent of damage already present and the current rate of progression of the disease are the most important indications of the future risk for glaucomatous damage.

Other critical risk factors that must be considered in the decision to initiate therapy include the level of IOP, central corneal thickness (CCT), age, race, and family history of glaucoma.

Other probable risk factors include myopia, systemic hypertension, systemic hypotension, nocturnal hypotension, vasospasm (associated with cold extremities, migraine, Raynaud's disease), sleep apnoea, and diabetes mellitus.

Some important issues to be taken into account for making decision to treat

- Psychosocial issues
- Patient's overall health
- Predicted life expectancy
- Current systemic medications
- Risk of medication side effects
- Degree of understanding of the disease and treatments
- Level of compliance, and
- Financial impact of treatment.

ESSENTIAL WORK UP BEFORE INITIATING THERAPY

Medical therapy once initiated will be life long and the ophthalmologist must ensure that a correct diagnosis has been made and rule out medical conditions which could be adversely affected by glaucoma medications, such as asthma, heart block, antihypertensive treatment, hypotension, diabetes, stroke, urinary stones, etc. Compliance to therapy, affordability of treatment and family history should be ascertained. In addition to routine ocular and systemic history taking, an assessment of the impact of visual function deterioration on activities of daily living should be done.

Diurnal IOP variation (Fig. 18.1), gonioscopy, stereoscopic disc evaluation/photographs and visual fields must be performed. The diurnal IOP measurement also helps in determining the timing of peak IOP spike in an individual patient and this information is used for setting an appropriate timing of glaucoma medication such that the peak IOP lowering effect of the drug blunts the IOP spike. If baseline IOP is

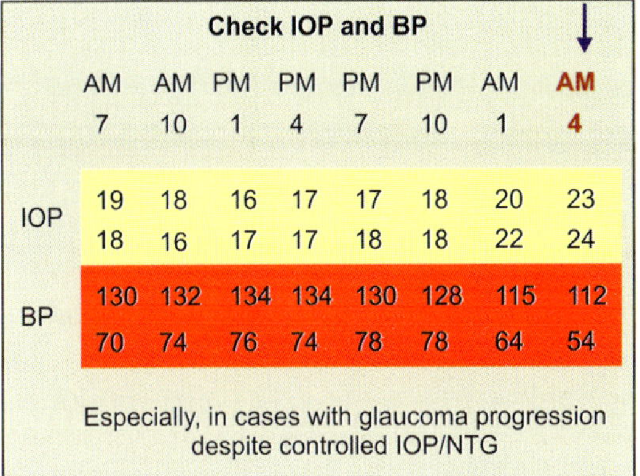

Fig. 18.1 *Diurnal IOP monitoring*

>30 mm Hg, it is reconfirmed once and the patient should be started on therapy without the need for performing a diurnal IOP recording.

Glaucoma suspects require a case to case risk-to-benefit analysis regarding when to begin treatment. The ocular hypertension treatment study (OHTS) provides guidelines for risk stratification. Therefore, one should be more aggressive in treating patients who are older, have thinner corneas, higher baseline IOP, and larger baseline cup: disc ratios.

Important factors to be considered before initiating treatment. Each treatment has its own inherent risks and benefits, which must be clearly discussed with the patient before initiating therapy. These include:

- Severity and type of glaucoma.
- Patient's compliance with treatment and his/her lifestyle
- Affordability of therapy.
- Patient's general health status and life expectancy.
- Individual patient risk factors, family history and access to healthcare delivery services.

GOALS AND STRATEGIES OF MEDICAL THERAPY FOR GLAUCOMA

GOALS OF MEDICAL THERAPY FOR GLAUCOMA

Glaucoma therapy is aimed at preventing further glaucomatous nerve damage. The basic goals of glaucoma therapy are (Table 18.1):

- To achieve target IOP and reduce IOP fluctuations with minimal possible medications
- To administer glaucoma medication which have the least side effects on the quality of life of the patient
- To achieve this treatment at an affordable and sustainable cost for the patient
- Monitor the structure and function of the optic nerve for further damage and adjust the target IOP to a lower level, if deterioration occurs.
- To treat non-IOP dependant systemic factors (systemic hypertension, low diastolic perfusion pressures [diastolic blood pressure minus IOP], diabetes, hyperlipidemia, vasospasm) which may contribute to the development and worsening of glaucomatous optic neuropathy.
- To educate and involve the patient and his family in the management of the disease process.

STRATEGIES OF MEDICAL THERAPY

Strategies of medical therapy, as mentioned earlier in the introduction, include:

- Medical therapy to lower intraocular pressure, and
- Medical therapy to address non-IOP dependent factors.

MEDIAL THERAPY TO LOWER INTRAOCULAR PRESSURE

Medical therapy to lower IOP can be discussed under two needs:

- Antiglaucoma medications (Table 18.1), and
- Principles and regimen of IOP lowering therapy

ANTIGLAUCOMA MEDICATIONS

Ideal medication is one that is effective, has minimal side effects, is cost-effective, and is easy to comply with. There is no ideal antiglaucoma drug at present, but the quest is on.

First-choice agent is the drug chosen on medical grounds.

First-line agent is selected on non-medical (usually cost) gounds.

Table 18.1 *Summary of ocular hypotensive medications*

Drug	*Mechanism of action*	*Efficacy*	*Local side effects*	*Systemic side effects*	*Peak effect, washout period*
Prostaglandin analogues. Latanoprost, bimatoprost, travoprost, unoprostone	Increase uveoscleral outflow by remodelling the extracellular matrix between the ciliary musculatures	Most efficacious of all topical antiglaucoma medications. Decrease IOP about 30–35% from baseline. Worldwide the first-line drug	Conjunctival hyperemia, stinging, hypertrichosis, trichomegaly, periocular skin pigmentation, uveitis, cystoid macular oedema in pseudophakes and aphakes	No known serious side effects. Some reports of transient flu-like symptoms, joint pains	2 weeks, 6 weeks
Beta blockers. Timolol, betaxolol (cardio-selective), levobunalol	Act on beta adrenergic receptor on the ciliary body and decrease aqueous production	Decrease IOP from 25–30% from baseline. Efficacy decreases over a period of time called as long-term tachyphylaxis	Ocular stinging, ocular hypoesthesia, epitheliopathy.	Side effects common on long-term instillation. Bradycardia, heart block, bronchospasm, hyperglycemia, depression, psychosis	4–6 weeks, 4–6 weeks
Alpha adrenergic agonists. Brimonidine, apraclonidine	Act on alpha adrenergic receptors on ciliary vasculature and decrease aqueous production and also increase uveoscleral outflow	20–25% decrease in IOP from baseline. Very efficacious as a prophylaxis to decrease post-laser IOP spike	Follicular conjunctivitis, associated periocular contact dermatitis, blepharoconjunctivitis, lid retraction.	Brimonidine crosses blood–brain barrier to cause systemic hypotension and drowsiness. It is thus contraindicated in children (<6 yrs, <6 kg)	2 weeks, 2 weeks
Cholinergic agonists. Pilocarpine	Increase trabecular outflow	Decrease IOP by 20–25%	Headache, brow ache, induced myopia, miosis, conjunctival hyperemia, iris cyst, uveitis, cystoid macular oedema, retinal detachment	Abdominal cramps, sweating, bronchospasm, diarrhoea	3 hours, 1 week
Carbonic anhydrase inhibitors. Dorzolamide, brinzolamide	Decrease aqueous production by inhibiting carbonic anhydrase enzyme in the ciliary processes	Decrease IOP by 20–25% from baseline	Stinging and burning sensation, corneal decompensation in Fuchs' cornea and post-keratoplasty eyes	Bitter taste in the mouth, rarely drug hypersensitivity	72 hrs, 1 week

Topical medications to treat glaucoma were first used in the 1870s, with the introduction of physostigmine and pilocarpine. Subsequently, other drugs categories have been added to the treatment armamentarium, including nonselective sympathomimetics in the 1920s [e.g., epinephrine, dipivefrin (later, the α-agonist apraclonidine in the early 1990s)], oral carbonic anhydrase inhibitors (e.g. acetazolamide) in the 1950s, and β-blockers (e.g. timolol and levobunolol) in the 1970s. Up until the late 1990s, β-blockers were the medical therapy of choice in the majority of newly diagnosed cases of open-angle glaucoma. In the mid-late 1990s, selective α_2-agonists (brimonidine), topical carbonic anhydrase inhibitors (dorzolamide and brinzolamide), and prostaglandin analogs (PGAs: latanoprost, travoprost, bimatoprost, unoprostone) were introduced. Combination products are also available (timolol-dorzolamide, timolol-latanoprost, timolol-travoprost, timolol-bimatoprost, timolol-brimonidine, and timolol-pilocarpine), but availability significantly varies from country to country. Since the late 1990s, PGAs have been considered the first-line agent for the majority of open-angle glaucomas.

Five classes of topical hypotensive medications summarized in Table 18.1 are:

- Prostaglandins
- Beta-blockers
- Selective (alpha-2) adrenergic agonists
- Carbonic anhydrase inhibitors (CAIs), and
- Cholinergics.

Newer topical hypotensive medications include:

- Rhokinase inhibitors and
- Omidenepag isopropyl

I. Prostaglandins analogues

Preparations

All drugs in this category are derivatives of prostaglandin F2a, and can be divided into three subcategories:

- *Prostaglandin analogues (PGAs).* Latanoprost (0.005%), travoprost (0.004%) and tafluoprost (0.0015%)
- *Prostamide.* Bimatoprost (lumigan 0.03% and 0.01%)
- *Ecosanoids.* Unoprostone isopropyl (rescula 0.15%).

Mechanism of action

These drugs have dual mechanism of action; increase both trabecular meshwork and uveoscleral outflow. These drugs cause extracellular matrix remodelling between longitudinal ciliary muscle fibre bundles. Alteration in matrix metalloproteinase secretion and opening of flow pathways increase uveoscleral outflow over time.

Indications

- Primary open-angle glaucoma including normal tension glaucoma
- Secondary open-angle glaucoma (pseudoexfoliation syndrome, pigment dispersion syndrome)
- *Chronic angle-closure glaucoma.* Increases the uveoscleral outflow by gaining access to the ciliary body either through the partially open part of the anterior chamber angle or through other routes, such as the posterior chamber between the iris and lens, the iris root itself, or the sclera.
- Limited efficacy in paediatric glaucomas.

Contraindications

Absolute contraindications. None

Relative contraindications. These are:

- Recent intraocular surgery
- History of herpetic keratitis
- Active uveitis.

Efficacy and dosage

- These drugs lower IOP on an average between 25 to 35% after 1 week of single, bedtime administration.
- Relatively flat IOP curves over 24 hours.
- Contact lenses should be removed before instillation of the eyedrops and may be reinserted after 15 minutes.

Adverse effects

- Conjunctival hyperemia (maximum with bimatoprost)
- Burning and itching
- Iris colour changes
- Hypertrichosis
- Periorbital skin hyperpigmentation

II. Beta adrenergic blockers

Depending on their selective receptor inhibition, beta blockers are classified as:

Selective. Betaxolol, atenolol and metoprolol are selective β1-blockers.

Non-selective. Timolol maleate, nadolol, befunolol, carteolol, penbutolol, labetalol, nipradilol are nonselective β-blockers.

Commercially available topical beta-blockers for ophthalmic use: timolol (maleate and hemihydrate), betaxolol, levobunolol, carteolol and metoprolol.

Mechanism of action

Beta-blockers antagonize β1 and β2 receptors in the ciliary body's nonpigmented epithelium and thereby reduce secretion of aqueous humor through an incompletely understood mechanism, which in turn lowers IOP.

Indications

- All forms of glaucoma.
- Beta-blockers are additive in combination with miotics, adrenergic agonists, both topical and systemic CAIs and prostaglandin analogs.

Contraindications

- Avoid beta-blockers in smokers and in those with a history of bronchospastic disorders.
- In diabetics as beta-blockers may mask the symptoms of hypoglycaemia.
- In patients with heart disease, heart block, or cardiac failure.

Efficacy and dosage

- Nonselective beta blockers lower IOP by 20–30%.
- One drop of timolol maleate 0.25% or 0.50% has its peak effect 2 h following administration and may last for 24 h.
- Residual effect of timolol on IOP may be detected for as long as 2–3 weeks, and beta blockade can be detected up to 1 month after discontinuation of the drug due to melanin binding, the "depot storage" effect.
- Timolol has little effect in sleeping patients because at night aqueous secretion is less than half that seen during daytime hours.

Short-term escape

- Seen in up to 20% of cases.
- Loss of initial IOP reduction within 2–3 weeks.
- May be due to an upregulation in the number of ocular beta receptors after initial complete blockade.

Long-term drift

- Loss of IOP control after many years of therapy, or even within 3 months.
- May be the result of drug tolerance or progression of the trabecular meshwork outflow problems.

Adverse effects

Both local and systemic adverse effects are known.

Ocular adverse effects include:

- Burning/pain/discomfort
- Hyperemia of conjunctiva
- Superficial punctate keratitis
- Corneal anaesthesia
- Allergic blepharoconjunctivitis
- Dry eye
- Hypotony

Systemic side effects are:

- Depression
- Anxiety
- Confusion/disorientation/hallucinations
- Fatigue/weakness/drowsiness
- Exacerbates myasthenia gravis
- Tinnitus
- Abnormal taste sensation
- Emotional lability
- Cerebrovascular accident
- Psychosis
- Bradycardia
- Raynaud's phenomenon
- Arrhythmia
- Heart failure
- Hypotension
- Hypertension
- Syncope
- Myocardial infarction
- Death
- Dyspnoea

- Status asthmaticus
- Pulmonary failure
- Apnoea, especially in children
- Maculopapular rash
- Alopecia
- Urticaria
- Abdominal cramping
- Impotence
- Altered response to hypoglycaemia

III. Alpha adrenergic agonists

Two topical alpha-adrenergic agonists are available for glaucoma therapy:

- *Apraclonidine.* Relatively nonselective for alpha-1 and alpha-2 receptors
- *Brimonidine.* More selective for alpha-2 than alpha-1 receptors. Brimonidine is 23 times more α_2 selective than apraclonidine and 12 times more selective than clonidine.

Mechanism of action

These drugs work by preventing the release of norepinephrine at presynaptic terminals. They both decrease aqueous production, and they may have some effect on episcleral venous pressure as well as uveoscleral outflow. Brimonidine may also affect conventional outflow in a positive manner.

Indications

- For acute prophylaxis of IOP elevation following argon laser trabeculoplasty, Nd:YAG and argon laser iridotomy, Nd:YAG capsulotomy, and cataract surgery.
- Mostly used as an adjunctive agent for most forms of glaucoma.

Contraindications

- Patients taking monoamine oxidase inhibitors (MAOIs) because they may precipitate a hypertensive crisis.
- Patients taking tricyclic antidepressants because of an increased risk of central nervous system-mediated depression.
- Brimonidine has been associated with respiratory and cardiac depression in infants and is contraindicated under the age of 2.

Efficacy and dosage

- These drugs lower intraocular pressure between 20 and 25%
- Dosed three times a day.

Adverse effects

The most frequent side effects reported with brimonidine are dry mouth, conjunctival blanching, systemic hypotension, fatigue, and drowsiness, especially in children. The brimonidine-purite formulations are preferred to brimonidine-benzalkonium chloride (BAC) formulations due to better tolerability while maintaining similar efficacy.

IV. Carbonic anhydrase inhibitors (CAIs)

Systemic CAIs. Acetazolamide, methazolamide and dichlorphenamide

Topical CAIs. Dorzolamide and brinzolamide

Mechanism of action

Both systemic and topical CAIs cause IOP reduction by a reduction in the accumulation of bicarbonate in the posterior chamber, with a decrease in sodium and associated fluid movement linked to the bicarbonate ion. High doses of acetazolamide bring about an additional decrease in IOP by relative metabolic acidosis. They decrease aqueous humour formation by direct antagonistic activity on ciliary epithelium carbonic anhydrase.

Indications

- Systemic CAIs are used where pressure reduction is needed on an immediate basis.
- Topical CAIs serve as reasonable first (especially in very young or very elderly) or second choice therapy for all forms of glaucoma.

Contraindications

- Patients with a history of kidney stones or other renal disease.
- Patients with liver disease
- Patients with cardiac disease
- Patients with Addison's disease
- Patients with severe chronic obstructive pulmonary disease
- Patients with sulfonamide allergy (sulfa cross-reactivity)

Efficacy and dosage

- They work to lower IOP throughout the 24 h day.
- The topical CAIs lower IOP about 20% and the oral CAIs closer to 30%.
- *Methazolamide* has a longer duration of action and is less bound to serum protein than is acetazolamide.
- *Acetazolamide* is the most commonly used, and is supplied in 125 or 250 mg tablets, or 500 mg sustained-release capsules. It may be dosed up to 250 mg four times daily or 500 mg SR capsules twice a day.
- Suggested frequency of instillation for dorzolamide 2% and brinzolamide 1% is three times daily.
- Patients on an adequate oral CAI dose are unlikely to have an additional advantage of a topical CAI.

Adverse effects

Oral CAIs. Malaise, fatigue, paresthesia, weight loss, depression, gastrointestinal distress, and nephrolithiasis.

Topical CAIs

- Stinging, discomfort, bitter taste and allergic conjunctivitis are common adverse effects with topical CAIs.
- Patients with compromised endothelial function may develop superficial punctate keratitis, corneal oedema, reversible or irreversible corneal decompensation, due to inhibition of Na/K ATPase and the bicarbonate dependent Mg-ATPase which use CA-II and CA-IV.
- Ocular surface irritation with dorzolamide may be a result of the drug's relative greater acidity (lower pH) when compared with that of brinzolamide.
- Brinzolamide suspension may cause more blurring than the dorzolamide solution.

V. Cholinergics (miotics; parasympathomimetic agents)

Preparations

The parasympathomimetics effectively lower IOP but are often poorly tolerated because of ocular side effects.

Miotics are subdivided into two classes based on mechanism of action:

- *Direct acting cholinergic agents.* Pilocarpine and carbachol
- *Indirect acting anti-cholinesterase agents.* Echothiophate iodide.

These days only ocular cholinergic agent used for therapeutic purpose world over is pilocarpine.

Mechanism of action

Pilocarpine lowers the intraocular pressure by constricting the ciliary body muscles that are connected to the scleral spur to open the trabecular meshwork mechanically and increase the outflow of aqueous humour through the conventional drainage pathways.

Indications

Pilocarpine 1 to 2% is used for the acute treatment of primary angle-closure glaucoma. It is most effective once the IOP has been reduced by aqueous suppressants and hyperosmotic agents and the blood flow to the ischaemic iris has been restored.

A diluted formulation of pilocarpine 0.1% is used in the work-up of patients with anisocoria to identify and increased sensitivity to cholinergic stimulation in Adie's tonic pupil.

Contraindications

These agents are contraindicated in patients aged over 40 years, with cataract, uveitis, and neovascular glaucoma.

Efficacy and dosage

- Pilocarpine 2% lowers IOP in 1 h and its effect lasts for 6–7 h.
- Generally dosed four times a day.

Adverse effects

Major systemic side effects of this group are intestinal cramps, bronchospasm, and cardiac irregularities.

Local side effects include stinging, lacrimation, pseudomyopia, browache and a miosed pupil, which can lead to difficulty in focusing and adapting from in dim light. Conjunctival thickening, iris cysts, cataract, and retinal detachment, may also be seen.

VI. Hyperosmotic agents

Hyperosmotic agents, such as oral glycerin and intravenous mannitol, are used to control acute episodes of elevated IOP.

Mechanism of action

These agents increase the blood osmolality which creates an osmotic gradient between the blood and the vitreous humour, drawing water from the vitreous cavity and reducing IOP. The larger the dose and the more rapid the administration, the greater the reduction in IOP because of the increased gradient.

Indications

- Initial treatment of acute and extreme elevation of IOP, including angle-closure glaucoma and certain secondary glaucomas.
- For preoperative preparation of select patients for intraocular surgery.

Contraindications

- Patients with well-established anuria, severe dehydration, frank or impending acute pulmonary oedema, severe cardiac decompensation.
- Hypersensitivity to any component of the preparations.

Efficacy and dosage

Glycerol

- Available as a 50% vol/vol (0.628 g/mL) solution for oral administration.
- The usual dose is 1 to 1.5 g/kg, which is about 2 to 3 mL/kg body weight.
- Begins to lower IOP after only approximately 10 minutes.

Mannitol

- Usual dose of mannitol for reduction of IOP is 0.5 to 2 g/kg of body weight, given as an intravenous infusion of a 20% solution over a period of 30 to 60 minutes.
- Intravenous mannitol has an onset of action within 45 minutes.

Adverse effects

- Nausea, vomiting, headache, backache, acute congestive heart failure, and myocardial infarction are common adverse effects. The rapid increase in extracellular volume and cardiac preload caused by hyperosmotic agents may precipitate or aggravate congestive heart.
- Hyperosmolality and electrolyte disturbances may cause various central nervous system side effects, including thirst, chills, fever, confusion, and disorientation.
- Oral glycerol should be used with caution in diabetic patients because the blood glucose may rise after metabolism of the drug.

VII. Rho-kinases inhibitors

Mechanism of action

These drugs lowers the IOP mainly by relaxing the cytoskeleton of trabecular meshwork and Schlemm's canal there by reducing the cell stiffness and increasing the conventional outflow. Netarsudil also has some neuro-protective role.

Preparations

Approved for clinical use are Ripasudil 0.4% to be used twice daily and netarsudil 0.02% to be used once daily.

Indication include: Primary open angle glaucoma, ocular hypertension and corneal endothelial dysfunction like Fuchs endothelial corneal dystrophy.

VIII. Omidenepag isopropyl 0.002% (ODPI)

Omidenepag Isopropyl (ODPI), a prodrug, it is activated by corneal esterases into a free acid form, Omidenepag isopropyl which binds to EP2 receptors and increases both trabecular and uveoscleral outflow by modulation of ECM and MMP. It is not inferior to Latanoprost 0.005%. Rather IOP reduction with ODPI is seen in patients non-responsive to Latanoprost.

Dose: Once daily dosage is required for adequate response.

Effectivity : In high IOP (22–34 mm Hg) and low IOP (16–22 mm Hg) a 4.9 mm Hg and 2.4 mm Hg reduction seen, respectively.

Adverse effects include: Conjunctival hyperemia (reversible) and macular edema (rarely).

Advantages over prostaglandins analogues include:

- Action via increasing both trabecular outflow and uveoscleral outflow.
- Improves deep superior sulcus.
- No hypertrichosis/hyperpigmentation of periocular skin and other peri-orbitopathic unlike prior PG analogues.

An ideal antiglaucoma drug

Maximum IOP lowering as monotherapy

- *Current status.* Prostaglandin class lowers IOP about 30%.

High responder rates to desired target IOP

- *Current status.* PGAs and beta-blockers have response rates (as monotherapies) of 50–70%. ***Flat 24 h IOP curves*** (less fluctuation) and diurnal and nocturnal control of IOP
- *Current status.* PGAs have fairly flat 24 h IOP curves; beta-blockers do not work at night.

No tachyphylaxis (short-term) or long-term drift

- *Current status:* PGAs have good long-term track records; some controversy about beta blocker "drift".

Increase ocular blood flow—ocular perfusion pressure

- *Current status.* Some evidences that topical carbonic anhydrase inhibitors (CAIs) may increase ocular blood flow and that PGAs and TCAIs may increase ocular perfusion pressure.

Disease modifying agents (e.g., "fix" the TM or other outflow pathways)

- *Current status.* None at the moment.

Neuroprotection by direct action on retinal ganglion cells

- *Current status.* Controversy regarding role of topical brimonidine as neuroprotective; oral memantine trials halted in early 2008 (failed to reach endpoint).

PRINCIPLES AND REGIMES OF MEDICAL THERAPY

Setting target IOP

Introduced by Paul Chandler in the 1950s, setting a target pressure was first recommended by the American Academy of Ophthalmology in its 1992 edition of the Preferred Practice Pattern for Primary Open Angle Glaucoma.

Target IOP is defined as "A range of acceptable IOP levels within which the progression of glaucomatous neuropathy will be halted/retarded". It is the specific level of pressure that, if achieved, will possibly prevent further optic nerve damage and is the IOP where the rate of loss of ganglion cell will almost equal the age-induced loss.

Target IOP is dependant on:

- *IOP level before treatment* (the lower the untreated IOP levels, the lower the target IOP should be.
- *Stage of glaucoma* (greater the pre-existing glaucoma damage, the lower the target IOP should be).
- Rate of progression during follow-up.
- Age and life expectancy (younger age requires lower target IOP).
- Presence of other risk factors, e.g. exfoliation syndrome.
- Family history of glaucoma.
- Systemic diseases (diabetes, HT, CAD, CVD)

There is no way to determine the pressure below which further optic nerve damage will be prevented in any particular patient, therefore, the initial target pressure is an estimate towards the ultimate goal of protecting the optic nerve. The target pressure is different among patients, and even in the same patient it may require recalculation in the course of the disease.

When initiating therapy, it is assumed that the measured pretreatment pressure range resulted in optic nerve damage, so, the initial target pressure selected is at least 20% lower than the pretreatment IOP.

As a general guideline, the IOP in any established case of glaucoma should always be kept below 18 mm Hg.

Specific target IOP can be set by classifying the disease based on severity of glaucomatous damage as follows:

- *Mild.* Glaucomatous optic nerve abnormalities with normal visual fields

  Target IOP. 20% IOP reduction from baseline values, keep IOP <18 mm Hg.

- *Moderate.* Visual field abnormalities in one hemifield but not within 5° of fixation
  Target IOP. 30% IOP reduction; set IOP below 15 mm Hg.
- *Severe.* Visual field abnormalities in either hemifields or field loss within 5° of fixation.
  Target IOP. 50% IOP reduction; set IOP below 13 mm Hg.

Diurnal fluctuation of IOP vis-a-vis target pressure

In addition to setting the target IOP, it is important to keep watch on the ***diurnal fluctuation of IOP***. The maximum IOP should always be kept below 18 mm Hg at all follow-up visits (AGIS study data) and the fluctuation of IOP (both diurnal and long-term variation) should be below 4 mm Hg.

The adequacy of the target pressure is periodically reassessed by comparing optic nerve status (quantitative assessments of the disc and nerve fibre layer, and visual field tests) with previous examinations. If progression occurs at the set target pressure, the target IOP should be lowered.

Tentatively assigned target pressure

Because of the uncertainties about what truly is the appropriate pressure for an individual, and because that pressure may change over time, we prefer the phrase, "Tentatively Assigned Target Pressure (TATP)". This stresses the need to re-evaluate this periodically and to acknowledge that it is an approximation.

Whom to treat?

Not every case of primary open-angle glaucoma, however, requires treatment.

- *True goal of glaucoma therapy* is not to lower IOP or to prevent progressive disc damage or visual field loss.
- *Primary goal of glaucoma treatment* is to preserve a patient's quality of life by preventing the development of functional visual impairment during the patient's lifetime, while minimizing any adverse effects of glaucoma treatment. Unfortunately, few studies have been carried out to evaluate real-life functional deficits in glaucoma.

Most patients are not bothered by early or even moderate amounts of glaucoma damage.

- Cases of early glaucoma in an elderly person may sometimes be treated best by observation in select cases, because even progressive changes may go undetected by the patient, and these patients are at significant risk of side effects from medication.
- Similarly, glaucoma therapy should be administered less aggressively in any patient who has a limited life expectancy.

Primary open-angle glaucoma is a bilateral disease, although it is often strikingly asymmetric. If damage is present in only one eye, it is important to first rule out secondary causes of unilateral open-angle glaucoma, which most commonly include pseudoexfoliation, traumatic angle recession, and corticosteroid-induced glaucoma. If secondary causes of glaucoma are excluded, the damage in one eye is predictive of damage in the other eye and treatment often is initiated in both eyes.

Initiating therapy

- Once the diagnosis of glaucoma has been confirmed, ocular hypotensive medications can be started, starting with one drug at a time. Therapy is usually started in worse eye (usually with higher IOP/more structural and functional damage) first. This is known as the "***one eye therapeutic trial***".
- A drug with at least 20% IOP lowering efficacy is chosen as the first-line therapy (usually a beta blocker or prostaglandin analogue). After the peak IOP reduction ability of that drug is reached, diurnal variation of IOP (IOP reading at every 3 h from early morning to late night, e.g. 7 am, 10 am, 1 pm, 4 pm, 7 pm, 10 pm) is evaluated to look for reduction in IOP and fluctuation.
- In eyes with ocular hypertension, if a decision has been made to treat and in cases with early glaucoma, topical β blocker therapy may be initiated as the first-line therapy provided there are no systemic contraindications.
- In an established open-angle glaucoma patient, once there is moderate/severe visual field damage, a prostaglandin analogue is preferred as it is more likely to achieve desired target IOP.

- In eyes with normal pressure glaucoma, prostaglandin analogues are the preferred choice to start therapy and beta blockers should be avoided as they are absorbed systemically and can lead to a decrease in optic nerve head perfusion pressure.
- In eyes with primary angle-closure glaucoma, the first step is to do a laser peripheral iridotomy, and then start with medical therapy as mentioned above.

Switching of therapy

- If the drug achieves the desired target IOP, it is continued and started in the second eye.
- If drug fails to reduce IOP by at least 20% from baseline or produces severe side effects, we switch to another class of drugs.
- However, if the first drug reduces IOP more than 20% from baseline but target IOP level is not reached, a second drug is added.
- A time interval of at least 5 minutes should be given before administering the second drug.
- In case IOP does not reach target IOP by three topical antiglaucoma medications, laser/ filtering surgery should be considered.

Combination therapy

If IOP is not at target with a single drug, a second drug is added. These two drugs should have different mechanism of action and the best combination is a prostaglandin analogue (which increases outflow) with a beta blocker (which decreases inflow).

Advantages. Using combination eyedrops with two drugs in the same bottle is a good choice, if more than one drug is required as it decreases number of eyedrops to be instilled into the eye, decreases preservative-induced conjunctival toxicity and increases compliance. The most important benefits of fixed-combination therapies are that they provide equivalent IOP reductions with the potential benefits of improved compliance, patient convenience, and cost savings. Also, fewer drops per day mean decreased exposure of the ocular surface to preservatives.

Disadvantage. A disadvantage that should be highlighted is that it is not possible to change the drug concentration or dosing schedule for one component medication independently of the other when using a fixed combination.

However, if adherence is improved by simplifying the regimen, the advantages of using a fixed combination outweigh this disadvantage.

Improving compliance

Non-compliance is a serious issue which leads to therapeutic failure and progression of optic neuropathy. It has been estimated that approximately 10% of all visual loss from glaucoma can be attributed to non-adherence to therapy. The major reason for non-compliance is that glaucoma is a chronic disease that requires lifetime therapy and is slowly progressive, therefore, patients do not notice immediate consequences, if they do not comply with treatment.

Therefore, a proper patient counselling about the disease process, the rationale for treatment and how drugs act, and the need of lifelong medication and follow-up cannot be over emphasized. At each follow-up, the patient should be questioned about possible systemic side effects which may lead to a discontinuation of medication by the patient. It is good to have printed cards for medication schedules, demonstrate the eyedrop administration technique and tailor dosing schedule to daily events.

Educating patient

Correct method to instill eyedrops

- The patient should be instructed to wash both hands, sit down on a chair or lie in bed. If seated, the head is tilted slightly backwards while gazing upward.
- The lower lid is gently pulled down with the nondominant hand to form a small concavity in which the drops will be placed.
- With dominant hand, the dispenser is held above this concavity. The bottle should be near enough to make sure that the drop will enter the eye and far enough so as not to touch it (2–5 cm).

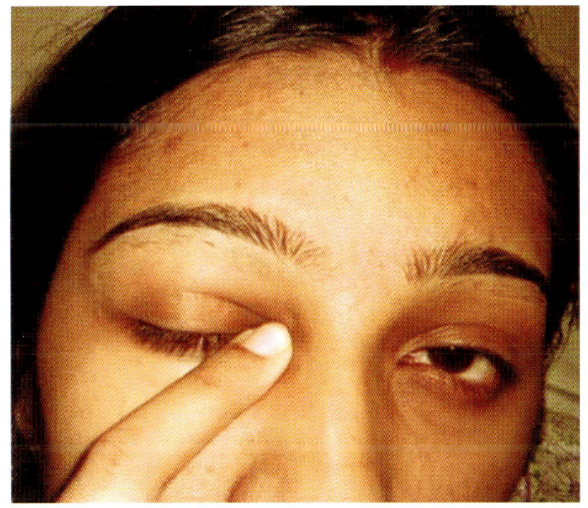

Fig. 18.2 *Nasolacrimal duct occlusion*

- Avoiding blinking and the body of the bottle is pressed so that a single drop falls into the eye.
- After application, lids should be kept closed (or digital compression be applied to the punctum; Fig. 18.2) for 1–2 minutes to minimize systemic absorption.
- The bottle cap should be replaced and any excess fluid wiped from the skin, especially when using prostaglandin medications that may darken the skin colour.

Practical points regarding topical medications

- The human tear volume is approximately 7 µl with a turnover rate of approximately 1 µl per minute. The use of topical drugs in the eyes doubles this rate.
- The spontaneous tear flow will cause complete washout of medication from conjunctival sac within 5 minutes.
- The volume of an eyedrop is 30 to 50 µl. Once a drop has been instilled in the conjunctival sac, only 20% manages to enter the eye, the rest either runs down the cheek or is drained through nasolacrimal duct.
- A substantial systemic absorption takes place through highly vascularized nasal mucosa.

Follow-up regimes

- In general, a patient with established glaucoma should be followed up every six months, however, the frequency of follow-up can be increased or decreased depending on the severity of disease and whether there is any progression or no over time.
- In stable patients with early disease, an yearly follow-up may be adequate, while in advanced cases or documented progression, a 3–4 monthly follow-up would be advised.

In addition to treating the ocular condition, the ophthalmologist should also focus on educating the patient to adopt a healthy lifestyle and take care of any systemic disease factors. Such measures include asking the patient to stop smoking, wear a loose tie, regular exercise, decrease weight, if obese, and meditation to decrease the stress associated with disease and improve the quality of life. For primary prevention and early detection, a checkup of other family members of the glaucoma patient is recommended.

Emerging trends in medical therapy

Novel agents have evolved as our understanding of the complex mechanisms involved in aqueous humour production and obstacles to aqueous outflow increases. Potential future candidates appear to act on enhancing trabecular meshwork outflow: the Rho-kinase inhibitors, ion-channel modulators and chelating agents. Work is also being done on other promising agents: serotonergics, melatonins, cannabinoids, adenosine agonists, components of the actomyosin system, nucleotide analogs and gene silencing. Methods to improve side effect profiles or efficacy of currently available therapies are also being developed. Novel drug delivery methods are being developed to address the challenge of drug adherence.

MEDICAL THERAPY TO ADRESS NON-IOP DEPENDENT FACTORS

Many non-IOP dependent factors are reported to contribute for causation of glaucomatous optic neuropathy (GON). Therefore, a thorough work up is essential for every patient of glaucoma so that the relevant non-IOP dependent factors can be addressed.

Figure 18.3 depicts the probable pathophysiological concept of GON. Based upon this concept, the measures to address non-IOP dependent

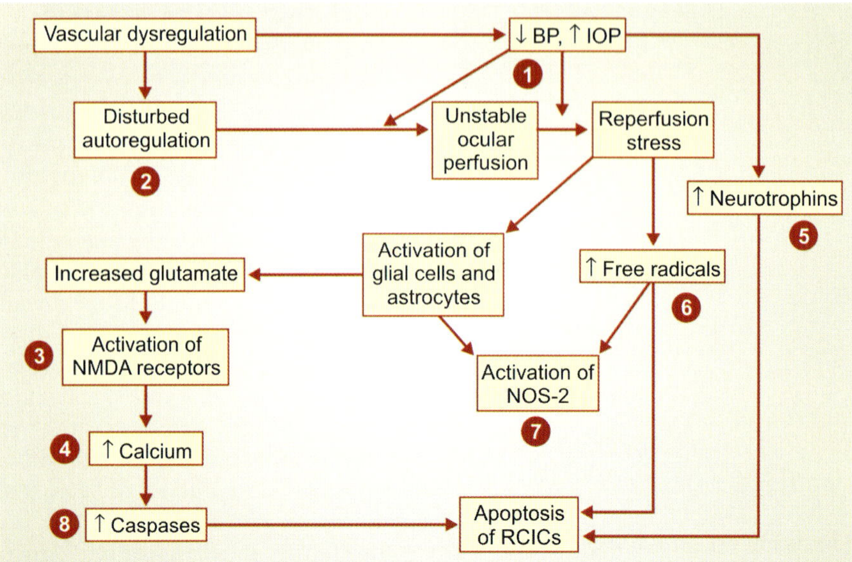

Fig. 18.3 *Role of non-IOP dependent factors in pathophysiology of glaucomatous optic neuropathy and interventional measures to address these factors (1, Measures to increase BP; 2, Measures to improve autoregulation; 3, NMDA receptor antagonists; 4, Calcium channel blockers; 5, Neurotrophins; 6, Free radical scavengers; 7, NOS inhibitors; and 8, Anti-apoptotic agents).*

factors in preventing GON, is highlighted in Fig. 18.3. Measures to address non-IOP dependent factors include:

I. Measures to improve ocular perfusion, and

II. Neuroprotective agents.

I. Measures to improve ocular perfusion

1. *Measures to increase systemic blood pressure*

Blood pressure can be increased by:

i. *Increasing salt intake* (1–5 g should be taken daily in the evening).

ii. *Low dose of fluorocortisone* (0.1 mg twice daily) is helpful in severe cases. Fluorocortisone is a mineralocorticoid that not only increases the blood pressure and reduces nocturnal dips but also indirectly improves the regulation of blood flow.

2. *Measures to improve vascular autoregulation*

i. *Non-pharmacological measures* to improve vascular autoregulation include avoiding cold, emotional stress and mechanical stress.

ii. *Pharmacological measures* include:

- *Carbonic anhydrase inhibitors* which increase as well as improve the regulation of ocular blood flow, and thus decrease the chances of reperfusion injury.
- *Low dose calcium channel blockers* (CCB) may improve the autoregulation. However, it may cause a further decrease in BP at night. Water-soluble CCBs act mainly at the optic nerve head by diffusing through the choroid.
- *Magnesium acts as a CCB* and helps in improving autoregulation when given in high doses.

II. Neuroprotective agents

Neuroprotection refers to mechanisms within nervous system which protect neurons from apoptosis or degeneration. It aims to protect undamaged and to rescue already damaged neurons from glaucoma insults to retinal ganglion cells.

Conventional anti-glaucoma drugs, like brimonidine and betaxolol, have been reported to have additional neuroprotective effect. Recently these drugs have not been shown to offer clinically significant neuroprotective effect. Presently, however, it has not been shown clinically that topical or oral neuroprotective agents are effective in preventing RGC death or in preserving the visual field in patients with open-angle glaucoma.

Neuroprotective agents being investigated to provide neuroprotection in glaucoma are:

1. ***NMDA receptor antagonists.*** Memantine is the most prominent neuroprotection agent in glaucoma. Selective receptor antagonists spare the normally firing neurons and blocks only the overexcited receptors. This is important for the normal functioning of brain. Memantine failed to demonstrate neuroprotection in phase III clinical trials.

2. ***Calcium channel blockers.*** These agents, like verapamil, nifedipine, have been found to be useful particularly in normal tension glaucoma. They block the calcium uptake and thus reduce the excitotoxicity. However, they may cause hypotension which may decrease the ocular prefusion pressure. Recent experimental evidence suggests that nilvadipine appears to have beneficial effects on different ocular structures without reducing ocular perfusion pressure. Due to its hydrophobic nature, nilvadipine has high permeability to the central nervous system, including the retina and has the highest antioxidant potency among calcium channel blockers.

Neuroprotective effect of another new calcium channel blocker—lomerizine, which increases blood flow velocity at optic nerve head level without causing systemic hypotension—has been positively evaluated in many experimental and clinical studies.

3. ***Neurotrophic factors.*** Blockage of retrograde flow of neurotrophins from brain to the retinal ganglion cells causes neuronal damage. The factors, like nerve growth factor, ciliary neurotrophic factor, and brain-derived factor, have been shown to reduce RGC death.

4. ***Antioxidants/free radical scavengers.*** Coenzyme Q10 is an important component of electron transport chain in mitochondria which potentiates energy production to overcome the consequences of excessive glutamate. It also acts as free radical scavenger. Other agents used are vitamin E, melatonin and ginkgo.

5. ***Nitric oxide synthatase inhibitors.*** Aminoguanidine, a potent inhibitor of inducible NOS 2, expressed over astrocytes, is being investigated. However, role in glaucoma is inconclusive.

6. ***Apoptosis inhibitors.*** Final pathway in RGC death is activation of caspases and apoptosis. Caspases 3 inhibitors increase survival of RGCs in many models of glaucoma. Anti-apoptotic factors are also being tried as nuroprotective agent.

LANDMARK GLAUCOMA STUDIES

OCULAR HYPERTENSION TREATMENT STUDY: LINKING IOP AND ONSET OF GLAUCOMA

Study group. Ocular hypertension treatment study (OHTS) enrolled 1,636 patients aged 40 to 80 years with ocular hypertension, i.e. normal visual fields, normal optic discs and untreated IOP of 24 to 32 mm Hg in one eye and 21 to 32 mm Hg in fellow eye.

Aim of the study was to determine, if anti-glaucoma drops delay or prevent glaucoma in ocular hypertensives.

Study design. The patients were initially randomized to observation or a stepped topical medical regimen; patients in observation group were offered medication after 7.5 years of follow-up.

Main outcome measures. Visual fields and stereoscopic optic disc photography.

Observations. After 10 years of follow-up, it was found that:

- Treatment reduced the risk of glaucoma by 50% (from 9.9 to 4.5%).
- The investigators used baseline risk factors, such as IOP, age, central corneal thickness, vertical cup-to-disc ratio, and pattern standard deviation, to establish low, medium and high-risk groups.
- The 10-year incidence of glaucoma was roughly linear, with treatment reducing it by about 50% in all three levels of risk. However, the absolute reduction was greatest in the high-risk group (from 42 to 19%) and least in the lowest-risk group (from 7 to 4%).

Practical considerations are:

- *Always take risk categories into account.* Patients with high risk may need early treatment whereas those with low risk may benefit only from observation.
- *Consider observation before treatment* in some patients as only 20% patients develop glaucoma and thus 80% are unnecessarily treated.

COLLABORATIVE INITIAL GLAUCOMA TREATMENT STUDY (CIGTS): TRABECULECTOMY VS. DRUGS FOR INITIAL THERAPY

Study group. The collaborative initial glaucoma study (CIGTS) enrolled 607 patients aged 25 to 75 years, with newly diagnosed open-angle glaucoma (OAG) and IOP of 20 mm Hg or greater; optic nerve damage and/or visual field loss in one or both eyes. Enrolled patients were randomized to initial treatment with stepped topical medication or trabeculectomy.

Study design. The CIGTS set an aggressive target IOP for each patient, according to baseline characteristics, and substantial and sustained IOP reduction was achieved in both treatment arms: roughly 35% with medication and 48% with surgery.

- The *medication arm* used a stepped regimen of topical medications, beginning with a single agent and adding drugs, if target IOP was not achieved or if visual field loss progressed.
- In the *surgical arm*, trabeculectomy was performed.
- In either arm, if treatment failed, the patient received argon laser trabeculoplasty (ALT).

Main outcome measures. Although visual fields were the primary outcome measure, the CIGTS was the first clinical glaucoma trial to include quality of life as an important outcome variable,

Observations include:

- Interim results from CIGTS showed no advantage overall.
- Later, subgroup analysis, however, revealed differences: Patients with moderate or advanced disease at the time of diagnosis had better results with surgery than with medication as initial treatment. Specifically, those who had a mean deviation of –10 dB or worse on the Humphrey Field Analyzer were more likely to show visual field progression, if initially treated with medicine.

Practical considerations are:

- *Consider surgery first in patients with moderate or advanced disease* as those who had a mean deviation of –10 dB or worse on the Humphrey Field Analyzer were more likely to show visual field progression, if initially treated with medicine.
- However, consider exceptions: African-Americans and diabetic patients do not fare as well as white patients with surgery first approach.
- *Filtering surgery is easier* before eyedrops are used. Surgeons reported that the pristine conjunctiva in patients who had not previously used eyedrops made filtering surgery technically easier than in patients who had used eyedrops prior to surgery.
- *Keep IOP steady.* CIGTS data showed that high IOP variability is unfavourable for glaucoma patients and that variability is greater with use of drops than after surgery.
- *Major surgical complications* are few. Although there were frequent minor complications right after trabeculectomy, CIGTS showed that few were serious, and all resolved without sequelae.

EARLY MANIFEST GLAUCOMA TRIAL: TREAT IOP EARLY, FOLLOW PROGRESS CLOSELY

Study group. Early manifest glaucoma trial (EMGT) conducted over a period of 7 to 11 years enrolled 255 patients, aged 50 to 80, with early-stage glaucoma in at least one eye defined as median visual field mean deviation of –4 dB and median IOP of 20 mm Hg.

Study design. The enrolled patients were randomized to initial treatment with a selective beta-blocker and ALT or left untreated until signs of progression appeared.

Main outcome measures. Visual fields and optic disc photographs.

Observations. It was found that every 1 mm Hg of IOP reduction was associated with a risk reduction of progression by 10 to 13%.

Practical considerations are:

- *Follow progression closely;* reset target as needed. It was found that it is beneficial to lower pressure in patients progressing quickly, even if IOP levels have been in the range of 15 to 18 mm Hg.
- *Persist in eking out the extra mm Hg.* Magnitude of treatment effect seen in the study should make the surgeons striving for a few extra millimetres of pressure lowering, as long as the side effects remain manageable.

COLLABORATIVE NORMAL-TENSION GLAUCOMA STUDY (CNTGS): IOP REDUCTION IMPORTANT EVEN FOR NORMOTENSIVES

Study group. Collaboration normal tension glaucoma study (CNTGS) enrolled 260 patients with normal-tension glaucoma (NTG) followed over five years. Entry criteria was eyes with either progressive NTG or NTG with field defects impinging on the point of fixation.

Study design. Patients were randomized to receive no therapy or IOP lowering by 30% with medication (pilocarpine or carbonic anhydrase inhibitor), laser, filtering surgery, or a combination.

Main outcome measures. Change from a three-field baseline in five of six follow-up visual fields.

Observations include:

- It was concluded that glaucoma progression was slower in the treated group than in the untreated group. However, over 50% of the patients did not show progression, so distinguishing progressive and non-progre-ssive disease is important.
- IOP could be lowered sufficiently in most of the cases with medications only and hence it was found that surgery may not be needed in these patients.

Practical considerations are:

- *Distinguish between progressive and non-progressive disease.* Progression in untreated NTG was highly variable, with a few patients deteriorating very rapidly without treatment and others at a moderate rate; but more than half did not have any demonstrable progression in five to seven years.
- *Surgery may not be necessary.* In CNTG, the goal was to lower pressure by 30%. It was possible to attain that goal in about half of the patients without surgery, using only laser and medical therapy (pilocarpine and systemic carbonic anhydrase inhibitors). With the medications available today, that pressure- lowering goal might be achieved without surgery in as many as 75 to 80%.
- *Double-check potential progression.* As visual field testing is subjective, especially with small increments of change, it is important to differentiate between testing variability and actual progression. Therefore, as many as five or six visual field confirmations were needed to avoid overdiagnosing decline.

ADVANCED GLAUCOMA INTERVENTION STUDY: EFFECT OF SEQUENCE IN SURGICAL PROCEDURES

Aim of Advanced Glaucoma Intervention Study (AGIS) was to assess the outcome of sequences of laser and surgical intervention in eyes that have failed on medical treatment.

Study group. AGIS included 591 patients who were on maximum tolerated medical therapy and baseline VA score 56 or better and baseline AGIS visual field score of 1–16.

Study design. They were randomized to receive ALT trabeculectomy-trabeculectomy (ATT) or trabeculectomy-ALT-trabeculectomy (TAT) and were followed up for 8–11 years.

Main outcome measures. Sustained decrease of visual field and sustained decrease of visual acuity.

Outcomes include:

- The outcomes were different between the two surgical sequences depending upon whether the patients were African-American or Caucasian. An analysis of sustained decrease of visual acuity showed that Caucasians did slightly worse and African-Americans did markedly worse, if they were randomized to TAT rather than ATT.

- According to visual field outcomes, Caucasians assigned to the ATT group fared better, while a worse outcome was again demonstrated for African-Americans.

Practical considerations are:
Take race into account when choosing therapy. It is important to choose the surgical approach according to ethnicity. For example, with some exceptions, first surgical option in African-American patients would be laser trabeculoplasty.

TUBE VS. TRABECULECTOMY STUDY: EXPANDING THE USE OF SHUNTS

Study group. Tube versus trabeculectomy (TVT) study enrolled 212 patients aged 18–85 years with prior cataract or glaucoma filtering surgery and uncontrolled glaucoma with IOP of 18 to 40 mm Hg on maximum tolerated medical therapy.

Study design. The enrolled patients were randomized to receive either tube shunt surgery and/or trabeculectomy with mitomycin C (MMC).

Main outcome measures. IOP, visual acuity, visual fields, surgical complications, glaucoma medications and treatment failure.

Observations include:

- After three months, both procedures produced sustained pressure reduction to the low teens throughout the five-year duration of the study. In addition, rates of visual loss and of late or serious postoperative complications were similar between the two treatment groups.
- However, tube shunt surgery had a higher long-term success rate (cumulative probability of failure at five years was 47% in the trabeculectomy group and 30% in the tube group).
- In addition, the shunts had a lower rate of early postoperative complications and of reoperation for glaucoma.
- In contrast, trabeculectomy plus MMC achieved better early pressure control (first three months) and less use of adjunctive medical therapy (first two years only).

Practical considerations are:
Put tubes in your armamentarium. TVT makes placing drainage shunts in cases preferable where trabeculectomy would have been as the first approach.

Assess the patient's unique needs. Factors, such as tolerance of medical therapy or willingness to undergo repeat glaucoma surgery, if needed, must be considered when choosing between the two procedures. In addition, the surgeon's experience and skill with each of the procedures are important considerations.

SUGGESTED READING

1. Asia Pacific Glaucoma guidelines, 2003-2004. Assessed at http://www.seagig.org/guidelines.php.
2. Brown MM, Brown GC, Spaeth GL. Improper topical self-administration of ocular medication among patients with glaucoma. Can J Ophthalmol 1984;19:2–5.
3. Chrai SS, Makoid MC, Eriksen SP, Robinson JR. Drop size and initial dosing frequency problems of topically applied ophthalmic drugs. J Pharm Sci 1974;63:333–38.
4. Danesh-Meyer HV. Neuroprotection in glaucoma: recent and future directions. Curr Opin Ophthalmol. 2011 Mar;22(2):78–86.
5. European Glaucoma Society: Terminology and Guidelines for Glaucoma. Ed 3. Published by the European Glaucoma Society. Assessed at http://www.eugs.org/eng/EGS_guidelines.asp.
6. Glaucoma diagnosis: Structure and function. In: Grave E, Wienereb R (eds). Kurger Publication: Hague, Netherlands; 2004.
7. Hodapp E, Parrish RK 2nd, Anderson DR. Clinical decisions in glaucoma. Mosby and Co: St Louis; 1993;63–92.
8. Jampel HD. Target pressure in glaucoma therapy. J Glaucoma 1997;6:133–38.
9. Leske MC, Heijl A, Hyman L, et al. Predictors of long-term glaucoma progression in the Early Manifest Glaucoma Trial. Ophthalmology 2007; 114(11):1965–72.
10. Maier P, Funk J, Schwarzer G, et al. Treatment of ocular hypertension and open-angle glaucoma:

meta-analysis of randomised controlled trials. Brit Med J 2005;331:134.
11. Nordstrom BL, Friedman DS, Mozaffari E, et al. Persistence and adherence with topical glaucoma therapy. Am J Ophthalmol 2005;140: 598–606.
12. Parikh R, Parikh S, Navin S, et al. Practical approach to medical management of glaucoma Indian J Ophthalmol 2008;56:223–30
13. Quigley HA. Proportion of those with open angleglaucoma who become blind. Ophthalmology 1999;106:2039–41.
14. Risk factors for progression of visual field abnormalities in normal tension glaucoma. Collaborative Normal Tension Glaucoma Study Group. Am J Ophthalmol 2003;136:820–829.
15. Sena DF, Lindsley K. Neuroprotection for treatment of glaucoma in adults. Cochrane Database
16. Singh K, Shrivastava A. Medical management of glaucoma: principles and practice. Indian J Ophthalmol 2011;59 Suppl:S88–92.
17. Cochrane Database Syst Rev. 2013 Feb 28;2: CD006539. doi: 10.1002/14651858. CD006539. pub3.
18. The myth of the glaucoma continuum. Paul Palmberg. In: Eye on the Bayou: New Concepts in Glaucoma, Cataract and Neuroophthalmology. Jonathan D. Nussdorf, Kugler Publications; 2006:83–87.
19. Zimmerman TJ, Kooner KS, Kandarakis AS, Ziegler LP. Improving the therapeutic index of topically applied ocular drugs. Arch Ophthalmol 1984;102:551–53.

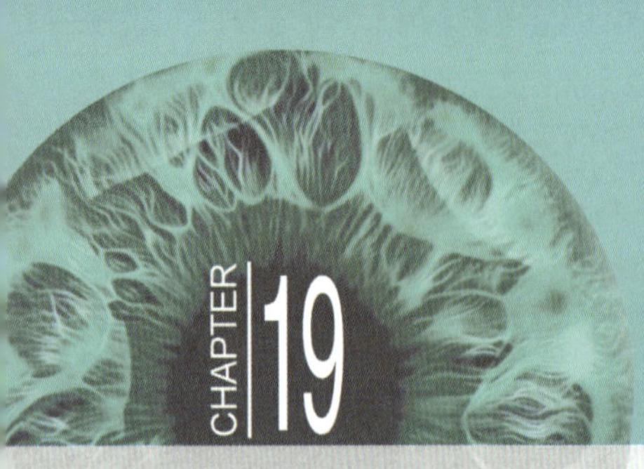

LASERS IN GLAUCOMA

INTRODUCTION

Glaucoma management has traditionally followed a stepwise algorithm that begins with topical medications and progresses to laser therapy, and if still the target intraocular pressure is not attained, then surgery is performed.

"Laser" is an acronym for Light Amplification by Stimulated Emission of Radiation. The development of the laser and its application in ophthalmology has been particularly important in glaucoma. Many types of lasers (xenon, krypton, argon, neodymium:yttrium aluminium-garnet (Nd:YAG), diode, excimer, titanium sapphire) have been used to treat glaucoma in various forms.

The application of lasers in glaucoma continues to evolve, with a trend towards primary and earlier intervention. Refinements in technology as well as clinical data has shown strong safety profiles and efficacies of newer laser modalities, which has led to an expanding role for lasers in the treatment of glaucoma.

BASIC TERMINOLOGIES

Basic terminologies associated with lasers are as below:

Continuous laser. If the output beam from the laser resembles light from a light bulb, it is called continuous wave laser. With electronic switches, continuous laser output can be turned on and off rapidly and precisely.

Pulsed laser. If the output from the laser is repetitive, with numerous repeated pulses generated by the system, each pulse with a short on-time and a longer off-time, it is called pulsed wave laser.

Q-switched laser. A Q-switched laser is a pulsed laser that contains a shutter-like device that does not allow emission of laser light until opened. Energy is built-up in a Q-switched laser and released by opening the device to produce a single, intense laser pulse.

Mode-locked laser. Lasers operate as a result of the resonant modes of the optical cavity that can affect the characteristics of the output beam.

When the phases of different frequency modes are synchronized, i.e. "locked together," the different modes will interfere with one another to generate a beat effect. The result is a laser output in the form of regularly spaced pulsations.

CLASSIFICATION OF LASER PROCEDURES

I. Lasers for outflow enhancement

a. Laser peripheral iridotomy
b. Peripheral iridoplasty
c. Laser pupilloplasty
d. Laser sphincterotomy and laser synaechiotomy
e. Goniophotocoagulation
f. Laser trabeculoplasty
  - Argon laser trabeculoplasty
  - Selective laser trabeculoplasty
  - Pattern laser trabeculoplasty
  - Micropulse diode laser trabeculoplasty
  - Titanium sapphire trabeculoplasty

g. Excimer laser trabeculotomy
h. Carbon dioxide assisted deep sclerotomy

II. Lasers for inflow reduction

a. Trans-scleral diode cyclophotocoagulation
b. Endoscopic cyclophotocoagulation

III. Postoperative lasers

a. Laser suturolysis
b. Laser goniopuncture
c. Laser reduction of dysesthetic blebs

LASERS FOR OUTFLOW ENHANCEMENT

LASER PERIPHERAL IRIDOTOMY

Laser peripheral iridotomy is the preferred procedure for treating angle-closure glaucoma caused by relative or absolute pupillary block.

Mechanism of action

Laser peripheral iridotomy (LPI) eliminates pupillary block by allowing the aqueous to pass directly from the posterior chamber into the anterior chamber, bypassing the pupil. The mechanism of action is chromophore independent and works well in all iris colours.

Indications and contraindications

Indications include:

Absolute indications

- Acute angle-closure glaucoma
- Primary angle-closure
- Primary angle-closure glaucoma
- Aphakic or pseudophakic pupillary block
- Occludable angle with acute angle-closure glaucoma in the fellow eye
- Luxated or subluxated crystalline lens
- Anterior chamber lens implant
- Nanophthalmos
- Pupillary block from silicone oil after vitrectomy
- Mixed-mechanism forms of glaucoma where IOP is maintained and filtering surgery can wait
- Pigment dispersion syndrome

Relative indications

- Younger patients, especially those who live some distance from medical care or who travel frequently or who need frequent dilation
- Narrow angles with positive provocative test
- Iris–trabecular contact demonstrated by compression gonioscopy

Contraindications include:

- Patients unable to cooperate
- Significant corneal oedema
- Very thick iris tissue
- Dilated pupil, unresponsive to miotics
- Flat anterior chamber
- Significant inflammation and/or neovascularization
- 360° synaechial closure

Patient preparation and technique

Patient preparation

Gonioscopy is done to assess the anterior chamber angle. IOP and intraocular inflammation are controlled. An informed consent is taken and the eye is pretreated with topical proparacaine 0.5%, pilocarpine 1%, and either apraclonidine (0.5% or 1%) or brimonidine (0.1%, 0.15%, or 0.2%).

Apraclonidine or brimonidine significantly reduces the risk of post-laser intraocular

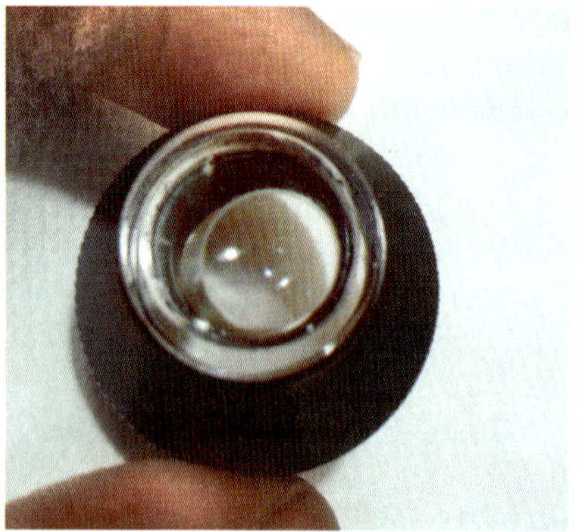

Fig. 19.1 *Abraham iridotomy lens with a Plano-convex button fused with the lens*

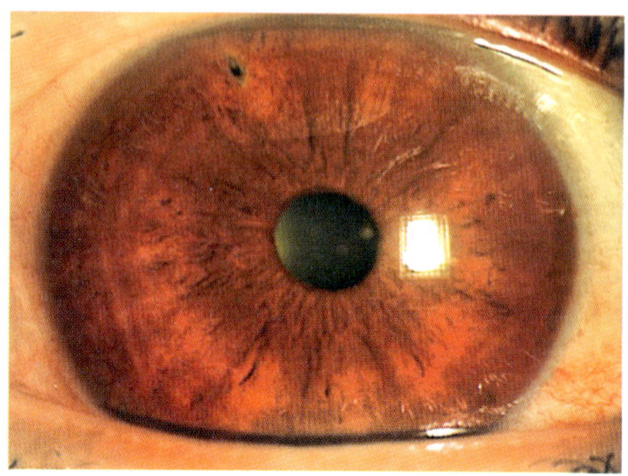

Fig. 19.2 *Laser iridotomy at 11 O'clock*

pressure spike. Pilocarpine is used to stretch the peripheral iris, making it thinner and easier to penetrate.

Technique of laser PI

Placement of iridotomy contact lens. After topical anaesthesia, the Abraham (Fig. 19.1) or Wise iridectomy contact lens is placed on the eye.

When the laser is used on the right eye, the contact lens should be held with the left hand, and *vice versa*. The plane of the contact lens must always be oriented parallel to the iris plane and the laser spot centred within the button. The laser beam should always be in sharp focus.

Nd:YAG laser PI. The Nd:YAG (laser of choice), LPI is done using the following settings:

- Mode: Q switches
- Power: 4–8 mJ
- Pulses/burst: 1–3
- Spot size: Fixed (50–100 microns)
- Laser duration 0.02–0.1

Argon laser PI. Argon laser is used for the angle-closure patients on anticoagulants, in a chronically inflamed eye, pretreating a spongy, thick, brown iris to minimize shredding with subsequent application of Nd:YAG energy, and in iridoplasty to break an attack of angle closure when it is difficult to create an initial LPI or the angle remains occluded or occludable after LPI.

Parameters for argon laser for a preparatory stretch burn are:

- Power: 200–600 mW
- Exposure time: 0.2–0.5 second
- Spot size: 200–500 microns

Parameters for argon laser for a penetration laser burn are:

- Power: 800–1000 mW
- Exposure time: 0.02 second
- Spot size: 50 microns

Important considerations during LPI are as below:

- *LPI should be performed in an area of iris normally covered by eyelid (Fig. 19.2).* Thin areas of iris, such as crypts or transillumination defects in pigment dispersion (after pilocarpine use), are preferable locations.
- *End point* is a pigment puff or a fluid gush, i.e. pigment epithelium storm, clear iris transillumination and visualization of lens.
- *Size of the iridotomy* created should be more than 150 microns (Fig. 19.2).
- *If corneal emphysema develops* during LPI, the procedure can be continued by asking the patient to look in a different direction. If the view to the iris is still limited after this manoeuvre, another site must be chosen.

Combined Nd:YAG and argon laser PI. In thick brown iris, YAG laser may fail in achieving adequate opening, then sequential combination of argon and Nd:YAG lasers is used in the same sitting. Initially argon laser 50 μ spot size 700 mW power and 0.1 second duration is used for about two-thirds of iris thickness with an approximate diameter of 300–500 μ and then

Nd:YAG laser—second laser with energy levels between 2 and 5 mJ in single pulse mode is used to create opening.

Post-laser management and complications

Post-laser management. Topical steroids are given four times a day for one to two weeks depending upon the inflammation. On follow-up visits, one should check the patency of iridotomy both on direct illumination and retroillumination and repeat the gonioscopy after withdrawal of pilocarpine (Fig. 19.3). Pupillary dilation may be required, if posterior synaechiae are suspected.

Complications include:

- Transient increase in pressure
- Iritis
- Iris bleed and/or hyphaema
- Corneal endothelial damage
- Focal cataract

LASER PERIPHERAL IRIDOPLASTY

Selected narrow angles may be widened by peripheral iridoplasty, particularly if the narrowing is not due to pupillary block. It consists of placing circumferential ring of non-penetrating contraction burns at far iris periphery just inside the limbus.

Mechanism of action

In iridoplasty, the laser causes thermal contraction of stromal collagen, which is primarily responsible for the immediate anatomical change. Later, proliferation of fibroblasts with the formation of a contraction membrane occurs.

Indications and contraindications

Indications include:

- Plateau iris
- For better outcome of laser trabeculoplasty in eyes with a plateau iris configuration.
- Adjunct for cases that retain an appositional closure of the filtering angle after LPI.
- Cases where an LPI cannot be initially created because of corneal oedema.
- Iris cyst
- Nanophthalmos

Contraindications include:

- Flat anterior chamber
- Excessive corneal oedema or opacification.

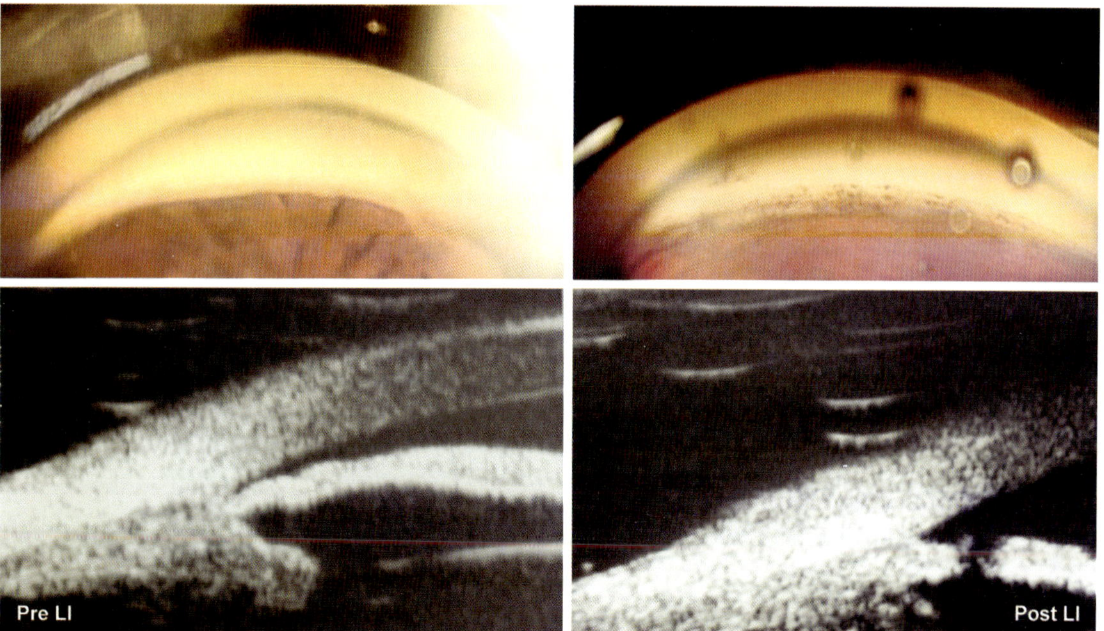

Fig. 19.3 *Gonioscopic opening of angle post-LPI confirmed by ultrasound biomicroscopy*

Patient preparation and technique

Patient preparation. An informed consent is taken and the eye is pretreated with topical proparacaine 0.5%, pilocarpine 1%, and either apraclonidine (0.5 or 1%) or brimonidine (0.1, 0.15, or 0.2%).

Technique

- *Abraham contact lens or Goldmann goniolens* is used so that the laser energy is delivered to the most peripheral portion of the iris that is accessible. Goldmann goniolens may be preferred as it provides better access to peripheral angle and allows to see the efficiency of contraction burns as they are being placed.
- *Laser parameters* for this procedure are long burns (0.5 second), large spot size (500 microns), and low power (200–350 mW).
- *Six spots* are placed per quadrant with 1000 microns (two laser spot) spacing (Fig. 19.4).
- *If bubble formation occurs*, energy application should be stopped in mid-pulse and the continuous-wave power should be decreased.
- *In cases of plateau iris or nanophthalmos*, the laser may need to be delivered even more peripherally using a goniolens. In such cases, the spot size should be reduced to 200 microns. Eyes with dark irides require less continuous-wave power than lighter irides.

Post-laser care and complications

Post-laser care. Post-laser regimen usually consists of topical steroids four times a day for a week. At the follow-up visit, gonioscopy is performed to re-examine the anterior chamber angle. Retreatment may be indicated in some cases and consists of either overlapping the spots or adding a row of applications to the initial treatment.

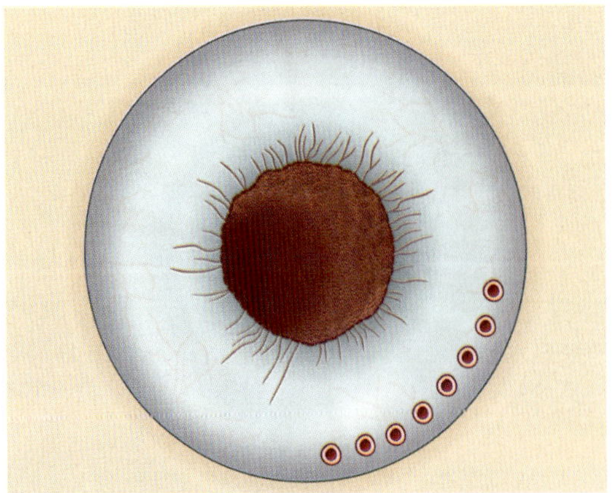

Fig. 19.4 *Patterns of burns that can be used for iridoplasty close to angle*

Complications include:

- Transient IOP elevation
- Mild iritis
- Synaechiae formation
- Corneal endothelial burns

GONIOPHOTOCOAGULATION

Goniophotocoagulation is used in neovascular glaucoma in conjunction with PRP in high risk situation. The goal of the treatment is the immediate ablation of vessels as they cross scleral spur. In first session, angle vessels are ablated and at 2–3-week intervals centrally located iris vessels are ablated. Argon laser is used with Power—200–500 mW, Spot size—100 mm, and duration—0.2 second.

LASER PUPILLOPLASTY

Laser pupilloplasty is used to dilate the rigid constricted pupil. The contraction burns applied near the pupillary portion of iris that contracts collagen fibres and then the pupil dilates. Indications are pupillary block glaucoma with cloudy cornea, pupillary block glaucoma in aphakia/pseudophakia or chronically constricted pupil. The spot size used is 200 mm, power—200–500 mW and duration—0.1–0.2 second.

LASER SPHINCTEROTOMY

Laser sphincterotomy is done with argon laser for transaction of iris sphincter using Wise lens with Spot size—50 mm, power 800–1500 mW and duration—0.01–0.02 sec. The power is reduced to 600–800 mW for posterior synaechiotomy.

LASER TRABECULOPLASTY

Argon laser trabeculoplasty (ALT)

The original laser trabeculoplasty procedure was described using a continuous wave argon laser (major peaks at 488 and 514 nm). ALT is the prototypical procedure against which other trabeculoplasty modalities are measured.

Mechanism of action

The exact mechanism by which the procedure works remains unknown, but it is believed that the laser energy applied to the trabecular meshwork initiates structural and/or physiologic changes that promote aqueous outflow. Local photocoagulation of directly treated trabecular tissue occurs along with an increased phagocytic activity of trabecular cells adjacent to treated areas. Changes in the extracellular matrix have also been noted after ALT due to an induction of matrix metalloproteinases.

Indications and contraindications

Indications include:

- Alternative to topical glaucoma medications as a first-line treatment for open-angle glaucoma (OAG).
- OAG (primary or secondary, e.g. pigmentary glaucoma, pseudoexfoliation glaucoma) patients uncontrolled on topical medications.
- OAG patients noncompliant with medications.

Contraindications

Absolute

Anterior chamber angle structures not visualized or identified or eyes with little or no trabecular meshwork pigmentation or distorted angle anatomy.

Relative

- Traumatic glaucoma, juvenile OAG, or glaucoma due to elevated episcleral venous pressure, due to poor response.
- Patient with advanced and rapidly progressive damage as these patients may require early surgery.

Patient preparation and technique

Patient preparation. An informed consent is taken and the eye is pretreated with topical proparacaine 0.5%, pilocarpine 1%, and either apraclonidine (0.5 or 1%) or brimonidine (0.1, 0.15 or 0.2%). Pilocarpine may improve the surgeon's access to angle structures. In patients with narrow angles, laser iridoplasty or a PI is performed prior to trabeculoplasty.

Technique of ALT is as below:

- *Standard parameters* of a 50-micron spot size and an exposure time of 0.1 second are usually employed. 50 spots are applied in 180° area, with two-spot area gap between the spots.
- *Using a goniolens or Ritch trabeculoplasty lens* (Fig. 19.5), argon green laser is applied at the junction of the pigmented and non-pigmented trabecular meshwork (Fig. 19.6).
- The desired end point is blanching of the trabecular meshwork or production of a tiny bubble. If a large bubble appears, the energy should be reduced.
- ALT procedure can also be performed with a diode laser. In this case, typical settings are 75-micron spot size, 0.1-second duration, and 600–1000 mW power.

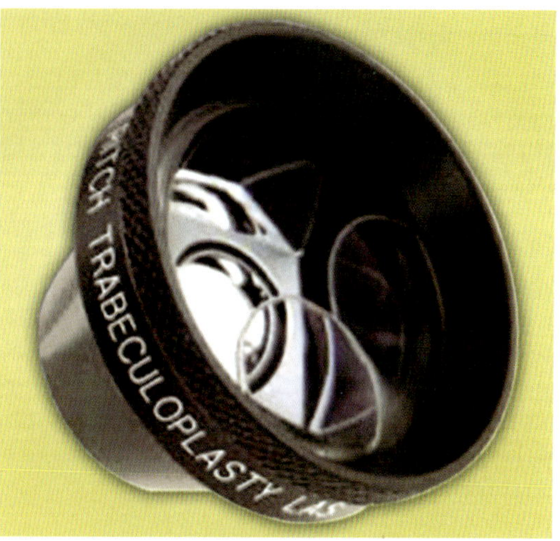

Fig. 19.5 *Ritch trabeculoplasty lens*

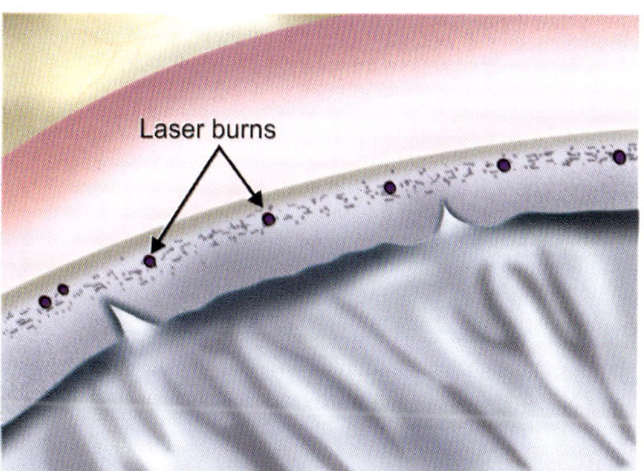

Fig. 19.6 *Laser burns to be applied at the junction of pigmented and non-pigmented trabecular meshwork for laser trabeculoplasty*

Post-laser management and complications

Post-laser management. Topical steroid, such as prednisolone acetate 1% four times a day, is prescribed for a week to control postoperative inflammation and patients are told to continue their IOP-lowering medications. The final IOP-lowering effect after ALT is expected about 1 month postoperatively. If IOP fails to fall another 180° can be lasered.

Complications include:

- Temporary or sustained IOP spikes
- Endothelial burns, if treatment is too anterior
- Peripheral anterior synaechiae, if treatment is too posterior
- Hyphaema

Selective laser trabeculoplasty

Selective laser trabeculoplasty (SLT) is a Q-switched 532 nm, frequency-doubled neodymium:yttrium aluminium-garnet (Nd:YAG) laser applied to the trabecular meshwork.

Mechanism of action

Laser produces selective photothermolysis, selective treatment of the pigmented trabecular meshwork cells. As a result, the fluence levels delivered to the trabecular meshwork are thousands of times lower than that achieved by ALT, resulting in decreased thermal damage to the trabecular meshwork.

Indications and contraindications

Indications

- Alternative to topical glaucoma medications as a first-line treatment for OAG
- OAG patients uncontrolled on topical medications
- OAG patients noncompliant with medications
- Patients with failed ALT treatment

Contraindications

- Inflammatory/uveitic glaucoma
- Primary or secondary angle-closure glaucoma
- Poor visualization of trabecular meshwork
- ICE syndrome

Patient preparation and technique

Patient preparation. Preoperatively, careful gonioscopy should be done to visualize the trabecular meshwork and plan the treatment area. After an informed consent, the eye should be pretreated with topical proparacaine 0.5%.

Technique of SLT is as below:

- *Goldmann, three-mirror goniolens* or *Latina SLT lens* (Fig. 19.7) is placed on the eye with methylcellulose.
- *Laser settings* are fixed except for the power. Spot size is 400 microns and pulse duration is 0.3 ns. The large spot size results in low fluences (mJ/cm^2). In more lightly pigmented angles, initial energy can be set at 0.8–1.0 mJ. In more heavily pigmented angles, the initial power can start off lower at 0.3–0.6 mJ.
- *Aiming beam is centred* over the trabecular meshwork and straddles the entire TM. The aiming beam will not be in sharp focus when the surgeon focuses on the trabecular meshwork to deliver treatment.
- *Small cavitation bubble* (champagne bubbles) formation is monitored with each pulse.
- *If a large bubble appears,* the power is reduced and titrated to produce the desired effect.

Post-laser management and complications

Post-laser management. NSAIDs are prescribed three to four times a day for three to five days.

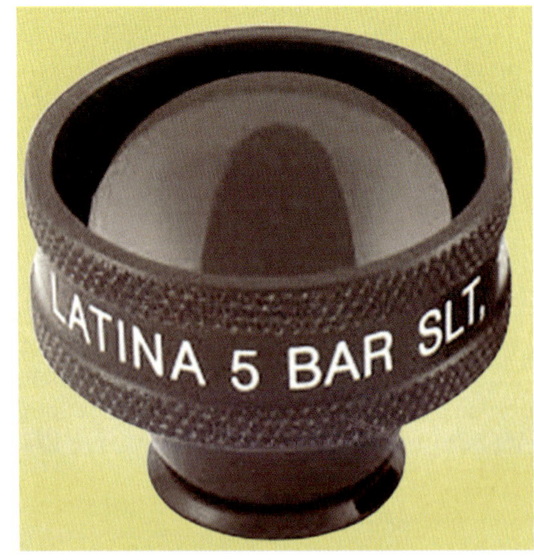

Fig. 19.7 *Latina SLT lens for selective laser trabeculoplasty*

Complications include:

- Transient IOP spike
- Mild iritis

Pattern laser trabeculoplasty

Pattern laser trabeculoplasty (PLT) using a 577 nm laser with computer-guided scanning technology (Pascal Streamline 577, Topcon Medical Laser Systems) appears to be an effective option for OAG. The software was initially introduced for the 532 nm pattern scanning laser and subsequently became available as an upgrade for the 577 nm laser.

In PLT, the laser delivers a treatment pattern of 39 spots of 100-micron each over 22.5° of arc (2.75 mm) and then rotates automatically so that the next pattern is precisely aligned and applied onto an untreated location. Because the treatment outcome is sub-visible, a computer-guided procedure provides automatic alignment of the patterns with no need for visible marks. PLT provides nearly uniform coverage of the trabecular meshwork with more than 1,000 spots of 100 μm in diameter.

Micropulse diode laser trabeculoplasty

Micropulse diode laser trabeculoplasty (MDLT) uses an 810-nm diode laser and includes the OcuLightSLx and IQ810 (Iridex Corporation, Mountain View, California, USA).

Each MDLT application delivers a train of 100 micropulses of 0.6 mJ, with a duration of 0.3 ms followed by an off period of 1.7 ms, each one having 100,000 times longer duration and 100,00 times lower power than the 0.6 mJ SLT's pulse. MDLT is slightly different from SLT as it aims at creating non-lethal temperature gradients at the pigmented cells, sufficient to produce inflammation, macrophages recruitment, release of cytokines and a biological cellular healing cascade leading to induction of cell division and metalloproteinases expression in the trabecular matrix. MDLT can interact with pigment laden cells, both in superficial and deep layers of trabecular meshwork.

The interpulse separation of MDLT is long enough to allow the temperature to return to baseline prior to the arrival of the next pulse and to prevent cumulative thermal rise and prevent the spread of coagulative heat to adjacent structures. As a consequence, MDLT is unlikely to produce micro-explosions, pigment dispersion and IOP spikes.

This laser also has other applications, such as trans-scleral cyclophotocoagulation, retinal photocoagulation and iridotomy.

Figure 19.8 shows a schematic diagram depicting spot size of various trabeculoplasty systems.

Titanium sapphire trabeculoplasty

Titanium sapphire laser trabeculoplasty (TLT) is currently undergoing Phase III trials and uses a 790 nm laser (SOLX, Inc., Waltham, Massachusetts, USA) that emits flash lamp-pumped, near-infrared energy in pulses that last 5–10 msec; a duration intermediate to ALT and SLT. TLT has been shown to provide deeper tissue penetration than the other lasers currently in use for trabeculoplasty without causing damage to the trabecular meshwork, and may therefore, be repeatable.

EXCIMER LASER TRABECULOTOMY

Ab interno excimer laser trabeculotomy (ELT) is useful both as a stand-alone procedure and in combination with cataract surgery.

Mechanism of action

ELT precisely excises tissue without causing thermal injury to or scarring of the surrounding

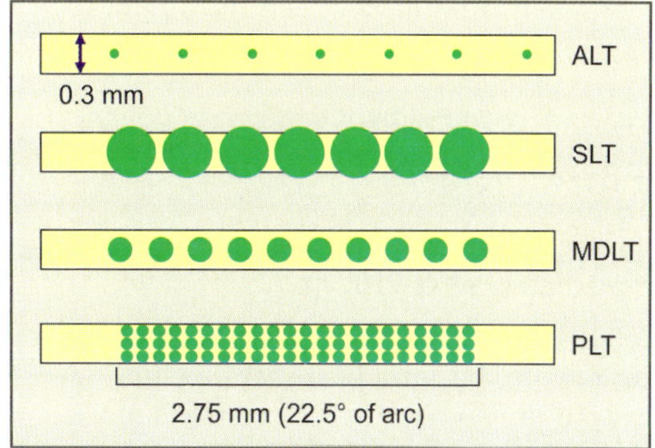

Fig. 19.8 *Schematic diagram showing spot size of various trabeculoplasty systems (ALT: Argon laser trabeculoplasty; SLT: Selective laser trabeculoplasty; MDLT: Micropulse diode laser trabeculoplasty; PLT: Pattern laser trabeculoplasty)*

tissue. This laser is designed to enhance outflow facility by creating microperforations in trabecular meshwork and inner wall of Schlemm's canal to access the outflow collector channels.

Indication and contraindication

Indication. Primary open-angle glaucoma

Contraindication. Angle-closure glaucoma

Patient preparation and technique

Patient preparation. A peribulbar block is required.

Technique of ELT is as below:

- The device utilizes a xenon chloride laser with a wavelength of 308 nm and pulsed delivery of 1.2 mJ over 80 ns duration.
- Aparacentesis is done and the anterior chamber is stabilized with a viscoelastic.
- To avoid the corneal absorption of laser radiation, an optical fibre is used to deliver the energy intracamerally. The fiberoptic probe is then advanced through the paracentesis and across the anterior chamber to contact the trabecular meshwork. The surgeon visualizes the placement through gonioscopy or via an endoscope.
- Pulsed photoablative energy is then applied.
- Generally, 10 sites are created in one or two inferior quadrants. A small amount of bloody reflux from Schlemm's canal confirms each opening's patency. The probe can then be removed from the eye and the viscoelastic is exchanged for balanced salt solution.

Post-laser management and complications

Postoperative care. Postoperatively, patients use topical antibiotics and steroid drops four times a day for 1 to 2 weeks. The IOP decreases immediately after ELT.

Complications. Intraoperative haemorrhage is common in the early postoperative period.

CARBON DIOXIDE LASER ASSISTED DEEP SCLERECTOMY

Deep sclerectomy is a continuously evolving procedure and could be an alternative to penetrating filtering glaucoma surgery. During the deep sclerectomy procedure after making conjunctival flap and then the partial thickness scleral flap, laser could be used to deroof Schlemm's canal by sclera bed ablation.

Type of laser used. Carbon diaoxide laser with wavelength 10,600 nm with spot size of 50 microns and power 100–500 mW.

Mechanism of action. The laser photoablates dry tissue and can remove the roof of the Schlemm's canal by uniform depth of ablation. It is important to achieve haemostasis by coagulation of tissue as the laser could be completely absorbed by even a single layer of water. It prevents accidental entry into the anterior chamber and cataract formation due to the procedure.

Complications

- Blood vessel, aqueous channels may be obstructed
- Scar formation
- Surgically induced astigmatism

LASERS FOR INFLOW REDUCTION

Laser cyclophotocoagulation can be done as:

I. *Trans-scleral laser cyclophotocoagulation* which is done by the following methods:

- Trans-scleral diode laser cyclophotocoagulation.
- Non-contact Nd:YAG laser cyclophotocoagulation
- Contact Nd:YAG laser cyclophotocoagulation

II. *Endoscopic cyclophotocoagulation*

TRANS-SCLERAL LASER PHOTOCOAGULATION

Trans-scleral Diode cyclophotocoagulation (TSCPC)

The diode laser is preferred for cyclophotocoagulation over other wavelengths since the melanin in the ciliary epithelium better absorbs this wavelength than others and hence causes more targeted destruction with less inflammation. So, 50% less energy is required as compared to Nd:YAG laser.

Mechanism of action

Aqueous humour is formed by a combination of ultrafiltration through fenestrated ciliary process capillaries and secretion by the pigmented and nonpigmented epithelium of the inner surface of the ciliary processes. TSCPC reduces aqueous humour production by coagulating proteins of the pigmented cells. Laser closes nearby capillaries and ablates the ciliary epithelium without destroying the ciliary body itself. This slows the aqueous humour production. The only eligibility requirement for treatment is that the eye must have some degree of functioning aqueous outflow. TSCPC then reduces aqueous inflow to match outflow, thereby reducing IOP.

Indications and contraindications

Indications

- Patients in whom multiple filtering surgeries have failed.
- Patients deemed to be at high risk for complications after or the failure of filtering surgery (e.g. individuals with aphakic glaucoma, neovascular glaucoma, or glaucoma after penetrating keratoplasty).
- Patients with low visual potential for whom an invasive procedure is not reasonable.

Contraindication. Uveitis

Patient preparation and technique

Patient preparation. Peribulbar or retrobulbar anaesthesia is required.

Technique of TSCPC is as below:

- *An 810 nm diode laser* (Iris Medical Instruments, Inc., Mountain View, CA) (Fig. 19.9) set initially at a duration of 2,000 milliseconds and a power of 2,000 mW is used for the first application. The energy is delivered via a handpiece with a 600 µm diameter quartz glass fibre called a G-probe.
- *The G-probe* (Fig. 19.10) is positioned with its anterior edge placed 1 mm posterior to the limbus with its footplate completely in contact with the ocular surface. To properly transmit energy, mild pressure must be applied to indent the conjunctiva and sclera.
- *Footplate is moved circumferentially* by one-half the probe's width after each application of laser energy. Traditionally, a row spots can be given with small gap (Fig. 19.11) the 3 and 9 O'clock positions are spared to avoid trauma to the long posterior ciliary vessels and nerves.
- *Power of each application of laser energy* is increased by 250 mW until an audible "pop" is heard, which indicates an overtreatment of the underlying tissue. At this point, one must decrease the power by 250 mW and complete the treatment at a setting near threshold.

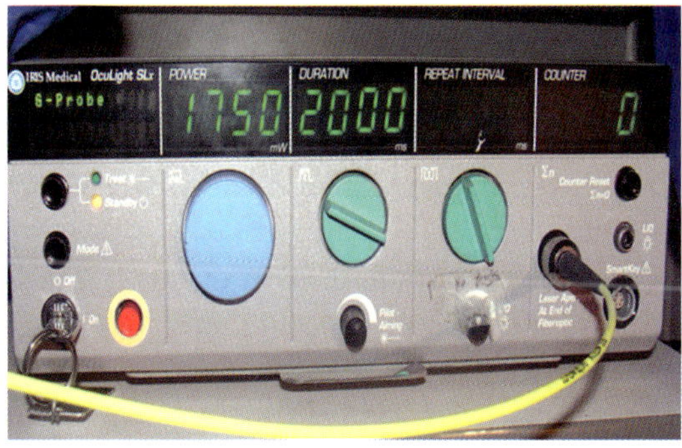

Fig. 19.9 *810 nm diode laser*

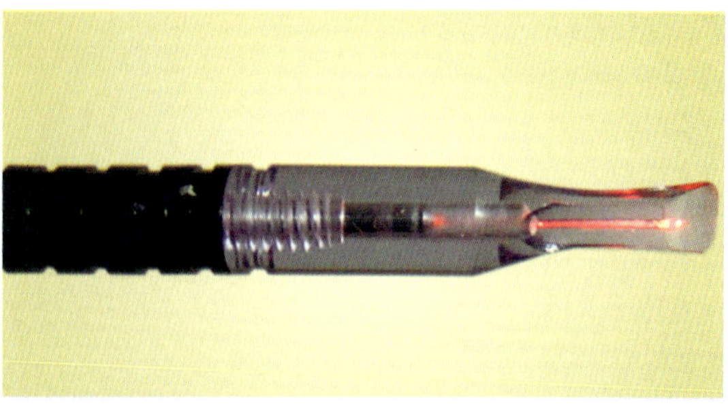

Fig. 19.10 *G-probe showing the head of the probe that is kept in contact with sclera near the limbus to perform trans-sclera photocoagulation*

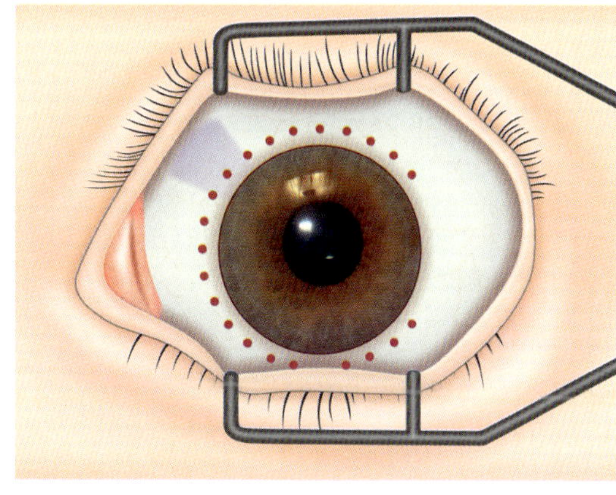

Fig. 19.11 *The row of spots that can be given with small gaps with the help of G-probe*

- *Each quadrant can accommodate five to six spots,* allowing for a total of 20 to 24 spots with a 360° treatment.
- *Care must be taken constantly to wet the ocular surface,* or overheating and burning of the conjunctiva and underlying tissues may occur.

Non-contact Nd:YAG laser cyclophotocoagulation

It delivers the laser energy by a slit-lamp delivery system and uses 1064 nm CW Nd:YAG laser. 8–9 spots per quadrant are placed 1–1.5 mm posterior to the limbus, sparing 3 and 9 O'clock positions.

Contact Nd:YAG laser cyclophotocoagulation

The probe is kept in contact with the conjunctiva. It uses less power than non-contact method. Settings used are 4–9 W power, duration of 0.5–0.7 second and 16–40 spots are placed.

Complications of trans-scleral photocoagulation

- Pain
- Inflammation (acute and chronic)
- IOP spikes
- Conjunctival burns
- Chemosis
- Subconjunctival haemorrhage
- Atonic pupil
- Hypotony/phthisis
- Decrease in or loss of vision
- Sympathetic ophthalmia

ENDOSCOPIC CYCLOPHOTOCOAGULATION

Endoscopic cyclophotocoagulation (ECP, Endo Optiks, Little Silver, New Jersey, USA) employs a fibreoptic cable to deliver pulsed, continuous-wave diode laser energy to the ciliary processes underdirect endoscopic visualization using a video monitor.

Mechanism of action

Endoscopic cyclophotocoagulation involves laser ablation of the ciliary body epithelium, which results in IOP reduction by decreasing the production of aqueous humour.

Indications and contraindications

Indications

Patients with refractory glaucomas, often having failed maximum tolerated medical therapy and prior glaucoma surgery. It is especially suitable for:

- Suited for eyes that have relatively good visual potential
- Suitable for patients who are on anticoagulation medications or are monocular.

Contraindications

Treating eyes with pseudoexfoliation is more difficult because the ciliary processes are smaller, aberrant and covered with white pseudoexfoliative material: Increase the power or move the tip of the endoprobe closer to the target tissue.

Patient preparation and technique

Patient preparation. Administration of acetazolamide prior to ECP may help to prevent a spike in IOP from underlying glaucoma, inflammation, or possible retained viscoelastic. Dilatation of the pupil is done with cyclopentolate 1% and phenylephrine 2.5%. A combination of topical and intracameral anaesthesia helps the patient tolerate the microscope light and reduces sensation in the ciliary body.

Technique of limbal approach

- This is *preferred because anterior vitrectomy* and associated risks for choroidal and retinal detachment are avoided.
- *Paracentesis* is created and the anterior chamber is filled with viscoelastic, which is further used to expand the nasal posterior sulcus. This viscoelastic expansion of the posterior chamber allows for easier approach to the pars plicata with the ECP probe.
- Entry into the anterior chamber at the temporal limbus is then made with 2.2 mm keratome.
- *20 gauge probe is inserted* through the clear cornea incision and into the posterior sulcus after orientation of the probe image outside of the eye (Fig. 19.12). At this time, the ciliary processes are viewed with the help of

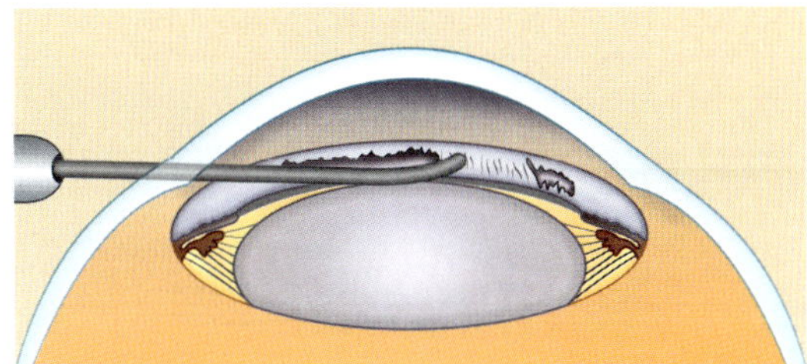

Fig. 19.12 *Probe placement through the clear corneal incision with endoscopic photocoagulation*

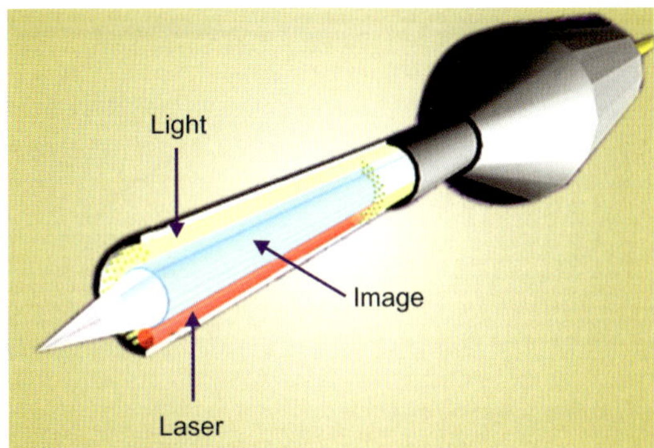

Fig. 19.13 *Endoscope for photocoagulation, the centre tube is for visualization and a parallel cable is for laser delivery at the tip*

endoscope (Fig. 19.13) on the monitor and treatment can begin.

- *Laser is set at continuous wave* and energy settings are 60–90 mW. Approximately 180° span of ciliary processes is photocoagulated.
- *Laser energy is applied to each process* until shrinkage and whitening occur. If excessive energy is used, the process explodes (or "pops") with bubble formation, leading to excessive inflammation and breakdown of the blood–aqueous barrier.
- After the nasal 180° of ciliary processes are treated, *a separate incision is created at the nasal limbus* in a similar fashion as above. The temporal ciliary processes are then photocoagulated for a total of 360°, if so desired.
- *Closure of the wounds* is done after the viscoelastic is flushed out using balanced salt solution irrigation of the anterior chamber.

Technique of pars plana approach. This approach is preferred in aphakic eyes with posterior synaechiae limiting access to the ciliary sulcus.

- An infusion port is inserted through the inferior pars plana and two superior entries are created for vitrectomy and illumination.
- Limited anterior vitrectomy is performed to allow adequate and safe access to all of the ciliary processes.
- The ECP probe is inserted through each superior entry for treatment of the opposite 180° of processes. There may be a few superior processes that cannot be accessed since the entry ports are not exactly 180° opposite each other.
- Laser cyclophotocoagulation is carried out with the same parameters and end points as described for the limbal approach.

Postoperative care and complications

Postoperative care. Patients are placed on a regimen of topical antibiotics, steroids, non-steroidal anti-inflammatory agents (NSAIDs), cycloplegics, and their preoperative glaucoma medications except for miotics and prostaglandin analogues since these may exacerbate intraocular inflammation or its sequelae.

Complications include:

- Elevated IOP
- Zonular damage
- Macular oedema
- Hypotony
- Retinal detachment

POSTOPERATIVE LASERS

LASER SUTUROLYSIS

These days trabeculectomy has "protected" scleral flaps fashioned using tight closure technique. For postoperative IOP control of these tight scleral flaps, a partial release of the flap by laser suture lysis (LSL) is done, which is performed a few days to a few weeks after surgery.

- *Argon or diode laser* is used to cut sutures without disrupting the conjunctiva.
- *Blumenthal (Fig. 9.14) or Hoskins (Fig. 19.15) suturolysis* lens is used to provide a clear view of the suture under the conjunctiva.

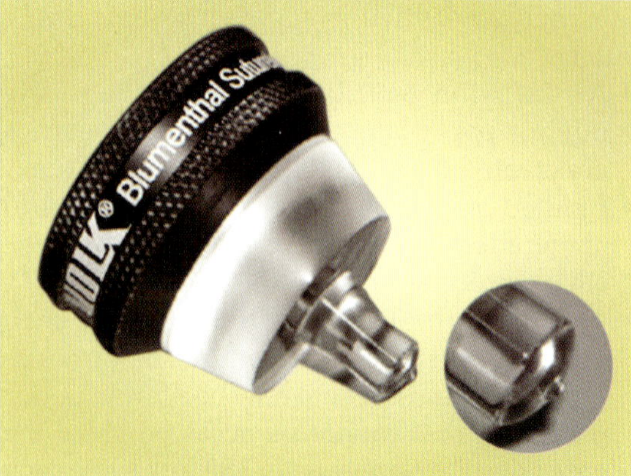

Fig. 19.14 *Blumenthal suturolysis lens where the tip of the lens is used to compress the conjunctiva to visualize the suture*

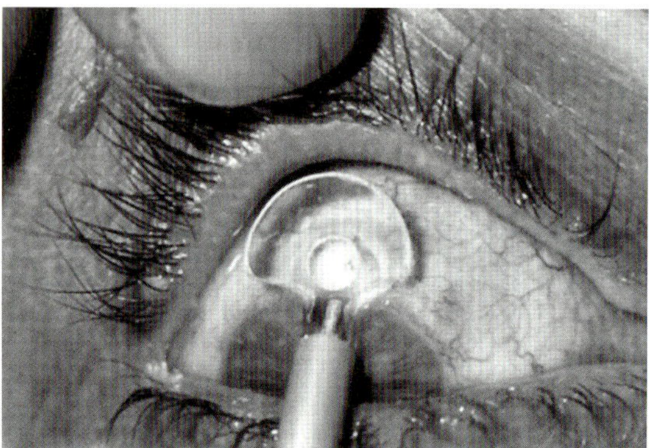

Fig. 19.15 *Hoskins lens that has a small convex lens that compresses the oedematous conjunctiva permitting a clear view of the tiny suture underneath the conjunctiva*

- *Parameters for treatment* depend on the thickness of the bleb and the type of laser that is used. Usually, an application of laser energy at a low power setting (50–100 mm at 300 mW) suffices. If the scleral flap sutures are tight and at least 4 mm long, visibility is better and cutting becomes easier. The laser beam cuts the suture in the middle and as the two ends of the same split the drainage from scleral flap could be improved (Fig. 19.16).

Contraindications include:

- Suture not visible through conjunction, and
- Thin and avascular conjunctiva due to MMC usage.

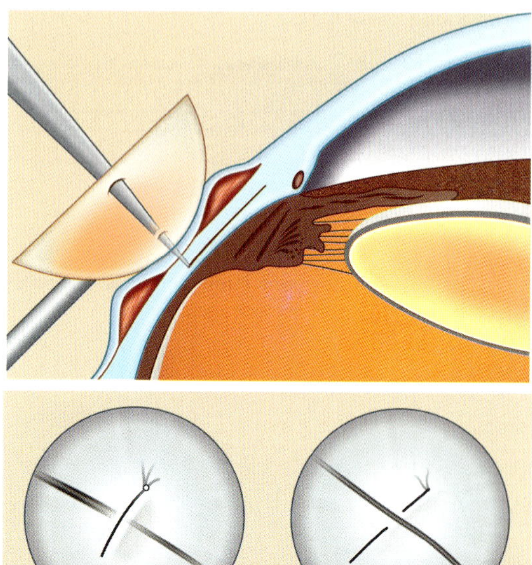

Fig. 19.16 *The laser beams cuts the suture in the middle and as the two ends of the same split, the drainage from scleral flap could be improved*

LASER GONIOPUNCTURE

Laser goniopuncture is a complementary adjunct to nonfiltering glaucoma surgery, such as deep sclerectomy, viscocanalostomy, and canaloplasty, contributing to intraocular pressure control and the avoidance of additional incisional surgery.

In these nonpenetrating surgeries, a trabeculo-Descemet window (TDW) is often created by the removal of overlying sclera and corneal stroma, which allows aqueous to flow from the anterior chamber into an intrascleral lake. The maintenance and long-term viability of the scleral lake is likely a significant factor in IOP control.

Laser goniopuncture has the potential to augment aqueous outflow through the TDW without additional incisional surgery by using the neodymium-doped:yttrium-aluminium-garnet (Nd:YAG) laser to puncture Descemet window creating one to several tiny holes or slits. It is performed within 6 to 8 weeks of surgery.

The anatomic target for goniopuncture is preferably Descemet's portion of the semitransparent TDW. Using a goniolens, beam is targeted approximately 150 to 200 μm anterior to Schwalbe's line choosing a thinner portion of the window and initially aiming centrally. Start with 3 mJ shots and later it can be intensified with multiple shots, 2 or 3 pulses per burst, and by gradually increasing the energy to generally no more than 5 or 6 mJ until the TDW is punctured. There is a risk of iris incarceration, but it is not very common.

Patients should be treated with anti-inflammatories for 7 to 14 days postprocedure.

LASER REDUCTION OF DYSESTHETIC BLEBS

Argon and Nd:YAG lasers are used to induce scarring and inflammation is dysesthetic, overfiltering blebs. The short-term outcome may be good because of shrinkage of bleb surface but long-term outcome is bad because of barotrauma which results in an ischaemic bleb. Holes and leaks are common complications.

SUGGESTED READING

1. Agrawal P, Dulku S, Nolan W, et al. The UK national cyclodiode laser survey. Eye 2011; 25: 168–73.
2. Babighian S, Caretti L, Tavolato M, et al. Excimer laser trabeculotomy vs 180° selective laser trabeculoplasty in primary open-angle glaucoma. A 2-year randomized, controlled trial. Eye 2010; 24:632–38.
3. Glaucoma Laser Trial (GLT). Results of argon laser trabeculoplasty versus topical medications. The Glaucoma Laser Trial Research Group. Ophthalmology 1990;97:1403–13.
4. Lima FE, Carvalho DM, Avila MP. Phacoemulsification and endoscopic cyclophotocoagulation as primary surgical procedure in coexisting cataract and glaucoma. Arq Bras Oftalmol 2010; 73:419–22.
5. Meyer JJ, Lawrence SD. What's new in laser treatment for glaucoma? Curr Opin Ophthalmol 2012;23:111–17.

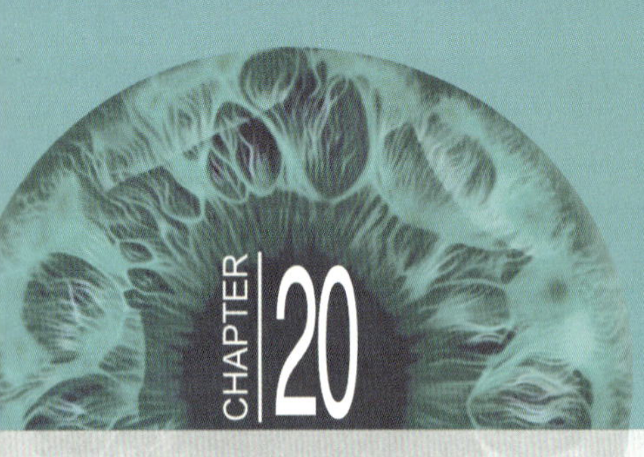

SURGICAL MANAGEMENT OF GLAUCOMA

INTRODUCTION AND CLASSIFICATION OF GLAUCOMA SURGERIES

INTRODUCTION

- *On the most fundamental level,* IOP-lowering surgeries decrease pressure either by inhibiting aqueous production or by enhancing its outflow.
- *Most glaucoma surgeries promote the aqueous outflow,* it is helpful to group them into extrascleral drainage (i.e. bleb-forming) procedures versus those that enhance physiologic outflow. Some surgeries are difficult to categorize, however, and may have more than one mechanism of action (e.g. canaloplasty).
- Both the enhancement of physiologic outflow and the bleb-forming procedures were first attempted more than 150 years ago, but great progress has been made since then.
- *Many new surgeries have been devised since 1856,* when von Graefe discovered that iridectomy is an effective surgical method for acute glaucoma treatment; the first glaucoma surgery reported in literature.
- Two years later, De Wecker presented sclerotomy as a procedure for chronic glaucoma.
- *Internal filtration* (cyclodialysis) was developed in 1900.
- *Ciliodestruction* was suggested, in 1932. A ciliarotomy is a surgical division of the ciliary zone in the treatment of glaucoma.
- *Four basic approaches,* relief of pupillary block, external filtration, internal filtration, and ciliodestruction, are still the valid techniques of glaucoma surgeries over 100 years later.
- Although majority of surgeries used nowadays were introduced in the 1960s, their roots can be traced to the work of surgeons in the 19th century.

- *Trabeculectomy*, in use since the mid-1960s, is the most effective glaucoma surgery in terms of intraocular pressure reduction but carries its own limitations.
- *Cairns trabeculectomy* (1968), ironically was initially conceived as a method of restoring physiologic outflow by removing the juxtacanalicular trabecular meshwork, but it ultimately became a sclerokeratectomy procedure that reduced IOP by permitting suprascleral fluid to escape and forming a bleb.
- *Goniotomy*. Probably a more important advance in the surgical restoration of physiology came in 1891, when Taylor performed goniotomy to remove the inner wall of the Schlemm's canal. Other advances were to follow, including sinusotomy, non-penetrating deep sclerectomy, viscocanalostomy, and canaloplasty.
- *Non-penetrating glaucoma surgeries* emerged at the same time when trabeculectomy was presented, but they are not used as commonly as trabeculectomy.
- *Molteno developed the first aqueous shunt* in 1967 to an external reservoir, initially using a juxtalimbal implant that was removed after a capsule formed. He eventually developed the (permanent) long tube implant that is very similar to the Molteno device used today.
- Since 1995, the majority of new surgeries have consisted of new implantable devices including SOLX, iStent, and Ex-PRESS shunt.

CLASSIFICATION OF GLAUCOMA SURGERIES

A. Based on type of glaucoma

The practical ways to group the surgical procedures required for particular type of glaucoma:

I. *Surgeries for congenital glaucoma*

Incisional angle surgery

- Goniotomy, and
- Trabeculotomy

Filtering operations

- Trabeculotomy with antimetabolites
- Combined trabeculotomy and trabeculectomy with anti-metabolites (standard procedure)

Glaucoma drainage devices (for refractory cases).

II. *Surgeries for primary open-angle glaucoma*

- Filtering operations
- Combined cataract and filtration surgeries
- Glaucoma drainage devices

III. *Surgeries for primary angle-closure glaucoma*

- Peripheral iridectomy
- Filtering operations
- Cataract surgery
- Combined cataract and filtration surgeries

IV. *Surgeries for secondary glaucomas*

Surgeries for the cause of glaucoma

- Lens extraction for lens-induced glaucomas.
- Vitrectomy for aqueous misdirection syndrome, glaucoma associated with vitreous prolapsed.
- Peripheral iridectomy for pupillary block.
- Goniosynaechiolysis.

V. *Surgeries for intractable glaucomas*

- Artificial drainage shunt operations
- Cyclodestructive procedures

B. Based on mechanism of lowering of IOP

Based on mechanism of lowering of IOP, the common glaucoma surgeries can be classified as below.

I. *Manipulation of aqueous outflow*

External filtration surgeries

- Free filtering operations
- Guarded filtering surgery (trabeculectomy)
- Non-penetrating filtration surgery

Internal filtration surgeries

Angle-based surgeries

- Goniotomy
- Trabeculotomy
- Goniosynaechiolysis

Canal-based surgeries

- Canaloplasty
- Trabectome
- Trabecular microbypass stent (iStent)

Widening of anterior chamber inlet

- Lens extraction

Pupillary block relief
- Surgical peripheral iridectomy

Glaucoma drainage devices

Valved devices
- Ahmed glaucoma valve (AGV)
- Krupin implant

Non-valved devices
- Molteno implant
- Baerveldt implant
- Schocket tube shunt
- ExPRESS glaucoma shunt

II. *Manipulation of aqueous inflow*

External procedures
- Cyclocryotherapy
- Cyclodiathermy
- Trans-scleral cyclophotocoagulation

Internal procedure

Endocyclophotocoagulation

COMMON GLAUCOMA SURGERIES

SURGICAL PERIPHERAL IRIDECTOMY

INDICATIONS

Therapeutic
- Acute angle-closure glaucoma
- Chronic angle-closure glaucoma
- Mixed mechanism glaucoma
- Phacomorphic glaucoma with an element of pupillary block
- Iris bombe

Prophylactic
- PAC
- Patients with silicone oil in eye (inferior iridectomy is done usually)
- Fellow eye of a patient with acute angle closure.

Diagnostic
- Plateau iris syndrome
- Malignant glaucoma

SURGICAL TECHNIQUE

1. *Incision*. A 4 mm limbal or preferably corneal incision is made with the help of razor blade fragment (Fig. 20.1A).

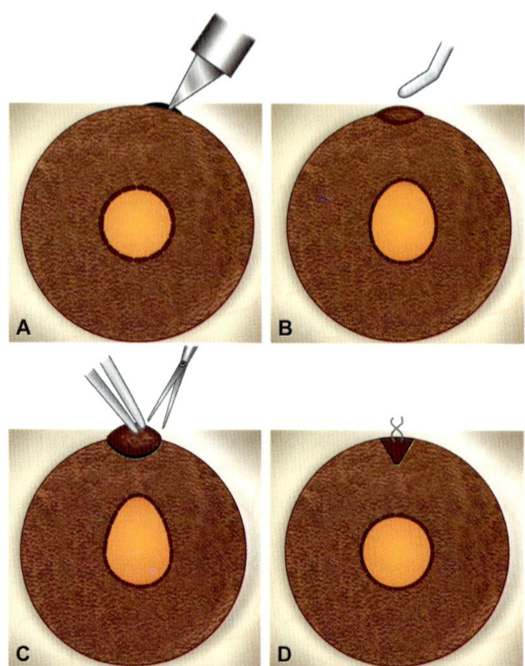

Fig. 20.1 *Technique of peripheral iridectomy: (A) Anterior limbal incision to open the anterior chamber; (B) Prolapse of peripheral iris by pressure at the posterior lip of the incision; (C) Excision of the prolapsed knuckle of the iris by Vannas scissors; (D) Suturing the wound*

2. *Iris prolapsed*. The posterior lip of the wound is depressed so that the iris prolapses. If the iris does not prolapse, it is grasped at the periphery with iris forceps (Fig. 20.1B).
3. *Iridectomy*. A small full thickness piece of iris is excised by Vannas scissors (Fig. 20.1C).
4. *Reposition of iris*. Iris is reposited back into the anterior chamber by stroking the lips of the wound or with iris repositors.
5. *Wound closure* is done with one or two 10-0 nylon sutures with buried knots (Fig. 20.1D).
6. *Subconjunctival injection* of dexamethasone 0.25 ml and gentamicin 0.5 ml is given.
7. *Patching of eye* is done with a sterile eye pad and sticking plaster.

GONIOTOMY AND TRABECULOTOMY

GONIOTOMY

Indications

It is an incisional angle surgery performed by internal approach for congenital glaucoma with relatively clear cornea.

Surgical Technique

1. In this procedure, a Barkan's goniotomy knife or a 25 G needle with bevel up is passed through the limbus on the temporal side (Fig. 20.2A). Under gonioscopic control (Swan-Jacob with handle or Barkan's operating lens) the knife is passed across the anterior chamber to the nasal part of the angle.
2. An incision is made in the angle approximately midway between root of the iris and Schwalbe's ring through approximately 75°. The knife is then withdrawn. Short sweeps of the needle or knife in one direction or the other will commonly produce a white line on the sclera as the iris drops backward (Fig. 20.2B).
3. If the angle is not seen well, the corneal epithelium may be scraped off using a blade or rubbed off after applying sterile glycerin.

Note. Although the procedure may have to be repeated, the eventual success rate is about 85%.

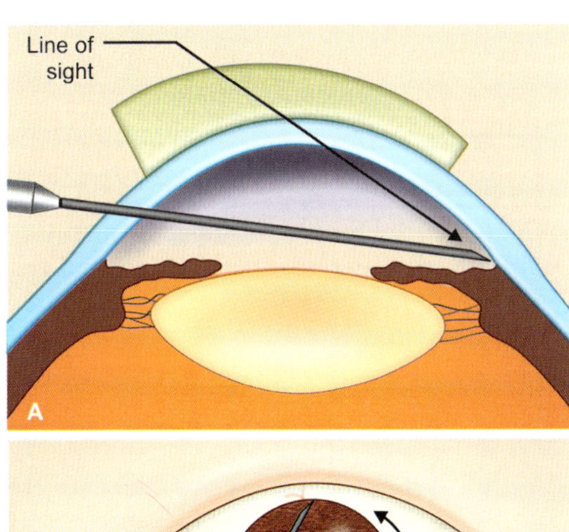

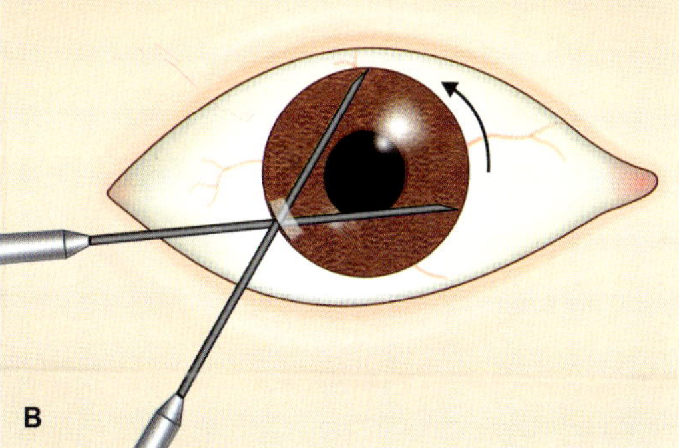

Fig. 20.2 *Technique of goniotomy: (A) Position of goniotomy knife in the angle under direct visualization; (B) Procedure of sweeping the knife in the angle*

TRABECULOTOMY

Indications

It is an incisional angle surgery performed by external approach:

1. Used when corneal clouding prevents visualization of the angle
2. In cases where goniotomy has failed.

Surgical Technique

1. In this, canal of Schlemm is exposed at about 12 O'clock position by a vertical scleral incision after making a conjunctival flap and partial thickness scleral flap.
2. The lower prong of Harm's trabeculotome is passed along the Schlemm's canal on one side and the upper prong is used as a guide (Fig. 20.3).
3. Then the trabeculotome is rotated so as to break the inner wall over one quarter of the canal. This is then repeated on the other side. The main difficulty in this operation is localization of the Schlemm's canal.

Illuminated microcatheter assisted circumferential trabeculotomy (IMCT)

The IMCT is a modified technique of trabeculotomy in which instead of rigid trabeculotome an illuminated microcatheter is introduced into

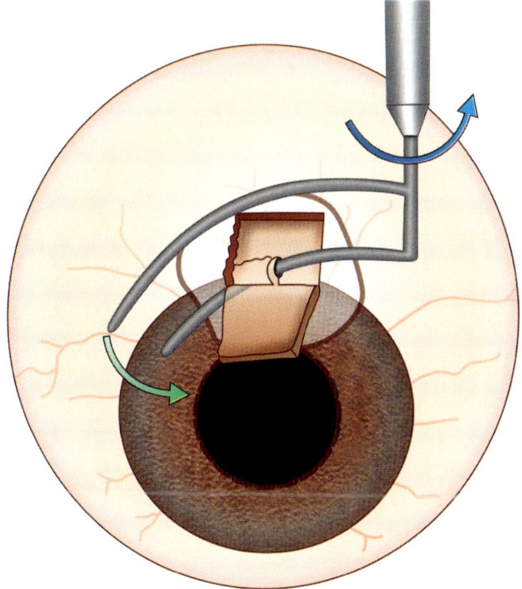

Fig. 20.3 *Trabeculotomy*

the Schlemm's canal and advanced through its whole circumference (360°). Then the two ends of the catheter are pulled in opposite directions like a purse-string, breaking through the trabecular meshwork to perform 360° trabeculotomy.

Advantages over conventional trabeculotomy/trabeculectomy includes:

- Overcomes problems associated with rigid instrumentation, bleb formation and mitomicin-C use.
- Avoids false passage formation.
- Treats entire circumference of the trabecular meshwork.
- Can be performed in cases with failed goniotomy/trabeculectomy.
- Can be performed in patients with hazy cornea.

FILTERING OPERATIONS

Filtering operations include external filtration surgeries and internal filtration surgeries.

EXTERNAL FILTRATION SURGERIES

External filtration surgeries can be grouped as below:

- *Free filtering operations.* Elliot's sclerocorneal trephining, punch sclerectomy, Scheie's thermosclerostomy and iridencleisis. All these are obsolute and just mentioned here for their historic importance.
- *Guarded filtering surgery.* Trabeculectomy (most commonly performed).
- *Non-penetrating filtration surgery.* Deep sclerectomy, viscocanalostomy.

TRABECULECTOMY

Indications

- Primary angle-closure glaucoma with peripheral anterior synaechial involving more than half of the angle.
- Primary open-angle glaucoma not controlled with medical and laser treatment.
- Congenital and developmental glaucomas where trabeculotomy and goniotomy fail.
- Secondary glaucomas where medical therapy is not effective.
- Patient intolerant or non-compliant to maximum medical therapy.

Relative contraindications

- *Blind eye*
  - Ciliary body ablation is a better option in a painful blind eye.
  - Risk of sympathetic ophthalmia should always be considered for any procedure on blind eye.
- *Rubeosis iridis*
  - Underlying problem should be addressed first.
  - Glaucoma drainage implant is a better option as peripheral iridectomy is not required.
- High-risk of failure and bleeding from iris.
- Active iritis
- Extensive conjunctival injury due to trauma or previous surgery (retinal detachment surgery).
- Extremely thin sclera due to extensive previous surgery or necrotizing scleritis.
- Failed filtration surgery with anti-metabolites
- Congenital glaucoma/aphakic glaucoma/uveitic glaucoma.

Surgical technique

1. *Initial steps* include peribulbar anaesthesia, painting, draping, exposure of eyeball and fixation with superior rectus suture or a corneal traction suture.
2. *Conjunctival flap* (Fig. 20.4A). A fornix-based or limbal-based conjunctival flap is fashioned and the underlying sclera is exposed. The Tenon's capsule is cleared away using a Tooke's knife, and haemostasis is achieved with a cautery.
3. *Scleral flap* (Fig. 20.4B). A partial thickness (usually half) limbal-based rectangular scleral flap of 5 × 5 mm size or triangular flap 3 × 3 mm size is reflected down towards the cornea.
4. *Excision of trabecular tissue* (Fig. 20.4B). A narrow strip (4 × 2 mm) of the exposed deeper sclera near the cornea containing the canal of Schlemm and trabecular meshwork is excised.
5. *Peripheral iridectomy* (Fig. 20.4C) is performed at 12 O'clock position with Vannas scissors.

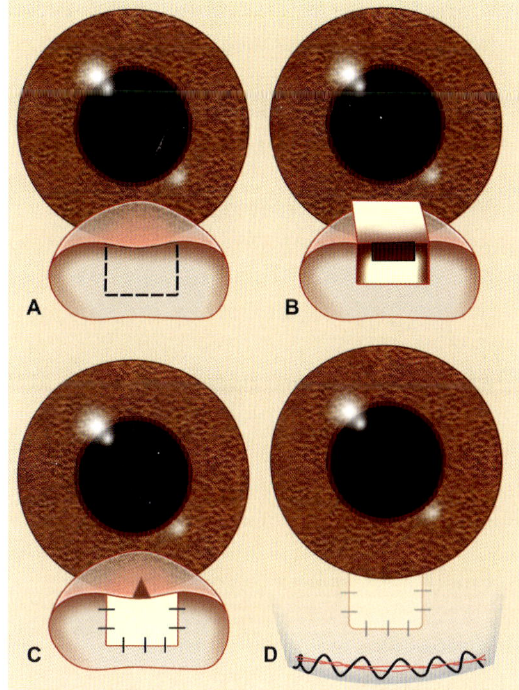

Fig. 20.4 *Steps of trabeculectomy*

6. *Closure*. The scleral flap is replaced and 10–0 nylon sutures are applied (fixed and releasable). Then the conjunctival flap is reposited and sutured with two interrupted sutures (in case of fornix-based flap) or continuous suture (in case of limbal-based flap) (Fig. 20.4D).
7. *Subconjunctival injections* of dexamethasone and gentamicin are given.
8. *Patching*. Eye is patched with a sterile eye pad and a green shield is applied over it.

Complications

Early complications

1. ***Buttonholing of conjunctiva.*** It may occur intraoperatively during preparation of conjunctival flap and postoperatively leads to leakage. Small perforations can be observed. However, if perforation is large and especially when anti-metabolites are being used, it should be used.

2. ***Hyphaema.*** It may be noted postoperatively. It generally resolves by itself within a week.

3. ***Shallow/flat anterior chamber.*** It may be associated with high IOP (pupillary block, malignant glaucoma) or low IOP (overfiltering blebs, leakage or choroidal detachment).

i. *Pupil block occurs* due to partial thickness peripheral iridectomy which is not patent. It is diagnosed, suggested by high IOP, flat bleb, negative Seidel's test and iris bombe formation. Treatment is Nd:YAG laser to remaining pigment epithelium and/or another laser iridotomy.

ii. *Over-filtration.* It can be either due to scleral flap leakage or bleb leakage due to conjunctival buttonholing or inadequate conjunctival closure. In it, IOP is low. In scleral flap leak, bleb is well formed and Seidel's test is negative. Initial treatment in eyes without iridocorneal touch involves pad and bandage with atropine and aqueous suppressants to promote spontaneous healing by reducing aqueous flow through fistula. In eyes with progressive shallowing and iridocorneal touch, anterior chamber reformation is required with air or sodium hyaluronate.

iii. *Malignant glaucoma/aqueous misdirection syndrome*, also known as ciliary-block glaucoma, is caused by blockage of aqueous flow at the pars plicata of ciliary body due to which it cannot take its normal route into anterior chamber and is forced backwards into vitreous. Typically, IOP is high with flat bleb and Seidel's negative test. Treatment : Initial treatment involves mydriatics (atropine and phenylephrine) to dilate ciliary ring, aqueous suppressants and intravenous mannitol, if IOP is very high. If medical treatment fails, Nd:YAG laser used via iridectomy or capsulotomy (in pseudophakic eyes) to disrupt anterior hyaloid face. In phakic eyes needle aspiration of the vitreous through pars plana vitrectomy is curative (also see pages 260–263).

iv. *Leakage.* In bleb leak, Seidel's test should be done to identify the site and size of leakage. Treatment options include pressure patch, bandaged contact lens, cyanoacrylate glue, autologous blood injection. If the leakage site is large, sliding conjunctival flap or AMT may be needed.

4. ***Underfiltration.*** These patients present with high IOP, flat bleb and a formed AC. Digital massage applied through lower lid may be useful. However, gonioscopy should be done prior to massage to ensure that sclerotomy is not blocked by the iris, lens or vitreous. If even after 7 days, digital massage fails, sequential suture lysis surgically or laser lysis using argon laser and special lenses, like Mendelkorn or Blumenthal, may be done.

5. *Postoperative endophthalmitis* may occur within first week. It should be treated by immediate intravitreal, intracameral and topical antibiotics. Vitrectomy may be required in non-responsive cases.

Late complications

1. *Chronic hypotony.* If IOP fails to rise even after 4–6 weeks, it is called late hypotony. Risk is more with the use of anti-metabolites. It may lead to hypotonous maculopathy. Treatment options are autologous blood injection, compression suture placement, reduction of the oversized bleb with cryotherapy or argon laser.
2. *Late leakage* is often due to thin walled blebs, more common with MMC application. Treatment is same as for early leakage. However, when these measures fail, surgical revision of the bleb may be needed.
3. *Encapsulated blebs*, also known as Tenon's cyst, occur usually during 2nd to 4th post-operative weeks and lead to failure of bleb and high IOP. It may start functioning adequately by itself, so aqueous suppressants may be tried for 4–6 weeks. However, if this fails, then surgical bleb revision should be done.
4. *Bleb failure.* Digital massage may be useful for around 3 months after surgery. However, later bleb needling may be done.
5. *Late infection.* Onset of infection occurs in subconjunctival space and then spreads to AC or vitreous cavity. Risk factors include thin walled blebs due to anti-metabolites, inferior blebs, diabetic patients, etc. It can be classified into three stages:
   - Stage 1: Blebitis
   - Stage 2: Stage 1 with AC exudation
   - Stage 3: Stage 2 with vitreous exudation.

   Treatment is topical antibiotics and if endophthalmitis develops, intravitreal injection and vitrectomy should be done, as per condition.
6. *Cataract formation* is also noted in some cases
7. *Other complications* include:
   - Cystoid macular oedema
   - Persistent uveitis, and
   - Hypotony maculopathy.

Prognosis with trabeculectomy surgery

Good prognosis is observed in patients with POAG, pseudoexfoliation, mixed mechanism glaucoma, prior clear cornea incision, and elderly.

Fair prognosis is observed in patients with JOAG, pigmentary, blunt trauma, steroid induced and middle age.

Poor prognosis occurs in patients with childhood glaucoma, neovascular, inflammatory, ICE syndrome, epithelial downgrowth, conjunctival scarring and young patients.

Antimetabolites in filtration surgery

Indications

It is recommended that anti-metabolites should be used for wound modulation, when any of the following risk factors for the failure of conventional trabeculectomy is present:

- Previous failed filtration surgery.
- Glaucoma-in-aphakia.
- Certain secondary glaucomas, e.g. inflammatory glaucoma, post-traumatic angle recession glaucoma, neovascular glaucoma and glaucomas associated with ICE syndrome.
- Patients treated with topical anti-glaucoma medications (particularly sympathomimetics) for over three years.
- Chronic cicatrizing conjunctival inflammation.

Antimetabolite agents

Either 5-fluorouracil (5-FU), 50 mg/ml for 5 minutes or mitomycin-C can be used.

- *Mitomycin-C* is only used at the time of surgery. A sponge soaked in 0.02% (2 mg in 10 ml) solution of mitomycin-C is placed at the site of filtration between the scleral and Tenon's capsule for 2 minutes, followed by a thorough irrigation with balanced salt solution.

- *Subconjunctival injection of 5-FU* can be given postoperatively, if the IOP rises at a later stage. 5 mg in 0.5 ml 180° away from the injection site is given along the HEALON-GV wall.

Complications

Complications with antimetabolites include hypotony, early and late wound leaks, epithelial damage, risk of infection, scleromalacia, and endothelial damage.

Sutureless trabeculectomy

Sutureless trabeculectomy can be done through a valvular sclerocorneal tunnel incision (4 × 4 mm size) using a specially designed Kelly Descemet's punch (Fig. 20.5). IOP reduction is inferior to that achieved with conventional trabeculectomy.

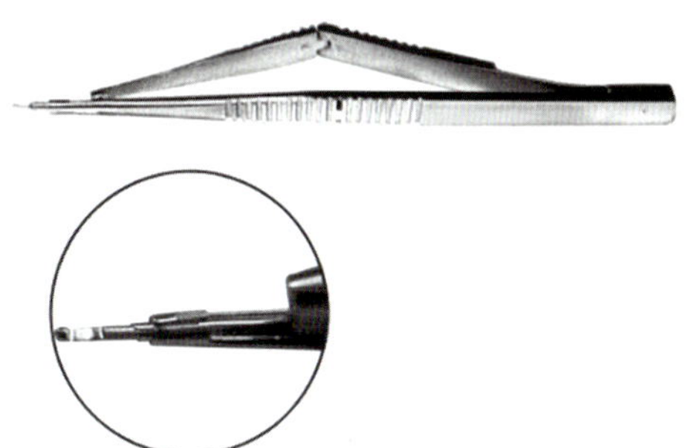

Fig. 20.5 *Kelly Descemet's punch*

NON-PENETRATING FILTRATION SURGERIES

Non-penetrating glaucoma surgery (NPGS) was introduced as a new surgical approach that would be safer than the standard filtering operation. In NPGS, there is no entry into the anterior chamber and no conjunctival bleb formation which eliminates the bleb related complications. These include:

- Sinusotomy
- Ab externo trabeculectomy
- Deep sclerectomy
- Viscocanalostomy

INDICATIONS, CONTRAINDICATIONS AND GOALS

Indications

- Open-angle glaucoma
- Glaucoma with high myopia
- Pigmentary glaucoma
- Pseudoexfoliation glaucoma
- Aphakic and pseudophakic glaucoma
- Congenital and juvenile glaucoma
- Sturge-Weber syndrome
- Aniridia and anterior segment dysgenesis.

Contraindications

Relative contraindications include narrow angle glaucoma, post-ALT, angle recession glaucoma, and late congenital glaucoma where mesodermal remnants reach Schwalbe's line.

Absolute contraindication is neovascular glaucoma.

Goals of NPGS

Goal of NPGS is to improve the outflow facility of aqueous humour but at the same time to maintain some resistance in the form of a membrane between anterior chamber and scleral dissection. This membrane is usually called trabeculo-Descemet's membrane.

SURGICAL TECHNIQUES

Sinusotomy

1. Corneal traction suture or superior rectus bridle suture is applied.
2. Conjunctival flap is made which can be fornix or limbal based.
3. Wet field cautery is done to achieve haemostasis.
4. Scleral flap 5 × 5 mm in size with one-third of scleral depth is dissected and extended into 1–1.5 mm cornea.
5. Removal of lamellar band of sclera and opening Schlemm's canal over 120° from 10 to 2 O'clock is then done, keeping inner wall of Schlemm's canal intact.
6. Suturing of scleral flap is then done with 10-0 nylon suture.
7. Conjunctiva is closed with 8-0 vicryl suture.

Ab externo trabeculectomy

1 to 4 steps are same as for sinusotomy.

5. Deep sclerectomy with unroofing of Schlemm's canal.

6. Inner wall of Schlemm's canal and juxtacanalicular trabecular meshwork removed.
7. Superficial scleral flap sutured to cover it.
8. Conjunctiva is closed with 8-0 vicryl suture.

Deep sclerectomy

Superior quadrant is preferred site.

1 to 4 steps are same as for sinusotomy.

5. *Deep scleral flap* measuring 4 × 4 mm (square in deep sclerectomy and parabolic in viscocanalostomy) is made leaving 10% of sclera above its upper margin (Fig. 20.6)
6. *Extension of the deeper scleral flap* is done into 1–1.5 mm of cornea and it leads to unroofing of the Schlemm's canal.
7. *Gentle pressure* on the floor of Schlemm's canal leads to detachment of Descemet's membrane from corneal stroma within the deep scleral flap.
8. *Deep scleral flap* is excised very close to its base
9. Schlemm's canal and juxtacanalicular trabecular meshwork is peeled off using blunt forceps.
10. Collagen implant or viscoelastics are used to maintain patency of the deep scleral bed.
11. Superficial scleral flap is then repositioned and sutured by 10-0 nylon suture.
12. Conjunctiva and Tenon's capsule are sutured in two layers using 8-0 vicryl.

Viscocanalostomy

1 to 6 steps till the deroofing of Schlemm's canal are similar to that of deep sclerectomy:

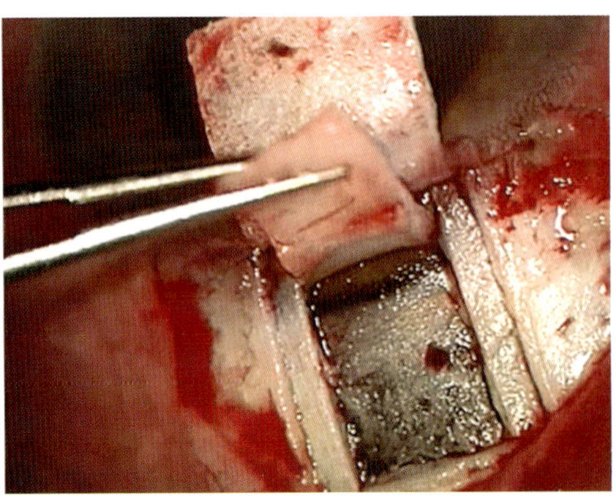

Fig. 20.6 *Deep scleral flap*

7. *Viscocanalostomy.* With the specific cannula, high molecular weight viscoelastic (e.g. Healon GV) is slowly injected into Schlemm's canal (Fig. 20.7). Cannula should not go beyond 1–1.5 mm from the ostia. Slow injection is repeated 6–7 times on each side.
8. *Trabeculo-Descemet's window* is created and rest of the steps as in deep sclerectomy are done.

Note. Injection of viscoelastic, probably ruptures the inner and outer walls of Schlemm's canal and these microruptures might also involve the juxtacanalicular trabecular meshwork facilitating aqueous outflow.

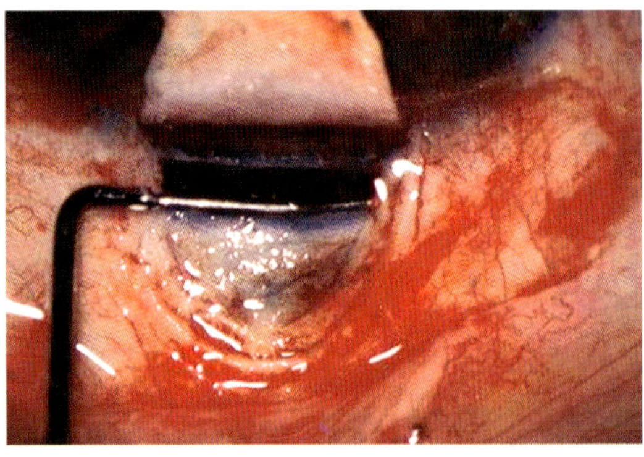

Fig. 20.7 *Viscocanalostomy*

COMPLICATIONS

Intraoperative complications

- Perforation of trabeculo-Descemet's membrane
- Haemorrhage during flap formation
- Malignant glaucoma

Postoperative complications

- Wound leak
- Hyphaema
- Choroidal detachment
- Hypotony
- Blebitis
- Shallow anterior chamber
- Implant displacement

INTERNAL FILTRATION PROCEDURES

ANGLE-BASED SURGERIES

Goniotomy

See page 322.

Trabeculotomy

See page 323.

CANAL-BASED PROCEDURES

Canal-based procedures, which restore filtration through Schlemm's canal, are designed to keep the normal anatomy instead of removing it and to be conjunctival bleb free, which should reduce the risk of long-term endophthalmitis and ocular hypotony. These procedures are indicated in POAG patients with normal angle anatomy. These procedures include:

- Canaloplasty
- Trabectome
- Trabecular micro-bypass stent (iStent)

Canaloplasty

Canaloplasty is designed to reestablish circumferential flow through Schlemm's canal, through which the aqueous in the eye usually drains.

- Superficial and deep scleral flaps are fashioned similar to deep sclerectomy (Fig. 20.8A and B).
- Deep flap is dissected to the plane of Schlemm's canal.
- Canaloplasty. A flexible fibreoptic cannula, with infrared beam at catheter's tip, is introduced into the Schlemm's canal to perform dilatation of the canal (Fig. 20.8C). After dilatation, the cannula is used to insert 10-0 prolene suture into the entire circumference of the canal and ends of suture are tied together to provide tension to the inner wall of canal and juxtacanalicular meshwork (Fig. 20.8D).
- A Descemet's window is made in the scleral bed so that aqueous can flow more easily into the canal.
- Scleral flaps are sutured tightly.

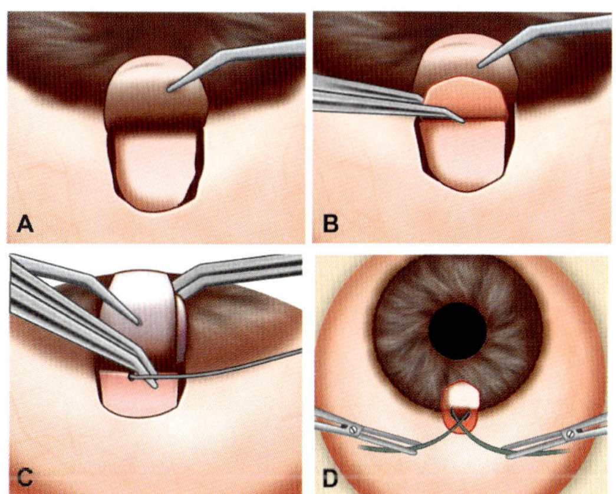

Fig. 20.8 *Steps of canaloplasty: (A and B) Fashioning of superficial and deep scleral flaps; (C) Introduction of flexible fibreoptic cannula in the Schlemm's canal; (D) Tying of prolene suture introduced in the Schlemm's canal*

Trabectome

The concept is similar in principle to ab interno trabeculotomy, the key difference being that a microelectrocautery device is used to ablate a strip of the trabecular meshwork and inner wall of Schlemm's canal, thus allowing direct access of aqueous to the collector channels (Figs 20.9A–D). This theoretically bypasses the main site of resistance to aqueous outflow and reestablishes the natural drainage passage way out of the eye.

Trabectome may be an excellent surgical option for patients who require postoperative IOPs in the mid-to-high teens. It can be used for primary open-angle, pigmentary, and pseudoexfoliative glaucoma. It can even be used in patients who had undergone previous filtering surgery (trabeculectomy or placement of a drainage tube). It can be performed alone or along with phacoemulsification (in the presence of operable cataract). When combined trabectome and cataract surgery are done then the ab interno trabeculotomy is completed before starting the phacoemulsification. This order of operation prevents the formation of phacoemulsification-related corneal oedema that could impair visualization of the angle structures.

iStent

Another new device that bypasses the trabecular meshwork and improves aqueous access to Schlemm's canal is the iStent, a MicroSnorkel (Figs 20.10A and B) that is inserted into Schlemm's canal. Introduced in 2007 and approved by the FDA in 2012, it is the smallest medical device ever made. Its tip is self-trephining and enters the trabecular meshwork ab interno. The metallic shunt builds on de Wecker's initial use of gold wire and removes

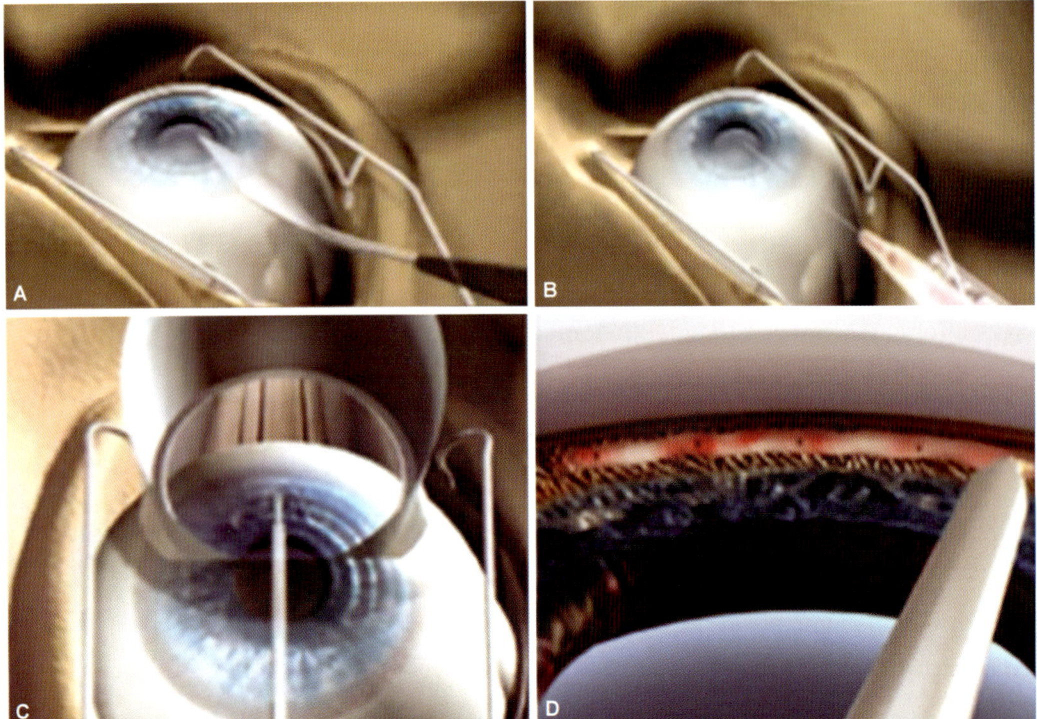

Fig. 20.9 *Steps of trabectome: (A) Entry through a clear corneal incision; (B) Inflation AC with a viscoelastic; (C and D) Small strip of diseased tissue being removed with an electrosurgical pulse to open access to the drainage system followed by irrigation with a saline solution to remove tissue debris; (treatment applied in 60–120° of angle)*

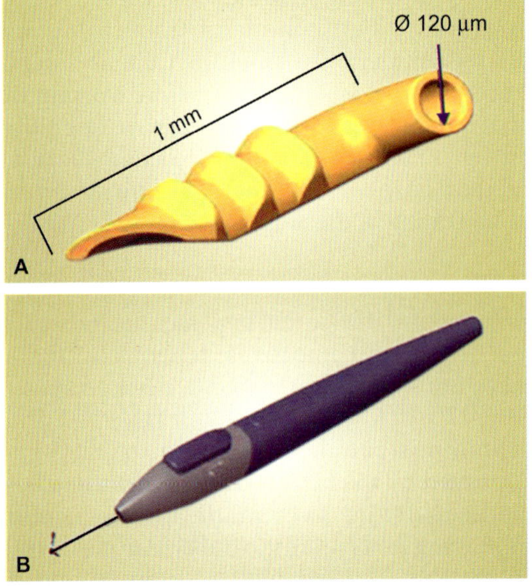

Fig. 20.10 *(A) Snorkel-shaped iStent; (B) iStent applicator*

resistance at the inner wall of the trabecular meshwork similarly to Taylor's goniotomy. It is possible that this microincisional surgical option will usher in a new era of surgical innovation.

COMBINED CATARACT AND FILTRATION SURGERIES

GENERAL CONSIDERATION

- In mild glaucoma cases, controlled on single topical anti-glaucoma medication, cataract extraction alone may control the IOP.
- Any angle-closure element, if present, peripheral iridectomy must be performed on table.
- In advanced glaucoma cases where macular split is impending (in 10-2 programme), trabeculectomy should be done first, cataract done later by temporal approach after a waiting period of at least 6 months.
- Combined procedure prevents a post-operative spike of IOP.

- It is generally less effective in controlling IOP over time compared to trabeculectomy alone. The newer small incision cataract surgeries and use of antifibrotic agents are, however, improving the surgical results, resembling trabeculectomy alone.
- Medical treatment for glaucoma may result in chronic miosis, and thus challenging cataract surgery through small pupil.
- Glaucoma patients may have coexisting pseudoexfoliation which increases the risk of zonular dehiscence and vitreous loss during cataract surgery.

INDICATIONS AND CONTRAINDICATIONS

Indications

Patients requiring more than two topical medications with significant cataract:

- Intolerance to medications with cataract requiring surgery
- Non-compliant patient, poor socioeconomic status
- One eyed patient with significant cataract and moderate glaucoma
- Moderate glaucoma controlled on 1–2 medications and requiring cataract surgery, to blunt the postoperative IOP spike which might damage already the sick optic nerve.
- AGIS demonstrated 78% risk of cataract post-trabeculectomy so any patient even with early cataract requiring trabeculectomy can undergo combined surgery provided the optic nerve damage is not advanced.

Relative contraindications

Combined surgery should be avoided in following situations:

- Glaucoma requiring very low target IOP.
- Advanced glaucoma with uncontrolled IOP and immediate need for successful IOP reduction.

TYPES OF COMBINED SURGERIES

Single site combined cataract and trabeculectomy

- SICS and trabeculectomy
- Phacotrabeculectomy

Two-site combined cataract and trabeculectomy

- SICS and trabeculectomy
- Phacoemulsification and trabeculectomy
- Various studies report two-site combined surgery to be more effective in lowering the IOP and better IOP control over a time period. But it is still a matter of debate as studies exist both in favour and against.

SURGICAL TECHNIQUE

Single site SICS and trabeculectomy

- A fornix-based conjunctival flap is made
- Scleral tunnel 5.5–7 mm in size is made superiorly. Flattened W incision is favoured as it results in secured wound and a good bleb formation postoperatively.
- Scleral tunnel is dissected using crescent knife as for regular SICS.
- Manual SICS is performed and IOL is inserted.
- Inner smaller scleral window is formed and PI done.
- Peak of the W is sutured followed by suturing of conjunctival flap.

Two-site SICS and trabeculectomy

- After making a conjunctival flap, scleral flap is dissected superiorly for trabeculectomy
- Temporal SICS is performed.
- Inner scleral window made, PI is done and trabeculectomy completed as usual.

Single site phacotrabeculectomy

- Scleral flap is dissected at the superior pole after making a conjunctival flap.
- Smaller scleral flap can be made, if foldable IOL is used.
- Phacoemulsification is performed through the base of the flap.
- After IOL insertion, a sclerostomy is performed
- Peripheral iridectomy is done and scleral flap sutured followed by suturing of conjunctival flap.

Two-site phaco and trabeculectomy

Same as SICS and trabeculectomy except that a temporal phacoemulsification is done.

COMPLICATIONS

- More severe anterior chamber inflammatory reaction compared to trabeculectomy alone. Two hypotheses responsible for this are:
  - Breakdown of blood–aqueous barrier lasts longer after combined surgery
  - Release of lens crystalline and lens epithelial cells into aqueous humour may upregulate the production of fibrogenic cytokines.
- Hyphaema
- Choroidal detachment
- Late complications, like posterior synaechiae and early posterior capsule opacification.

ARTIFICIAL DRAINAGE SHUNT OPERATIONS

GENERAL CONSIDERATIONS

Artificial drainage shunts, or the so-called glaucoma valve implants, are devices which allow aqueous outflow by creating a communication between the anterior chamber and sub-Tenon's space. The operation using glaucoma valve implant is also called Seton operation.

Indications and contraindications

Indications

These are mainly reserved for intractable glaucomas or those unlikely to respond to the conventional filtration surgery. Such cases include:

- Neovascular glaucoma
- Penetrating keratoplasty with glaucoma
- Retinal detachment surgery with glaucoma
- Iridocorneal endothelial syndrome
- Traumatic glaucoma
- Uveitic glaucoma
- Open-angle glaucoma with failed trabeculectomy
- Epithelial downgrowth
- Refractory infantile glaucoma
- Sturge-Weber syndrome

Contraindications

Absolute

- Eyes with severe scleral or sclera-limbal thinning
- Extensive fibrosis of conjunctiva
- Ciliary block glaucoma

Relative

- Vitreous in anterior chamber
- Intraocular silicone oil: Implant, if required, is placed in inferotemporal quadrant.

Parts and material of a drainage device

Parts of a drainage device are:

- *Silicone tube:* Implanted into AC
- *Plate/disc:* Kept beneath the conjunctiva and Tenon's capsule.

Material of the plate may be:

- *Polypropylene.* Ahmed and Molteno implants
- *Silicone.* Baerveldt, Krupin implant

Surgical procedure: basic principles

- *Priming of the valve* is done by injecting isotonic saline into the tube.
- *Traction suture* is applied for adequate surgical exposure.
- *Preferred site* is superotemporal quadrant followed by inferotemporal. Increased risk of diplopia is present, if superonasal site is used.
- *Isolation and identification of recti muscles* is then done gently.
- *Dissection of partial thickness scleral flap* to cover the tube is carried out.
- *Tucking the plate into sub-Tenon's space and suturing onto sclera* is done using 7-0/8-0 silk sutures about 8 mm posterior to limbus except nasally where distance is kept 6 mm. In non-valved devices, two-stage implantation is adopted to avoid postoperative hypotony. Tube is inserted 6–8 weeks following positioning of external plate to allow formation of fibrous capsule around the plate. More commonly, tube lumen is occluded with absorbable suture like vicryl.
- *Paracentesis into anterior chamber* is done and viscoelastics injected.
- *Insertion of tube in anterior chanber.* Track for entry of tube into anterior chamber is created using 23 or 22 gauge needle. Tube is inserted parallel to the plane of iris and positioned between cornea and iris avoiding corneal touch and it should be 2–3 mm into anterior chamber. The tube is sutured to the sclera and is covered with partial thickness scleral flap or donor sclera.

- *Conjunctiva is sutured* with 8-0 vicryl.
- *Viscoelastics can be left in anterior chamber* since it flows freely through the tube in a few hours.

Postoperative phases

I. *Hypotensive phase*

- It lasts from day 1 to 3–4 weeks after surgery. IOP is <10 mm Hg.
- Diffuse and thick-walled bleb is present with minimally engorged vessels and low IOP.

II. *Hypertensive phase*

- Starts from 3 to 6 weeks after surgery and lasts for 4 to 6 months.
- More common with Ahmed glaucoma valve.
- Inflamed and dome-shaped bleb is seen with high IOP.
- Treatment involves antiglaucoma medications and digital massage, if IOP >21 mmHg.
- If not responsive to above, needling can be done or 5-FU injected subconjunctivally in the opposite quadrant.

III. *Stable phase*

The IOP stabilizes in the early teens.

Complications

- Hypotony due to overfiltration, wound leak or choroidal effusions.
- Tube obstruction. It manifests with high IOP with deep anterior chamber. Obstruction is caused by blood, fibrin, vitreous or iris plug or related to tight external ligature around the tube.
- Tube retraction from the anterior chamber may occur in some cases.
- Diplopia. More common with the Baerveldt implant due to its larger size.
- Corneal decompensation may occur when tube is touching endothelium.
- Tube and end plate exposure is also reported in some cases.
- Suprachoroidal haemorrhage is also reported.
- Late failure of valve.
- Endophthalmitis, though rare, but may occur.

COMMON GLAUCOMA DRAINAGE DEVICES

I. Glaucoma drainage devices with no resistance

These devices do not offer any resistance to aqueous outflow.

1. ***Single plate Molteno implant.*** It was the earliest implant device. In this implant, silicone tube is attached to a polypropylene end plate.
2. ***Double plate Molteno implant.*** In this implant, a second end plate is attached to the right or left of the original end plate, thus doubling its surface area (270 mm^2). It is placed 8–10 mm away from limbus in medial and lateral quadrants with connecting silicone tube passing over superior rectus muscle. Second and third generation Molteno implants incorporate a biological valve.
3. ***Baerveldt implant*** (Fig. 20.11). This implant is constructed entirely of medical grade silicone with an episcleral plate with different surface areas (250 or 350 mm^2). The silicone plate is barium impregnated to increase ultrasound resolution and identification using CT scan, X-ray. This also leads to a thin, durable and flexible

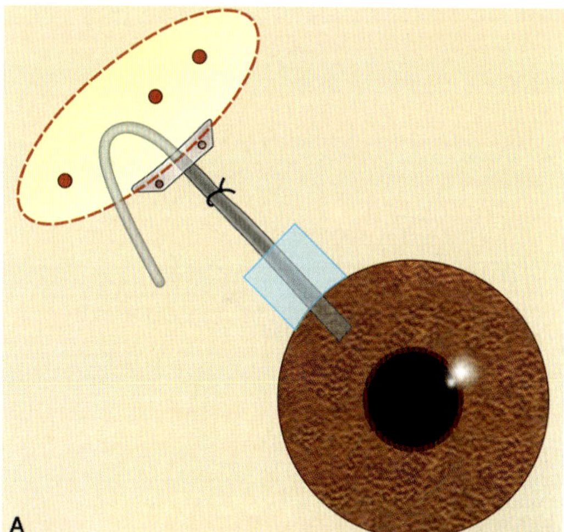

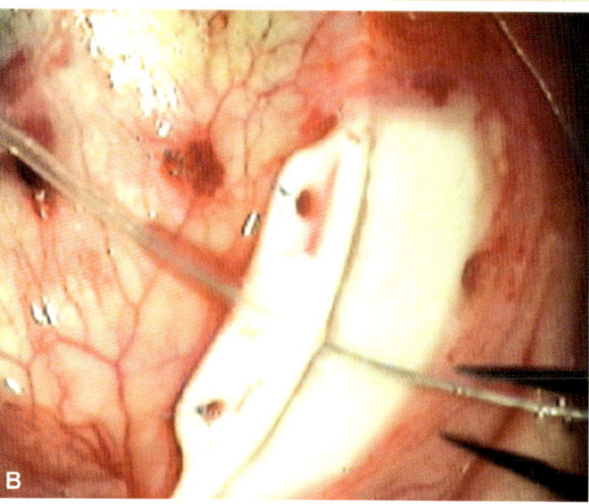

Fig. 20.11 *Baerveldt implant in position*

implant. The wings are placed under rectus muscle insertion in superotemporal quadrant. Proximal portion of the plate has a flange with large fixation holes to allow the growth of fibrous tissues which aids in scleral fixation (Figs 20.11A and B).

4. ***Schocket implant.*** The implant comprises of a silastic tube used for nasolacrimal intubation (Fig. 20.12A). An opening is made in the centre by cutting with spring scissors (Fig. 20.12B). One end of the implant is inserted into the AC, while the other end is tucked underneath a No. 20 retinal-encircling band placed underneath the rectus muscles (Fig. 20.12C). The material can be assembled in most operating rooms.

5. ***ExPRESS R50.*** ExPRESS stands for "excessive pressure regulating shunt system" (Fig. 20.13).

It is a single piece, stainless steel, translimbal implant that is placed with the help of an inserter. ExPRESS shunt was developed to shunt fluid from inside the eye to under the conjunctiva. Because there was a tendency for the shunt to erode through the conjunctiva, surgeons started placing the ExPRESS shunt under a partial-thickness scleral flap as a modification of trabeculectomy. Many glaucoma surgeons also use the ExPRESS glaucoma filtration device implanted underneath a scleral flap, not for superior IOP reduction (it reduces IOP to a similar level as trabeculectomy), but for a more favourable safety and postoperative recovery profile than standard trabeculectomy.

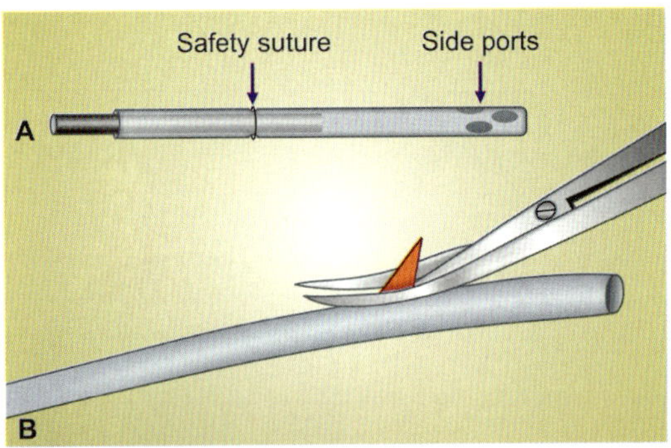

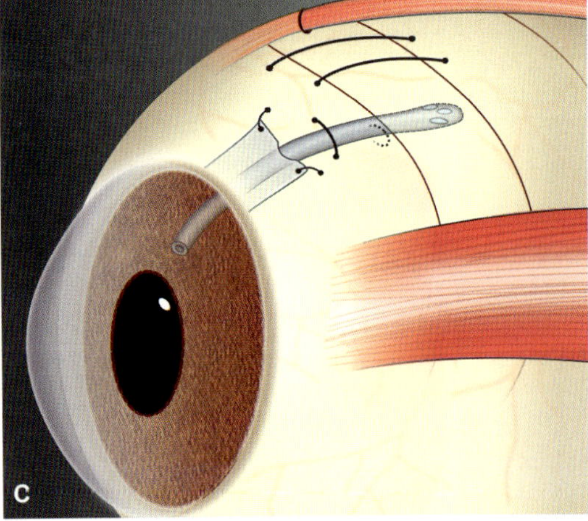

Fig. 20.12 (A) Schocket implant; (B) Making an opening in the centre of implant; (C) Placement of one end of implant in the anterior chamber and other underneath the encircling band

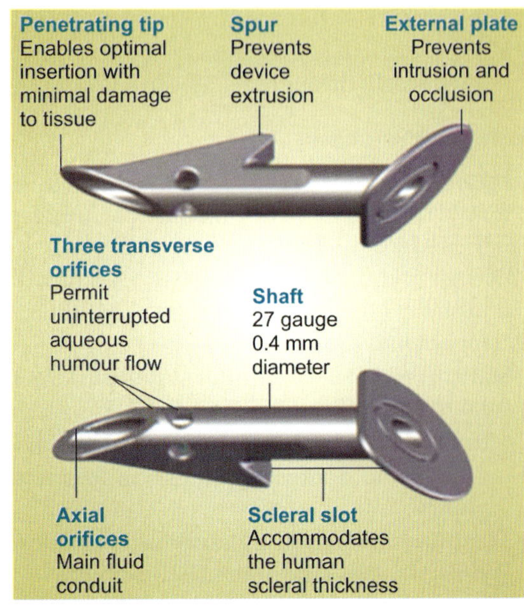

Fig. 20.13 ExPRESS glaucoma filtration device

II. Flow restricted drainage devices

1. ***Ahmed glaucoma valve.*** It has a silicone tube and a polypropylene body. The end plate measures 185 mm^2. The valve consists of thin silicone elastomer membranes (8 mm long × 7 mm wide) that create a venturi-shaped chamber. The inlet cross-section of the chamber is wider than the outlet (Bernoulli principle), with a resultant pressure differential between the anterior chamber and the bleb. The valve is designed to open when IOP is 8 mm Hg.

2. ***Krupin slit valve.*** It has a silicone tube with a slit valve attached to a silicone oval end plate. surface area of the end plate is 180 mm^2. The opening pressure of the slit valve is designed to be 11–14 mm Hg, and the closing pressure is designed to be 2 mm Hg.

III. Glaucoma drainage devices with variable resistance

These are modifications of the original Molteno implant and the Baerveldt implant (Fig. 20.14). They incorporate a resistance mechanism dependent on tissue apposition to limit flow.

1. ***Molteno dual bridge device*** (Molteno with a pressure ridge). Initial drainage area is limited by dividing the top portion of the plate into two separate spaces with a thin V-shaped ridge. Aqueous encounters resistance from the overlying conjunctiva while flowing over the ridge.
2. ***Baerveldt bioseal implant.*** It consists of a flap overhanging the silicone tube at its insertion into the end plate.

IV. Glaucoma devices in pipeline

1. ***CyPass Micro-Stent.*** CyPass (transcend), is made from a biocompatible material (polyimide) and features a unique delivery system. The CyPass is a micro-implantable device, 6 mm in length, with a small lumen of 300 μm (Fig. 20.15). It allows for an ab interno surgical approach, which spares the conjunctiva, does not penetrate the sclera and leaves the trabecular meshwork intact.
2. ***EyePass bidirectional glaucoma implant.*** The EyePass bidirectional glaucoma implant (GMP Vision Solutions, Inc.) consists of a dual 6.0 mm

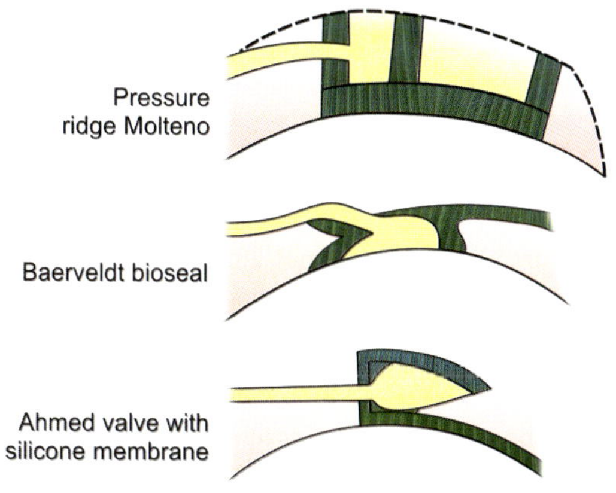

Fig. 20.14 *Glaucoma devices with variable resistance*

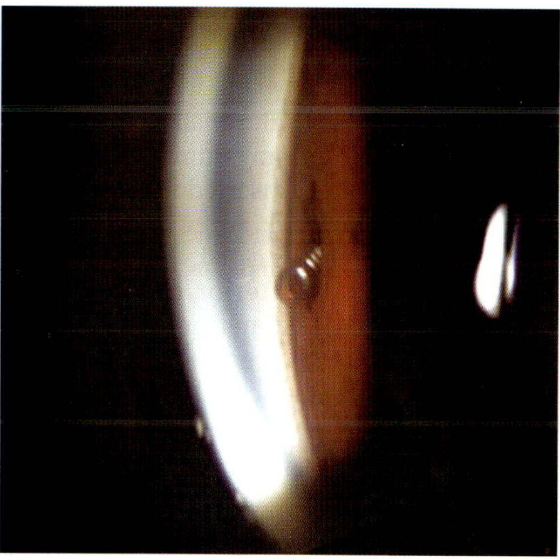

Fig. 20.15 *CyPass micro-stent*

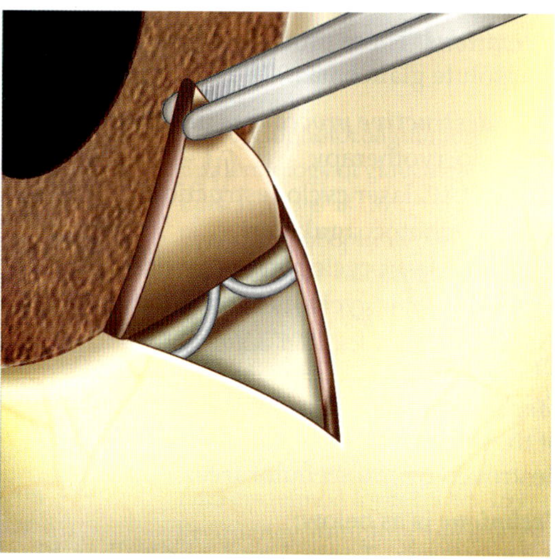

Fig. 20.16 *EyePass bidirectional glaucoma implants*

long silicone tube bonded at 1 end for less than 1.0 mm, creating a Y-shape (Fig. 20.16)

It can be used as a stand alone procedure or in combination with cataract surgery. After a fornix-based superomedial conjunctival dissection, a two-third thickness triangular scleral flap of with a 4.0 mm basis is dissected. Before the Schlemm's canal is unroofed, clear corneal cataract surgery is performed. This is followed by the Schlemm's canal unroofing by dissecting a second scleral flap or by opening the canal with small Vannas scissors. Before the